Psoriasis and Psoriatic Arthritis

Pathophysiology, Therapeutic Intervention, and Complementary Medicine

Psoriasis and Psoriatic Arthritis

Pathophysiology, Therapeutic Intervention, and Complementary Medicine

Edited by

Siba P. Raychaudhuri
University of California Davis, School of Medicine
and Veterans Affairs Medical Center Sacramento, CA

Smriti K. Raychaudhuri
University of California Davis, School of Medicine
and Veterans Affairs Medical Center Sacramento, CA

Debasis Bagchi
University of Houston College of Pharmacy, Houston, TX, USA

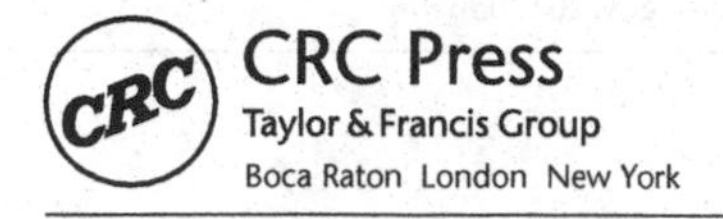

CRC Press is an imprint of the
Taylor & Francis Group, an **informa** business

CRC Press
Taylor & Francis Group
6000 Broken Sound Parkway NW, Suite 300
Boca Raton, FL 33487-2742

First issued in paperback 2021

ISBN 13: 978-1-03-209586-8 (pbk)
ISBN 13: 978-1-4987-5606-8 (hbk)

Publisher's Note
The publisher has gone to great lengths to ensure the quality of this reprint but points out that some imperfections in the original copies may be apparent.

Library of Congress Cataloging-in-Publication Data

Names: Raychaudhuri, Siba P., editor. | Kundu-Raychaudhuri, Smriti K., editor. |
Bagchi, Debasis, 1954- editor.
Title: Psoriasis and psoriatic arthritis : pathophysiology, therapeutic intervention, and
complementary medicine / [edited by] Siba P. Raychaudhuri, Smriti K. Raychaudhuri & Debasis Bagchi.
Other titles: Psoriasis and psoriatic arthritis (Raychaudhuri)
Description: Boca Raton, FL : CRC Press/Taylor & Francis Group, 2018. |
Includes bibliographical references.
Identifiers: LCCN 2017036704 | ISBN 9781498756068 (hardback)
Subjects: | MESH: Psoriasis--therapy | Arthritis, Psoriatic--therapy | Psoriasis--epidemiology |
Arthritis, Psoriatic--epidemiology | Complementary Therapies
Classification: LCC RL321 | NLM WR 205 | DDC 616.5/26--dc23
LC record available at https://lccn.loc.gov/2017036704

Visit the Taylor & Francis Web site at
http://www.taylorandfrancis.com

and the CRC Press Web site at
http://www.crcpress.com

To my late beloved friend and colleague, Pinaki Ranjan Khan (Bhaduri). I always see him in his smiling face, my great friend, philosopher, and guide. May Almighty God bless him always.

Debasis Bagchi

To my parents, Durga Pada and Bilwabasani Roychowdhury, my sister, Dr. Moitrayee Roychowdhury, and my brothers, Dr. Debi Prasad & Vwani Prasad Roychowdhury.

Siba P. Raychaudhuri

To my parents, Mrityunjoy and Uma Kundu, and to my daughters, Blossom, Gunjari and Genea.

Smriti K. Raychaudhuri

Contents

Preface

Psoriasis is a lifelong chronic autoimmune disorder, a chronic heterogeneous skin pathophysiology characterized by thick, scaly skin lesions and accompanied by massive inflammation, extensive hyperproliferation of keratinocytes, scaly plaques, and erythema. In psoriasis lesions, skin cells (keratinocytes) grow too quickly, resulting in thick, white, silvery, or red patches on the skin. Generally, skin cells grow gradually and flake off about every 4 weeks. New skin cells grow to replace the outer layers of the skin as they shed. However, in psoriasis, new skin cells move rapidly to the surface of the skin in days rather than weeks. They build up and form thick patches known as plaques. The patches range in size from small to large. They most often appear on the elbows, scalp, feet, knees, hands, or lower back, or as the more embarrassing flaking of the skin and/or patches on the face. Generally, psoriasis is most common in adults, but teenagers and children can also suffer from it.

Psoriasis is not just a skin condition; it begins underneath the skin. It is a chronic disease of the immune system. Psoriasis is frequently associated with a severe form of arthritis. In other words, psoriatic arthritis is a chronic form of inflammatory arthritis accompanied by psoriasis. Psoriasis and psoriatic arthritis together are considered psoriatic diseases. Several comorbidities are associated with psoriatic disease, such as type 2 diabetes, metabolic syndrome, cardiovascular disease, and depression.

Several pharmaceutical therapeutics and treatment options are available for psoriasis and psoriatic arthritis. This book demonstrates a significant number of treatment modalities available for psoriasis and psoriatic arthritis. Currently, nutraceuticals and functional food-based formulations are becoming popular for almost every medical condition. Here we have invited several leading authorities to contribute their opinion on nutraceuticals and functional food-based therapy for psoriasis and psoriatic arthritis.

A total of 21 chapters have been compiled in this book involving global leaders in the field. The first two sections present an extensive discussion of the epidemiology, genetics, pathogenesis, and inflammatory sequences of psoriasis; the association of the metabolic syndrome; angiogenesis and the roles of adhesion molecules; the regulatory role of Th17 cells; and the nerve growth factor and its receptor system.

Section III emphasizes the clinical profiles, including the clinical spectrum of psoriasis and spondyloarthritis, comorbidities in psoriatic arthritis.

Section IV, Part A, highlights the treatment regimen in seven discrete chapters, including the current treatment recommendations for psoriasis, the management of psoriatic arthritis, intricate aspects and the role of IL-23/IL-17 inhibitors, the roles of disease-modifying antirheumatic drugs, topical therapies, JAK-STAT pathophysiology, and finally, the concept of total care, which is a multidisciplinary approach for the management of psoriatic disease.

Section IV, Part B, includes three classic chapters highlighting the beneficial roles of nutraceutical components, herbal products, and the impact of nutrition and dietary supplements on psoriasis pathology. Bioactive whey extract has demonstrated the presence of growth factors, active peptides, and immunoglobulins that block skin inflammation by inhibiting the actions of tumor necrosis factor-alpha and inflammatory cascade at the molecular level. Several antioxidants, including alpha lipoic acid, N-acetyl cysteine, glutathione, curcumin and turmeric, astaxanthin, and several structurally diverse antioxidants, demonstrate a potential natural therapeutic strategy for psoriasis. Nutraceutical therapeutic options are far less expensive and not associated with adverse side effects.

Section V provides a commentary from the editors' desk, discussing the final take-home message for the readers.

The editors sincerely thank all the eminent authors and contributors in this book, and more importantly, the editors thank Randy Brehm and Sylvester O'Gilvie for their cooperation and assistance. We sincerely hope that our readers enjoy reading this book.

Siba P. Raychaudhuri
Smriti K. Raychaudhuri
Debasis Bagchi

Editors

Siba P. Raychaudhuri, MD, FACP, FACR, is the chief of the Rheumatology Division at the VA Medical Center in Sacramento, California, and a senior faculty in the Division of Rheumatology, Allergy and Clinical Immunology at the University of California, Davis. Dr. Raychaudhuri is a dermatologist, rheumatologist, and immunologist. He has an extensive background in translational research that extends back to his fellowship period at Stanford University, California. Dr. Raychaudhuri's research group works in arthritis, human autoimmune diseases, cell biology, the nerve growth factor, and animal models of human diseases. His research group has dissected the regulatory role of the nerve growth factor and its receptor system in cell trafficking, angiogenesis, the growth and survival of keratinocytes, T cells, and fibroblast-like synovium. These observations have provided new insights into the pathogenesis of psoriasis, psoriatic arthritis, rheumatoid arthritis, and osteoarthritis. Dr. Raychaudhuri's research over the last three decades has promoted significant insight into and understanding of the cytokine network in autoimmune arthritis, which includes the regulatory roles of RANTES, fractalkine, IL-9, IL-17, and IL-22 in psoriasis, psoriatic arthritis, and rheumatoid arthritis.

Smriti K. Raychaudhuri, MD, is a professor of medicine and medical microbiology at California Northstate University College of Medicine. She is also the director of the Cellular and Clinical Immunology Research Laboratory at the Sacramento VA Medical Center, California. Dr. Raychaudhuri earned her MD in 1987 from the All India Institute of Medical Sciences, Delhi and received her postdoctoral training in immunology at Stanford University, California. She conducted clinical trials on immune-based therapy for HIV at Stanford University. Currently, her research group works on the pathogenesis of autoimmune diseases, with a focus on elucidating the cytokine network and cell trafficking in psoriasis and psoriatic arthritis.

Debasis Bagchi, PhD, MACN, CNS, MAIChE, received his PhD in medicinal chemistry in 1982. He is the chief scientific officer at Cepham Research Center, Piscataway, New Jersey; a professor in the Department of Pharmacological and Pharmaceutical Sciences at the University of Houston College of Pharmacy, Texas; and an adjunct faculty at Texas Southern University, Houston. He served as the senior vice president of research and development of InterHealth Nutraceuticals Inc., Benicia, California, from 1998 until February 2011, and then as director of innovation and clinical affairs at Iovate Health Sciences, Oakville, Ontario, until June 2013. Dr. Bagchi received the Master of American College of Nutrition Award in October 2010. He is a past chairman of the International Society of Nutraceuticals and Functional Foods, a past president of the American College of Nutrition, Clearwater, Florida, and a past chair of the Nutraceuticals and Functional Foods Division of the Institute of Food Technologists, Chicago. He is serving as a distinguished advisor on the Japanese Institute for Health Food Standards, Tokyo. Dr. Bagchi is a member of the Study Section and Peer Review Committee of the National Institutes of Health, Bethesda, Maryland. He has 324 papers in peer-reviewed journals, 30 books, and 19 patents. Dr. Bagchi is also a member of the Society of Toxicology, a member of the New York Academy of Sciences, a fellow of the Nutrition Research Academy, and a member of the TCE stakeholder Committee of the Wright-Patterson Air Force Base, Ohio. Dr. Bagchi is the associate editor of the *Journal of Functional Foods*, the *Journal of the American College of Nutrition*, and *Archives of Medical and Biomedical Research*, and he also serves on the editorial boards of numerous peer-reviewed journals, including *Antioxidants & Redox Signaling*, *Cancer Letters*, *Toxicology Mechanisms and Methods*, and *The Original Internist* among other journals.

Contributors

Amita Aggarwal
Department of Clinical Immunology
Sanjay Gandhi Postgraduate Institute of Medical Sciences
Lucknow, India

Maria J. Antonelli
MetroHealth Medical Center/Case Western Reserve University
Cleveland, Ohio

Debasis Bagchi
Department of Pharmacological and Pharmaceutical Sciences
University of Houston College of Pharmacy
Houston, Texas
and
Cepham Inc.
Piscataway, New Jersey

Subhashis Banerjee
Bristol-Myers Squibb
Princeton, New Jersey

Soumya D. Chakravarty
Division of Rheumatology
Drexel University College of Medicine
Philadelphia, Pennsylvania
and
Janssen Scientific Affairs, LLC
Horsham, Pennsylvania

Vinod Chandran
Department of Medicine
Division of Rheumatology
University of Toronto
Toronto, Ontario, Canada

Andrea Chaparro
Rheumatology and Clinical Immunology
Military Hospital/EMNG
Bogota, Colombia

Jayson Chen
Product Safety Laboratories
Dayton, New Jersey

Deep Dutta
Department of Endocrinology
Venkateshwar Hospitals
Dwarka, New Delhi, India

Joerg Ermann
Division of Rheumatology, Immunology and Allergy
Department of Medicine
Brigham and Women's Hospital
and
Harvard Medical School
Boston, Massachusetts

Dipyaman Ganguly
IICB-Translational Research Unit of Excellence (TRUE) and Division of Cancer Biology and Inflammatory Disorders
CSIR-Indian Institute of Chemical Biology
Kolkata, India

Latika Gupta
Department of Clinical Immunology
Sanjay Gandhi Postgraduate Institute of Medical Sciences
Lucknow, India

Asmita Hazra
Department of Biochemistry
Christian Medical College Vellore
Vellore, Tamil Nadu, India

Andrzej P. Herman
Laboratory of Molecular Biology
Kielanowski Institute of Animal Physiology and Nutrition
Polish Academy of Sciences
Warsaw, Poland

Anna Herman
Faculty of Cosmetology
Academy of Cosmetics and Health Care
Warsaw, Poland

Urmila Jarouliya
School of Studies in Biotechnology
Jiwaji University
Gwalior, Madhya Pradesh, India

Raj K. Keservani
School of Pharmaceutical Sciences
Rajiv Gandhi Proudyogiki Vishwavidyalaya
Bhopal, Madhya Pradesh, India

Adarsh M. B.
Post-Graduate Institute of Medical Education and Research (PGIMER)
Chandigarh, Panjab, India

Chelsea Ma
Department of Dermatology
School of Medicine
University of California
Davis, California

Marina Magrey
MetroHealth Medical Center/Case Western Reserve University
Cleveland, Ohio

Saptarshi Mandal
Department of Transfusion Medicine and Blood Bank
All India Institute of Medical Sciences Jodhpur
Jodhpur, Rajasthan, India

Emanual Maverakis
Department of Dermatology
School of Medicine
University of California
Davis, California

Philip Mease
Swedish Medical Center and University of Washington
Seattle, Washington

Odete Mendes
Product Safety Laboratories
Dayton, New Jersey

Satinath Mukhopadhyay
Department of Endocrinology
Institute of Postgraduate Medical Education and Research (IPGMER) and Seth Sukhlal Karnani Memorial (SSKM) Hospital
Kolkata, India

Remy Pollock
Psoriatic Arthritis Program
Center for Prognosis Studies in the Rheumatic Diseases
Toronto Western Hospital
Toronto, Ontario, Canada

Sanchita Raychaudhuri
Harvard College
Molecular and Cellular Biology
Cambridge, Massachusetts

Siba P. Raychaudhuri
VA Sacramento Medical Center
Department of Veterans Affairs
Northern California Health Care System
Mather, California
and
Department of Medicine
Division of Rheumatology, Allergy and Clinical Immunology
School of Medicine
University of California
Davis, California

Smriti K. Raychaudhuri
VA Sacramento Medical Center
Department of Veterans Affairs
Northern California Health Care System
Mather, California

Debashis Sarkar
Department of Dermatology and Venereology
MGM Medical College and LSK Hospital
Kishanganj, India

Aman Sharma
Clinical Immunology and Rheumatology Services
Department of Internal Medicine
Postgraduate Institute of Medical Education and Research
Chandigarh, India

Mithila Shitut
Product Safety Laboratories
Dayton, New Jersey

Michael Sticherling
Hautklinik Universitätsklinikum Erlangen
Erlangen, Germany

Anand Swaroop
Cepham Inc.
Piscataway, New Jersey

Rafael Valle Oñate
Colombian Clinic of Rheumatology
Military Hospital/EMNG
Bogota, Colombia
and
Brigham and Women's Hospital
Harvard University
Boston, Massachusetts

Reason Wilken
Department of Dermatology
School of Medicine
University of California
Davis, California

Section I

Disease Epidemiology and Genetics

1 Epidemiology of Psoriasis and Psoriatic Arthritis

Adarsh M. B. and Aman Sharma

CONTENTS

1.1 INTRODUCTION

Psoriasis (PsO), the great dermatologic mystery, has been known since the days of Hippocrates and is one of the oldest maladies. From that dark era when it was a social stigma, with people being kept in isolation, the modern-day treatment instills confidence of good treatment outcomes. From the historical use of arsenic and boiled viper, we have reached a stage where the therapeutic armamentarium has expanded to include an increasing array of biological agents. Still, a lot needs to be done, and thus the quest to know continues. Epidemiological aspects play a crucial role in describing any disease. These help in analyzing the distribution as well as determinants of a disease. Epidemiological studies have often helped in policy making on disease prevention and treatment.

1.2 PREVALENCE OF PSORIASIS

The prevalence of PsO in most of the population is around 0.5%–5%.[1,2] It has been reported to be 4.2% in Norway,[1] 2.8% in Italy,[3] 0.47% in China,[4] and 0.34% in Japan[2] in various population-based studies. The prevalence is higher in clinic-based studies, with PsO accounting for up to 8% of patients. The prevalence of PsO was found to be higher among young women in a Norwegian population survey. The onset of PsO was also early among females in this population,[1] while in most other studies, the prevalence of PsO was higher among males.[4,5]

1.3 INCIDENCE AND PREVALENCE OF PSORIATIC ARTHRITIS

Since the time Alibert described an arthritis associated with PsO, psoriatic arthritis (PsA) has evoked curiosity in numerous minds. It is a chronic inflammatory arthritis characterized by enthesitis, spinal involvement, and nail changes. Against the initial belief of a relatively benign nature, it is now accepted that it can be as crippling and chronic as rheumatoid arthritis (RA), with up to one-third of patients developing erosions within the first year of the disease. Based on the population surveyed and the methods used (registry based or population based), the prevalence rates vary. The prevalence of PsA in registry-based studies varies from 0.19% in the United Kingdom[6] to 0.74% in a Latin American population.[7] The prevalence in population-based studies was reported to be 0.47% in the Czech Republic,[8] 0.25% in the United States,[9] and 0.13% in Norway.[10] The incidence rate was 6.9/100,000 in the Norwegian study. Studies in the Asian population are lacking, except for a single Chinese study that reported a low prevalence of 0.02%.[11] As in the case of PsO, there is a male predominance in PsA, with a male-to-female ratio of 1.2–2:1 in various studies,[7,10,12] with the onset of arthritis in the third or fourth decade.[7]

1.4 CLASSIFICATION CRITERIA OF PSORIATIC ARTHRITIS

The evolution of criteria used in the classification of PsA over the years hints at the ongoing efforts to develop the most suitable criteria. One reason for the difference in incidence of PsA in various epidemiological studies is the use of different classification criteria. Since the first criteria proposed by Moll and Wright, which was simple and based on clinical variables alone, the criteria evolved through Bennette, Vasey, Gladman, the European Spondyloarthropathy Study Group (ESSG), McGonagle, and the latest Classification Criteria for Psoriatic Arthritis (CASPAR). Except for the Bennette criteria, none of the others used synovial fluid assessment or synovial biopsy as a variable. It was ESSG criteria that introduced the family history of PsO into the criteria for the first time. The CASPAR, which were formed as the result of an international collaboration, have a sensitivity and specificity above 90% in most of the validation studies.[13,14] Although the recent Assessment of Spondyloarthritis Society (ASAS) criteria for peripheral spondyloarthropathy can be used to classify PsA, when compared with CASPAR, it has a low sensitivity (48% vs. 89%).[15] Some authors suggest giving a differential weight to the variables in CASPAR, especially those of present PsO and a past history of PsO, as well as defining the musculoskeletal symptoms to improve it. Most of the current epidemiological studies and clinical trials on PsA use CASPAR.

1.5 CLINICAL CHARACTERISTICS AND PREVALENCE OF PSORIATIC ARTHRITIS IN PSORIASIS

The prevalence of PsA among PsO patients varies widely. The variation is due to the different criteria used, the geographic area, and the investigator (rheumatologist or dermatologist). It varies from 1% to 48%.[16–19] The prevalence is lower among the Asian population, with most studies reporting a prevalence of less than 10%.[16,20,21] In an Indian study, the prevalence was 8.7%.[20] The annual incidence rate of developing arthritis in a PsO cohort, which was followed for a duration of 4 years, was 1.87 per 100 person-years.[22] In a multicentric clinic-based cross-sectional study in Europe, the incidence rate was found to be 74 per 1000 persons, and it remained constant after PsO diagnosis.[23] The prevalence of arthritis was 20% at 30 years in the same study. The cumulative incidence of PsA was 1.7%, 3.1%, and 5.1% at 5, 10, and 20 years of PsO diagnosis, respectively.[24] Subclinical arthritis with capsular distension and periarticular edema has been shown on MRI in 68% of PsO patients.[25] Arthritis is most common among patients with plaque-type PsO compared with the guttate or pustular type.[16,26,27] In most series, including that by Moll and Wright,[28] the most common presentation of PsA is assymetrical oligoarthritis.[10,27,29,30] However, many studies in the Asian population have reported polyarthritis, either symmetrical or asymmetrical, as the most common pattern of involvement.[20,26] The presence of polyarthritis itself has been shown to be a predictor for erosive disease.[12] The incidence of spinal involvement varies among various populations and is reported to be higher in the Asian population than in the Western population.[20,21,26,31] Arthritis mutilans is seen in less than 5% of patients.[10,27] It has also been observed that PsA patients with early-onset PsO have fewer skin lesions and less joint involvement at presentation and a higher frequency of spondyloarthropathy.

1.6 RISK FACTORS FOR THE DEVELOPMENT OF PSORIATIC ARTHRITIS IN PSORIASIS

Patients with PsA have severe scalp involvement, skin disease, and nail changes.[30,32] Nail dystrophy, intergluteal/perianal PsO, and scalp lesions have also been shown to be associated with PsA.[24] Among the Asian population, Indian ethnicity has been suggested as a risk factor for the development of PsA.[31] Patients with PsA have a higher mortality than the general population. High disease burden, as suggested by an elevated erythrocyte sedimentation rate (ESR) and erosive disease, is a predictor of mortality in PsA.[33]

1.7 GENETIC EPIDEMIOLOGY OF PSORIASIS AND PSORIATIC ARTHRITIS

Both PsO and PsA have a multifactorial pattern of inheritance. Most of the initial evidence for the genetic predisposition of a disease comes from twin studies. In PsO, the risk is three times more in monozygotes than in heterozygotes.[34] There have not been many studies done in twins. Moll and Wright described PsA among monozygotic twins in a set of triplets. Among the population-based studies, the sibling recurrence risk for PsO varies between 4 and 10.[35] The lifetime risk for PsO, as calculated by Swanbeck et al., was 0.04 if no parent was affected and 0.65 if both were affected.[36] For PsA, the sibling recurrence rate is substantially higher than that for PsO. In the United Kingdom, the sibling recurrence risk was calculated to be 55 based on the prevalence rates for PsA.[35] The estimated heritability for PsO is 60%–90%. Although most of the time inheritance is multifactorial, an autosomal pattern has also been shown. It has also been seen that affected children with PsO are more likely to have an affected father than an affected mother, and this is attributed to genetic imprinting.[37] Considering human leukocyte antigen (HLA) studies, type I PsO (onset less than 40 years) had a stronger HLA association with HLA-Cw6 and HLA-DR7 than type II PsO. Early-onset and more severe PsO has been associated with HLA-Cw*0602.[38] A candidate region was identified in chromosome 16 in a genome-wide scan for PsA.[39] PsA patients with early-onset PsO have a stronger HLA association. HLA-Cw*0602 has been shown to be associated with PsA. HLA-B27 is more common with back involvement, while HLA-B37 and HLA-B38 are more common with peripheral arthritis.[40]

1.8 ROLE OF SCREENING TOOLS

Undiagnosed PsA among patients with PsO varies from 4.9% to 85% in various studies highlighting the unmet need for having a sensitive screening tool for diagnosing PsA in patients with PsO. Many such screening tools have been developed, but their utility rests on the sensitivity, as well as the ease of administration. This includes the Psoriatic Arthritis Screening and Evaluation (PASE) tool, the Psoriasis Epidemiology Screening Tool (PEST), the Toronto Psoriatic Arthritis Screen (ToPAS), and Early Arthritis for Psoriasis Patients (EARP) questionnaires. The PASE questionnaire had a sensitivity and specificity of 82% and 73% at a cutoff score of 47,[41] while they were 76% and 76% at a score of 44.[42] Although the PASE score correlated with the disease severity and treatment response, the complexity of its administration made it less attractive. The sensitivity and specificity of the PEST questionnaire were 92% and 78%,[43] while those of ToPAS were 87% and 93%[44] and those of EARP were 85% and 92%.[45] In the COMPAQ study, EARP was found to have the greatest sensitivity, while ToPAS II had the highest specificity among the four questionnaires.[46] The ease of doing EARP makes it more attractive. The use of these screening questionnaires may help in early identification, and thereby in early initiation of treatment.

1.9 EPIDEMIOLOGY OF METABOLIC SYNDROME AND CARDIOVASCULAR DISEASE RISK FACTORS IN PSORIATIC ARTHRITIS AND PSORIASIS

Being chronic inflammatory conditions, PsO and PsA predispose to metabolic syndrome and coronary events. This is brought about by endothelial dysfunction,[47] accelerated atherogenesis, increased insulin resistance, and hyperleptinemia.[48] The prevalence of diabetes mellitus, systemic hypertension, obesity, and dyslipidemia was found to be higher in PsO, with an odds ratio of around 2 for each of these factors.[2,5,49,50] The incidence of metabolic syndrome was reported to be 59% in an Indian PsA cohort.[51] The adjusted relative risk for myocardial infarction was 3.1 in a study,[50] although higher rates of obesity and smoking might have had confounding effects in these PsO patients.[49] The chronic inflammatory state in PsO appears to play a part in the development of metabolic syndrome. Early identification of these comorbidities will help to decrease morbidity in these patients.

To conclude, there are varying prevalence rates of PsO and PsA among various populations. The incidence and prevalence of PsA among PsO also vary significantly. Part of this difference is due to the different classification criteria used. The increasing use of CASPAR has brought some uniformity in recent times. There is a need to have better screening strategies for the early diagnosis of PsA. There is also an unmet need to have a uniform screening strategy for metabolic syndrome in these patients.

REFERENCES

1. Olsen, Grjibovski, Magnus, Tambs, and Harris. 2005. Psoriasis in Norway as observed in a population-based Norwegian twin panel. *Br J Dermatol* 153:346–51.
2. Kubota, Kamijima, Sato et al. 2015. Epidemiology of psoriasis and palmoplantar pustulosis: A nationwide study using the Japanese national claims database. *BMJ Open* 5:e006450.
3. Saraceno, Mannheimer, and Chimenti. 2008. Regional distribution of psoriasis in Italy. *J Eur Acad Dermatol Venereol* 22:324–9.
4. Ding, Wang, Shen et al. 2012. Prevalence of psoriasis in China: A population-based study in six cities. *Eur J Dermatol* 22:663–7.
5. Cohen, Gilutz, Henkin et al. 2007. Psoriasis and the metabolic syndrome. *Acta Derm Venereol* 87:506–9.
6. Ogdie, Langan, Love et al. 2013. Prevalence and treatment patterns of psoriatic arthritis in the UK. *Rheumatology (Oxford)* 52:568–75.
7. Soriano, Rosa, Velozo et al. 2011. Incidence and prevalence of psoriatic arthritis in Buenos Aires, Argentina: A 6-year health management organization-based study. *Rheumatology (Oxford)* 50:729–34.
8. Hanova, Pavelka, Holcatova, and Pikhart. 2010. Incidence and prevalence of psoriatic arthritis, ankylosing spondylitis, and reactive arthritis in the first descriptive population-based study in the Czech Republic. *Scand J Rheumatol* 39:310–7.
9. Gelfand, Gladman, Mease et al. 2005. Epidemiology of psoriatic arthritis in the population of the United States. *J Am Acad Dermatol* 53:573.
10. Nossent and Gran. 2009. Epidemiological and clinical characteristics of psoriatic arthritis in northern Norway. *Scand J Rheumatol* 38:251–5.
11. Li, Sun, Ren et al. 2012. Epidemiology of eight common rheumatic diseases in China: A large-scale cross-sectional survey in Beijing. *Rheumatology (Oxford)* 51:721–9.
12. Queiro-Silva, Torre-Alonso, Tinture-Eguren, and Lopez-Lagunas. 2003. A polyarticular onset predicts erosive and deforming disease in psoriatic arthritis. *Ann Rheum Dis* 62:68–70.
13. Leung, Tam, Ho et al. 2010. Evaluation of the CASPAR criteria for psoriatic arthritis in the Chinese population. *Rheumatology (Oxford)* 49:112–5.
14. Tillett, Costa, Jadon et al. 2012. The ClASsification for Psoriatic ARthritis (CASPAR) criteria—A retrospective feasibility, sensitivity, and specificity study. *J Rheumatol* 39:154–6.
15. van den Berg, van Gaalen, van der Helm-van Mil, Huizinga, and van der Heijde. 2012. Performance of classification criteria for peripheral spondyloarthritis and psoriatic arthritis in the Leiden Early Arthritis cohort. *Ann Rheum Dis* 71:1366–9.
16. Kawada, Tezuka, Nakamizo et al. 2003. A survey of psoriasis patients in Japan from 1982 to 2001. *J Dermatol Sci* 31:59–64.

17. Alenius, Stenberg, Stenlund, Lundblad, and Dahlqvist. 2002. Inflammatory joint manifestations are prevalent in psoriasis: Prevalence study of joint and axial involvement in psoriatic patients, and evaluation of a psoriatic and arthritic questionnaire. *J Rheumatol* 29:2577–82.
18. Mease, Gladman, Papp et al. 2013. Prevalence of rheumatologist-diagnosed psoriatic arthritis in patients with psoriasis in European/North American dermatology clinics. *J Am Acad Dermatol* 69:729–35.
19. Carneiro, Paula, and Martins. 2012. Psoriatic arthritis in patients with psoriasis: Evaluation of clinical and epidemiological features in 133 patients followed at the University Hospital of Brasilia. *An Bras Dermatol* 87:539–44.
20. Kumar, Sharma, and Dogra. 2014. Prevalence and clinical patterns of psoriatic arthritis in Indian patients with psoriasis. *Indian J Dermatol Venereol Leprol* 80:15–23.
21. Baek, Yoo, Shin et al. 2000. Spondylitis is the most common pattern of psoriatic arthritis in Korea. *Rheumatol Int* 19:89–94.
22. Eder, Chandran, Shen et al. 2011. Incidence of arthritis in a prospective cohort of psoriasis patients. *Arthritis Care Res (Hoboken)* 63:619–22.
23. Christophers, Barker, Griffiths et al. 2010. The risk of psoriatic arthritis remains constant following initial diagnosis of psoriasis among patients seen in European dermatology clinics. *J Eur Acad Dermatol Venereol* 24:548–54.
24. Wilson, Icen, Crowson et al. 2009. Incidence and clinical predictors of psoriatic arthritis in patients with psoriasis: A population-based study. *Arthritis Rheum* 61:233–9.
25. Offidani, Cellini, Valeri, and Giovagnoni. 1998. Subclinical joint involvement in psoriasis: Magnetic resonance imaging and x-ray findings. *Acta Derm Venereol* 78:463–5.
26. Rather, Nisa, and Arif. 2015. The pattern of psoriatic arthritis in Kashmir: A 6-year prospective study. *N Am J Med Sci* 7:356–61.
27. Kane, Stafford, Bresnihan, and FitzGerald. 2003. A prospective, clinical and radiological study of early psoriatic arthritis: An early synovitis clinic experience. *Rheumatology (Oxford)* 42:1460–8.
28. Moll and Wright. 1973. Psoriatic arthritis. *Semin Arthritis Rheum* 3:55–78.
29. Veale, Rogers, and Fitzgerald. 1994. Classification of clinical subsets in psoriatic arthritis. *Br J Rheumatol* 33:133–8.
30. Yang, Qu, Tian et al. 2011. Prevalence and characteristics of psoriatic arthritis in Chinese patients with psoriasis. *J Eur Acad Dermatol Venereol* 25:1409–14.
31. Thumboo, Tham, Tay et al. 1997. Patterns of psoriatic arthritis in Orientals. *J Rheumatol* 24:1949–53.
32. Elkayam, Ophir, Yaron, and Caspi. 2000. Psoriatic arthritis: Interrelationships between skin and joint manifestations related to onset, course and distribution. *Clin Rheumatol* 19:301–5.
33. Gladman, Farewell, Wong, and Husted. 1998. Mortality studies in psoriatic arthritis: Results from a single outpatient center. II. Prognostic indicators for death. *Arthritis Rheum* 41:1103–10.
34. Elder, Nair, Guo et al. 1994. The genetics of psoriasis. *Arch Dermatol* 130:216–24.
35. Rahman and Elder. 2005. Genetic epidemiology of psoriasis and psoriatic arthritis. *Ann Rheum Dis* 64 (Suppl 2):ii37–9; discussion ii40–1.
36. Swanbeck, Inerot, Martinsson, et al. 1997. Genetic counselling in psoriasis: Empirical data on psoriasis among first-degree relatives of 3095 psoriatic probands. *Br J Dermatol* 137:939–42.
37. Rahman, Gladman, Schentag, and Petronis. 1999. Excessive paternal transmission in psoriatic arthritis. *Arthritis Rheum* 42:1228–31.
38. Gudjonsson, Karason, Antonsdottir et al. 2002. HLA-Cw6-positive and HLA-Cw6-negative patients with psoriasis vulgaris have distinct clinical features. *J Invest Dermatol* 118:362–5.
39. Karason, Gudjonsson, Upmanyu et al. 2003. A susceptibility gene for psoriatic arthritis maps to chromosome 16q: Evidence for imprinting. *Am J Hum Genet* 72:125–31.
40. Gladman, Anhorn, Schachter, and Mervart. 1986. HLA antigens in psoriatic arthritis. *J Rheumatol* 13:586–92.
41. Husni, Meyer, Cohen, Mody, and Qureshi. 2007. The PASE questionnaire: Pilot-testing a psoriatic arthritis screening and evaluation tool. *J Am Acad Dermatol* 57:581–7.
42. Dominguez, Husni, Holt, Tyler, and Qureshi. 2009. Validity, reliability, and sensitivity-to-change properties of the psoriatic arthritis screening and evaluation questionnaire. *Arch Dermatol Res* 301:573–9.
43. Ibrahim, Buch, Lawson, Waxman, and Helliwell. 2009. Evaluation of an existing screening tool for psoriatic arthritis in people with psoriasis and the development of a new instrument: The Psoriasis Epidemiology Screening Tool (PEST) questionnaire. *Clin Exp Rheumatol* 27:469–74.
44. Gladman, Schentag, Tom et al. 2009. Development and initial validation of a screening questionnaire for psoriatic arthritis: The Toronto Psoriatic Arthritis Screen (ToPAS). *Ann Rheum Dis* 68:497–501.

45. Tinazzi, Adami, Zanolin et al. 2012. The early psoriatic arthritis screening questionnaire: A simple and fast method for the identification of arthritis in patients with psoriasis. *Rheumatology (Oxford)* 51:2058–63.
46. Mishra, Kancharla, Dogra, and Sharma. 2017. Comparison of the four validated psoriatic arthritis screening tools in diagnosing psoriatic arthritis in patients with psoriasis (COMPAQ Study). *Br J Dermatol* 176:765–70.
47. Sharma, Reddy, Sharma, Dogra, and Vijayvergiya. 2016. Study of endothelial dysfunction in patients of psoriatic arthritis by flow mediated and nitroglycerine mediated dilatation of brachial artery. *Int J Rheum Dis* 19:300–4.
48. Chen, Wu, Shen et al. 2008. Psoriasis independently associated with hyperleptinemia contributing to metabolic syndrome. *Arch Dermatol* 144:1571–5.
49. Sommer, Jenisch, Suchan, Christophers, and Weichenthal. 2006. Increased prevalence of the metabolic syndrome in patients with moderate to severe psoriasis. *Arch Dermatol Res* 298:321–8.
50. Gelfand, Neimann, Shin et al. 2006. Risk of myocardial infarction in patients with psoriasis. *JAMA* 296:1735–41.
51. Sharma, Gopalakrishnan, Kumar, Vijayvergiya, and Dogra. 2013. Metabolic syndrome in psoriatic arthritis patients: A cross-sectional study. *Int J Rheum Dis* 16:667–73.

2 Genetics of Psoriasis and Psoriatic Arthritis

Remy Pollock and Vinod Chandran

CONTENTS

2.1 INTRODUCTION: THE PHENOTYPES

2.1.1 Psoriasis

Psoriasis is a common, chronic immune-mediated skin disease that affects 0.6%–6.5% of Europeans and 3.15% of North Americans [1]. Although it is not often considered life threatening, psoriasis has a major impact on the quality of life and is associated with significant morbidity, comorbidity, and mortality [2]. It has been estimated that psoriasis places an annual burden on health care systems and society of approximately $112 billion in the United States alone [3]. Psoriasis follows an unpredictable and variable clinical course characterized by periods of high and low disease activity [4]. It presents most commonly, in 85%–90% of patients, as chronic plaque psoriasis, which is characterized by symmetrical, silvery-white, scaly plaques. These plaques result from hyperproliferation of the epidermis, incomplete differentiation of keratinocytes, and infiltration of the epidermis and papillary dermis by activated immune cells. Plaques can present anywhere on the body, but are most commonly found on the trunk, limbs, scalp, elbows, and knees, and in the body folds [5]. Other forms of psoriasis include guttate psoriasis, palmoplantar psoriasis, and psoriatic erythroderma.

2.1.2 Psoriatic Arthritis

Psoriasis is often accompanied by inflammation of a number of other organ systems, not just the skin. It can target diverse tissues such as the gut, eye, and musculoskeletal system, resulting in the associated features of inflammatory bowel disease, uveitis, and most commonly, arthritis [1,4]. The specific form of arthritis that develops in psoriasis patients is known as psoriatic arthritis (PsA), which has been recognized as a clinical entity distinct from rheumatoid arthritis since 1964 [6]. PsA usually manifests in the third or fourth decade of life, and develops after psoriasis onset in the majority (~70%) of cases [7]. The overall prevalence of PsA among psoriasis patients is estimated to be 30%, while its prevalence in the general population varies widely between ethnicities, ranging from as low as 0.00001% in Japan to 0.25% in the United States and 0.42% in Italy [1]. PsA is classified as a spondyloarthritis, making it closely related to ankylosing spondylitis, reactive arthritis, inflammatory bowel disease–associated arthritis, juvenile idiopathic arthritis, enthesitis-related arthritis, and undifferentiated spondyloarthritis. PsA has several manifestations that typify this group of diseases, including axial arthritis, asymmetric peripheral arthritis, enthesitis, dactylitis, and skin and joint disease, and a strong association with the human leukocyte antigen (HLA) B allele *HLA-B*27*. Like psoriasis, PsA follows a variable disease course and is characterized by periods of remissions and flares. However, periods of remission are short, lasting on average 2.6 years, and relapses are common [8,9]. Overall, PsA is a chronic, progressive disease that can lead to joint damage, disability, increased mortality, reduced quality of life and function, and a long list of comorbidities, including cardiovascular disease, type 2 diabetes, neurologic conditions, gastrointestinal disorders, and liver disease [10,11].

2.1.3 Onset of Psoriasis and Psoriatic Arthritis

It is well known that environmental exposures can trigger psoriasis and PsA. Environmental factors that appear to influence the onset of psoriasis include physical trauma to the skin (known as the Koebner phenomenon), which can result in the appearance of plaques directly at the site of trauma; emotional stress; viral and bacterial infections; humidity; cold weather; diet; obesity; smoking; and certain medications [1,12]. Environmental risk factors associated with the development of PsA include trauma to the joints and bone (known as the deep Koebner phenomenon), heavy lifting, infections, changing residence, and rubella vaccination [13–15]. Although these numerous environmental factors are significantly associated with both psoriasis and PsA, the strength of these associations is generally quite weak, and as a result, they explain only a small proportion of disease risk. Therefore, environment cannot be the sole cause of psoriasis and PsA, and additional factors, such as genetics and the interaction of genes with environmental risk factors, likely explain the origins of these complex diseases.

This chapter aims to review the current state of knowledge pertaining to the genetics of psoriasis and PsA, including the evidence of a heritable component of each disease, and review the genes and variants associated with psoriasis and PsA both within and outside of the major histocompatibility complex (MHC), and how they relate to disease pathogenesis. We also review evidence for gene–gene and gene–environment interactions, and variants associated with response to therapy (pharmacogenetics). Finally, we discuss the challenges of studying the genetics of these complex overlapping diseases, the future of genetic investigations, and their potential clinical applications.

2.2 EVIDENCE OF A GENETIC COMPONENT AND MODE OF INHERITANCE

2.2.1 Psoriasis

Any discussion of genetics must begin with reviewing the evidence of a familial component to the disease in question. It has long been recognized that there is a strong familial component to psoriasis, as evidenced by family and twin studies. Family studies typically estimate the recurrence risk ratio of a disease (λ), a measure of familial aggregation defined as the prevalence of disease among relatives of a proband compared with the prevalence among the general population [16]. In large population-based epidemiological studies of psoriasis, the recurrence risk ratio specifically among first-degree relatives of psoriasis patients (λ_1) was estimated to be between 4 and 13, and among siblings of psoriasis patients (λ_s), it was estimated to be between 4 and 10 [5,17–19]. Although these estimates provide some evidence of a heritable component to disease, they cannot conclusively rule out the effect of a shared environment among affected family members, which could contribute to the familial aggregation observed.

Twin studies compare disease concordance rates between genetically identical monozygotic (MZ) and dizygotic (DZ) twins. Studies in psoriasis have shown a concordance rate ranging from 20% to 70% among MZ twins and 9% to 20% among DZ twins, indicating a higher risk of disease among the more genetically similar MZ twins [20–23]. Although these numbers still reflect both shared genes and a shared environment, twin studies do enable the dissection of phenotypic variation into additive genetic effects, dominant genetic effects, common (shared) environmental effects, and random (nonshared) environmental effects. Broad-sense heritability (H^2) is defined as the proportion of phenotypic variance that can be explained by all genetic effects (additive and dominant), and it has been estimated to be quite high relative to other complex diseases, ranging from 60% to 90% [18], which suggests that shared genetics plays a much larger role than shared environment in the above estimates for psoriasis.

2.2.2 Psoriatic Arthritis

Family studies suggest an even stronger genetic contribution to the risk of PsA than psoriasis. In 1973, Moll and Wright first estimated λ_1 for PsA to be 55 [24]. Subsequent studies have estimated λ_1 for PsA to be 40, and the more specific λ_s for PsA to be 30.4 [25,26]. Interestingly, the first estimate was derived from the Icelandic genealogical database, which was used to create family trees of individuals identified to have PsA, and in the same study, the λ_1 for rheumatoid arthritis was estimated to be 2.78, suggesting that the genetic burden may be much greater in PsA [25]. Only one twin study has been performed in PsA to date, and it found the disease concordance rates among MZ and DZ twins to be 10% and 3.8%, respectively, using Moll and Wright's diagnostic criteria, and 11% and 5%, respectively, using the Classification Criteria for Psoriatic Arthritis (CASPAR) [27]. Unfortunately, it is difficult to dissect the contributions of genetics and shared environment, as this study was underpowered to accurately estimate heritability.

2.2.3 Mode of Inheritance

From analysis of pedigrees and family studies, it is possible to determine the mode of inheritance of psoriasis and PsA. Although it has been previously proposed that psoriasis follows a dominant or recessive pattern of simple Mendelian genetics, these patterns seem limited to only certain families who represent the exception rather than the rule. Overall, in most families psoriasis shows no clear pattern of inheritance, having a tendency to disappear and reappear within pedigrees, which is more consistent with a multifactorial pattern of inheritance [28]. Similarly, in PsA, family studies using the Icelandic genealogical database demonstrated that the relative risk of PsA in first-, second-, third-, and fourth-degree relatives declined from 39 to 12, 3.6, and 2.3, respectively. This observed "dose–response" decrease of more than a factor of 2 for each degree of relatedness is consistent with multifactorial inheritance and the presence of multiple, interacting susceptibility genes [16,17]. A parent-of-origin effect manifesting as an increased risk and severity of disease during male compared with female transmission has also been observed for both psoriasis and PsA, which provides further evidence of non-Mendelian inheritance mechanisms, such as genomic imprinting, operating in these diseases [29–31].

2.3 GENETICS OF PSORIASIS

2.3.1 Definition of Disease Phenotype

The majority of studies in psoriasis have sought to determine genetic associations with its most common clinical form, chronic plaque psoriasis, as opposed to the less common forms of guttate, flexural/inverse, erythrodermic, and pustular psoriasis. To further decrease disease heterogeneity, many studies have also focused on early-onset (type 1) psoriasis, which appears before the age of 40 and is thought to have a stronger genetic component than late-onset (type 2) psoriasis, which is thought to be largely environmental [32].

2.3.2 Linkage Studies

Genome-wide linkage studies constitute some of the earliest genetic investigations in psoriasis. These studies identified microsatellite markers associated with psoriasis by analyzing their cosegregation with affected individuals within families, and characterized psoriasis susceptibility loci *PSORS1* through *PSORS10* [33]. *PSORS1*, an 80–200 kb region on chromosome 6p21.3, is the strongest and most important genetic determinant of psoriasis, accounting for approximately one-third of the heritability [34]. Several genes within this region, including MHC gene *HLA-C*, corneodesmosin (*CDSN*), and coiled coil alpha helical rod protein 1 (*CCHCR1*), were hypothesized to drive the association [35,36]. There is now sufficient evidence to suggest that *HLA-C*, and specifically the *C*0602* allele, is the primary association in different populations [37,38]. Interestingly, the association of *HLA-C*0602* with psoriasis appears to be limited to type 1 psoriasis [39], is strongest with guttate psoriasis [40] and the Koebner phenomenon, and is associated with familial aggregation and more severe disease [41]. *PSORS2* was mapped to 17q24–25, which contains candidate genes involved in the immune system and atopic dermatitis, such as *RUNX1, RAPTOR, SLC9A3R1, NAT9,* and *TBCD* [32]. The remaining *PSORS* loci were mapped to various regions throughout the genome, such as 4q34 (*PSORS3*, candidate gene *IRF2*), 1q21 (*PSORS4*, candidate genes *LOR, FLG, PGLYRP3* and *4*, and *S100* family genes in the epidermal differentiation complex), 3q21 (*PSORS5*, candidate genes *SLC12A8, CSTA,* and *ZNF148*), 19p13 (*PSORS6*, candidate gene *JUNB*), 1p32 (*PSORS7*, candidate genes *PTPN22* and *IL23R*), 16q (*PSORS8*, candidate genes *CX3CL1, CXCR3,* and *CARD15*), 4q31 (*PSORS9*, candidate gene *IL15*), and 18p11 (*PSORS10*), as reviewed in [32,42].

2.3.3 Major Histocompatibility Complex Class I Genes

While successful in identifying several candidate psoriasis susceptibility regions, linkage studies have limited power to detect genes with modest effect compared with genetic association studies [32]. The first genetic association studies in psoriasis were performed in the 1970s and took a candidate gene approach, examining the gene-dense MHC region, which contains numerous genes with important immune functions [43,44]. Psoriasis was found to be associated with HLA Class I genes *HLA-C* and *HLA-B*; however, the association with *HLA-B*, particularly alleles *B*13, B*37,* and *B*57,* was later found to be due to extended haplotypes, resulting in linkage disequilibrium (LD) with *HLA-C* [45]. Subsequent studies have identified additional *HLA-B* alleles that appear to be associated with psoriasis independently of *HLA-C*, such as *HLA-B*38* and *B*39* [46]. Genes proximal to the HLA region have also been investigated—however, such investigations have been hampered by the strong LD that extends throughout MHC Class I, which has made the identification of independent effects of susceptibility loci difficult. Nonetheless, studies of the highly polymorphic MHC Class I chain-related gene A (*MICA*), located 100 kb centromeric to *HLA-B*, suggested an independent association between *MICA*016* and psoriasis [47]. Studies that have imputed the *HLA-C*0602* genotype before adjusting for its presence in conditional regression analyses have found two significant, independent association signals within the C6orf10 locus (rs2073048) and at a locus 30 kb centromeric to *HLA-B* and 16 kb telomeric to *MICA* (rs13437088), which were also significant in a Han Chinese population [48,49]. However, a later imputation study found no apparent risk of psoriasis conferred by *MICA* [50].

2.3.4 Genes Outside of the Major Histocompatibility Complex

Candidate gene and genome-wide association studies (GWASs) have also uncovered associations between psoriasis and genes residing outside of the MHC. For example, β defensins (*DEFB*), angiotensin-converting enzyme (*ACE*), and vitamin D receptor (*VDR*) have all been associated with psoriasis in candidate gene studies. *DEFB* genes map to three clusters on chromosomes 8p23.1, 20p13, and 20q11.1, and encode small antimicrobial peptides [51]. An increased copy number of *DEFB4* has been associated with psoriasis in a study of 190 Dutch psoriasis patients and 303 controls [52]. Angiotensin-converting enzyme, encoded by the *ACE* gene on chromosome 17, controls arterial vasoconstriction and has been associated with type 2 diabetes, hypertension, Alzheimer's disease [53], and psoriasis, although associations with psoriasis are conflicting [54–59]. A meta-analysis confirmed that the homozygous I/I genotype and I allele increased risk of psoriasis, while the heterozygous I/D genotype decreased risk in Asian but not Caucasian populations [57]. Similarly, the association of variants within the vitamin D receptor has been studied in psoriasis with conflicting results [60–66]. In this case, meta-analyses have confirmed the lack of significant association with VDR gene variants and psoriasis patients overall [67].

The number of associations with psoriasis found outside the MHC increased dramatically after the introduction of technology to perform GWASs (Table 2.1). GWASs test the association of hundreds of thousands of common single-nucleotide polymorphisms (SNPs) (variants with a minor allele frequency of ≥5%) in unrelated cases compared with controls, with larger sample sizes increasing the statistical power to detect associations with smaller effect sizes [68]. The first clear association with psoriasis identified by GWASs was a known association with an SNP in the 3′ untranslated region (UTR), and targeted resequencing identified an additional association 60 kb upstream of *IL12B* (rs3212227 and rs6887695, respectively) [69]. *IL12B* encodes the p40 subunit common to both *IL12* and *IL23* cytokines. The association with *IL12B* has since been replicated in other studies [70–72], and meta-analysis has confirmed that both SNPs are significantly associated with psoriasis [73].

GWASs have also uncovered associations with genes within the late cornified envelope (*LCE*) cluster spanning a 320 kb region within the epidermal differentiation complex in *PSORS4* [70,71,74]. In particular, the *LCE3* cluster, encompassing five genes (*LCE3A*, *3B*, *3C*, *3D*, and *3E*) that are known to be aberrantly expressed in psoriatic lesions, harbors genetic variants that significantly differ between psoriasis patients and controls. A GWAS of patients from a Han Chinese population linked *LCE3A* variants rs4845454 and rs1886734 and *LCE3D* variants rs4112788 and rs4085613 with psoriasis [71], while a sequencing study further implicated missense variants within *LCE3D* with psoriasis susceptibility [75]. Allelic dosage of *LCE3D* variants appears to influence psoriasis severity, with individuals with moderate to severe psoriasis showing a higher frequency of homozygosity for *LCE3D* risk alleles than individuals with mild psoriasis [76]. Furthermore, these variants are in LD with a deletion of *LCE3B* and *LCE3C* (*LCE3C_LCE3B-del*), which has also been associated with psoriasis susceptibility, occurring at a significantly higher frequency in psoriasis patients

TABLE 2.1
Genes Associated with Chronic Plaque Psoriasis in GWASs

Gene/Locus	Chromosome	Variant	Odds Ratio (95% CI)	*p* Value	Reference
IL12B	5q33	rs3212227	0.64 (0.56–0.73)	7.85×10^{-10}	69
LCE3A	1q21	rs4845454	0.76 (0.72–0.80)	4.35×10^{-29}	71
LCE3A	1q21	rs1886734	0.76 (0.73–0.80)	2.18×10^{-28}	71
LCE3D	1q21	rs4112788	0.77 (0.74–0.81)	7.13×10^{-27}	71
LCE3D	1q21	rs4085613	0.76 (0.72–0.80)	6.69×10^{-30}	71
HLA-C	6p21	rs10484554	2.8 (2.4–3.3)	1.80×10^{-39}	70
HCP5	6p21	rs2395029	4.1	2.13×10^{-26}	70
LHFP-COG6	13q14	rs7993214	0.71	2.00×10^{-6}	70
15q21	15q21	rs3803369	1.43	2.90×10^{-5}	70
3p24	3p24	rs6809854	1.14 (1.04–1.26)	1.12×10^{-7}	72
IL28RA	1p36	rs4649203	1.13 (1.05–1.22)	6.89×10^{-8}	72
REL	2p16	rs702873	1.12 (1.04–1.20)	3.59×10^{-9}	72
IFIH1	2q24	rs17716942	1.29 (1.17–1.43)	1.06×10^{-13}	72
ERAP1	5q15	rs27524	1.13 (1.05–1.22)	2.56×10^{-11}	72
TRAF3IP2	6p21	rs240993	1.25 (1.16–1.34)	5.29×10^{-20}	72
NFKBIA	14q13	rs8016947	1.19 (1.11–1.27)	1.52×10^{-11}	72
TYK2	19p13	rs12720356	1.40 (1.23–1.61)	4.04×10^{-11}	72
IL23R	1p31	rs11209026	1.49 (1.27–1.74)	7.13×10^{-7}	72
IL23A	12q13	rs2066808	1.49 (1.28–1.73)	2.49×10^{-7}	72
IL13	5q31	rs20541	1.12 (1.02–1.24)	2.32×10^{-2}	72
TNIP1	5q33	rs1024995	1.27 (1.14–1.44)	3.92×10^{-5}	72
TNFAIP3	6q23	rs610604	1.22 (1.13–1.32)	6.54×10^{-7}	72
ZNF313	20q13	rs2235617	1.20 (1.11–1.30)	1.65×10^{-6}	72
CDKAL1	6p22	rs6908425	0.88 (0.77–1.00)	3.10×10^{-2}	82
PTPN22	1p13	rs3789604	0.86 (0.75–0.98)	1.30×10^{-2}	82
ADAM33	20p13	rs597980	1.10 (0.99–1.22)	3.00×10^{-2}	82
NOS2	17q11	rs4795067	1.19	4.00×10^{-11}	85
FBXL19	16p11	rs10782001	1.16	9.00×10^{-10}	85
PSMA6-NFKBIA	14q13	rs12586317	1.15	2.00×10^{-8}	85
RNF114	20q13	rs495337	1.19	1.00×10^{-6}	85

Note: CI, confidence interval.

(63%–72%) than in controls (49%–69%) [71,77,78]. This finding has been replicated in several independent populations, including German, Dutch, Spanish, and Chinese populations [77,79–81].

Other psoriasis susceptibility genes identified in GWASs in patients of European and Chinese origin include *HCP5* (rs2395029), which had the strongest association in one study [70], and has no known function but is associated with a low viral set point in HIV infection; genes called lipoma HMGIC fusion partner (*LHFP*), and conserved oligomeric Golgi complex component 6 (*COG6*) on chromosome 13q13; signal peptide peptidase-like 2a (*SPPL2A*); loci on 15q21 [70] and 3p24; *IL28RA*; *REL*; *IFIH1*; *ERAP1*; *TRAF3IP2*; *NFKBIA*; *TYK2* [72]; interleukin 23 receptor subunit (*IL23R*); p19 subunit of IL23 (*IL23A*); *IL13*; *TNIP1*; *TNFAIP3*; *ZNF313* [72]; *CDKAL1*; *PTPN22*; and *ADAM33* [82]. Several of these associations have been replicated in independent studies, including *IL23R*, *IL23A*, *TNFAIP3*, *TNIP* [83], *IL13* [48], and *TRAF3IP2* [84]. Meta-analysis of two GWASs and subsequent replication in three independent cohorts identified additional psoriasis susceptibility loci at *NOS2*, *FBXL19*, *PSMA6-NFKBIA*, and *RNF114* [48,84,85]. A multistage replication study of the Chinese GWAS also identified additional susceptibility loci at *PTTG1*, *CSMD1*,

GJB2, *SERPINB8*, and *ZNF816A*, although only *ZNF816A* and *GJB2* showed evidence for association with the German replication cohort, which did not hold when combined with an American replication cohort [83].

2.3.5 Genetic Associations with Psoriasis Subtypes

While most studies have focused on the most common form of psoriasis, chronic plaque psoriasis, and early-onset type 1 psoriasis, the genetic underpinnings of other subtypes are beginning to be elucidated. Generalized pustular psoriasis (GPP) is a rare form characterized by acute, subacute, or chronic sterile pustular eruptions that occur in patients with or without psoriasis vulgaris. GPP is occasionally life threatening, involving fever and other systemic manifestations, and can be triggered by factors such as infections, pregnancy, hypocalcemia, and drugs [86]. Interestingly, in contrast to the multifactorial genetic architecture of psoriasis vulgaris, an autosomal recessive inheritance pattern of GPP has been reported in several Tunisian families. Linkage and sequencing studies revealed an association with a 1.2 Mb region on 2q13–14.1 containing a homozygous mutation in *IL36RN* (p.L27P), which reduces the stability of the encoded protein, decreasing its expression and potency, and leading to pro-inflammatory signaling [87]. Thus far, 17 different mutations in *IL36RN* have been associated with GPP in patients from Africa, Europe, and Asia [86,88,89], some of which cause sporadic GPP [90]. These mutations are thought to be specifically associated with GPP without psoriasis vulgaris, as they are found in significantly higher frequency in these patients compared with patients with GPP and psoriasis vulgaris [86,91,92]. Other mutations associated with sporadic GPP occur in the coding region of *CARD14* (p.Glu138Ala) [93], a scaffolding protein important in NFκB activation and the gene underlying the association at *PSORS2*, as well as *AP1S3*, which encodes the AP-1 complex small subunit [94]. Furthermore, the unique genetic underpinnings of late-onset psoriasis (type 2 psoriasis, >40 years) are also beginning to be understood. Unlike type 1 and guttate psoriasis, type 2 psoriasis is not strongly associated with *HLA-C*0602* [68], but is associated with variants within the *IL1B* gene on chromosome 2q14.1 [95]. The genetic heterogeneity found between different psoriasis subtypes suggests different pathogenic mechanisms underlying these variable clinical phenotypes.

2.3.6 Pathogenic Insights from Genetic Studies

Genetic associations with psoriasis vulgaris can give us important clues into the pathophysiology of the disease. The genes identified thus far suggest that psoriasis results from dysfunction of both the epidermis and immune system. In particular, based on their functions, susceptibility genes can be assembled into those that play a role in skin barrier function, and both the innate and adaptive immune systems [96].

Genes that implicate dysregulation of skin barrier function include the *LCE* family, which encode proteins expressed in the upper strata of the epidermis, the stratum corneum, and are crucial to normal epidermal differentiation. It has been speculated that mutations in *LCE* genes cause abnormal differentiation observed in psoriatic skin lesions [77]. However, variants within the *S100* genes are in LD with *LCE3C_LCE3B-del* and may be responsible for the association with this region, and their functions are fitting, as they encode chemoattractants expressed during epithelial barrier injury [97]. It has also been hypothesized that the loss of *LCE3C* and *LCE3B* expression may lead to insufficient LCE protein expression, resulting in an imperfect repair response following barrier disruption and activation of the immune system [74]. Alternatively, loss of important epidermal-specific enhancers within the *LCE3C_LCE3B-del* deletion may contribute to psoriasis [97]. *DEFB* genes encode antimicrobial peptides, one of which, *DEFB4*, is dramatically reduced in expression in psoriasis, while others show increased expression in psoriatic keratinocytes upon stimulation with Th1 or Th17 cytokines [98]. These antimicrobial peptides function in the attraction of T cells and immature dendritic cells to the skin, serving as a link between the innate and adaptive immune systems [99]. Finally, *GJB2* encodes connexin 26, a gap junction protein expressed at high levels in psoriatic keratinocytes [100], that can mediate ATP release and indirectly regulate epidermal differentiation and inflammation in psoriasis [101].

In addition to the association with β defensin genes, several other genetic associations point toward a role for innate immunity in psoriasis. NFκB is a key regulator of the innate immune response. It is stimulated by cytokines such as tumor necrosis factor (TNF), IL1, and IL17, and can trigger the expression of several inflammatory genes [96]. NFκB signaling is complex, involving several proteins, many of which have been found to be associated with psoriasis in recent GWASs, including *TNFAIP3*, *TNIP1*, *TRAF3IP2*, *REL*, *NFKBIA*, *FBXL19*, *NOS2*, *CARD14*, *CARM1*, *UBE2L3*, and *IFIH1* [33]. These proteins all function in the activation or inhibition of NFκB or its functions. *IFIH1*, an RNA helicase, is also involved in activating interferons (IFNs). Similarly, *TYK2* is a tyrosine kinase involved in activating type 1 IFN signaling. Finally, associations with the *MICA* gene further suggest the involvement of natural killer (NK) cells, as *MICA* encodes a cellular or metabolic stress-induced ligand of the activating NK, NKT, and T-cell receptor NKG2D. The role of innate immune cells such as NK or NKT cells in psoriasis has not yet been defined; however, it is possible that they play a role given their capacity to secrete inflammatory cytokines such as TNFα, IFNγ, and IL22 [102].

The strongest evidence implicating the adaptive immune system in psoriasis pathogenesis is the strong association with *HLA-C*0602*, which encodes an important peptide presentation protein expressed on the surface on almost all nucleated cells. It was suggested that this specific *HLA-C* allele was responsible for presenting an epitope present in type 1 keratins, which would function as an autoantigen that is cross-reactive with streptococcal protein M, serving to trigger an autoimmune response mediated by CD8+ T cells, which recognize this MHC Class I molecule [103]. More recent evidence suggests that other endogenous proteins may serve as autoantigens in psoriasis, such as the melanocyte-produced protein ADAMTSL5 [104] and the antimicrobial peptide cathelicidin (LL37) [105]. Further genetic evidence implicating antigen presentation in psoriasis pathogenesis is the association with *ERAP1*, which functions in trimming peptides within the endoplasmic reticulum for presentation by HLA Class I molecules.

Several other associations identified by GWASs also implicate adaptive immunity in psoriasis, particularly the Th17/IL23 axis. Th17 cells, which are maintained by IL23 signaling, play an important role in mediating activation of the innate and adaptive immune systems. GWASs have identified *IL12B*, which encodes the p40 subunit of *IL23*, *IL23A*, which encodes its p19 subunit, *IL23R*, which encodes a subunit of the IL23 receptor, and *RNF114*, which is involved in T-cell activation [48,69,72,106–108]. Variants in these genes may result in dysfunctional IL23 signaling, perhaps serving to enhance Th17 cell expansion [109]. *TRAF3IP2*, also identified by GWASs, plays an important role in signaling downstream of the IL17 receptor through NFκB signaling, which may result in the upregulation of pro-inflammatory genes [109–111]. Lastly, TYK2 has also been shown to be able to stimulate the transcription of IL17 [112].

2.4 GENETICS OF PSORIATIC ARTHRITIS

2.4.1 Definition of Disease Phenotype

Early genetic studies of PsA were performed on patients satisfying the diagnostic criteria proposed by Moll and Wright: the presence of psoriasis and inflammatory arthritis (peripheral and/or sacroiliitis or spondylitis), and the absence of rheumatoid factor on serological tests [113]. More recent studies, particularly those performed after the CASPAR were published, have tended to use these criteria instead [32]. The CASPAR define PsA as the presence of inflammatory articular disease of the joint, spine, or entheses, and ≥3 points from the following: current psoriasis (2 points) or family history (1 point) or personal history (1 point) of psoriasis, psoriatic nail dystrophy, rheumatoid factor negativity, dactylitis, and radiographic evidence of juxta-articular new bone formation

(1 point each) [114]. While establishing a more specific definition of PsA, the CASPAR still allow for substantial heterogeneity among patients, which likely still reflects a diversity of pathogenic alterations and underlying susceptibility genes [96].

Since most PsA patients have concomitant psoriasis, in any discussion of the genetics of PsA it must also be clarified whether the associations presented are those specific to skin disease, joint disease, or both. Currently, the most widely accepted paradigm of PsA as a "disease within a disease" is supported by the finding that the majority of genes associated with skin disease in psoriasis are also associated with PsA, reflecting perhaps the shared skin disease phenotype, or the pleiotropic effects of the same susceptibility genes on both skin and joint manifestations of the disease. In addition, the finding of additional susceptibility genes associated specifically with PsA, and not psoriasis alone, further supports this model. Taken together, these findings demonstrate that the genes related to psoriatic skin disease are merely a subset of those related to PsA overall [115]. The following two sections review the shared genetic associations between psoriasis and PsA, and the associations that appear to be specific to joint disease in PsA.

2.4.2 Genes Associated with Psoriatic Arthritis and Psoriasis

Most genetic associations identified in psoriasis thus far have also been found to be significantly associated with PsA. This holds true for even the strongest psoriasis susceptibility locus, *HLA-C*0602*, which was shown to be significantly increased in frequency in PsA patients compared with the general population, but significantly decreased in frequency in PsA patients compared with patients with psoriasis alone [116,117]. However, other studies report equal frequencies of *HLA-C*0602* in PsA and psoriasis patients [17,118]. Other psoriasis HLA susceptibility alleles, such as *HLA-B*1302* and *B*5701*, are also associated with both psoriasis and PsA across various populations [41,119–121], although these alleles form haplotypes with *HLA-C*0602*, and thus associations are likely due to LD with *HLA-C*. Near the HLA region, associations with the *TNFA* –238 polymorphism and both psoriasis and PsA have been reported and confirmed by meta-analysis [122].

Outside of the MHC, the copy number variation (CNV) in the *LCE* cluster associated with psoriasis, *LCE3C_LCE3B-del*, is also associated with PsA in British, Italian, and Spanish populations [123,124], but not in German or Tunisian cohorts of PsA patients [79,125]. Meta-analysis of the association with *LCE3C_LCE3B-del* suggests that it is indeed a susceptibility locus for PsA, as well as for psoriasis [126]. Candidate gene association studies, GWASs, and meta-analyses have found significant or at least nominally significant associations with known or newly identified psoriasis susceptibility loci *HCP5, IL12B, TRAF3IP2, TNIP1, LCE, IL23A, IL23R, IFIH1, ERAP1, REL, RUNX3, NOS2, FBXL19, RNF114*, and *PSMA6-NFKBIA* [70,73,76,84,126–140]. In addition, a locus on chromosome 4q27 containing *IL2* and *IL21* genes, previously associated with PsA but not psoriasis in a small GWAS, was later found to be associated with psoriasis as well [70,141]. These findings emphasize the strong genetic overlap between psoriasis and PsA.

2.4.3 Genes Associated with Psoriatic Arthritis but not Psoriasis without Arthritis

Despite the genetic overlap between psoriasis and PsA, the substantially higher heritability estimates for PsA suggest the presence of additional risk loci associated specifically with psoriatic joint manifestations and not skin manifestations [142]. Although numbering far fewer than the shared associations, several PsA-specific associations have been characterized (Table 2.2). The strongest and most notable of these is *HLA-B*27*, a known marker of the spondyloarthritis family of diseases to which PsA belongs. The association with *B*27* is evident when comparing PsA patients with both psoriasis patients and healthy controls. The frequency of *B*27* among PsA patients is much lower (20%–35%) than that among ankylosing spondylitis patients (80%–95%) [143], indicating that even though it is the strongest PsA-specific genetic marker to date, it contributes only a small proportion of the overall genetic risk of PsA. *B*27* has consistently been shown to be associated with

TABLE 2.2
Genes Differentially Associated with PsA and Psoriasis without Arthritis

Gene/Locus	Chromosome	Allele/Variants	Odds Ratio (95% CI)	*p* Value	Reference
HLA-B	6p21	*B*27*	5.17	1.00×10^{-4}	117
HLA-B	6p21	*B*08*	1.61	9.00×10^{-3}	117
HLA-B	6p21	*B*38*	1.65	2.60×10^{-2}	117
HLA-B	6p21	*B*3901*	3.74 (1.99–7.01)	1.00×10^{-4}	144
HLA-C	6p21	*C*06*	0.58	2.00×10^{-4}	117
RNF39	6p22	rs1150735	n/a	2.65×10^{-6}	151
KIR	19q13	*KIR2DS2*	1.25 (1.01–1.54)	4.40×10^{-2}	152
IL13	5q31	rs1800925, rs848	1.28	4.50×10^{-2}	138
IL12B	5q33	rs2082412	n/a	4.00×10^{-2}	136
FBXL19	16p11	rs10782001	1.12	2.20×10^{-2}	85
IL23R	1p31	rs11209026	0.52 (0.35–0.77)	8.30×10^{-2}	70
TRAF3IP2	6q21	rs33980500	1.57 (1.38–1.78)	4.57×10^{-12}	84
REL	2p16	rs13017599	1.27 (1.18–1.35)	1.18×10^{-8}	128
PTPN22	1p13	rs2476601	1.32	1.49×10^{-9}	154
NOS2	17q11	rs4795067	1.22	5.27×10^{-9}	154
ZNF816A	19q13	rs9304742	n/a	1.00×10^{-2}	136
ADAMTS9-MAGI1	3p14	26 kb deletion	1.48 (1.21–1.82)	5.97×10^{-5}	155

Note: CI, confidence interval; n/a, not available.

PsA and significantly differentiates PsA and psoriasis patients [117,144]. Other alleles of *HLA-B*, such as *B*08*, *B*38*, and *B*39*, have also been consistently associated with PsA but not psoriasis [46,117,144–146]. Interestingly, a fine mapping study of the MHC region confirmed the association of PsA with *HLA-B*27*, and pinpointed it to a specific amino acid residue at position 45 of the *HLA-B* gene (Glu45), which is contained within *B*27*, *B*38*, and *B*39* and confers a stronger risk for PsA compared with these alleles [50]. Conversely, *HLA-C*0602* is associated with PsA compared with controls, but this association is not as strong as with psoriasis alone, and in fact, it is significantly more frequent in psoriasis than PsA patients. *HLA-C*0602* is thus more strongly associated with skin disease, and appears to be "protective" toward the development of joint disease. *HLA-C*12* is also associated with PsA, but this association appears to be due to its strong LD with *HLA-B*38* [117].

Genes located near the MHC, such as *MICA*, and in particular the *MICA* transmembrane GCT trinucleotide repeat polymorphism A9, were shown to be associated specifically with PsA and not psoriasis independently of *HLA-C* in a Spanish PsA cohort [147,148]. Similar results were found in Jewish [149] and Croatian [150] cohorts. Further studies in a Canadian cohort revealed that the same A9-containing alleles associated with PsA were also associated with psoriasis and were in LD with the primary associations at *HLA-B* and *HLA-C*, but homozygosity for *MICA*00801* increased the risk of PsA compared with psoriasis when the two groups were directly compared [47]. However, a large fine mapping and imputation study of the MHC also failed to demonstrate independent associations between alleles of *MICA* and both PsA and psoriasis [50]. SNPs 1.5 kb upstream of the *RNF39* locus were also identified by high-resolution mapping of the MHC to be associated with PsA compared with controls after conditioning on HLA risk alleles [151].

Genes outside of the MHC that are significantly associated with PsA compared with psoriasis patients include the killer cell immunoglobulin-like receptors (KIRs), a polygenic and polymorphic cluster of genes located on chromosome 19q13.4. Specifically, the *KIR2DS2* locus, which encodes an activating NK cell surface receptor, is associated with PsA compared with controls and compared with patients with psoriasis alone [152]. Two variants within the *IL13* gene on chromosome

5q31, originally reported in psoriasis GWASs [48,72], were found to be specifically associated with PsA [129], particularly when compared with patients with psoriasis alone [138]. Variants within *IL12B* and *FBXL19* were also found in psoriasis GWASs to be associated with both psoriasis and PsA; however, in both cases the associations were stronger with the subgroup of PsA patients, and indeed, both genes significantly differentiated PsA and psoriasis patients when compared directly [48,85,136]. Similarly, several variants within *IL23R* [133], as well as *TRAF3IP2* [84,127] and *REL* [128], have been associated with both psoriasis and PsA, with the association of PsA with certain SNPs being stronger than that of both controls and psoriasis patients [153]. The rs2476601 variant within the *PTPN22* locus and the rs4795067 variant within the *NOS2* locus were recently found to be associated with PsA compared with controls and psoriasis patients, but were not significant in psoriasis patients compared with controls [154]. Furthermore, a Chinese study showed that markers within the *ZNF816A* gene were associated with PsA compared with psoriasis patients [136]. Lastly, a large study from Spain discovered and replicated an association of PsA with a 26 kb intergenic deletion of chromosome 3p14.1 between the *ADAMTS9-MAGI1* genes. This deletion was found in significantly lower frequency in psoriasis patients than in PsA patients [155]. On the other hand, in a meta-analysis of psoriasis GWASs, variants within *LCE3C/B* and *TNFRSF9* were found to be specifically associated with psoriasis patients who did not develop PsA, suggesting that like *HLA-C*0602*, they serve as a protective factor for the development of joint disease [156].

For some genes outside of the MHC, a direct comparison has never been made or direct comparisons have found no significant differences between groups. However, if these genes are more strongly associated with PsA than psoriasis, they are nonetheless considered to be legitimate PsA-specific associations, as the association with psoriasis may be due to the presence of undiagnosed PsA, compounded with the fact that many patients will eventually develop PsA within the psoriasis group. Examples of such genes include the immunoglobulin (Ig) heavy-chain HS 1,2-A enhancer region, which was found to be associated with psoriasis and PsA patients in Italians; however, the odds ratio reported (OR = 3.68) was larger for PsA [157]. An intergenic region in 5q31 marked by index SNP rs715285 was also found to be more strongly associated with PsA but only nominally associated with psoriasis, and this was independent of the known association with *IL13*, which resides in the same region [158]. Other genes that appear to be strongly associated with PsA but their association with psoriasis is unknown include *CARD15*, which was identified in a genome-wide linkage study of PsA when conditioned on paternal inheritance only and has been shown to be associated with PsA compared with controls [159,160].

2.4.4 Genetic Associations with Disease Expression

Genetic associations with age of disease onset or disease expression have focused mainly on HLA risk alleles. With regard to age of onset, *HLA-C*0602* positivity in PsA patients has been found to decrease age of onset of skin disease, but increase the time interval between the onset of psoriasis and the onset of joint disease, whereas *HLA-B*27* or *B*39* positivity shortens this interval, as *B*27* in particular is associated with an earlier age of arthritis onset [144,161]. *B*27* is also associated with axial disease in PsA patients, as well as a greater burden of articular damage [162], whereas *B*38* and *B*39* are associated with peripheral polyarthritis [143]. Unsurprisingly, *B*27* is strongly associated with symmetrical sacroiliitis in ankylosing spondylitis, as well as symmetrical sacroiliitis in PsA, as opposed to the more common asymmetric sacroiliitis, which is associated with *B*08* [163]. Clinically detectable enthesitis in PsA is associated with *B*2705* and *C*0102*, which together form a haplotype, but this association is lost in multivariable analyses, suggesting that another gene present in the haplotype drives the association with enthesitis [163]. Joint deformity and fusion is associated with the haplotype *HLA-B*0801-HLA-C*0701*, while dactylitis is associated with *B*27*, particularly the *B*2705-C*0102* haplotype, as well as the *B*0801-C*0701* haplotype. Finally, after grouping PsA patients into tertiles based on a novel continuous severity score that takes into account enthesitis, sacroiliitis, dactylitis, joint deformity, erosion, fusion, and osteolysis [162], it was found that the top tertile (i.e., severe disease) was associated with *B*27-C*02*, *B*37-C*06*, and *B*08-C*07* haplotypes [163]. Other studies have suggested that *C*0602* and *DRB1*07* carriage are associated with milder disease with fewer involved or damaged joints [164].

2.4.5 Pathogenic Insights from Genetic Studies

Genetic studies in PsA can also give us some clues into the pathogenesis of joint disease. The overlapping genetic associations between psoriasis and PsA suggest that the two diseases have several pathogenic mechanisms in common, including the involvement of innate and adaptive immunity. Innate immune pathways implicated in PsA include NFκB and interferon signaling, via the association of PsA with genes such as *MICA*, *KIR2DS2*, *TNIP1*, *REL*, *TYK2*, and *FBXL19* [33]. With regard to adaptive immune pathways, such as Th17 signaling, a few significant associations exist, including *IL12B*, *TRAF3IP2*, *IL23A*, *IL23R*, and *STAT3* [84,127,135,165,166]. Associations with other Th17-related genes, such as *IL17A*, *IL17RA*, *IL17RD*, and *IL17R*, could not be demonstrated or replicated [167]. This does not imply an insignificant role for Th17 signaling in PsA, as Th17 cells are known to be increased in the blood of PsA patients, correlate with disease activity [168], and stimulate osteoclastogenesis and bone erosions in joints [169]. The efficacy of IL12/23 p40 and IL17 monoclonal antibodies in PsA further supports a role for the Th17 pathway in PsA pathogenesis.

The best evidence for the involvement of adaptive immunity in PsA comes from the association with *HLA-B*27*; however, the pathogenic role of *B*27* in PsA remains unclear. Hypotheses regarding its role include the arthritogenic peptide hypothesis, the *B*27* misfolding hypothesis, and the *B*27*-free heavy-chain and homodimer hypothesis [170–172]. The arthritogenic peptide hypothesis postulates that *B*27* binds and presents shared arthritogenic peptides from disease-causing pathogens to CD8+ T cells, and these peptides are also cross-reactive to a self-peptide that can also be bound and presented by *B*27*. If this binding is mediated by particular amino acid residues contained within the HLA-B binding pocket, such as Glu45, this might explain the strong association with Glu45 and the alleles *B*27*, *B*38*, and *B*39* [50]. However, no arthritogenic peptides have been identified in PsA, and animal studies suggest that CD8+ T cells are not required for disease [173]. The misfolding hypothesis postulates that misfolded *B*27* heavy chains accumulate in the endoplasmic reticulum, chronically stimulating a stress response that leads to the release of inflammatory cytokines that trigger the innate immune response [172]. Some animal studies support this hypothesis [174], whereas others have shown that reversal of the accumulation of misfolded heavy chains has no effect on disease phenotype [175]. The *B*27*-free heavy-chain and homodimer hypothesis postulates that both the innate and adaptive immune systems are triggered by misfolded *B*27* molecules on the cell surface via their interactions with various immunoregulatory receptors, which could include the KIRs and/or the leukocyte immunoglobulin-like receptors (LILRs) [170–172]. This theory is supported by the finding of an enrichment of KIR3DL2+ CD4+ T cells producing IL17 after stimulation with *B*27* homodimers in the peripheral blood and synovial fluid of PsA patients [176].

2.5 EPISTASIS AND GENE–ENVIRONMENT INTERACTIONS

Gene products do not function in isolation, but interact with each other to form complex molecular networks. Genetic variants themselves also interact, in that the risk of developing a disease conferred by one variant can be conditioned by the presence of other variants in the genome [42]. Although there are few examples of such genetic interactions, called epistasis, in humans, a few examples have been characterized in psoriasis. In a Chinese population, the combination of risk alleles in both the MHC and *LCE* genes increased psoriasis risk by 26-fold, while the combination of risk alleles in the MHC and *IL12B* increased risk 36-fold relative to noncarriers [177]. Interaction between the MHC and *LCE* was also found in a Dutch study, but not in other studies from China [81,178], or studies in Spanish, Italian, American, German, or Tunisian populations [77,79,125]. An epistatic interaction between the functionally linked *ERAP1* gene and the *HLA-C*06* allele has also been found to increase psoriasis risk [72]. As previously described, ERAP1 functions in the processing of peptides that are to be presented by the HLA Class I molecules, and contributes to the susceptibility to another HLA Class I–associated disease, ankylosing spondylitis [179]. Epistatic interactions between *LCE3C/3D* and other psoriasis risk alleles (*IL23R, IL13, TNIP1/ANXA6, IL12B, CDKAL1, HLA-C, TNFAIP3, IL23A/STAT2*, and *ZNF313*) have also been investigated but yielded no evidence of any significant interaction after multiple testing correction [180].

In addition to interacting with other genes, risk variants can also interact with environmental factors to influence disease susceptibility. Smoking is a well-characterized, dose-dependent risk factor for the development of psoriasis [181], but interestingly, it is also associated with a delay in the time to PsA onset if smoking begins after psoriasis onset or a decrease in time to PsA onset if smoking begins before psoriasis onset [182]. This relationship between smoking and PsA is further influenced by variants within the *IL13* locus. However, the nature of this influence is contentious. One study found that the minor alleles of rs1800925*T, rs20541*A, and rs848*A showed a protective association with PsA but not psoriasis patients compared with controls, and this protective association was negated by smoking [129]. However, another study comparing PsA and psoriasis patients directly found that rs1800925*T and rs848*A were indeed protective, and smoking combined with rs1800925*T carriers became even more protective against PsA [138].

2.6 PHARMACOGENETICS OF PSORIASIS AND PSORIATIC ARTHRITIS

Of the various drugs used to treat psoriasis and PsA, the genetic factors underlying clinical responsiveness, including efficacy and toxicity, have been studied mainly for systemic agents such as methotrexate (MTX), acitretin, and biologics such as tumor necrosis alpha inhibitors (TNFi) and interleukin 12/23 inhibitors (IL12/23i). The aim of these studies is to identify sequence variants that can be used to predict in individual patients which drug will produce the best response with minimal side effects [28]. Of the systemic agents, MTX is the most extensively researched, as it is often used as first-line therapy for both psoriasis and PsA, but has variable efficacy and causes gastrointestinal and hepatotoxicity in approximately 30% of patients [183]. MTX is transported into cells and functions to inhibit enzymes involved in the folate, purine, and pyrimidine pathways, although its exact mechanism of action in psoriatic disease is poorly understood. Pharmacogenetic studies of MTX have taken a candidate gene approach and examined genes involved in its intracellular uptake (*ABCC1* and *ABCG2*) and metabolism (*FPGS, GGH, MTHFR*, and *ATIC*). In psoriasis patients, improved response was associated with SNPs in ATP binding cassette superfamily transporter genes *ABCC1* and *ABCG2* [184]. No association was found with genes involved in MTX metabolism [185]. Toxicity has been associated with SNPs in *ABCC1*, as well as the reduced folate carrier 1 gene (*RFC1*) [186] and thymidylate synthase (*TYMS*), although associations with the latter have shown conflicting results [186–188]. In PsA patients, variants within dihydrofolate reductase (*DHFR*), the enzyme that is directly inhibited by MTX and responsible for converting dihydrofolate to tetrahydrofolate, have been associated with improved response, while SNPs within *MTHFR* were associated with hepatotoxicity [189]. Poor response to acitretin, another systemic agent used in psoriasis, is associated with a variant at position 460 of the vascular endothelial growth factor gene (*VEGF*) [190].

Of the biologic drugs, TNFi are the most extensively researched. A study of both psoriasis and PsA patients from Toronto and Michigan demonstrated an association of the *TNFAIP3* rs610604*G allele and the haplotype *TNFAIP3* rs610604*G-rs2230926*T with response to TNFi, including etanercept, infliximab, and adalimumab, in Michigan patients, but not in Toronto patients [191]. Another study in a Greek population of psoriasis patients showed an association between variants in *TNFA* (rs1799724*CC) and *TNFRSF1B* (rs1061622*TT) and a positive response to etanercept, defined as a >75% reduction in the Psoriasis Area and Severity Index (PASI) score after 6 months, but not infliximab or adalimumab. This may be explained by slight differences in their modes of action, as etanercept binds the soluble form of TNFα, while adalimumab and infliximab bind transmembrane TNFα. *TNFA-TNFRSF1B* haplotypes (rs1799724-rs1061622 CT, CG, and TG) are also associated with response to TNFi [192]. In studies of PsA patients, the *TNFA* –308GG genotype was associated with better TNFi response than the AA or AG genotypes [193], and the *TNFRSF10A* rs20575*CC genotype was associated with a response to infliximab at 6 months, while *TNFR1A* rs767455*AA was associated with a response at 3 months [194]. Interestingly, epistatic interactions between *HLA-C*06* and *LCE* and *PDE3A* and *SLCO1C1* genotypes have also been associated with clinical improvement in psoriasis patients treated with TNFi [193]. Recently, GWASs have also yielded hits associated with clinical response to TNFi in *TNFAIP3* [191]. Lastly, in addition to response to TNFi, response to the IL12/23 inhibitor ustekinumab has been investigated. Ustekinumab is a monoclonal antibody that targets the shared p40 subunit of IL12/23. A more rapid and increased response to ustekinumab has been found in a single study of psoriasis patients who are *HLA-C*06* positive [195].

Overall, pharmacogenetic studies performed thus far have tended to use small sample sizes, meaning that they may be underpowered to detect significant associations. In addition, few studies have been independently replicated, and have failed to account for potential confounding factors that may affect drug response, such as alcohol consumption, stress, and body mass index [28,142], so there is a chance that initially reported associations represent false positives.

2.7 CHALLENGES AND FUTURE PERSPECTIVES

There are several challenges in the investigation of the genetics of psoriatic disease highlighted in the above-mentioned studies. This section discusses these challenges and offers future perspectives in their context. The first challenge is delineating the risk factors specific to skin and joint disease. Although heritability estimates of PsA are much higher than those for psoriasis, relatively fewer PsA-specific risk factors have been identified. Studies that directly compare psoriasis and PsA patients are ideal for this purpose; however, few have been performed thus far, as many studies have compared PsA patients with healthy controls. Even in direct comparisons of psoriasis and PsA patients, there is the possibility that PsA patients will be misclassified into the psoriasis group if they are not examined by a rheumatologist to identify the presence of PsA, which would reduce the power to identify significant associations. Moreover, because even those psoriasis patients without PsA at the time of the study might subsequently develop PsA, it has been suggested that cohort studies and more sophisticated statistical analyses, such as time-to-event analysis, are perhaps more appropriate than the current case-control studies [196]. However, cohort studies of sufficient sample size and appropriate periodic phenotyping are difficult to perform and prohibitively expensive.

A second challenge in the study of psoriasis and PsA genetics is the problem of missing heritability. The studies performed thus far, including GWASs, have characterized a small proportion of the genetic variance in psoriasis and PsA risk. It has been estimated that only 22% and 46% of psoriasis heritability can be explained by variants identified by GWASs in Caucasian and Chinese subjects, respectively [197,198]. The remaining "missing" heritability could be attributable to several factors. It has been suggested that GWAS sample sizes may have been too small, and thus the studies underpowered to detect significant associations with variants with small odds ratios. However, variants with such weak effects would not contribute much to the overall heritability. Highly deleterious rare variants (those with minor allele frequencies of <1%) with large effect sizes, which are not represented on GWAS chips but can be identified through techniques such as next-generation sequencing, exome sequencing, targeted resequencing, and exome chips, have also been proposed to contribute to missing heritability. A targeted resequencing study identified 15 rare variants in exon 4 of the *CARD14* gene, which were present in as few as a single individual [199]. However, overall, the evidence for the involvement of rare variants is still limited [75,200].

Additional CNVs may theoretically contribute, as few genome-wide CNV studies have been performed to explore this possibility in psoriatic disease due to technical difficulties in testing for CNVs. Heritable epigenetic phenomena, including genomic imprinting, may also play a role, as evidenced by studies that consistently demonstrate a paternal parent-of-origin effect on disease susceptibility and expression [29–31], which is thought to be mediated by epigenetics. Lastly, it is also possible that additional susceptibility genes exist that affect risk only in certain contexts, for instance, only in the presence of other susceptibility genes (epistasis), or only after exposure to a particular environmental trigger (gene–environment interactions). There is already some evidence for significant epistatic and gene–environment interactions in psoriasis and PsA, and there might be more to be discovered.

A third challenge is characterizing the functional relevance of the variants identified thus far. Only a small fraction of psoriasis susceptibility loci identified, including *IL23R* and *CARD14*, are located within coding regions, and thus may have rather straightforward causal effects on protein structure or function [93,201,202]. The remaining loci are located outside coding regions, such as in promoters, enhancers, or repressors, where they may function to alter the expression of nearby genes or even genes megabases away. Such expression quantitative trait loci (eQTL) can be identified by correlating SNPs with gene expression data generated from homogeneous and relevant cell types [142]. Bioinformatic tools such as the Encyclopedia of DNA Elements (ENCODE) database may also help to provide clues into the functions of these variants and allow us to generate hypotheses that can be experimentally tested using new techniques, such as chromosome conformation capture to identify interactions between far-apart genes, or CRISPR/Cas9 to confirm the causal nature of variants in cellular or animal models [142].

A comprehensive understanding of the genetics of psoriasis and PsA promises to be beneficial to future clinical practice by enabling personalized medicine. Genetic information may one day help us to forecast clinical phenotype and disease course, helping us to predict which patients are destined to develop severe psoriasis and PsA. Advances in pharmacogenetics will help us to identify patients who will respond well or poorly to particular treatments, which will help guide clinical decision making and expedite appropriate treatment [68]. In these respects, it is unlikely that a single genetic marker will achieve high enough accuracy, and it is more likely that a multimarker genetic panel will provide superior accuracy in a clinical setting [203]. Studies aiming to validate multiple variants for risk prediction have thus far shown improved risk prediction over single variants [180,204], and additional studies in this subject are ongoing.

2.8 CONCLUSIONS

A large proportion of the overall risk of psoriasis and PsA is determined by genetic factors. Several of these factors have been characterized, the strongest of which remain the long-known associations with MHC genes *HLA-C*06* for skin disease and *HLA-B*27* for joint disease. Several other variants scattered throughout the genome, identified through a combination of candidate gene and genome-wide linkage and association studies, contribute a small but significant amount to the overall risk of psoriasis and PsA. Genetic studies have helped to improve our understanding of the pathogenesis of these diseases, allowing us to model them as diseases resulting from a combination of defects in skin barrier function, and innate and adaptive immune processes. Genetic studies also give us insight into the relationship between skin and joint disease, with many common associations reflecting the shared skin pathology of psoriasis and PsA, or perhaps suggesting pleiotropy, as well as emerging evidence of novel associations specific to joint disease beyond the MHC. Studies in the immediate future will focus on refining genetic association signals for clinical use in personalized medicine through validation studies, as well as the functional annotation of validated associations to determine their causal roles in the pathogenesis of disease.

REFERENCES

1. Chandran V, Raychaudhuri SP. Geoepidemiology and environmental factors of psoriasis and psoriatic arthritis. *J Autoimmun* 2010; 34(3):J314–J321.
2. Oliveira Mde F, Rocha Bde O, Duarte GV. Psoriasis: Classical and emerging comorbidities. *An Bras Dermatol* 2015; 90(1):9–20.
3. Brezinski EA, Dhillon JS, Armstrong AW. Economic burden of psoriasis in the United States: A systematic review. *JAMA Dermatol* 2015; 151(6):651–658.
4. Naldi L, Gambini D. The clinical spectrum of psoriasis. *Clin Dermatol* 2007; 25(6):510–518.
5. Langley RG, Krueger GG, Griffiths CE. Psoriasis: Epidemiology, clinical features, and quality of life. *Ann Rheum Dis* 2005; 64 (Suppl 2):ii18–23; discussion ii24–25.
6. Eder L, Gladman DD. Psoriatic arthritis: Phenotypic variance and nosology. *Curr Rheumatol Rep* 2013; 15(3):316.
7. Gladman DD. Clinical, radiological, and functional assessment in psoriatic arthritis: Is it different from other inflammatory joint diseases? *Ann Rheum Dis* 2006; 65 (Suppl 3):iii22–24.
8. Gladman DD, Hing EN, Schentag CT, Cook RJ. Remission in psoriatic arthritis. *J Rheumatol* 2001; 28(5):1045–1048.
9. Cantini F, Niccoli L, Nannini C, Cassara E, Pasquetti P, Olivieri I et al. Criteria, frequency, and duration of clinical remission in psoriatic arthritis patients with peripheral involvement requiring second-line drugs. *J Rheumatol Suppl* 2009; 83:78–80.
10. Gladman DD, Antoni C, Mease P, Clegg DO, Nash P. Psoriatic arthritis: Epidemiology, clinical features, course, and outcome. *Ann Rheum Dis* 2005; 64 (Suppl 2):ii14–17.
11. Husted JA, Thavaneswaran A, Chandran V, Eder L, Rosen CF, Cook RJ et al. Cardiovascular and other comorbidities in patients with psoriatic arthritis: A comparison with patients with psoriasis. *Arthritis Care Res (Hoboken)* 2011; 63(12):1729–1735.
12. Nestle FO, Kaplan DH, Barker J. Psoriasis. *N Engl J Med* 2009; 361(5):496–509.
13. Eder L, Law T, Chandran V, Shanmugarajah S, Shen H, Rosen CF et al. Association between environmental factors and onset of psoriatic arthritis in patients with psoriasis. *Arthritis Care Res (Hoboken)* 2011; 63(8):1091–1097.
14. Pattison E, Harrison BJ, Griffiths CE, Silman AJ, Bruce IN. Environmental risk factors for the development of psoriatic arthritis: Results from a case-control study. *Ann Rheum Dis* 2008; 67(5):672–676.
15. Tey HL, Ee HL, Tan AS, Theng TS, Wong SN, Khoo SW. Risk factors associated with having psoriatic arthritis in patients with cutaneous psoriasis. *J Dermatol* 2010; 37(5):426–430.
16. Risch N. Linkage strategies for genetically complex traits. I. Multilocus models. *Am J Hum Genet* 1990; 46(2):222–228.
17. Rahman P, Elder JT. Genetic epidemiology of psoriasis and psoriatic arthritis. *Ann Rheum Dis* 2005; 64 (Suppl 2):ii37–39; discussion ii40–31.
18. Elder JT, Nair RP, Guo SW, Henseler T, Christophers E, Voorhees JJ. The genetics of psoriasis. *Arch Dermatol* 1994; 130(2):216–224.
19. Di Lernia V, Ficarelli E, Lallas A, Ricci C. Familial aggregation of moderate to severe plaque psoriasis. *Clin Exp Dermatol* 2014; 39(7):801–805.
20. Brandrup F, Holm N, Grunnet N, Henningsen K, Hansen HE. Psoriasis in monozygotic twins: Variations in expression in individuals with identical genetic constitution. *Acta Derm Venereol* 1982; 62(3):229–236.
21. Duffy DL, Spelman LS, Martin NG. Psoriasis in Australian twins. *J Am Acad Dermatol* 1993; 29(3):428–434.
22. Farber EM, Nall ML, Watson W. Natural history of psoriasis in 61 twin pairs. *Arch Dermatol* 1974; 109(2):207–211.
23. Lonnberg AS, Skov L, Skytthe A, Kyvik KO, Pedersen OB, Thomsen SF. Heritability of psoriasis in a large twin sample. *Br J Dermatol* 2013; 169(2):412–416.
24. Moll JM, Wright V. Familial occurrence of psoriatic arthritis. *Ann Rheum Dis* 1973; 32(3):181–201.
25. Karason A, Love TJ, Gudbjornsson B. A strong heritability of psoriatic arthritis over four generations—The Reykjavik Psoriatic Arthritis Study. *Rheumatology (Oxford)* 2009; 48(11):1424–1428.
26. Chandran V, Schentag CT, Brockbank JE, Pellett FJ, Shanmugarajah S, Toloza SM et al. Familial aggregation of psoriatic arthritis. *Ann Rheum Dis* 2009; 68(5):664–667.
27. Pedersen OB, Svendsen AJ, Ejstrup L, Skytthe A, Junker P. On the heritability of psoriatic arthritis. Disease concordance among monozygotic and dizygotic twins. *Ann Rheum Dis* 2008; 67(10):1417–1421.

28. Hebert HL, Ali FR, Bowes J, Griffiths CE, Barton A, Warren RB. Genetic susceptibility to psoriasis and psoriatic arthritis: Implications for therapy. *Br J Dermatol* 2012; 166(3):474–482.
29. Pollock RA, Thavaneswaran A, Pellett F, Chandran V, Petronis A, Rahman P et al. Further evidence supporting a parent-of-origin effect in psoriatic disease. *Arthritis Care Res (Hoboken)* 2015; 67(11):1586–1590.
30. Rahman P, Gladman DD, Schentag CT, Petronis A. Excessive paternal transmission in psoriatic arthritis. *Arthritis Rheum* 1999; 42(6):1228–1231.
31. Burden AD, Javed S, Bailey M, Hodgins M, Connor M, Tillman D. Genetics of psoriasis: Paternal inheritance and a locus on chromosome 6p. *J Invest Dermatol* 1998; 110(6):958–960.
32. Chandran V. The genetics of psoriasis and psoriatic arthritis. *Clin Rev Allergy Immunol* 2013; 44(2):149–156.
33. O'Rielly DD, Rahman P. Genetic, epigenetic and pharmacogenetic aspects of psoriasis and psoriatic arthritis. *Rheum Dis Clin North Am* 2015; 41(4):623–642.
34. Trembath RC, Clough RL, Rosbotham JL, Jones AB, Camp RD, Frodsham A et al. Identification of a major susceptibility locus on chromosome 6p and evidence for further disease loci revealed by a two stage genome-wide search in psoriasis. *Hum Mol Genet* 1997; 6(5):813–820.
35. Oka A, Tamiya G, Tomizawa M, Ota M, Katsuyama Y, Makino S et al. Association analysis using refined microsatellite markers localizes a susceptibility locus for psoriasis vulgaris within a 111 kb segment telomeric to the HLA-C gene. *Hum Mol Genet* 1999; 8(12):2165–2170.
36. Tazi Ahnini R, Camp NJ, Cork MJ, Mee JB, Keohane SG, Duff GW et al. Novel genetic association between the corneodesmosin (MHC S) gene and susceptibility to psoriasis. *Hum Mol Genet* 1999; 8(6):1135–1140.
37. Nair RP, Stuart PE, Nistor I, Hiremagalore R, Chia NV, Jenisch S et al. Sequence and haplotype analysis supports HLA-C as the psoriasis susceptibility 1 gene. *Am J Hum Genet* 2006; 78(5):827–851.
38. Fan X, Yang S, Huang W, Wang ZM, Sun LD, Liang YH et al. Fine mapping of the psoriasis susceptibility locus PSORS1 supports HLA-C as the susceptibility gene in the Han Chinese population. *PLoS Genet* 2008; 4(3):e1000038.
39. Allen MH, Ameen H, Veal C, Evans J, Ramrakha-Jones VS, Marsland AM et al. The major psoriasis susceptibility locus PSORS1 is not a risk factor for late-onset psoriasis. *J Invest Dermatol* 2005; 124(1):103–106.
40. Asumalahti K, Ameen M, Suomela S, Hagforsen E, Michaelsson G, Evans J et al. Genetic analysis of PSORS1 distinguishes guttate psoriasis and palmoplantar pustulosis. *J Invest Dermatol* 2003; 120(4):627–632.
41. Gudjonsson JE, Karason A, Runarsdottir EH, Antonsdottir AA, Hauksson VB, Jonsson HH et al. Distinct clinical differences between HLA-Cw*0602 positive and negative psoriasis patients—An analysis of 1019 HLA-C- and HLA-B-typed patients. *J Invest Dermatol* 2006; 126(4):740–745.
42. Puig L, Julia A, Marsal S. The pathogenesis and genetics of psoriasis. *Actas Dermosifiliogr* 2014; 105(6):535–545.
43. White SH, Newcomer VD, Mickey MR, Terasaki PI. Disturbance of HL-A antigen frequency in psoriasis. *N Engl J Med* 1972; 287(15):740–743.
44. Russell TJ, Schultes LM, Kuban DJ. Histocompatibility (HL-A) antigens associated with psoriasis. *N Engl J Med* 1972; 287(15):738–740.
45. Jenisch S, Henseler T, Nair RP, Guo SW, Westphal E, Stuart P et al. Linkage analysis of human leukocyte antigen (HLA) markers in familial psoriasis: Strong disequilibrium effects provide evidence for a major determinant in the HLA-B/-C region. *Am J Hum Genet* 1998; 63(1):191–199.
46. Gladman DD, Anhorn KA, Schachter RK, Mervart H. HLA antigens in psoriatic arthritis. *J Rheumatol* 1986; 13(3):586–592.
47. Pollock R, Chandran V, Barrett J, Eder L, Pellett F, Yao C et al. Differential major histocompatibility complex class I chain-related A allele associations with skin and joint manifestations of psoriatic disease. *Tissue Antigens* 2011; 77(6):554–561.
48. Nair RP, Duffin KC, Helms C, Ding J, Stuart PE, Goldgar D et al. Genome-wide scan reveals association of psoriasis with IL-23 and NF-kappaB pathways. *Nat Genet* 2009; 41(2):199–204.
49. Feng BJ, Sun LD, Soltani-Arabshahi R, Bowcock AM, Nair RP, Stuart P et al. Multiple loci within the major histocompatibility complex confer risk of psoriasis. *PLoS Genet* 2009; 5(8):e1000606.
50. Okada Y, Han B, Tsoi LC, Stuart PE, Ellinghaus E, Tejasvi T et al. Fine mapping major histocompatibility complex associations in psoriasis and its clinical subtypes. *Am J Hum Genet* 2014; 95(2):162–172.
51. Ganz T. Defensins: Antimicrobial peptides of innate immunity. *Nat Rev Immunol* 2003; 3(9):710–720.

52. Hollox EJ, Huffmeier U, Zeeuwen PL, Palla R, Lascorz J, Rodijk-Olthuis D et al. Psoriasis is associated with increased beta-defensin genomic copy number. *Nat Genet* 2008; 40(1):23–25.
53. Crisan D, Carr J. Angiotensin I-converting enzyme: Genotype and disease associations. *J Mol Diagn* 2000; 2(3):105–115.
54. Ozkur M, Erbagci Z, Nacak M, Tuncel AA, Alasehirli B, Aynacioglu AS. Association of insertion/deletion polymorphism of the angiotensin-converting enzyme gene with psoriasis. *Br J Dermatol* 2004; 151(4):792–795.
55. Chang YC, Wu WM, Chen CH, Lee SH, Hong HS, Hsu LA. Association between the insertion/deletion polymorphism of the angiotensin I-converting enzyme gene and risk for psoriasis in a Chinese population in Taiwan. *Br J Dermatol* 2007; 156(4):642–645.
56. Weger W, Hofer A, Wolf P, El-Shabrawi Y, Renner W, Kerl H et al. The angiotensin-converting enzyme insertion/deletion and the endothelin -134 3A/4A gene polymorphisms in patients with chronic plaque psoriasis. *Exp Dermatol* 2007; 16(12):993–998.
57. Liu T, Han Y, Lu L. Angiotensin-converting enzyme gene polymorphisms and the risk of psoriasis: A meta-analysis. *Clin Exp Dermatol* 2013; 38(4):352–358; quiz 359.
58. Veletza S, Karpouzis A, Giassakis G, Caridha R, Papaioakim M. Assessment of insertion/deletion polymorphism of the angiotensin converting enzyme gene in psoriasis. *J Dermatol Sci* 2008; 49(1):85–87.
59. Coto-Segura P, Alvarez V, Soto-Sanchez J, Morales B, Coto E, Santos-Juanes J. Lack of association between angiotensin I-converting enzyme insertion/deletion polymorphism and psoriasis or psoriatic arthritis in Spain. *Int J Dermatol* 2009; 48(12):1320–1323.
60. Park BS, Park JS, Lee DY, Youn JI, Kim IG. Vitamin D receptor polymorphism is associated with psoriasis. *J Invest Dermatol* 1999; 112(1):113–116.
61. Okita H, Ohtsuka T, Yamakage A, Yamazaki S. Polymorphism of the vitamin D(3) receptor in patients with psoriasis. *Arch Dermatol Res* 2002; 294(4):159–162.
62. Lee DY, Park BS, Choi KH, Jeon JH, Cho KH, Song KY et al. Vitamin D receptor genotypes are not associated with clinical response to calcipotriol in Korean psoriasis patients. *Arch Dermatol Res* 2002; 294(1–2):1–5.
63. Kaya TI, Erdal ME, Tursen U, Camdeviren H, Gunduz O, Soylemez F et al. Association between vitamin D receptor gene polymorphism and psoriasis among the Turkish population. *Arch Dermatol Res* 2002; 294(6):286–289.
64. Saeki H, Asano N, Tsunemi Y, Takekoshi T, Kishimoto M, Mitsui H et al. Polymorphisms of vitamin D receptor gene in Japanese patients with psoriasis vulgaris. *J Dermatol Sci* 2002; 30(2):167–171.
65. Ruggiero M, Gulisano M, Peruzzi B, Giomi B, Caproni M, Fabbri P et al. Vitamin D receptor gene polymorphism is not associated with psoriasis in the Italian Caucasian population. *J Dermatol Sci* 2004; 35(1):68–70.
66. Halsall JA, Osborne JE, Pringle JH, Hutchinson PE. Vitamin D receptor gene polymorphisms, particularly the novel A-1012G promoter polymorphism, are associated with vitamin D3 responsiveness and non-familial susceptibility in psoriasis. *Pharmacogenet Genomics* 2005; 15(5):349–355.
67. Stefanic M, Rucevic I, Barisic-Drusko V. Meta-analysis of vitamin D receptor polymorphisms and psoriasis risk. *Int J Dermatol* 2013; 52(6):705–710.
68. Mahil SK, Capon F, Barker JN. Genetics of psoriasis. *Dermatol Clin* 2015; 33(1):1–11.
69. Cargill M, Schrodi SJ, Chang M, Garcia VE, Brandon R, Callis KP et al. A large-scale genetic association study confirms IL12B and leads to the identification of IL23R as psoriasis-risk genes. *Am J Hum Genet* 2007; 80(2):273–290.
70. Liu Y, Helms C, Liao W, Zaba LC, Duan S, Gardner J et al. A genome-wide association study of psoriasis and psoriatic arthritis identifies new disease loci. *PLoS Genet* 2008; 4(3):e1000041.
71. Zhang XJ, Huang W, Yang S, Sun LD, Zhang FY, Zhu QX et al. Psoriasis genome-wide association study identifies susceptibility variants within LCE gene cluster at 1q21. *Nat Genet* 2009; 41(2): 205–210.
72. Genetic Analysis of Psoriasis C, the Wellcome Trust Case Control C, Strange A, Capon F, Spencer CC, Knight J et al. A genome-wide association study identifies new psoriasis susceptibility loci and an interaction between HLA-C and ERAP1. *Nat Genet* 2010; 42(11):985–990.
73. Zhu KJ, Zhu CY, Shi G, Fan YM. Meta-analysis of IL12B polymorphisms (rs3212227, rs6887695) with psoriasis and psoriatic arthritis. *Rheumatol Int* 2013; 33(7):1785–1790.
74. Shen C, Gao J, Yin X, Sheng Y, Sun L, Cui Y et al. Association of the late cornified envelope-3 genes with psoriasis and psoriatic arthritis: A systematic review. *J Genet Genomics* 2015; 42(2):49–56.
75. Tang H, Jin X, Li Y, Jiang H, Tang X, Yang X et al. A large-scale screen for coding variants predisposing to psoriasis. *Nat Genet* 2014; 46(1):45–50.

76. Julia A, Tortosa R, Hernanz JM, Canete JD, Fonseca E, Ferrandiz C et al. Risk variants for psoriasis vulgaris in a large case-control collection and association with clinical subphenotypes. *Hum Mol Genet* 2012; 21(20):4549–4557.
77. de Cid R, Riveira-Munoz E, Zeeuwen PL, Robarge J, Liao W, Dannhauser EN et al. Deletion of the late cornified envelope LCE3B and LCE3C genes as a susceptibility factor for psoriasis. *Nat Genet* 2009; 41(2):211–215.
78. Coin LJ, Cao D, Ren J, Zuo X, Sun L, Yang S et al. An exome sequencing pipeline for identifying and genotyping common CNVs associated with disease with application to psoriasis. *Bioinformatics* 2012; 28(18):i370–i374.
79. Huffmeier U, Bergboer JG, Becker T, Armour JA, Traupe H, Estivill X et al. Replication of LCE3C-LCE3B CNV as a risk factor for psoriasis and analysis of interaction with other genetic risk factors. *J Invest Dermatol* 2010; 130(4):979–984.
80. Coto E, Santos-Juanes J, Coto-Segura P, Diaz M, Soto J, Queiro R et al. Mutation analysis of the LCE3B/LCE3C genes in psoriasis. *BMC Med Genet* 2010; 11:45.
81. Xu L, Li Y, Zhang X, Sun H, Sun D, Jia X et al. Deletion of LCE3C and LCE3B genes is associated with psoriasis in a northern Chinese population. *Br J Dermatol* 2011; 165(4):882–887.
82. Li Y, Liao W, Chang M, Schrodi SJ, Bui N, Catanese JJ et al. Further genetic evidence for three psoriasis-risk genes: ADAM33, CDKAL1, and PTPN22. *J Invest Dermatol* 2009; 129(3):629–634.
83. Sun LD, Cheng H, Wang ZX, Zhang AP, Wang PG, Xu JH et al. Association analyses identify six new psoriasis susceptibility loci in the Chinese population. *Nat Genet* 2010; 42(11):1005–1009.
84. Ellinghaus E, Ellinghaus D, Stuart PE, Nair RP, Debrus S, Raelson JV et al. Genome-wide association study identifies a psoriasis susceptibility locus at TRAF3IP2. *Nat Genet* 2010; 42(11):991–995.
85. Stuart PE, Nair RP, Ellinghaus E, Ding J, Tejasvi T, Gudjonsson JE et al. Genome-wide association analysis identifies three psoriasis susceptibility loci. *Nat Genet* 2010; 42(11):1000–1004.
86. Sugiura K. The genetic background of generalized pustular psoriasis: IL36RN mutations and CARD14 gain-of-function variants. *J Dermatol Sci* 2014; 74(3):187–192.
87. Marrakchi S, Guigue P, Renshaw BR, Puel A, Pei XY, Fraitag S et al. Interleukin-36-receptor antagonist deficiency and generalized pustular psoriasis. *N Engl J Med* 2011; 365(7):620–628.
88. Li X, Chen M, Fu X, Zhang Q, Wang Z, Yu G et al. Mutation analysis of the IL36RN gene in Chinese patients with generalized pustular psoriasis with/without psoriasis vulgaris. *J Dermatol Sci* 2014; 76(2):132–138.
89. Hayashi M, Nakayama T, Hirota T, Saeki H, Nobeyama Y, Ito T et al. Novel IL36RN gene mutation revealed by analysis of 8 Japanese patients with generalized pustular psoriasis. *J Dermatol Sci* 2014; 76(3):267–269.
90. Onoufriadis A, Simpson MA, Pink AE, Di Meglio P, Smith CH, Pullabhatla V et al. Mutations in IL36RN/IL1F5 are associated with the severe episodic inflammatory skin disease known as generalized pustular psoriasis. *Am J Hum Genet* 2011; 89(3):432–437.
91. Sugiura K, Takemoto A, Yamaguchi M, Takahashi H, Shoda Y, Mitsuma T et al. The majority of generalized pustular psoriasis without psoriasis vulgaris is caused by deficiency of interleukin-36 receptor antagonist. *J Invest Dermatol* 2013; 133(11):2514–2521.
92. Korber A, Mossner R, Renner R, Sticht H, Wilsmann-Theis D, Schulz P et al. Mutations in IL36RN in patients with generalized pustular psoriasis. *J Invest Dermatol* 2013; 133(11):2634–2637.
93. Jordan CT, Cao L, Roberson ED, Pierson KC, Yang CF, Joyce CE et al. PSORS2 is due to mutations in CARD14. *Am J Hum Genet* 2012; 90(5):784–795.
94. Setta-Kaffetzi N, Simpson MA, Navarini AA, Patel VM, Lu HC, Allen MH et al. AP1S3 mutations are associated with pustular psoriasis and impaired Toll-like receptor 3 trafficking. *Am J Hum Genet* 2014; 94(5):790–797.
95. Hebert HL, Bowes J, Smith RL, McHugh NJ, Barker JN, Griffiths CE et al. Polymorphisms in IL-1B distinguish between psoriasis of early and late onset. *J Invest Dermatol* 2014; 134(5):1459–1462.
96. O'Rielly DD, Rahman P. Genetics of susceptibility and treatment response in psoriatic arthritis. *Nat Rev Rheumatol* 2011; 7(12):718–732.
97. de Guzman Strong C, Conlan S, Deming CB, Cheng J, Sears KE, Segre JA. A milieu of regulatory elements in the epidermal differentiation complex syntenic block: Implications for atopic dermatitis and psoriasis. *Hum Mol Genet* 2010; 19(8):1453–1460.
98. Niyonsaba F, Ogawa H, Nagaoka I. Human beta-defensin-2 functions as a chemotactic agent for tumour necrosis factor-alpha-treated human neutrophils. *Immunology* 2004; 111(3):273–281.
99. Yang D, Chertov O, Bykovskaia SN, Chen Q, Buffo MJ, Shogan J et al. Beta-defensins: Linking innate and adaptive immunity through dendritic and T cell CCR6. *Science* 1999; 286(5439):525–528.

100. Labarthe MP, Bosco D, Saurat JH, Meda P, Salomon D. Upregulation of connexin 26 between keratinocytes of psoriatic lesions. *J Invest Dermatol* 1998; 111(1):72–76.
101. Djalilian AR, McGaughey D, Patel S, Seo EY, Yang C, Cheng J et al. Connexin 26 regulates epidermal barrier and wound remodeling and promotes psoriasiform response. *J Clin Invest* 2006; 116(5):1243–1253.
102. Harden JL, Krueger JG, Bowcock AM. The immunogenetics of psoriasis: A comprehensive review. *J Autoimmun* 2015; 64:66–73.
103. Valdimarsson H, Karason A, Gudjonsson JE. Psoriasis: A complex clinical and genetic disorder. *Curr Rheumatol Rep* 2004; 6(4):314–316.
104. Arakawa A, Siewert K, Stohr J, Besgen P, Kim SM, Ruhl G et al. Melanocyte antigen triggers autoimmunity in human psoriasis. *J Exp Med* 2015; 212(13):2203–2212.
105. Lande R, Botti E, Jandus C, Dojcinovic D, Fanelli G, Conrad C et al. The antimicrobial peptide LL37 is a T-cell autoantigen in psoriasis. *Nat Commun* 2014; 5:5621.
106. Capon F, Bijlmakers MJ, Wolf N, Quaranta M, Huffmeier U, Allen M et al. Identification of ZNF313/RNF114 as a novel psoriasis susceptibility gene. *Hum Mol Genet* 2008; 17(13):1938–1945.
107. Capon F, Di Meglio P, Szaub J, Prescott NJ, Dunster C, Baumber L et al. Sequence variants in the genes for the interleukin-23 receptor (IL23R) and its ligand (IL12B) confer protection against psoriasis. *Hum Genet* 2007; 122(2):201–206.
108. Smith RL, Warren RB, Eyre S, Ho P, Ke X, Young HS et al. Polymorphisms in the IL-12beta and IL-23R genes are associated with psoriasis of early onset in a UK cohort. *J Invest Dermatol* 2008; 128(5):1325–1327.
109. Di Cesare A, Di Meglio P, Nestle FO. The IL-23/Th17 axis in the immunopathogenesis of psoriasis. *J Invest Dermatol* 2009; 129(6):1339–1350.
110. Blumberg H, Dinh H, Dean C Jr., Trueblood ES, Bailey K, Shows D et al. IL-1RL2 and its ligands contribute to the cytokine network in psoriasis. *J Immunol* 2010; 185(7):4354–4362.
111. Rahman P, Sun S, Peddle L, Snelgrove T, Melay W, Greenwood C et al. Association between the interleukin-1 family gene cluster and psoriatic arthritis. *Arthritis Rheum* 2006; 54(7):2321–2325.
112. Oyamada A, Ikebe H, Itsumi M, Saiwai H, Okada S, Shimoda K et al. Tyrosine kinase 2 plays critical roles in the pathogenic CD4 T cell responses for the development of experimental autoimmune encephalomyelitis. *J Immunol* 2009; 183(11):7539–7546.
113. Moll JM, Wright V. Psoriatic arthritis. *Semin Arthritis Rheum* 1973; 3(1):55–78.
114. Taylor W, Gladman D, Helliwell P, Marchesoni A, Mease P, Mielants H et al. Classification criteria for psoriatic arthritis: Development of new criteria from a large international study. *Arthritis Rheum* 2006; 54(8):2665–2673.
115. Castelino M, Barton A. Genetic susceptibility factors for psoriatic arthritis. *Curr Opin Rheumatol* 2010; 22(2):152–156.
116. Ho PY, Barton A, Worthington J, Plant D, Griffiths CE, Young HS et al. Investigating the role of the HLA-Cw*06 and HLA-DRB1 genes in susceptibility to psoriatic arthritis: Comparison with psoriasis and undifferentiated inflammatory arthritis. *Ann Rheum Dis* 2008; 67(5):677–682.
117. Eder L, Chandran V, Pellet F, Shanmugarajah S, Rosen CF, Bull SB et al. Human leucocyte antigen risk alleles for psoriatic arthritis among patients with psoriasis. *Ann Rheum Dis* 2012; 71(1):50–55.
118. Szczerkowska Dobosz A, Rebala K, Szczerkowska Z, Nedoszytko B. HLA-C locus alleles distribution in patients from northern Poland with psoriatic arthritis—Preliminary report. *Int J Immunogenet* 2005; 32(6):389–391.
119. Ferrandiz C, Pujol RM, Garcia-Patos V, Bordas X, Smandia JA. Psoriasis of early and late onset: A clinical and epidemiologic study from Spain. *J Am Acad Dermatol* 2002; 46(6):867–873.
120. Fernandez-Torres RM, Paradela S, Fonseca E. Psoriasis in patients older than 65 years. A comparative study with younger adult psoriatic patients. *J Nutr Health Aging* 2012; 16(6):586–591.
121. Armesto S, Santos-Juanes J, Galache-Osuna C, Martinez-Camblor P, Coto E, Coto-Segura P. Psoriasis and type 2 diabetes risk among psoriatic patients in a Spanish population. *Australas J Dermatol* 2012; 53(2):128–130.
122. Rahman P, Siannis F, Butt C, Farewell V, Peddle L, Pellett F et al. TNFalpha polymorphisms and risk of psoriatic arthritis. *Ann Rheum Dis* 2006; 65(7):919–923.
123. Bowes J, Flynn E, Ho P, Aly B, Morgan AW, Marzo-Ortega H et al. Variants in linkage disequilibrium with the late cornified envelope gene cluster deletion are associated with susceptibility to psoriatic arthritis. *Ann Rheum Dis* 2010; 69(12):2199–2203.

124. Docampo E, Rabionet R, Riveira-Munoz E, Escaramis G, Julia A, Marsal S et al. Deletion of the late cornified envelope genes, LCE3C and LCE3B, is associated with rheumatoid arthritis. *Arthritis Rheum* 2010; 62(5):1246–1251.
125. Chiraz BS, Myriam A, Ines Z, Catherine J, Fatma B, Ilhem C et al. Deletion of late cornified envelope genes, LCE3C_LCE3B-del, is not associated with psoriatic arthritis in Tunisian patients. *Mol Biol Rep* 2014; 41(6):4141–4146.
126. Docampo E, Giardina E, Riveira-Munoz E, de Cid R, Escaramis G, Perricone C et al. Deletion of LCE3C and LCE3B is a susceptibility factor for psoriatic arthritis: A study in Spanish and Italian populations and meta-analysis. *Arthritis Rheum* 2011; 63(7):1860–1865.
127. Huffmeier U, Uebe S, Ekici AB, Bowes J, Giardina E, Korendowych E et al. Common variants at TRAF3IP2 are associated with susceptibility to psoriatic arthritis and psoriasis. *Nat Genet* 2010; 42(11):996–999.
128. Ellinghaus E, Stuart PE, Ellinghaus D, Nair RP, Debrus S, Raelson JV et al. Genome-wide meta-analysis of psoriatic arthritis identifies susceptibility locus at REL. *J Invest Dermatol* 2012; 132(4):1133–1140.
129. Duffin KC, Freeny IC, Schrodi SJ, Wong B, Feng BJ, Soltani-Arabshahi R et al. Association between IL13 polymorphisms and psoriatic arthritis is modified by smoking. *J Invest Dermatol* 2009; 129(12): 2777–2783.
130. Huffmeier U, Lascorz J, Bohm B, Lohmann J, Wendler J, Mossner R et al. Genetic variants of the IL-23R pathway: Association with psoriatic arthritis and psoriasis vulgaris, but no specific risk factor for arthritis. *J Invest Dermatol* 2009; 129(2):355–358.
131. Filer C, Ho P, Smith RL, Griffiths C, Young HS, Worthington J et al. Investigation of association of the IL12B and IL23R genes with psoriatic arthritis. *Arthritis Rheum* 2008; 58(12):3705–3709.
132. Jadon D, Tillett W, Wallis D, Cavill C, Bowes J, Waldron N et al. Exploring ankylosing spondylitis-associated ERAP1, IL23R and IL12B gene polymorphisms in subphenotypes of psoriatic arthritis. *Rheumatology (Oxford)* 2013; 52(2):261–266.
133. Eiris N, Gonzalez-Lara L, Santos-Juanes J, Queiro R, Coto E, Coto-Segura P. Genetic variation at IL12B, IL23R and IL23A is associated with psoriasis severity, psoriatic arthritis and type 2 diabetes mellitus. *J Dermatol Sci* 2014; 75(3):167–172.
134. Rahman P, Inman RD, Maksymowych WP, Reeve JP, Peddle L, Gladman DD. Association of interleukin 23 receptor variants with psoriatic arthritis. *J Rheumatol* 2009; 36(1):137–140.
135. Bowes J, Orozco G, Flynn E, Ho P, Brier R, Marzo-Ortega H et al. Confirmation of TNIP1 and IL23A as susceptibility loci for psoriatic arthritis. *Ann Rheum Dis* 2011; 70(9):1641–1644.
136. Yang Q, Liu H, Qu L, Fu X, Yu Y, Yu G et al. Investigation of 20 non-HLA (human leucocyte antigen) psoriasis susceptibility loci in Chinese patients with psoriatic arthritis and psoriasis vulgaris. *Br J Dermatol* 2013; 168(5):1060–1065.
137. Bowes J, Ho P, Flynn E, Ali F, Marzo-Ortega H, Coates LC et al. Comprehensive assessment of rheumatoid arthritis susceptibility loci in a large psoriatic arthritis cohort. *Ann Rheum Dis* 2012; 71(8):1350–1354.
138. Eder L, Chandran V, Pellett F, Pollock R, Shanmugarajah S, Rosen CF et al. IL13 gene polymorphism is a marker for psoriatic arthritis among psoriasis patients. *Ann Rheum Dis* 2011; 70(9):1594–1598.
139. Bowes J, Eyre S, Flynn E, Ho P, Salah S, Warren RB et al. Evidence to support IL-13 as a risk locus for psoriatic arthritis but not psoriasis vulgaris. *Ann Rheum Dis* 2011; 70(6):1016–1019.
140. Apel M, Uebe S, Bowes J, Giardina E, Korendowych E, Juneblad K et al. Variants in RUNX3 contribute to susceptibility to psoriatic arthritis, exhibiting further common ground with ankylosing spondylitis. *Arthritis Rheum* 2013; 65(5):1224–1231.
141. Warren RB, Smith RL, Flynn E, Bowes J, Consortium U, Eyre S et al. A systematic investigation of confirmed autoimmune loci in early-onset psoriasis reveals an association with IL2/IL21. *Br J Dermatol* 2011; 164(3):660–664.
142. Budu-Aggrey A, Bowes J, Barton A. Identifying a novel locus for psoriatic arthritis. *Rheumatology (Oxford)* 2016; 55(1):25–32.
143. Queiro R, Morante I, Cabezas I, Acasuso B. HLA-B27 and psoriatic disease: A modern view of an old relationship. *Rheumatology (Oxford)* 2016; 55(2):221–229.
144. Winchester R, Minevich G, Steshenko V, Kirby B, Kane D, Greenberg DA et al. HLA associations reveal genetic heterogeneity in psoriatic arthritis and in the psoriasis phenotype. *Arthritis Rheum* 2012; 64(4):1134–1144.
145. Armstrong RD, Panayi GS, Welsh KI. Histocompatibility antigens in psoriasis, psoriatic arthropathy, and ankylosing spondylitis. *Ann Rheum Dis* 1983; 42(2):142–146.

146. Queiro-Silva R, Torre-Alonso JC, Tinture-Eguren T, Lopez-Lagunas I. The effect of HLA-DR antigens on the susceptibility to, and clinical expression of psoriatic arthritis. *Scand J Rheumatol* 2004; 33(5):318–322.
147. Gonzalez S, Martinez-Borra J, Torre-Alonso JC, Gonzalez-Roces S, Sanchez del Rio J, Rodriguez Perez A et al. The MICA-A9 triplet repeat polymorphism in the transmembrane region confers additional susceptibility to the development of psoriatic arthritis and is independent of the association of Cw*0602 in psoriasis. *Arthritis Rheum* 1999; 42(5):1010–1016.
148. Gonzalez S, Martinez-Borra J, Lopez-Vazquez A, Garcia-Fernandez S, Torre-Alonso JC, Lopez-Larrea C. MICA rather than MICB, TNFA, or HLA-DRB1 is associated with susceptibility to psoriatic arthritis. *J Rheumatol* 2002; 29(5):973–978.
149. Gonzalez S, Brautbar C, Martinez-Borra J, Lopez-Vazquez A, Segal R, Blanco-Gelaz MA et al. Polymorphism in MICA rather than HLA-B/C genes is associated with psoriatic arthritis in the Jewish population. *Hum Immunol* 2001; 62(6):632–638.
150. Grubic Z, Peric P, Eeeuk-Jelicic E, Zunec R, Stingl K, Curkovic B et al. The MICA-A4 triplet repeats polymorphism in the transmembrane region confers additional risk for development of psoriatic arthritis in the Croatian population. *Eur J Immunogenet* 2004; 31(2):93–98.
151. Rahman P, Roslin NM, Pellett FJ, Lemire M, Greenwood CM, Beyene J et al. High resolution mapping in the major histocompatibility complex region identifies multiple independent novel loci for psoriatic arthritis. *Ann Rheum Dis* 2011; 70(4):690–694.
152. Chandran V, Bull SB, Pellett FJ, Ayearst R, Pollock RA, Gladman DD. Killer-cell immunoglobulin-like receptor gene polymorphisms and susceptibility to psoriatic arthritis. *Rheumatology (Oxford)* 2014; 53(2):233–239.
153. Stuart PE, Nair RP, Tsoi LC, Tejasvi T, Das S, Kang HM et al. Genome-wide association analysis of psoriatic arthritis and cutaneous psoriasis reveals differences in their genetic architecture. *Am J Hum Genet* 2015; 97(6):816–836.
154. Bowes J, Loehr S, Budu-Aggrey A, Uebe S, Bruce IN, Feletar M et al. PTPN22 is associated with susceptibility to psoriatic arthritis but not psoriasis: Evidence for a further PsA-specific risk locus. *Ann Rheum Dis* 2015; 74(10):1882–1885.
155. Julia A, Pinto JA, Gratacos J, Queiro R, Ferrandiz C, Fonseca E et al. A deletion at ADAMTS9-MAGI1 locus is associated with psoriatic arthritis risk. *Ann Rheum Dis* 2015; 74(10):1875–1881.
156. Coto E, Santos-Juanes J, Coto-Segura P, Alvarez V. New psoriasis susceptibility genes: Momentum for skin-barrier disruption. *J Invest Dermatol* 2011; 131(5):1003–1005.
157. Cianci R, Giambra V, Mattioli C, Esposito M, Cammarota G, Scibilia G et al. Increased frequency of Ig heavy-chain HS1,2-A enhancer *2 allele in dermatitis herpetiformis, plaque psoriasis, and psoriatic arthritis. *J Invest Dermatol* 2008; 128(8):1920–1924.
158. Bowes J, Budu-Aggrey A, Huffmeier U, Uebe S, Steel K, Hebert HL et al. Dense genotyping of immune-related susceptibility loci reveals new insights into the genetics of psoriatic arthritis. *Nat Commun* 2015; 6:6046.
159. Karason A, Gudjonsson JE, Upmanyu R, Antonsdottir AA, Hauksson VB, Runasdottir EH et al. A susceptibility gene for psoriatic arthritis maps to chromosome 16q: Evidence for imprinting. *Am J Hum Genet* 2003; 72(1):125–131.
160. Rahman P, Bartlett S, Siannis F, Pellett FJ, Farewell VT, Peddle L et al. CARD15: A pleiotropic autoimmune gene that confers susceptibility to psoriatic arthritis. *Am J Hum Genet* 2003; 73(3):677–681.
161. Queiro R, Torre JC, Gonzalez S, Lopez-Larrea C, Tinture T, Lopez-Lagunas I. HLA antigens may influence the age of onset of psoriasis and psoriatic arthritis. *J Rheumatol* 2003; 30(3):505–507.
162. Haroon M, Winchester R, Giles JT, Heffernan E, FitzGerald O. Certain class I HLA alleles and haplotypes implicated in susceptibility play a role in determining specific features of the psoriatic arthritis phenotype. *Ann Rheum Dis* 2016; 75(1):155–162.
163. FitzGerald O, Haroon M, Giles JT, Winchester R. Concepts of pathogenesis in psoriatic arthritis: Genotype determines clinical phenotype. *Arthritis Res Ther* 2015; 17:115.
164. Ho PY, Barton A, Worthington J, Thomson W, Silman AJ, Bruce IN. HLA-Cw6 and HLA-DRB1*07 together are associated with less severe joint disease in psoriatic arthritis. *Ann Rheum Dis* 2007; 66(6):807–811.
165. Zhu KJ, Zhu CY, Shi G, Fan YM. Association of IL23R polymorphisms with psoriasis and psoriatic arthritis: A meta-analysis. *Inflamm Res* 2012; 61(10):1149–1154.
166. Cenit MC, Ortego-Centeno N, Raya E, Callejas JL, Garcia-Hernandez FJ, Castillo-Palma MJ et al. Influence of the STAT3 genetic variants in the susceptibility to psoriatic arthritis and Behcet's disease. *Hum Immunol* 2013; 74(2):230–233.

167. Catanoso MG, Boiardi L, Macchioni P, Garagnani P, Sazzini M, De Fanti S et al. IL-23A, IL-23R, IL-17A and IL-17R polymorphisms in different psoriatic arthritis clinical manifestations in the northern Italian population. *Rheumatol Int* 2013; 33(5):1165–1176.
168. Leipe J, Grunke M, Dechant C, Reindl C, Kerzendorf U, Schulze-Koops H et al. Role of Th17 cells in human autoimmune arthritis. *Arthritis Rheum* 2010; 62(10):2876–2885.
169. van Kuijk AW, Reinders-Blankert P, Smeets TJ, Dijkmans BA, Tak PP. Detailed analysis of the cell infiltrate and the expression of mediators of synovial inflammation and joint destruction in the synovium of patients with psoriatic arthritis: Implications for treatment. *Ann Rheum Dis* 2006; 65(12):1551–1557.
170. McHugh K, Bowness P. The link between HLA-B27 and SpA—New ideas on an old problem. *Rheumatology (Oxford)* 2012; 51(9):1529–1539.
171. Robinson PC, Brown MA. The genetics of ankylosing spondylitis and axial spondyloarthritis. *Rheum Dis Clin North Am* 2012; 38(3):539–553.
172. Colbert RA, Tran TM, Layh-Schmitt G. HLA-B27 misfolding and ankylosing spondylitis. *Mol Immunol* 2014; 57(1):44–51.
173. May E, Dorris ML, Satumtira N, Iqbal I, Rehman MI, Lightfoot E et al. CD8 alpha beta T cells are not essential to the pathogenesis of arthritis or colitis in HLA-B27 transgenic rats. *J Immunol* 2003; 170(2):1099–1105.
174. Khare SD, Hansen J, Luthra HS, David CS. HLA-B27 heavy chains contribute to spontaneous inflammatory disease in B27/human beta2-microglobulin (beta2m) double transgenic mice with disrupted mouse beta2m. *J Clin Invest* 1996; 98(12):2746–2755.
175. Tran TM, Dorris ML, Satumtira N, Richardson JA, Hammer RE, Shang J et al. Additional human beta2-microglobulin curbs HLA-B27 misfolding and promotes arthritis and spondylitis without colitis in male HLA-B27-transgenic rats. *Arthritis Rheum* 2006; 54(4):1317–1327.
176. Bowness P, Ridley A, Shaw J, Chan AT, Wong-Baeza I, Fleming M et al. Th17 cells expressing KIR3DL2+ and responsive to HLA-B27 homodimers are increased in ankylosing spondylitis. *J Immunol* 2011; 186(4):2672–2680.
177. Zheng HF, Zuo XB, Lu WS, Li Y, Cheng H, Zhu KJ et al. Variants in MHC, LCE and IL12B have epistatic effects on psoriasis risk in Chinese population. *J Dermatol Sci* 2011; 61(2):124–128.
178. Li M, Wu Y, Chen G, Yang Y, Zhou D, Zhang Z et al. Deletion of the late cornified envelope genes LCE3C and LCE3B is associated with psoriasis in a Chinese population. *J Invest Dermatol* 2011; 131(8):1639–1643.
179. Australo-Anglo-American Spondyloarthritis C, Reveille JD, Sims AM, Danoy P, Evans DM, Leo P et al. Genome-wide association study of ankylosing spondylitis identifies non-MHC susceptibility loci. *Nat Genet* 2010; 42(2):123–127.
180. Chen H, Poon A, Yeung C, Helms C, Pons J, Bowcock AM et al. A genetic risk score combining ten psoriasis risk loci improves disease prediction. *PLoS One* 2011; 6(4):e19454.
181. Setty AR, Curhan G, Choi HK. Smoking and the risk of psoriasis in women: Nurses' Health Study II. *Am J Med* 2007; 120(11):953–959.
182. Rakkhit T, Wong B, Nelson TS et al. Time to development of psoriatic arthritis decreases with smoking prior to psoriasis onset and increases with smoking after psoriasis onset. *J Invest Dermatol* 2007; 127(Suppl 1):S52.
183. Warren RB, Chalmers RJ, Griffiths CE, Menter A. Methotrexate for psoriasis in the era of biological therapy. *Clin Exp Dermatol* 2008; 33(5):551–554.
184. Warren RB, Smith RL, Campalani E, Eyre S, Smith CH, Barker JN et al. Genetic variation in efflux transporters influences outcome to methotrexate therapy in patients with psoriasis. *J Invest Dermatol* 2008; 128(8):1925–1929.
185. Warren RB, Smith RL, Campalani E, Eyre S, Smith CH, Barker JN et al. Outcomes of methotrexate therapy for psoriasis and relationship to genetic polymorphisms. *Br J Dermatol* 2009; 160(2): 438–441.
186. Campalani E, Arenas M, Marinaki AM, Lewis CM, Barker JN, Smith CH. Polymorphisms in folate, pyrimidine, and purine metabolism are associated with efficacy and toxicity of methotrexate in psoriasis. *J Invest Dermatol* 2007; 127(8):1860–1867.
187. Mandola MV, Stoehlmacher J, Muller-Weeks S, Cesarone G, Yu MC, Lenz HJ et al. A novel single nucleotide polymorphism within the 5′ tandem repeat polymorphism of the thymidylate synthase gene abolishes USF-1 binding and alters transcriptional activity. *Cancer Res* 2003; 63(11):2898–2904.
188. Gusella M, Bolzonella C, Crepaldi G, Ferrazzi E, Padrini R. A novel G/C single-nucleotide polymorphism in the double 28-bp repeat thymidylate synthase allele. *Pharmacogenomics J* 2006; 6(6):421–424.

189. Xiao H, Xu J, Zhou X, Stankovich J, Pan F, Zhang Z et al. Associations between the genetic polymorphisms of MTHFR and outcomes of methotrexate treatment in rheumatoid arthritis. *Clin Exp Rheumatol* 2010; 28(5):728–733.
190. Young HS, Summers AM, Read IR, Fairhurst DA, Plant DJ, Campalani E et al. Interaction between genetic control of vascular endothelial growth factor production and retinoid responsiveness in psoriasis. *J Invest Dermatol* 2006; 126(2):453–459.
191. Tejasvi T, Stuart PE, Chandran V, Voorhees JJ, Gladman DD, Rahman P et al. TNFAIP3 gene polymorphisms are associated with response to TNF blockade in psoriasis. *J Invest Dermatol* 2012; 132 (3 Pt 1):593–600.
192. Vasilopoulos Y, Manolika M, Zafiriou E, Sarafidou T, Bagiatis V, Kruger-Krasagaki S et al. Pharmacogenetic analysis of TNF, TNFRSF1A, and TNFRSF1B gene polymorphisms and prediction of response to anti-TNF therapy in psoriasis patients in the Greek population. *Mol Diagn Ther* 2012; 16(1):29–34.
193. Batalla A, Coto E, Gonzalez-Fernandez D, Gonzalez-Lara L, Gomez J, Santos-Juanes J et al. The Cw6 and late-cornified envelope genotype plays a significant role in anti-tumor necrosis factor response among psoriatic patients. *Pharmacogenet Genomics* 2015; 25(6):313–316.
194. Morales-Lara MJ, Canete JD, Torres-Moreno D, Hernandez MV, Pedrero F, Celis R et al. Effects of polymorphisms in TRAILR1 and TNFR1A on the response to anti-TNF therapies in patients with rheumatoid and psoriatic arthritis. *Joint Bone Spine* 2012; 79(6):591–596.
195. Talamonti M, Botti E, Galluzzo M, Teoli M, Spallone G, Bavetta M et al. Pharmacogenetics of psoriasis: HLA-Cw6 but not LCE3B/3C deletion nor TNFAIP3 polymorphism predisposes to clinical response to interleukin 12/23 blocker ustekinumab. *Br J Dermatol* 2013; 169(2):458–463.
196. Eder L, Chandran V, Gladman DD. What have we learned about genetic susceptibility in psoriasis and psoriatic arthritis? *Curr Opin Rheumatol* 2015; 27(1):91–98.
197. Tsoi LC, Spain SL, Knight J, Ellinghaus E, Stuart PE, Capon F et al. Identification of 15 new psoriasis susceptibility loci highlights the role of innate immunity. *Nat Genet* 2012; 44(12):1341–1348.
198. Jiang L, Liu L, Cheng Y, Lin Y, Shen C, Zhu C et al. More heritability probably captured by psoriasis genome-wide association study in Han Chinese. *Gene* 2015; 573(1):46–49.
199. Jordan CT, Cao L, Roberson ED, Duan S, Helms CA, Nair RP et al. Rare and common variants in CARD14, encoding an epidermal regulator of NF-kappaB, in psoriasis. *Am J Hum Genet* 2012; 90(5):796–808.
200. Hunt KA, Mistry V, Bockett NA, Ahmad T, Ban M, Barker JN et al. Negligible impact of rare autoimmune-locus coding-region variants on missing heritability. *Nature* 2013; 498(7453):232–235.
201. Di Meglio P, Villanova F, Napolitano L, Tosi I, Terranova Barberio M, Mak RK et al. The IL23R A/Gln381 allele promotes IL-23 unresponsiveness in human memory T-helper 17 cells and impairs Th17 responses in psoriasis patients. *J Invest Dermatol* 2013; 133(10):2381–2389.
202. Sarin R, Wu X, Abraham C. Inflammatory disease protective R381Q IL23 receptor polymorphism results in decreased primary CD4+ and CD8+ human T-cell functional responses. *Proc Natl Acad Sci U S A* 2011; 108(23):9560–9565.
203. Reveille JD. Genetics of spondyloarthritis—Beyond the MHC. *Nat Rev Rheumatol* 2012; 8(5):296–304.
204. Kang J, Kugathasan S, Georges M, Zhao H, Cho JH, Consortium NIG. Improved risk prediction for Crohn's disease with a multi-locus approach. *Hum Mol Genet* 2011; 20(12):2435–2442.

Section II

Pathogenesis

3 Inflammation in Psoriasis and Psoriatic Arthritis

Latika Gupta and Amita Aggarwal

CONTENTS

3.1 INTRODUCTION

Psoriatic arthritis (PsA) is a clinically heterogeneous disease of the skin, joint, enthesis, and bone. Psoriasis and PsA form different ends of the same disease spectrum, although recent literature has brought to light subtle differences in the genetics and pathogenesis among two of these diseases [1]. In the past, psoriasis was thought to be a disorder of unregulated keratinocyte proliferation, as evidenced by the increased thickness of the layers of the epidermis and the increased turnover of the cells. However, now it is evident that it is a chronic immune-inflammatory disease that drives the increased keratinocyte proliferation.

Although the exact cause of psoriasis is not known, it is thought to result from a complex interaction of genetic, environmental, and epigenetic factors that drive the immune-mediated inflammation (Figure 3.1). The major players include innate immune cells, Th17 cells, and interleukin (IL)-23/IL-17 cytokines [2–4]. Being a class I major histocompatibility complex (MHC)–associated disease, it has been proposed that tissue-specific factors lead to local inflammation, and that this results in failure of peripheral tolerance that permits MHC class I positive T cells to gain access to the tissue following their activation by dendritic cells (DCs) in the lymphoid system [5]. Psoriasis is thought to have a greater adaptive immune component, as seen by its excellent response to T-cell-based

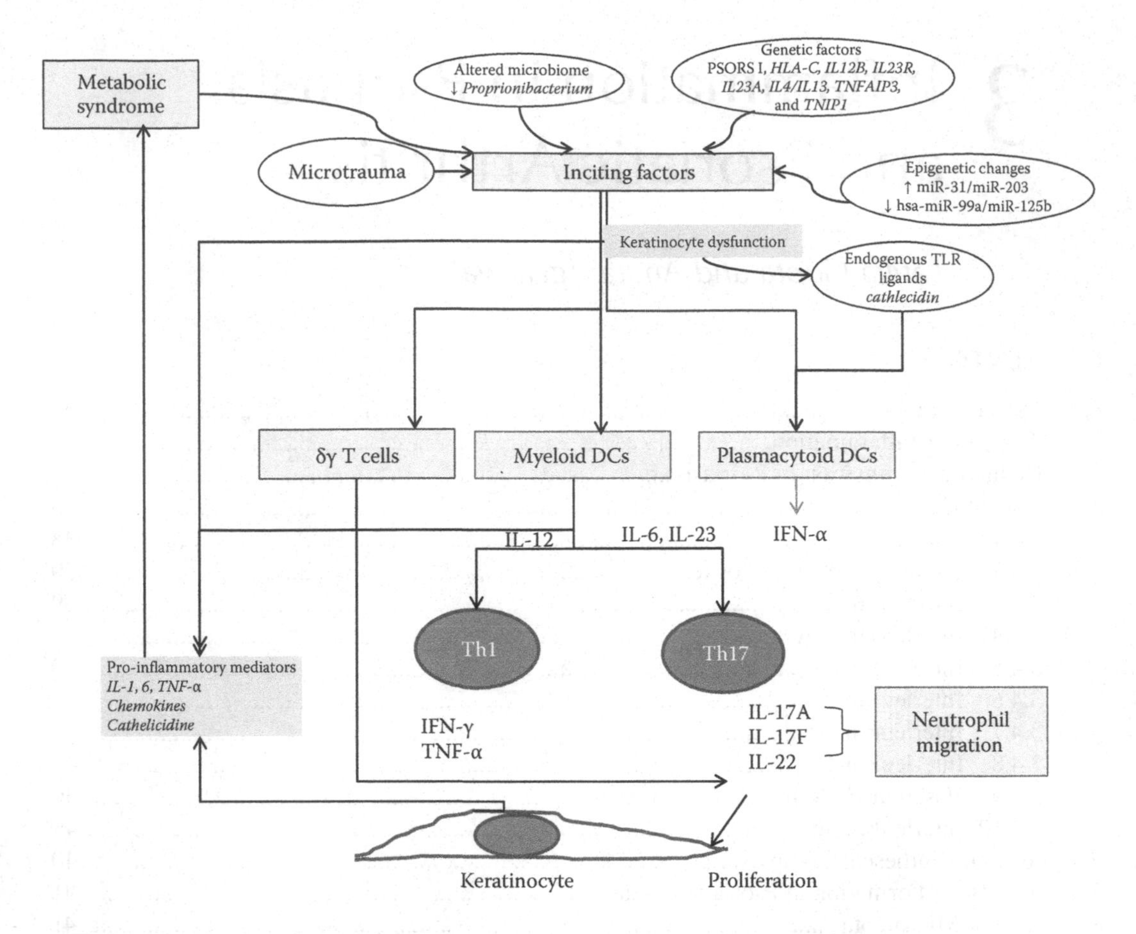

FIGURE 3.1 Multiple factors, like stress, trauma, microbes, genetic predisposition, and epigenetic changes, lead to keratinocyte dysfunction. Keratinocytes produce cathelicidin, which binds to DNA and activates pDCs via TLR-9 to produce IFN-α. In addition, the inciting agents can also activate monocytes, leading to the production of pro-inflammatory cytokines. Pro-inflammatory cytokines and the activated DCs skew the naïve T cells toward Th1 and Th17. IL-17- and IL-22-induced chemokine production leads to neutrophil migration to the epidermis, where neutrophils can form a microabscess. In addition, pro-inflammatory cytokines induce keratinocyte proliferation. Obesity and metabolic syndrome may act as an inciting agent or may help in the perpetuation of inflammation.

therapies, while nail, bone, and joint diseases respond better to cytokine-based therapies, highlighting the role of innate immune activation in them.

Understanding the pathogenesis may help us to design better-targeted therapies. This chapter provides an overview of pathogenesis and inflammation. The subsequent chapters provide detailed information on specific pathways.

3.2 TRIGGERS OF INFLAMMATION

The exact trigger in psoriasis is unknown. Streptococcal infection can trigger guttate psoriasis, possibly through molecular mimicry of M protein of the bacterial cell wall with keratin. The cathelicidin (LL-37), an antimicrobial peptide, is overexpressed in psoriatic skin lesions; its binding to self-DNA can activate DCs via Toll-like receptor (TLR)-9 and may act as the trigger for a break in peripheral tolerance in psoriasis. The TLR-7/8 agonist imiquimod can induce a psoriasis-like skin disease in mice through production of interferon (IFN)-α by plasmacytoid dendritic cells (pDCs).

This further strengthens the case for TLR activation from any microbial or endogenous insult being the inciting event in the pathogenesis of psoriasis [1,6].

Psoriasis often develops at sites of trauma (called the Koebner phenomenon). Patients with PsA also have a history of preceding trauma more often than those with other inflammatory arthritides, like rheumatoid arthritis. Rubella vaccination, house moving, recurrent oral ulcers, and bone fractures have also been deemed to be risk factors for the development of psoriasis and related arthritides [7]. The recent proposition to classify psoriasis and PsA as MHC-I-opathy further strengthens the case for a causal link to preceding trauma [8]. Smoking, on the other hand, is protective for psoriasis in individuals carrying the human leukocyte antigen (HLA)-*C*06* allele [5,9].

3.3 CELLULAR INFLAMMATION IN PSORIASIS

The classical psoriatic skin lesion is characterized by hyperkeratosis, parakeratosis, and an increased depth of rete pegs, along with inflammatory cells (DCs, macrophages, and T cells in the dermis), while the epidermis shows a significant neutrophilic infiltration with a sprinkling of T cells [10]. Neutrophils accumulate in a perivascular fashion in early psoriasis lesions and then migrate to the epidermis, where their collection manifests as pustules, which are called Munro's microabscesses. The neutrophils are also the key cells that secrete IL-17, which plays an important role in the perpetuation of the inflammatory response.

Infiltration by T lymphocytes is a consistent finding in skin biopsies from patients with psoriasis. They constitute a significant fraction of dermal mononuclear inflammatory cell infiltrate. CD8+ T cells predominate in the epidermis; most of these express addressins that promote homing to the skin. Interestingly, clonal restriction of resident memory epidermal T cells seems limited to the CD8 compartment. This finding might suggest a link between viral or self-antigens in the epidermis and psoriasis, since endogenous and viral antigens are typically presented to CD8 T cells, and not CD4 T cells, via MHC class I [11]. Synovial fluid evaluation in PsA also shows that the CD8+ T-cell population dominates compared with CD4+ T cells. Cytokines secreted by CD8+ T cells activate synovial fibroblast, leading to the release of cytokines and matrix metalloproteinases, which cause synovitis.

In the dermis, CD4+ T-cell predominance is seen. Most T cells in skin lesions have a memory phenotype and express cutaneous lymphocyte antigen (CLA), the skin addressin, suggesting that they are exposed to antigen in the skin. In contrast, only 10% of circulating T lymphocytes are CLA+ [12].

NK cells constitute 5%–8% of the cellular infiltrate in psoriasis, more so in the mid- and papillary dermis. Some recent studies have shown lower CD57 expression in NK cells in patients, suggesting skewing to an immature phenotype. Immature NK cells produce more cytokines (IFN-γ) and have a heightened response to IL-2 stimulation. They also exhibit a higher degranulation capacity and greater turnover, lending support to their possible active participation in the ongoing inflammation in psoriasis [12].

Lesional skin is infiltrated by macrophages and DCs. The DCs show an activated phenotype with expression of CD80, CD83, and CD86. DCs in psoriasis plaques exhibit decreased migration in response to normal stimuli. The CD18 hypomorphic mouse model highlights a critical role for macrophages in the development of psoriasis. Depletion of macrophages reverses psoriasiform lesions in mice models [13].

Langerhans cells are immature dendritic cells (iDCs), and have been found in psoriasis lesions, sometimes in increased abundance. Healed lesions and uninvolved skin lack mature DCs, explaining why previous studies have shown that DCs from psoriatic lesions could activate T cells, while those from uninvolved skin failed to do so. pDCs, albeit a minor DC subset in skin lesions, produce large amounts of IFN-α when activated. Upregulation of IFN-α has been detected in early psoriatic lesions. In addition, in a mouse xenograft model of psoriasis, the development of psoriatic lesions was dependent on IFN-α production by pDCs. In contrast, activated or mature myeloid DCs are known to be major producers of IL-12 and IL-23, and thus strong polarizers of T-cell responses to the Th1 phenotype [14].

Recent data also suggests a role for innate lymphoid cells (ILC) in the pathogenesis of psoriasis via IL-22 production. The ILC-3 subset expresses the NKp44 receptor, as well as the CCR6 chemokine, and produces IL-17 [3].

The role of T cells in the onset and perpetuation of inflammation in psoriasis is well established. Therapies that block T-cell activation or induce T-cell death, such as alefacept (an inhibitor of the T-cell-activating interaction between LFA3 on antigen-presenting cells and CD2 on T cells), have been effective for psoriasis. In addition, the injection of T cells from psoriatic skin lesions can induce psoriatic features in nonlesional human skin transplanted onto severe combined immunodeficient (SCID) mice. This happens only with CD4+ T-cell transfer and not with CD8+ T cells, suggesting a dominant role of the former in the pathogenesis [15,16].

Both Th17 and Th1 subsets of CD4 T cells and, to a lesser extent, Th22 cells have been implicated in psoriasis. Early investigational studies presumed a dominating role for Th1 cells; however, after the description of Th17 cells, they are now believed to be the major players. Th17 cells develop in psoriatic skin under the polarizing effects of IL-1, IL-6, transforming growth factor (TGF)-β, and IL-23 produced by inflammatory DCs. The activation of Th17 cells by IL-23 stimulates these cells to produce IL-17A and IL-22, cytokines that promote keratinocyte activation and growth. Ustekinumab, a highly effective drug that is currently in use for psoriasis, is a monoclonal antibody that binds to IL-23, leading to the death of Th17 cells. In PsA, CD8+ IL-17-producing cells are a major source of IL-17 in comparison with rheumatoid arthritis. CD8+ IL-17-producing cells show good correlation with acute phase reactants, as well as Doppler ultrasound scores for synovitis [12].

Th1 cells produce an array of pro-inflammatory cytokines, including IFN-γ, IL-2, and TNF-α, and contribute to the amplification of inflammation. IFN-γ, the prototypic cytokine produced by these cells, can promote psoriasis-like changes in nonlesional psoriatic skin [17].

Failure of regulation of activation of T cells by regulatory T cells also contributes to continued inflammation. CD18 knockout mice that are deficient in regulatory T cells develop skin lesions of psoriasis. Additionally, defects in the suppressive function of regulatory T cells have been found in psoriasis lesions [13].

A role for epidermal keratinocytes as triggers for the initiation of psoriasis is a subject of much debate. Keratinocyte-derived antimicrobial peptides (AMPs), including β defensins, cathelicidins, and psoriasin (S100A7), are upregulated in psoriatic epidermis early in the course of lesion development. AMPs have both chemoattractant and immunomodulatory effects on DCs and T cells and may contribute to cutaneous inflammation. One theory on the initiation of psoriasis involves the upregulation of the AMP cathelicidin LL-37 in skin. LL-37 may bind self-DNA and stimulate the production of IFN-α by pDCs through TLR-9. LL-37 has also been shown to be antigenic in psoriasis; LL-37 stimulates both CD4 and CD8 T cells in an HLA-restricted manner. Vitamin D analogues have an immunomodulatory function, and seek to target this pathway in psoriasis [18].

3.4 ROLE OF CYTOKINES

3.4.1 Interferon-α

Type 1 IFN pathways are upregulated in early lesions of psoriasis. IFN-α present in psoriatic skin is largely derived from pDCs. Systemic treatment with IFN-α can exacerbate psoriasis, and topical imiquimod (which induces local IFN-α production) has led to the development of psoriasis in humans and psoriasis-like disease in mice. Psoriasis-like disease develops in mice that lack the repressors of IFN-α signaling [17].

3.4.2 Tumor Necrosis Factor-α

Activated DCs, Th17 and Th1 cells, and keratinocytes in psoriatic skin produce TNF-α and respond to its effects. Elevated levels of TNF-α are found in lesional skin of psoriatic patients. The dramatic clinical improvement of psoriasis with anti-TNF agents further lends support to the role of TNF-α in the pathogenesis of psoriasis [19].

3.4.3 Interleukin-23

IL-23 is the cytokine responsible for the proliferation and survival of Th17 cells, which is an increasingly important T-cell subset in many autoimmune diseases, including psoriasis and Crohn's disease. IL-23 is produced by myeloid DCs and at low levels by keratinocytes on TLR stimulation. Polymorphisms in the IL-23 receptor, p40 and p19 subunits of IL-23, increase susceptibility to psoriasis, highlighting the importance of the IL-17/IL-23 axis in inflammation in psoriasis. Apart from ustekinumab, biologic agents that selectively block IL-23; tildrakizumab, guselkumab, and BI 655066 have shown benefit in small trials [19–21].

3.4.4 Interleukin-17A

IL-17A, a cytokine produced by Th17 cells, is elevated in skin lesions of psoriasis and the serum of patients with psoriasis. IL-17A is involved in the activation and recruitment of neutrophils, the enhancement of angiogenesis, and the promotion of the release of other inflammatory cytokines (TNF-α, IL-1, and IL-6). IL-17A can also directly activate keratinocytes and induce cytokine release. Secukinumab, an anti-IL-17A monoclonal antibody, has shown efficacy results equivalent to or better than those of other available biologic agents for moderate to severe plaque psoriasis. Phase II trials have also demonstrated the efficacy of another anti-IL-17 monoclonal antibody (ixekizumab) and an anti-IL-17 receptor antibody (brodalumab) in psoriasis [22,23].

3.4.5 Interleukin-12

IL-12 is produced by activated myeloid DCs. This cytokine promotes the differentiation of Th1 cells, which are considered important in the pathogenesis of psoriasis. Indirect evidence for a contributory role for IL-12 in psoriasis comes from findings of increased Th1 cells and IFN-γ (a product of Th1 cells) in psoriatic skin. However, a study surprisingly failed to detect the upregulation of the p35 subunit of IL-12 in psoriatic skin. It is possible that ustekinumab, an effective biologic agent for psoriasis that targets both IL-12 and IL-23, may function primarily through the drug's effects on the IL-23 pathway [17,24].

3.4.6 Interleukin-22

IL-22 is produced by Th17 and Th22 cells. It stimulates the growth and activation of keratinocytes and has little effect on immune cells. In keratinocytes, it signals via STAT3 to cause cell hyperproliferation, secretion of AMPs, and production of matrix metalloproteinases that support increased cell mobility. IL-22 levels are increased in the blood of patients with psoriasis and in psoriatic plaques. Treatment of psoriasis decreases these levels. Molecular therapies that target IL-22 are in clinical trials [17,25].

3.4.7 Interleukin-20

IL-20 production by keratinocytes plays an important synergistic role downstream of IL-22. IL-20 is highly expressed in psoriatic skin and promotes alterations in epidermal thickness, maturation defects, and upregulation of AMPs. Blocking IL-20 in a SCID xenotransplant model of psoriasis induces the resolution of psoriasis and blocks initiation of the disease [17].

3.4.8 Interleukin-13

Associations between PsA and IL-13 have been replicated in two independent studies. Both studies failed to identify association with psoriasis alone [26,27].

3.4.9 Vascular Endothelial Growth Factor

Endothelial cells within psoriatic plaques express elevated levels of vascular endothelial growth factor (VEGF), prostaglandins, and nitric oxide. All these contribute to leaky and tortuous vessels in psoriatic skin. In addition, transgenic mice overexpressing VEGF in the epidermis have been found to develop psoriasiform skin changes. Activated vasculature promotes the attraction and transmigration of the leukocytes discussed above. Antiangiogenic agents have actually demonstrated some success in psoriasis patients, but more investigation is needed [17].

3.4.10 Interleukin-36

IL-36 is a set of cytokines belonging to the IL-1 family, which includes three agonists, namely, IL-36α, IL-36β, and IL-36γ, and an IL-36 receptor antagonist (IL-36Ra). Agonistic IL-36 receptor (IL-36R) ligation leads to intracellular signals similar to those induced by IL-1. Epithelial cells constitutively express IL-36 agonists and IL-36Ra, where they act as primary defense mechanisms at the skin barrier. Knockout data from transgenic mice suggest that IL-36, in contrast to IL-1, is not involved in the development of experimental arthritis [28].

Transgenic overexpression of IL-36α in keratinocytes is associated with the development of psoriasis-like lesions. Also, mutations in the *IL36RN* gene in patients with a deficiency in IL-36Ra (DITRA) who have nonfunctional IL-36Ra protein develop generalized pustular psoriasis. The stark absence of arthritis in DITRA compared with IL-1Ra deficiency (DIRA) highlights how IL-36 uncouples the inflammation in the skin and joint in psoriatic diseases [28].

3.5 SYNOVIO-ENTHESEAL COMPLEX

Enthesitis is considered a key feature of PsA. The enthesis is the attachment site of the joint capsule, tendon, or ligament to bone. MRI studies have shown that inflammation at the enthesis is more widespread than originally thought, involving the bone, synovium, and several contiguous structures. The concept of a synovio-entheseal complex (SEC) has been proposed, in which, in health, the synovium provides nourishment and lubrication to the entheseal fibrocartilage. When a mechanically stressed enthesis is injured, the associated inflammatory reaction would be manifested in the juxtaposed synovium. In a collagen-induced arthritis murine model, enthesitis and entheseal new bone formation were dependent on IL-23 and IL-22 contributed by double-negative T cells and γδ T cells [29]. The findings of increased vascularity at entheseal sites, particularly at places of microdamage and ensuing repair, suggest that local trauma may drive the entheseal inflammatory response. A recent report describing the development of unifocal PsA in identical twins following site-specific injury further provides additional support that biomechanical strain can trigger altered bone remodeling in a genetically susceptible host [30].

Ultrasound studies in psoriasis have shown that subclinical enthesitis of large insertions is common in psoriasis [31]. It is believed that the entheses may be the site of origin for the inflammatory response in PsA in contrast to rheumatoid arthritis, where inflammation originates in the synovium. However, there is no consensus on this issue to date.

3.6 NEW BONE FORMATION IN PSORIATIC DISEASES

New bone formation in PsA differs from that in other conditions, as it is centered at entheseal sites only. Psoriasis patients without arthritis have also been seen to manifest new bone formation, suggesting a continuum of bone alterations from psoriasis to PsA. Recent data suggest that the IL-23/IL-17 pathway is directly involved in altered bone phenotypes in PsA. IL-17 and IL-22 are produced from CD8+ IL-17+ T cells, γδ T cells, and type 3 ILCs apart from Th17 and Th22 cells. However, the role of these cells in bone remodeling is not yet clear. Overexpression of IL-22 leads to transcriptomic signatures of osteoproliferation and new bone formation, while IL-17 upregulates genes involved in inflammation and bone resorption [32].

Earlier studies implicated alterations in TNF-α and related cytokines in new bone formation. However, TNF-α suppresses bone formation by inducing DKK1 and sclerostin (SOST), inhibitors of the Wnt signaling pathway [33]. Since the TNF-α blockade does not have a significant impact on the formation of syndesmophytes or osteophytes, it is unlikely to play a major role in new bone formation [34,35].

3.7 ROLE OF MICROBIOTA

The microbiome affects the local milieu, as well as the immune system. Different bacteria serve different functions, ranging from scavenging on dead and decaying cells to the production of natural oils, or restriction of pathogenic bacteria by competition for nutrients. The microbiota on the surface of psoriatic skin differs from unaffected areas, as well as from those of healthy controls, apart from variation accounted for by factors like the part of the body and whether the skin there is moist or dry. Microbial diversity is higher in the cast of microbes inhabiting psoriatic plaques than in controls. Abundance of the *Propionibacterium* genus was highest in healthy skin, followed by unaffected skin from psoriasis patients, and then psoriatic lesions, suggesting that their abundance is low in inflammatory milieus. Eczema, a disease partly similar to psoriasis, has *Staphylococcus aureus* colonization in both healthy and eczematous skin of 90% of affected children [36].

3.8 NONAUTOIMMUNE MECHANISMS IN PATHOGENESIS

The Koebner phenomenon suggests the role of microtrauma in skin disease. The presence of changes at the bone–synovium–entheses organ on MRI reflects a role of microtrauma in enthesitis, arthritis, and nail changes. The DBA/1 mice model established that enthesitis can be precipitated in aging male mice when housed under crowded conditions, which induced fighting and trauma [37].

Dermal DCs (DDCs) lie in close contact with sensory neurons. Upon TLR stimulation, these DDCs release IL-23 and induce inflammation. These effects are mediated via activation of ion channels TRPV1 and NaV1.8, and the ablation of these ion channels can completely abrogate the ensuing inflammation [20].

Hence, multiple nonimmune events, like infections, trauma, and nerve cells, are required to modulate the inflammatory response in a genetically predisposed host.

3.9 ADIPOKINES AND METABOLIC SYNDROME

Metabolic syndrome is two to three times more prevalent in patients with psoriasis than in the general population. The association is stronger for those with severe psoriasis than for patients with milder disease. Increased diabetes mellitus and cardiovascular risk are unavoidable accompaniments, and this also translates into reduced life expectancy in psoriasis. These observations have been followed by various speculations on possible pathogenic connections between the two entities [38].

In obesity, M1-type macrophages and T cells infiltrate the hypertrophic and damaged adipose tissue. Soluble mediators from these adipokines result in a systemic subclinical inflammatory state, as reflected by elevated C-reactive protein. Differences in susceptibility loci for psoriasis and metabolic syndrome make coinheritance a less plausible explanation [5].

Inflammation could be the forerunner of accelerated atherosclerosis, as seen in rheumatoid arthritis and lupus. In such a case, the extent of metabolic disturbances parallels the duration of inflammation and should be reversed with treatment as well.

Indirect evidence weakly supports this hypothesis, as myocardial infarction risk is lower in psoriasis patients receiving systemic antipsoriatic drugs [39]. However, the metabolic side effects of antipsoriatic drugs, like weight gain with anti-TNF inhibitors and hyperlipidemia from acitretin, preclude an unbiased assessment.

Does obesity predispose to psoriasis? Some studies have demonstrated that obesity frequently occurs prior to the onset of psoriasis and identified obesity as being an independent risk factor for the development of psoriasis [40]. Moreover, there is evidence that body weight reduction improves skin disease and also therapy response in these patients (the latter being not completely explainable by pharmacokinetic aspects) [41]. Obesity worsens skin inflammation in murine models, establishing the latter hypothesis more firmly. This underlying mechanism could be mediated by adipokines.

Adipokines are soluble mediators released from adipocytes and surrounding cells, such as macrophages. Some adipokines, like resistin, chemerin, fetuin-A, TNF-α, IL-1β, and IL-6, drive insulin resistance, dyslipidemia, vascular dysfunction, and immune cell tissue infiltration and activation. It seems plausible that they promote skin inflammation as well. On the other hand, adiponectin and omentin exert anti-inflammatory, insulin-sensitizing, antiatherogenic, and fat mass–reducing effects. However, their levels are often decreased in psoriasis, reflecting a poor metabolic state [42].

3.10 WHAT DRIVES PSORIASIS TO PSORIATIC ARTHRITIS?

Approximately 30% of psoriasis patients develop arthritis, but the events that underlie this transition are poorly understood. In a proteomic study that compared skin biopsies from psoriasis patients with and without PsA, periostin (POSTN) and inhibition of β5 integrin (ITGB5) were identified as biomarkers of arthritis. The two molecules are crucial in the transmigration and chemotaxis of inflammatory cells [43].

PsA is therefore a disease of remarkable clinical, prognostic, and functional heterogeneity. It seems probable that unifying molecular pathways would not suffice to explain each of these diverse manifestations. A complex interaction of environmental triggers, like microbes, trauma, and genetic predisposition shape the immune inflammation. The heterogeneity in clinical features and pathogenic pathways is mirrored by the response to targeted therapies. IL-17-targeted therapies work better for the skin, while anti-TNF biologics work equally well for the joints and skin disease.

All this translates into a felt need for better insights into mechanisms driving disease in each tissue compartment, as offering targeted therapies for a better quality of life may be the future in psoriasis and associated diseases.

REFERENCES

1. Krueger JG, Bowcock A. Psoriasis pathophysiology: Current concepts of pathogenesis. *Ann Rheum Dis* 2005;64(S2):ii30–6.
2. Shikhagaie MM, Germar K, Bal SM, Ros XR, Spits H. Innate lymphoid cells in autoimmunity: Emerging regulators in rheumatic diseases. *Nat Rev Rheumatol* 2017;13:164–73.
3. Villanova F, Flutter B, Tosi I, Grys K, Sreeneebus H, Perera GK et al. Characterization of innate lymphoid cells in human skin and blood demonstrates increase of NKp44+ ILC3 in psoriasis. *J Invest Dermatol* 2014;134:984–91.
4. Ward NL, Umetsu DT. A new player on the psoriasis block: IL-17A- and IL-22-producing innate lymphoid cells. *J Invest Dermatol* 2014;134:2305–7.

5. Bowcock AM, Krueger JG. Getting under the skin: The immunogenetics of psoriasis. *Nat Rev Immunol* 2005;5:699–711.
6. Ben Salem C, Hmouda H, Bouraoui K. Psoriasis. *N Engl J Med* 2009;361:1710.
7. Takeshita J, Grewal S, Langan SM, Mehta NN, Ogdie A, Van Voorhees AS et al. Psoriasis and comorbid diseases: Epidemiology. *J Am Acad Dermatol* 2017;76:377–90.
8. McGonagle D, Aydin SZ, Gül A, Mahr A, Direskeneli H. "MHC-I-opathy"-unified concept for spondyloarthritis and Behçet disease. *Nat Rev Rheumatol* 2015;11:731–40.
9. Eder L, Shanmugarajah S, Thavaneswaran A, Chandran V, Rosen CF, Cook RJ et al. The association between smoking and the development of psoriatic arthritis among psoriasis patients. *Ann Rheum Dis* 2011;71:219–24.
10. Grove GL. Epidermal cell kinetics in psoriasis. *Int J Dermatol* 1979;18:111–22.
11. Di Meglio P, Villanova F, Navarini AA, Mylonas A, Tosi I, Nestle FO et al. Targeting CD8(+) T cells prevents psoriasis development. *J Allergy Clin Immunol* 2016;138:274–6.e6.
12. Cai Y, Fleming C, Yan J. New insights of T cells in the pathogenesis of psoriasis. *Cell Mol Immunol* 2012;9:302–9.
13. Wang H, Peters T, Sindrilaru A, Scharffetter-Kochanek K. Key role of macrophages in the pathogenesis of CD18 hypomorphic murine model of psoriasis. *J Invest Dermatol* 2009;129:1100–14.
14. Jariwala SP. The role of dendritic cells in the immunopathogenesis of psoriasis. *Arch Dermatol Res* 2007;299:359–66.
15. Wagner EF, Schonthaler HB, Guinea-Viniegra J, Tschachler E. Psoriasis: What we have learned from mouse models. *Nat Rev Rheumatol* 2010;6:704–14.
16. Kundu-Raychaudhuri S, Datta-Mitra A, Abria CJ, Peters J, Raychaudhuri SP. Severe combined immunodeficiency mouse-psoriatic human skin xenograft model: A modern tool connecting bench to bedside. *Indian J Dermatol Venereol Leprol* 2014;80:204–13.
17. Baliwag J, Barnes DH, Johnston A. Cytokines in psoriasis. *Cytokine* 2015;73:342–50.
18. Morizane S, Yamasaki K, Mühleisen B, Kotol PF, Murakami M, Aoyama Y et al. Cathelicidin antimicrobial peptide LL-37 in psoriasis enables keratinocyte reactivity against TLR9 ligands. *J Invest Dermatol* 2012;132:135–43.
19. McInnes IB. Cytokine targeting in psoriasis and psoriatic arthritis: Beyond TNFalpha. *Ernst Scher Res Found Workshop* 2006;56:29–44.
20. Riol-Blanco L, Ordovas-Montanes J, Perro M, Naval E, Thiriot A, Alvarez D et al. Nociceptive sensory neurons drive interleukin-23-mediated psoriasiform skin inflammation. *Nature* 2014;510:157–61.
21. Langley R, Thaci D, Papp K, Riedl E, Reich K, Shames R. MK-3222, an anti–IL-23p19 humanized monoclonal antibody, provides significant improvement in psoriasis over 52 weeks of treatment that is maintained after discontinuation of dosing. *J Am Acad Dermatol* 2014;70:AB176.
22. Leonardi C, Matheson R, Zachariae C, Cameron G, Li L, Edson-Heredia E et al. Anti-interleukin-17 monoclonal antibody ixekizumab in chronic plaque psoriasis. *N Engl J Med* 2012;366:1190–9.
23. Papp KA, Leonardi C, Menter A, Ortonne J-P, Krueger JG, Kricorian G et al. Brodalumab, an anti-interleukin-17-receptor antibody for psoriasis. *N Engl J Med* 2012;366:1181–9.
24. Campa M, Mansouri B, Warren R, Menter A. A review of biologic therapies targeting IL-23 and IL-17 for use in moderate-to-severe plaque psoriasis. *Dermatol Ther* 2015;6:1–12.
25. Hao J-Q. Targeting interleukin-22 in psoriasis. *Inflammation* 2014;37:94–9.
26. Swindell WR, Xing X, Stuart PE, Chen CS, Aphale A, Nair RP et al. Heterogeneity of inflammatory and cytokine networks in chronic plaque psoriasis. *PloS One* 2012;7:e34594.
27. Cancino-Díaz JC, Reyes-Maldonado E, Bañuelos-Pánuco CA, Jiménez-Zamudio L, García-Latorre E, León-Dorantes G et al. Interleukin-13 receptor in psoriatic keratinocytes: Overexpression of the mRNA and underexpression of the protein. *J Invest Dermatol* 2002;119:1114–20.
28. Dietrich D, Gabay C. Inflammation: IL-36 has proinflammatory effects in skin but not in joints. *Nat Rev Rheumatol* 2014;10:639–40.
29. Sherlock JP, Joyce-Shaikh B, Turner SP, Chao C-C, Sathe M, Grein J et al. IL-23 induces spondyloarthropathy by acting on ROR-γt+ CD3+CD4-CD8- entheseal resident T cells. *Nat Med* 2012;18:1069–76.
30. Ng J, Tan AL, McGonagle D. Unifocal psoriatic arthritis development in identical twins following site specific injury: Evidence supporting biomechanical triggering events in genetically susceptible hosts. *Ann Rheum Dis* 2015;74:948–9.
31. van der Ven M, Karreman M, Weel A, Tchetverikov I, Vis M, Nijsten T et al. FRI0562 ultrasound enthesitis in primary care psoriasis patients with musculoskeletal complaints. *Ann Rheum Dis* 2015;74(S2):631.
32. Smith JA, Colbert RA. Review: The interleukin-23/interleukin-17 axis in spondyloarthritis pathogenesis: Th17 and beyond. *Arthritis Rheumatol* 2014;66:231–41.

33. Osta B, Benedetti G, Miossec P. Classical and paradoxical effects of TNF-α on bone homeostasis. *Front Immunol* 2014;5:48.
34. Baraliakos X, Listing J, Rudwaleit M, Haibel H, Brandt J, Sieper J et al. Progression of radiographic damage in patients with ankylosing spondylitis: Defining the central role of syndesmophytes. *Ann Rheum Dis* 2007;66:910–5.
35. van Tok M, van Duivenvoorde L, Kramer I, Ingold P, Knaup V, Taurog J, Kolbinger F, Baeten D. Anti-IL-17A, but not anti-TNF, can halt pathological new bone formation in experimental spondyloarthritis [abstract]. *Arthritis Rheumatol* 2016;68(S10). Available from http://acrabstracts.org/abstract/anti-il-17a-but-not-anti-tnf-can-halt-pathological-new-bone-formation-in-experimental-spondyloarthritis/.
36. Trivedi B. Microbiome: The surface brigade. *Nature* 2012;492:S60–1.
37. Lories R, Matthys P, de Vlam K, Derese I, Luyten F. Ankylosing enthesitis, dactylitis, and onychoperiostitis in male DBA/1 mice: A model of psoriatic arthritis. *Ann Rheum Dis* 2004;63:595–8.
38. Nakajima H, Nakajima K, Tarutani M, Morishige R, Sano S. Kinetics of circulating Th17 cytokines and adipokines in psoriasis patients. *Arch Dermatol Res* 2011;303:451–5.
39. Ogdie A, Yu Y, Haynes K, Love TJ, Maliha S, Jiang Y et al. Risk of major cardiovascular events in patients with psoriatic arthritis, psoriasis and rheumatoid arthritis: A population-based cohort study. *Ann Rheum Dis* 2015;74:326–32.
40. Kumar S, Han J, Li T, Curhan G, Choi HK, Qureshi AA. Obesity, waist circumference, weight change, and the risk of psoriasis in US women. *J Eur Acad Dermatol Venereol* 2013;27:1293–8.
41. Sandoval LF, Pierce A, Davis SA, Feldman SR. Improved psoriasis with weight loss: The role of behavioural factors. *Br J Dermatol* 2015;172:826–7.
42. Abella V, Scotece M, Conde J, López V, Lazzaro V, Pino J et al. Adipokines, metabolic syndrome and rheumatic diseases. *J Immunol Res* 2014;2014:343746.
43. Cretu D, Liang K, Saraon P, Batruch I, Diamandis EP, Chandran V. Quantitative tandem mass-spectrometry of skin tissue reveals putative psoriatic arthritis biomarkers. *Clin Proteomics* 2015;12:1.

4 Psoriasis and Diabetes: An Unholy Alliance

Satinath Mukhopadhyay, Deep Dutta, and Dipyaman Ganguly

CONTENTS

4.1 INTRODUCTION

Psoriasis is a chronic autoimmune disorder, having an underlying genetic basis, that is triggered by environmental factors and characterized by patchy scaly skin lesions, which can involve any part of the body, but more commonly the extensor regions [1]. It has been associated with various other disorders, most commonly psoriatic arthritis (30%), followed by depression, cardiovascular disease, obesity, and Crohn's disease [1]. Psoriasis is not an uncommon disorder; a prevalence of 2%–4%, with a peak incidence between 15 and 25 years age and without any sex predilection, has been reported. The incidence of psoriasis goes up as we move away from the equator, a trend similar to that seen with multiple sclerosis [2]. Psoriasis has been repeatedly linked with various other autoimmune disorders, including inflammatory bowel disease and spondyloarthropathies.

Recent studies have identified a link between psoriasis, obesity, and diabetes. Diabetes is a spectrum disorder, having autoimmunity at one end and insulin resistance at the other. Beta cell dysfunction and loss are the end points of disease pathogenesis of diabetes, irrespective of the starting point being autoimmunity against pancreatic beta cells or insulin resistance at the peripheral target tissues, namely, adipose tissue, skeletal and cardiac muscles, and liver. This chapter explores the relationship between psoriasis and diabetes at the levels of epidemiology, pathogenetic mechanisms, and treatment outcomes.

4.2 EPIDEMIOLOGIC DATA

Longitudinal and prospective studies from the United States and Denmark have found that patients with psoriasis, especially those with the more severe forms, have a higher risk of developing diabetes [3–5]. In the Danish population-based study, a total of 52,613 patients with psoriasis, including 6,784 having severe disease, were identified from the national population registry of 4,614,807 individuals [4]. The incidence of new-onset diabetes was 6.93% (6.63–7.25) and 9.65% (8.68–10.73) in patients with psoriasis and severe psoriasis, respectively, which was significantly higher than that of the rest of the population (3.67 [confidence interval {CI} 3.65–3.69]), which translated to *incidence rate ratios* of 1.49 (CI 1.43–1.56) and 2.13 (1.91–2.37) for those with mild and severe psoriasis, respectively [4]. Another population-based study from Germany evaluating 87,964 type 2 diabetes mellitus (T2DM) patients aged 40 years or older with 72,148 matched nondiabetic controls revealed that a total of 3.4% of patients with T2DM and 2.8% of matched controls developed psoriasis within 10 years of follow-up, resulting in a hazard ratio (HR) of 1.18 (95% CI 1.08–1.29) for diabetes patients developing psoriasis, which is significantly higher and in line with the previously cited Danish study [6]. In a much smaller cohort of 77 patients of chronic plaque psoriasis and 92 age- and sex-matched controls reported from western India, the occurrences of impaired fasting glucose, impaired glucose tolerance, and T2DM were 5.2%, 9.1%, and 32.5%, respectively; the corresponding prevalence rates in the control population being 6.5%, 3.3%, and 15.2% respectively [7]. In a similar study from Turkey, 18.6% of persons with psoriasis had dysglycemia, compared with only 2.5% in the matched control group [8]. In other smaller studies from India, the occurrence of dysglycemia in patients with psoriasis has been reported to range from 20% to 30% [9,10].

It has to be realized that the relationship between psoriasis and diabetes in epidemiologic studies is bidirectional. In a study involving female nurses with psoriasis, the relative risk of developing diabetes was 1.63 (95% CI 1.25–2.12), whereas in another population-based nested analysis of 1061 diabetic patients in the United Kingdom, a 1.31 (95% CI 1.13–1.51) times increased relative risk of developing psoriasis was reported [11,12]. This is especially concerning as with the worsening diabetes global pandemic, the burden of psoriasis is likely to increase exponentially in the near future.

However, it must be highlighted that not all epidemiologic data have documented a positive link between psoriasis and type 2 diabetes. Analysis of the National Health and Nutrition Examination Survey (NHANES) database indicated that psoriasis was positively associated with overweight and obesity, and waist circumference, but not diabetes [13]. The reason for these conflicting results could be methodological, that is, inadequate population size, information bias, and inadequate adjustments for covariates. The situation is somewhat reminiscent of the one surrounding the contribution of maternal obesity and/or gestational diabetes mellitus (GDM) on fetal macrosomia. While most studies show a strong association between GDM and fetal macrosomia, others incriminate maternal obesity as the key factor, irrespective of the presence or absence of GDM.

4.3 INFLAMMATORY CROSSROADS OF PSORIASIS AND DIABETES

Psoriasis is an inflammatory disease of the skin that has a strong autoimmune component, although the identity of the relevant autoantigens remains far from clear. Keratinocytes in the psoriatic plaque drive the recruitment of immune cells by expressing antimicrobial peptides, chemokines, and growth factors, thereby serving both as the initiator tissue and as the target organ in the disease process [14]. Increased systemic inflammation (increased circulating levels of tumor necrosis factor-α [TNF-α] and interleukins [ILs] 6, 8, and 11), which occurs in psoriasis, is also linked with insulin resistance, endothelial dysfunction, and dyslipidemia, each of them playing an important role in the development of dysglycemia [15]. This is supported by the observation that TNF-α inhibitors and IL6 blockers, used for the treatment of psoriasis, are associated with an improvement in insulin resistance and a favorable impact on glycemia in these patients [16].

A primary defect in the regulatory T-cell function has been implicated in the development of psoriasis [4]. The innate immunity, especially the invariant natural killer T (iNKT) cells, has been implicated in the pathogenesis of psoriasis [2]. Obesity is also associated with increased systemic inflammation and activation of innate immunity [17]. Obesity has been linked to both decreased number and function of natural killer (NK) cells, especially the variant iNKT cells [12]. iNKT cells, often referred to as the "Swiss knife" of the immune system, have a major immunoregulatory function. They can produce multiple cytokines in a short period of time, directing the immune response toward a pro-inflammatory (Th1 or Th17) or anti-inflammatory (Th2) response, depending on the tissue of origin of the immune activation process [18].

4.4 T-HELPER 17 RESPONSE IN PSORIASIS AND DIABETES

Effector T cells that produce IL-17 and IL-22, namely, CD4+ Th17 cells and γδ T cells (DG2), have a major role in psoriatic inflammation. IL-23, a cytokine released by dendritic cells and critical for the maintenance of IL-17-producing T cells, is also an important player in the pathogenetic process [19,20] (Figure 4.1). This T-cell-dominant autoimmune process presupposes a critical role of aberrant activation of antigen-presenting cells, like dendritic cells [21,22]. Biologic therapies using monoclonal antibodies to IL-17 (secukinumab and ixekizumab) and IL-23 (ustekinumab and tildrakizumab) are under clinical trial in psoriasis [23], apart from more innate pro-inflammatory cytokines, like TNF-α (adalimumab, etanercept, and ustekinumab) [24].

The important role of the Th17 response and the involvement of dendritic cells are well appreciated in both type 1 and type 2 diabetes. In the context of the syndromic concurrence of psoriasis and type 2 diabetes, a growing body of literature reporting a role of the Th17 response in metabolic syndrome components, including systemic insulin resistance, provides a lot of support. Patients with type 2 diabetes show higher serum levels of IL-6, IL-1β, and TGF-β [25], all of which are important for Th17 differentiation [26,27]. It has been reported that peripheral blood of type 2 diabetes patients shows elevated Th17 cells and a gene signature for a Th17 response [28]. In another study, it was found that among obese individuals, diabetics had higher levels of circulating Th17 cytokines [29]. Thus, a dominant Th17 response may constitute an important pathogenetic mechanism linking psoriasis and diabetes. Of interest here, metformin, the first-line antihyperglycemic drug, has been shown to ameliorate disease in a preclinical model of inflammatory bowel disease by inhibiting the Th17 immune response [30], thus further supporting this notion. However, it remains to be validated if a dominant Th17 response actually underlies insulin resistance in psoriatic patients.

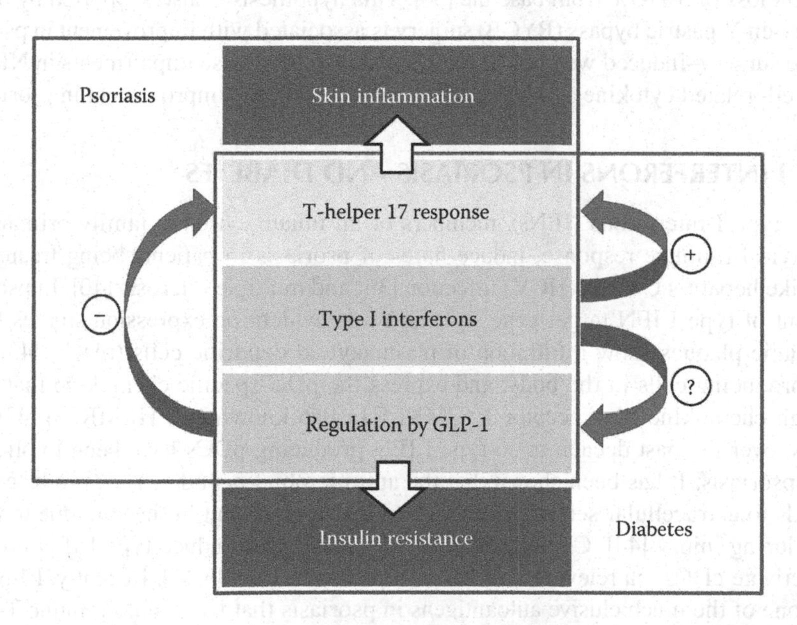

FIGURE 4.1 Plausible pathogenetic mechanisms underlying the concurrence of psoriasis and diabetes. Concurrence may result from several shared pathogenetic nodes in psoriasis and diabetes, two apparently discrete clinical contexts. Both T-helper 17 response and type I IFN induction are critical pathways involved in psoriasis pathogenesis. Recent studies have found the involvement of them in the pathogenesis of diabetes as well. On the other hand, GLP-1 and GLP-1R agonists are known insulin secretion enhancers, but recent studies have found a regulatory role in the Th17 response and a therapeutic role in psoriasis.

4.5 INCRETINS, PSORIASIS, AND DIABETES

Incretin molecules accentuate glucose-mediated insulin release from the pancreatic beta cells. They are small peptides released from the gastrointestinal tract, the most important of them being glucagon-like peptide 1 (GLP-1). GLP-1 analogues are approved agents for managing type 2 diabetes with the added benefits of causing significant weight loss in obese patients with diabetes. GLP-1 receptors (GLP-1Rs) are widely distributed in the human body. Apart from the gastrointestinal tract from where it is released and islets of pancreas, GLP-1R has been identified in the kidneys, brain, heart, and T and B lymphocytes in mice and humans [31–33]. Incretin molecules have a role in T-cell migration, maturation, and activation. In a small study in patients of type 2 diabetes with psoriasis, 6 weeks therapy of GLP-1 analogues was associated with improvement in skin lesions of psoriasis, accompanied by a decrease in iNKT cells in the psoriatic skin plaques and a simultaneous increase in circulating levels of iNKT cells [30]. In keeping with the above observation, the GLP-1R antagonist exendin 9 has been shown to block the modulation of iNKT cell cytokine production by GLP-1 [30,34]. In another study, the treatment of seven patients with type 2 diabetes and psoriasis with the GLP-1 agonist liraglutide resulted in improvement in the clinical severity of psoriasis, along with a decrease in dermal $\gamma\delta$ T-cell number and IL-17 expression [35]. Exenatide, another GLP-1 agonist, has also been shown to be beneficial in the resolution of skin lesions of psoriasis [36].

Various immunomodulatory roles have been attributed to GLP-1 and its analogues (GLP-1a), like inhibition of chemokine-induced migration of CD4+ lymphocytes. GLP-1 promotes activation of the transcription factor CREB, which regulates the expression of anti-inflammatory genes, such as IL-10 [36]. The permissive effect of GLP-1a on CREB-induced production of anti-inflammatory proteins may have a role in psoriasis-ameloriating effects of this class of drugs [30].

It is interesting to note that the weight loss induced by GLP-1a-like liraglutide may also contribute to the improvement in psoriasis. This is because in all the small studies where GLP-1a has been evaluated with regards to psoriasis, improvement in psoriasis was consistently associated with significant weight loss of 3%–5% from baseline [30]. This hypothesis is also supported by the observation that Roux-en-Y gastric bypass (RYGB) surgery is associated with improvement in psoriasis [37]. This bariatric surgery–induced weight loss has been shown to reverse impairments in NK cell activity and NK cell–related cytokine synthesis, which may explain the improvement in psoriasis [38].

4.6 TYPE I INTERFERONS IN PSORIASIS AND DIABETES

Interestingly, type I interferons (IFNs), members of an innate cytokine family primarily responsible for antiviral immune response, induce flares of psoriasis in patients being treated for other conditions, like hepatitis C virus (HCV) infection [39] and multiple sclerosis [40]. In psoriatic skin, an enrichment of type I IFN target gene signature was evident on expression studies [41]. Newly formed psoriatic plaques show infiltration of plasmacytoid dendritic cells (pDCs) [42], the major type I IFN-producing cells in the body, and express the pDC-specific chemokine that can recruit pDCs through chemokine-like receptor 1 (CMKLR1; also known as CHEMR23) [43]. Based on these studies, over the past decade or so type I IFN-producing pDCs have been implicated in the initiation of psoriasis. It has been shown that the antimicrobial peptide LL37, produced by keratinocytes, binds to extracellular self-origin DNA and RNA, abundant in the skin due to normal cell turnover or during injury [44]. Complexes of LL37–nucleic acid induce type I IFN production by pDCs and activate cDCs via relevant Toll-like receptors (TLRs) [45,46]. Recently, LL37 had been found to be one of the much elusive autoantigens in psoriasis that led to autoimmune T-cell activation [47]. Other skin-derived antimicrobial peptides have also been implicated in similar innate immune activation in psoriasis [48]. Accordingly, relevant TLRs, as well as type I IFNs, are potential therapeutic targets in psoriasis [49–51].

A critical role of type I IFN induction in the context of insulin resistance is also notable from relevant literature. Most important, a clinical association is noted from the development of insulin resistance in patients receiving type I IFNs as a therapy against HCV infection. More direct evidence comes from studies reporting infiltration of pDCs in the visceral adipose tissue (VAT) of obese individuals [52–54]. Induction of type I IFNs via TLR activation in situ that contribute to polarization of VAT-recruited macrophages to a pro-inflammatory phenotype has been documented [55]. Chemerin, the pDC-specific chemokine, is also associated with clinical parameters of metabolic syndrome [56], and genetic deficiency of this chemokine prevents the development of type 2 diabetes in a preclinical model [57]. In obese individuals, VAT-expressed chemerin was shown to drive pDC recruitment [58], quite akin to psoriatic pathogenesis.

Thus, yet another shared pathogenetic node between psoriasis and diabetes is the induction of type I IFNs. Circumstantial evidence also comes from the predisposition of metabolic syndrome components in systemic lupus erythematosus [56], another autoimmune disease again critically dependent on pDC-derived type I IFNs [57]. Recent studies showing an antidiabetogenic effect of hydroxychloroquine bring further support to this notion [58,59], as the major mechanism of action of hydroxychloroquine is through inhibition of endosomally located TLRs, like TLR9 and TLR7, which are the most important mediators of type I IFN induction in pDCs. Future studies that look for systemic induction of type I IFNs in patients with psoriasis, who develop concomitant systemic insulin resistance, will enable confirmation of the proposed type I IFN connection between psoriasis and diabetes.

4.7 DIABETES IN PSORIASIS

Globally, only one in every two patients with diabetes actually knows that they have diabetes. Even in patients who know they have diabetes, less than half of them achieve the HbA1c targets of <7%. Hence, we have a long way to go in terms of ensuring good glycemic control in patients with diabetes. It is important to highlight here that the glycemic control in patients of psoriasis with diabetes is even worse than in patients who have diabetes without psoriasis. Diabetes in psoriasis is complicated by the increased occurrence of other comorbidities and depression, which has a significant impact on the quality of life of the individual [60]. The psychosocial symptoms associated with psoriasis may have an adverse impact on medication compliance, which may have an impact on long-term glycemic control. Glucocorticoids are commonly used in the management of psoriasis, which per se is associated with the increased occurrence of diabetes, as well as having an adverse impact on glycemic control in patients with preexisting diabetes. Of note, hydroxychloroquine has been recently approved by the Drug Controller General of India (DCGI) for the treatment of type 2 diabetes not controlled with other oral agents.

4.8 FUTURE DIRECTION AND CONCLUSIONS

The current data from preclinical as well as small isolated uncontrolled clinical studies have suggested a pathogenic link between psoriasis and type 2 diabetes. GLP-1a used in the treatment has been documented to be beneficial in reducing skin lesions of psoriasis. While there appears to be an urgent need for a large-scale multicentric clinical trial evaluating the role of GLP-1a in the treatment of psoriasis, GLP-1 agonists can be attractive options for the treatment of persons with type 2 diabetes and psoriasis, as this group of drugs can ameliorate both hyperglycemia and psoriasis. In fact, GLP-1a should be the preferred second-line antidiabetes agent after metformin for managing diabetes in patients with psoriasis.

REFERENCES

1. Hwang ST, Nijsten T, Elder JT. Recent highlights in psoriasis research. *J Invest Dermatol* 2017;137: 550–556.
2. Sticherling M. Psoriasis and autoimmunity. *Autoimmun Rev* 2016;15:1167–1170.

3. Azfar RS, Seminara NM, Shin DB, Troxel AB, Margolis DJ, Gelfand JM. Increased risk of diabetes mellitus and likelihood of receiving diabetes mellitus treatment in patients with psoriasis. *Arch Dermatol* 2012;148(9):995–1000.
4. Khalid U, Hansen PR, Gislason GH et al. Psoriasis and new-onset diabetes mellitus: A Danish nationwide cohort study. *Diabetes Care* 2013;36(8):2402–2407.
5. Li W, Han J, Hu FB, Curhan GC, Qureshi AA. Psoriasis and risk of type 2 diabetes among women and men in the United States: A population-based cohort study. *J Invest Dermatol* 2012;132(2):291–298.
6. Jacob L, Kostev K. Psoriasis risk in patients with type 2 diabetes in German primary care practices. *Prim Care Diabetes* 2017;11(1):52–56.
7. Pereira RR, Amladi ST, Varthakavi PK. A study of the prevalence of diabetes, insulin resistance, lipid abnormalities, and cardiovascular risk factors in patients with chronic plaque psoriasis. *Indian J Dermatol* 2011;56(5):520–526.
8. Ucak S, Ekmekci TR, Basat O, Koslu A, Altuntas Y. Comparison of various insulin sensitivity indices in psoriatic patients and their relationship with type of psoriasis. *J Eur Acad Dermatol Venereol* 2006;20(5):517–522.
9. Nigam P, Dayal SG. Diabetic status in psoriasis. *Indian J Dermatol Venereol Leprol* 1979;45:171–174.
10. Sundharam A, Singh R, Agarwal PS. Psoriasis and diabetes mellitus. *Indian J Dermatol Venereol Leprol* 1980;46:158–162.
11. Qureshi AA, Choi HK, Setty AR et al. Psoriasis and the risk of diabetes and hypertension: A prospective study of US female nurses. *Arch Dermatol* 2009;145:379–382.
12. Brauchli YB, Jick SS, Meier CR. Psoriasis and the risk of incident diabetes mellitus: A population-based study. *Br J Dermatol* 2008;159:1331–1337.
13. Casagrande SS, Menke A, Cowie CC. No association between psoriasis and diabetes in the U.S. population. *Diabetes Res Clin Pract* 2014;104:e58–e60.
14. Blauvelt A. T-helper 17 cells in psoriatic plaques and additional genetic links between IL-23 and psoriasis. *J Invest Dermatol* 2008;128(5):1064–1067.
15. Cohen AD, Dreiher J, Shapiro Y et al. Psoriasis and diabetes: A population based cross sectional study. *J Eur Acad Dermatol Venereol* 2008;22:585–589.
16. Al-Mutairi N, Shabaan D. Effects of tumor necrosis factor α inhibitors extend beyond psoriasis: Insulin sensitivity in psoriasis patients with type 2 diabetes mellitus. *Cutis* 2016;97(3):235–241.
17. Lynch LA, O'Connell JM, Kwasnik AK, Cawood TJ, O'Farrelly C, O'Shea DB. Are natural killer cells protecting the metabolically healthy obese patient? *Obesity (Silver Spring)* 2009;17:601–605.
18. Hogan AE, Tobin AM, Ahern T et al. Glucagon-like peptide-1 (GLP-1) and the regulation of human invariant natural killer T cells: Lessons from obesity, diabetes and psoriasis. *Diabetologia* 2011;54(11):2745–2754.
19. Cai Y, Shen X, Ding C, Qi C, Li K, Li X, Jala VR, Zhang HG, Wang T, Zheng J, Yan J. Pivotal role of dermal IL-17-producing γδ T cells in skin inflammation. *Immunity* 2011;35:596–610.
20. Gaffen SL, Jain R, Garg AV, Cua DJ. The IL-23-IL-17 immune axis: From mechanisms to therapeutic testing. *Nat Rev Immunol* 2014;14(9):585–600.
21. Zaba LC, Fuentes-Duculan J, Eungdamrong NJ, Abello MV, Novitskaya I, Pierson KC, Gonzalez J, Krueger JG, Lowes MA. Psoriasis is characterized by accumulation of immunostimulatory and Th1/Th17 cell-polarizing myeloid dendritic cells. *J Invest Dermatol* 2009;129(1):79–88.
22. Ganguly D, Haak S, Sisirak V, Reizis B. The role of dendritic cells in autoimmunity. *Nat Rev Immunol* 2013;13(8):566–577.
23. Campa M, Mansouri B, Warren R, Menter A. A review of biologic therapies targeting IL-23 and IL-17 for use in moderate-to-severe plaque psoriasis. *Dermatol Ther (Heidelb)* 2016;6(1):1–12.
24. Richter L, Vujic I, Sesti A, Monshi B, Sanlorenzo M, Posch C, Rappersberger K. Etanercept, adalimumab, and ustekinumab in psoriasis: Analysis of 209 treatment series in Austria. *J Dtsch Dermatol Ges* 2017;15(3):309–317.
25. Herder C, Zierer A, Koenig W, Roden M, Meisinger C, Thorand B. Transforming growth factor-beta1 and incident type 2 diabetes: Results from the MONICA/KORA case-cohort study, 1984–2002. *Diabetes Care* 2009;32:1921–1923.
26. Yang L, Anderson DE, Baecher-Allan C, Hastings WD, Bettelli E, Oukka M, Kuchroo VK, Hafler DA. IL-21 and TGF-beta are required for differentiation of human T(H)17 cells. *Nature* 2008;454:350–352.
27. Acosta-Rodriguez EV, Napolitani G, Lanzavecchia A, Sallusto F. Interleukins 1beta and 6 but not transforming growth factor-beta are essential for the differentiation of interleukin 17-producing human T helper cells. *Nat Immunol* 2007;8:942–949.

28. Jagannathan-Bogdan M, McDonnell ME, Shin H, Rehman Q, Hasturk H, Apovian CM, Nikolajczyk BS. Elevated proinflammatory cytokine production by a skewed T cell compartment requires monocytes and promotes inflammation in type 2 diabetes. *J Immunol* 2011;186(2):1162–1172.
29. Ip B, Cilfone NA, Belkina AC et al. Th17 cytokines differentiate obesity from obesity-associated type 2 diabetes and promote TNFα production. *Obesity (Silver Spring)* 2016;24(1):102–112.
30. Lee SY, Lee SH, Yang EJ, Kim EK, Kim JK, Shin DY, Cho ML. Metformin ameliorates inflammatory bowel disease by suppression of the STAT3 signaling pathway and regulation of the between Th17/Treg balance. *PLoS One* 2015;10(9):e0135858.
31. Hadjiyanni I, Baggio LL, Poussier P, Drucker DJ. Exendin-4 modulates diabetes onset in nonobese diabetic mice. *Endocrinology* 2008;149:1338–1349.
32. Hadjiyanni I, Siminovitch KA, Danska JS, Drucker DJ. Glucagon-like peptide-1 receptor signalling selectively regulates murine lymphocyte proliferation and maintenance of peripheral regulatory T cells. *Diabetologia* 2010;53:730–740.
33. Marx N, Burgmaier M, Heinz P et al. Glucagon-like peptide-1(1-37) inhibits chemokine-induced migration of human CD4-positive lymphocytes. *Cell Mol Life Sci* 2010;67:3549–3555.
34. Buysschaert M, Baeck M, Preumont V, Marot L, Hendrickx E, Van Belle A, Dumoutier L. Improvement of psoriasis during glucagon like peptide 1 analogue therapy in type 2 diabetes is associated with decreasing dermal γδ T cell number: A prospective case series study. *Br J Dermatol* 2014;171:15561.
35. Buysschaert M, Tennstedt D, Preumont V. Improvement of psoriasis during exenatide treatment in a patient with diabetes. *Diabetes Metab* 2012;38:868.
36. Mellett M, Atzei P, Jackson R, O'Neill LA, Moynagh PN. Mal mediates TLR-induced activation of CREB and expression of IL-10. *J Immunol* 2011;186:4925–4935.
37. Hossler EW, Maroon MS, Mowad CM. Gastric bypass surgery improves psoriasis. *J Am Acad Dermatol* 2011;65:198–200.
38. Moulin CM, Marguti I, Peron JPS, Halpern A, Rizzo LV. Bariatric surgery reverses natural killer (NK) cell activity and NK-related cytokine synthesis impairment induced by morbid obesity. *Obes Surg* 2011;21:112–118.
39. Erkek E, Karaduman A, Akcan Y, Sökmensüer C, Bükülmez G. Psoriasis associated with HCV and exacerbated by interferon alpha: Complete clearance with acitretin during interferon alpha treatment for chronic active hepatitis. *Dermatology* 2000;201(2):179–181.
40. Amschler K, Meyersburg D, Kitze B, Schön MP, Mössner R. Onset of psoriasis upon interferon beta treatment in a multiple sclerosis patient. *Eur J Dermatol* 2016;26(2):211–212.
41. Van der Fits L, van der Wel LI, Laman JD, Prens EP, Verschuren MCM. In psoriasis lesional skin the type I interferon signaling pathway is activated, whereas interferon-alpha sensitivity is unaltered. *J Invest Dermatol* 2004;122(1):51–60.
42. Nestle FO, Conrad C, Tun-Kyi A, Homey B, Gombert M, Boyman O, Burg G, Liu YJ, Gilliet M. Plasmacytoid predendritic cells initiate psoriasis through interferon-a production. *J Exp Med* 2005;202:135–143.
43. Albanesi C, Scarponi C, Pallotta S et al. Chemerin expression marks early psoriatic skin lesions and correlates with plasmacytoid dendritic cell recruitment. *J Exp Med* 2009;206:249–258.
44. Lande R, Gregorio J, Facchinetti V et al. Plasmacytoid dendritic cells sense self-DNA coupled with antimicrobial peptide. *Nature* 2007;449(7162):564–569.
45. Ganguly D, Chamilos G, Lande R, Gregorio J, Meller S, Facchinetti V, Homey B, Barrat FJ, Zal T, Gilliet M. Self-RNA-antimicrobial peptide complexes activate human dendritic cells through TLR7 and TLR8. *J Exp Med* 2009;206(9):1983–1994.
46. Lande R, Botti E, Jandus C et al. The antimicrobial peptide LL37 is a T-cell autoantigen in psoriasis. *Nat Commun* 2014;5:5621.
47. Lande R, Chamilos G, Ganguly D, Demaria O, Frasca L, Durr S, Conrad C, Schröder J, Gilliet M. Cationic antimicrobial peptides in psoriatic skin cooperate to break innate tolerance to self-DNA. *Eur J Immunol* 2015;45(1):203–213.
48. Jiang W, Zhu FG, Bhagat L, Yu D, Tang JX, Kandimalla ER, La Monica N, Agrawal S. A Toll-like receptor 7, 8, and 9 antagonist inhibits Th1 and Th17 responses and inflammasome activation in a model of IL-23-induced psoriasis. *J Invest Dermatol* 2013;133(7):1777–1784.
49. Yao Y, Richman L, Morehouse C et al. Type I interferon: Potential therapeutic target for psoriasis? *PLoS One* 2008;3:e2737.
50. Bissonnette R, Papp K, Maari C et al. A randomized, double-blind, placebo-controlled, phase I study of MEDI-545, an anti-interferon-alfa monoclonal antibody, in subjects with chronic psoriasis. *J Am Acad Dermatol* 2010;62:427–436.

51. Stefanovic-Racic M, Yang X, Turner MS et al. Dendritic cells promote macrophage infiltration and comprise a substantial proportion of obesity-associated increases in CD11c+ cells in adipose tissue and liver. *Diabetes* 2012;61:2330–2339.
52. Bertola A, Ciucci T, Rousseau D et al. Identification of adipose tissue dendritic cells correlated with obesity-associated insulin-resistance and inducing Th17 responses in mice and patients. *Diabetes* 2012;61:2238–2247.
53. Ghosh AR, Bhattacharya R, Bhattacharya S et al. Adipose recruitment and activation of plasmacytoid dendritic cells fuel metaflammation. *Diabetes* 2016;65(11):3440–3452.
54. Li Y, Shi B, Li S. Association between serum chemerin concentrations and clinical indices in obesity or metabolic syndrome: A meta-analysis. *PLoS One* 2014;9:e113915.
55. Ernst MC, Haidl ID, Zúñiga LA et al. Disruption of the chemokine-like receptor-1 (CMKLR1) gene is associated with reduced adiposity and glucose intolerance. *Endocrinology* 2012;153:672–682.
56. Parker B, Bruce I. SLE and metabolic syndrome. *Lupus* 2013;22:1259–1266.
57. Sisirak V, Ganguly D, Lewis KL, Couillault C, Tanaka L, Bolland S, D'Agati V, Elkon KB, Reizis B. Genetic evidence for the role of plasmacytoid dendritic cells in systemic lupus erythematosus. *J Exp Med* 2014;211(10):1969–1976.
58. Wasko MC, McClure CK, Kelsey SF, Huber K, Orchard T, Toledo FG. Antidiabetogenic effects of hydroxychloroquine on insulin sensitivity and beta cell function: A randomised trial. *Diabetologia* 2015;58:2336–2343.
59. Chen YM, Lin CH, Lan TH, Chen HH, Chang SN, Chen YH, Wang JS, Hung WT, Lan JL, Chen DY. Hydroxychloroquine reduces risk of incident diabetes mellitus in lupus patients in a dose-dependent manner: A population-based cohort study. *Rheumatology (Oxford)* 2015;54(7):1244–1249.
60. Schwandt A, Bergis D, Dapp A, Ebner S, Jehle PM, Köppen S, Risse A, Zimny S, Holl RW. Psoriasis and diabetes: A multicenter study in 222078 type 2 diabetes patients reveals high levels of depression. *J Diabetes Res* 2015;2015:792968.

5 Angiogenesis and Roles of Adhesion Molecules in Psoriatic Disease

Asmita Hazra and Saptarshi Mandal

CONTENTS

5.1 INTRODUCTION

In the field of research related to the process of blood vessel formation, several terms are encountered frequently: *angiogenesis*, *vasculogenesis*, *arteriogenesis*, and *vascular remodeling*. Vasculogenesis is the process of de novo blood vessel assembly from unstructured precursors. It is common during embryonic development but is also known to happen postnatally. Angiogenesis, on the other hand, is the process of new vessel formation from preexisting vessels. The term *arteriogenesis* may be used to mean further development (after vasculogenesis or angiogenesis) of vessels through steps like stabilization, identity specification, and growth in diameter and wall thickness to become a mature vessel. However, arteriogenesis is sometimes also used in a narrower sense of development of collateral vessels in response to arterial occlusion.

Vascular remodeling is a general term for the process of structural changes that can happen during or after vessel formation as a part of vasculogenesis, angiogenesis, or arteriogenesis. These structural changes may include changes in size, shape, composition, maturation, or specification of vessel type toward vein or artery. Remodeling can take place in an individual vessel or a whole network, with some vessels becoming stabilized or strengthened and some vessels regressed or pruned.

The majority of the angiogenesis research centers around the study of endothelial cell differentiation, proliferation, and organization in relation to other cell types. The endothelial cells form a continuous layer named the intima or endothelium (literally inner lining) that lines the inside of vertebrate blood vessels. Endothelial cells are absent in invertebrates who have "open circulation" of the hemolymph, directly bathing the tissues. Endothelial cells, the mural layers outside them, and circulating immune cells and coagulation and kinin cascades, and so forth, have coevolved into a sophisticated machinery that maintains this barrier between blood and the tissue, and yet maintains perfusion and exchanges all through life. Endothelial cells in vitro are capable of forming tubes by themselves if cultured on Matrigel or a similar three-dimensional (3-D) scaffold of extracellular matrix (ECM).

Angiogenesis research originally received the most attention through the anticancer drug industry. However, angiogenesis is also a central part of more common processes, like wound healing and chronic inflammation. Aberrant angiogenesis gives rise to many different diseases in different contexts. Psoriasis is one such disease, which includes angiogenesis in its core pathogenesis.

5.1.1 Types of Angiogenesis

The main two types of angiogenesis, in terms of mechanism, are (1) sprouting and (2) nonsprouting types. Nonsprouting angiogenesis is an umbrella that includes many types: (2a) intussusception, (2b) transluminal bridging, (2c) intercalation, (2d) elongation, (2e) glomeruloid body formation, (2f) vascular mimicry, (2g) vascular cooption, (2h) "mother vessel" formation, and (2i) vascular malformation (VM).

5.1.1.1 Sprouting Angiogenesis

It is the best known and probably the most common type of angiogenesis that involves sprouts, that is, new capillary branches with a free tip growing outward from the abluminal surface of preexisting vessels. Endothelial sprouts act as new branch points and are usually abundant in angiogenic vessels in inflammation or tumors. Sprouts are broadest at their base, taper toward a blind ending, and are headed by a single nondividing "tip cell," which throws out multiple filopodia, giving a budding, sprout-like look. Sprouting can encroach into previously avascular tissue. The sprouting process is usually accompanied by local vasodilation, increased vascular permeability, and cell proliferation. The process is slow, requiring more than 24 h to develop new sprouts and at least 3–5 days for sprouts to anastomose into capillary loops with lumen and be integrated into the vascular system (Djonov et al. 2003). The mechanism of sprouting angiogenesis is described in Section 5.1.2.

5.1.1.2 Nonsprouting Angiogenesis

5.1.1.2.1 Intussusceptive Angiogenesis

Intussusception, or splitting-type, angiogenesis is one of the most well-known types of nonsprouting angiogenesis that can also give rise to branching. It was discovered in the 1980s. This process of angiogenesis is also fairly common. It occurs by a multistep process of forming intraluminal tissue pillars with a connective tissue core. The pillars are commonly generated by the fusion of folds of the vessel wall projecting inward from opposite sides into the vascular lumen (for alternative mechanisms, see Section 5.1.1.3). Eventually, several pillars increase in size and fuse with each other, splitting up the initial capillary into multiple branches that remain anastomosed. Pillar formation may take 4–5 h but may be faster (about 1 h) at higher blood flow (Djonov et al. 2003). Thus, in contrast to sprouting, which needs several days for extensive proliferation of endothelial cells, intussusception can occur in the virtual absence of endothelial cell proliferation at low vascular permeability levels, and often requires only 4–5 h to complete. It was thought that only already vascularized tissue can obtain higher vessel density with intussusception, but not nonvascular tissue, unlike sprouting. However, recent research (Kilarski and GerWins 2009) showed that during wound healing, myofibroblastic tension can pull preexisting vessels into the tissue void. The pulled vessels can then grow by elongation or intussusception or sprouting.

5.1.1.2.2 Transluminal Bridging

It is somewhat similar to intussusception in that it also causes splitting of the lumen. However, here partitioning of the lumen is initially by thin endothelial cell projections alone, rather than endothelium-wrapped connective tissue pillars that form in intussusception. But eventually, the partitions would be invaded by connective tissue. Transluminal bridging eventually produces capillary size vessels, which are not hyperpermeable.

5.1.1.2.3 Intercalation

It is a type of nonbranching angiogenesis. Intercalation means incorporation of new endothelial cells in patches, followed by rearrangement of endothelial cells, leading to an increase in surface area and other dimensions. It usually happens through the incorporation of circulating endothelial progenitor cells (EPCs). It can also involve the incorporation of tumor cells or trophoblasts, which could give rise to a mosaic vessel with vascular mimicry. It may involve transendothelial migration and mural insertion of circulating pericyte progenitors. Vessel fusion, sometimes called "homing" in embryology, may also be grouped by some authors under this category.

5.1.1.2.4 Elongation Angiogenesis

It is one of the lesser known types of angiogenesis that is also of a nonbranching nature. It is seen in the endometrium during the proliferative phase of the menstrual cycle (Gambino et al. 2002) and in psoriatic skin plaques and nail folds, and psoriatic arthritis (PsA) (Creamer et al. 2002b; Veale et al. 2005). It is described in detail in Section 5.2.2.1. Angiogenesis in psoriatic skin and its mechanism are further discussed in Section 5.2.5, especially under subsection 5.2.5.1.

5.1.1.2.5 Glomeruloid Body Formation

Glomeruloid bodies are closely associated loops of microvessels surrounded by a variably thickened basement membrane within which a limited number of pericytes are embedded. It happens commonly in intracranial tumors, especially high-grade glioma and meningiomas, but also in a wide variety of other tumors. Glomeruloid angiogenesis is dependent on high levels of soluble or small forms of vascular endothelial growth factor (VEGF) (see Section 5.2.5.1) and regresses in their absence. It should not be confused with angiogenesis in the renal glomerulus, where a capillary loop splits by intussusception, whereas glomeruloid angiogenesis in intracranial lesions is possibly nonbranching. Controversies exist regarding whether the later stages of glomeruloid formations are similar to convoluted version elongation or involve vessel-within-vessel formation, for example, those forming within dilated mother vessels, which can happen through processes somewhat similar to those for intussusception. Although glomeruloid bodies look structurally hyperpermeable, they are underperfused; thus, actual leaking of transudate is low.

5.1.1.2.6 *Vascular Mimicry*

Some tumor cells, monocytes, and trophoblasts are capable of incorporating or intercalating into a mosaic vessel or sometimes replace an entire segment of a vessel. The incorporating cells often show an endothelial-like phenotype and sometimes also develop mural layers through mimicry. These phenomena are called vascular mimicry.

5.1.1.2.7 *Vascular Co-Option*

Tumor cells often migrate to host organ blood vessels and initiate blood vessel–dependent tumor growth, as opposed to classic angiogenesis, co-opting and cuffing around adjacent vessels. It is more frequently observed in cancer of densely vascularized organs, including the brain, lung, and liver, where the primary tumor cells co-opt the adjacent quiescent blood vessels of the host tissue.

5.1.1.2.8 *Mother Vessel Formation*

These are VEGF-dependent, highly permeable, dilated, thin-walled, serpentine, strongly VEGF receptor (VEGFR)–positive sinusoids with very few pericytes and a thin basement membrane that develop from preexisting venules or capillaries (e.g., those co-opted by a tumor) within hours of exposure to high-level VEGF, especially VEGF165. This involves a three-step process of (1) degradation of noncompliant basement membrane, (2) mural or pericyte detachment, and (3) extensive rapid enlargement through vesiculovacuolar fusion in the endothelial cells, usually leading to a three- to fivefold increase in cross-sectional area.

5.1.1.2.9 *Vascular Malformations*

VM in the field of angiogenesis refers to vessels that are different from normal arteries and veins, with an inappropriately large size and thinner asymmetric muscular coat, and may be found sporadically in nonmalignant skin or brain vessels and in tumor vessels. VM may form through an intermediate mother vessel stage. VMs retain the large size of their mother vessels and acquire again the smooth muscle cell layer. They are not supposed to be permeable to plasma proteins (unlike the mother vessel). Moreover, unlike glomeruloid bodies and mother vessels, VMs persist indefinitely in a low-VEGF environment, although their lining endothelium is maintained by paracrine VEGFA secreted by neighboring mural cells. They are likely to be resistant to systemic anti-VEGF therapy.

5.1.1.3 Other Types of Angiogenesis

The distinction between angiogenesis, vasculogenesis, arteriogenesis, and remodeling may sometimes get blurred. For example, intercalation, that is, incorporation of circulating EPCs and possibly other hematopoietic progenitors (e.g., pericyte progenitor cells [PPCs]) into a preexisting vessel wall, is a common mechanism that is sometimes considered a form of postnatal vasculogenesis but may also be considered angiogenesis or constitute a part of angiogenesis. Progenitors can also be recruited from the adventitia of an existing vessel, especially arteries, to participate in another type of angiogenesis or arteriogenesis related to repair for damaged vessels. Intercalation can sometimes also be used to mean vascular fusion (homing in embryology), which is more vascular remodeling than angiogenesis.

Intussusception is described above in simple terms, and the most well-known example of infolding is mentioned as the mechanism of intravascular pillar formation. But actually, there are many different mechanisms described in the literature (Patan 2013), for example, pillar formation by folding of the vessel wall, connection of adjacent pillars, "in situ loop formation," pillar formation by connection of opposing intraluminal tissue folds, segmentation, apposition, recanalization of the thrombotic vein by remodeling, and arterial recanalization through fibroblastic invasion, followed by pillar formation. Segmentation, apposition, and recanalization are relatively more common in adult angiogenesis and are based on intra- and extravascular fibrin deposits.

5.1.2 Overview of Angiogenic Mechanisms

Sprouting (a type of branching) angiogenesis is the most understood type of angiogenic model. Although angiogenesis in psoriatic skin mostly follows the elongation type, angiogenesis in PsA possibly also involves other modes of angiogenesis/remodeling. It would be worthwhile to get an overview of its mechanism.

Normal endothelial cells in a stable vessel are quiescent and form a monolayer of "phalanx" cells. They rarely proliferate and do not migrate out of the basement membrane layer, which they share with the pericytes. Their need for proliferation is less (about 1 in 1000 cells) because of their low apoptosis frequency. "Angiogenic stimuli"–like hypoxia, inflammation, soluble angiogenic mediators, metabolic and mechanical stress, or programmed tissue remodeling act on endothelial cells. Endothelial cells become "activated" and initiate the process of angiogenesis, which may include a cascade of events. The activated endothelial cells take up either of the two phenotypes. One phenotype is tip cells, which are dominant endothelial cells. They are selected by lateral inhibition (Notch signaling) and lead the tips of sprouts. Tip cells stay individual; do not divide, but have long filopodia that help in pathfinding and migration; and eventually fuse with opposite tip cells (with the help of a myeloid bridge cell) during anastomosis formation. The other phenotype is stalk cells that follow the tip cell and initially make a solid cord or column by proliferation and later form the lumen.

Below is a simplified example schema for sprouting angiogenesis. The steps may temporally overlap, shuffle, or have other variations:

> Perturbation of the vascular quiescent state (by a tilt in the pro- and antiangiogenic balance) → angiogenic stimulus sensing and endothelial activation → release of proteases and degradation of the basement membrane (matrix metalloproteinase [MMP] and tissue inhibitors of metalloproteinases [TIMP] imbalance, plasmin, etc.) → detachment of pericytes from endothelial cells (shift from Ang1 to Ang2 angiopoietin signaling) → signaling between endothelial cells (mainly Notch and VEGF signaling) to form active tip cells and stalk cells → development of new sprouts starting with podosome rosette invading through the basement membranes → tip cells' filopodia guided by spatial cues → endothelial stalk cell proliferation into solid cords → guidance of opposing tip cells by myeloid bridge cells → anastomosis followed by lumen formation in the fused cords → fusion of sprouts to generate connectivity → establishment of flow → extravasation of immune cells (amplifying angiogenesis) and supportive cells (dampening angiogenesis) → stabilization (basement membrane deposition, ensheathing by mural cells, e.g., pericytes, smooth muscle cells, progenitor cells, telocytes, and fibroblasts) → diameter and branching pattern remodeling → regression of disconnected sprouts → vascular type (e.g., venous or arterial or lymphatic) identity establishment

Maintaining the quiescence of the endothelium is far from a passive process. Homeostatic low-level autocrine signaling of VEGF, Ang1, Notch, and fibroblast growth factor (FGF) maintains the quiescent phalanx cell phenotype (Welti et al. 2013). Low-level baseline signaling is important, as shifting the balance of this signaling in either direction can activate the endothelial cell. For example, a higher level of Notch activation activates the Wnt pathway, which produces a proliferating stalk cell phenotype. Stable laminar perfusion through a vessel keeps endothelial cell metabolism at a low level by Krüppel-like factor (KLF) 2–mediated repression of glycolytic enzymes, such as fructose-2,6-bisphosphatase 3 (PFKFB3). The quiescence also includes inputs from homeobox transcription factors, for example, HOX D10, HOX A5, and Gax (growth arrest homeobox or mesenchyme homeobox [Meox2]), which suppress NFkB signaling that is downstream of many pro-angiogenic signals. The basement membrane around the endothelial layer, especially ECM molecule laminin α4 (but not α5), is capable of suppressing tip cell formation by inducing Notch signaling. The oxygen sensing machinery described below is part of the homeostatic mechanism that also fine-tunes the vessel shape to optimize tissue perfusion and oxygen levels.

The initiation of angiogenesis generally involves sensing of the angiogenic stimulus formed by a shift in the balance of the local vessel homeostatic milieu toward a "pro-angiogenic" state. The angiogenic signal can be a rapid release of pre-stored and sequestered molecules, or local new synthesis and secretion of agonists as, for example, growth factors like VEGFs, angiopoietins, FGFs, and other signaling molecules like chemokines, alarmins, and so forth. The release can be from a dormant state bound to the ECM or from storage granules of cells that may concentrate them, for example, mast cells, neutrophils, and platelets. Inflammatory cells, especially myeloid cells, described later, can play the role of the vessel destabilization event, as well as an angiogenic signal generation event or its amplification. Whatever the route of initiation, the endothelial activation involves turning on an "angiogenic switch" (cooperative molecular on–off event rather than a gradual event) in the endothelial cells, which amplify and maintain the expression of the players of the angiogenic cascade. The sprouting part of the angiogenesis has many mechanistic similarities to epithelial-to-mesenchymal transition (EMT) and has been dubbed endothelial-to-mesenchymal transition (EndMT) and is mediated partly by the Snail/Slug family of transcription factors, which are Notch and NFkB targets. The sprouting endothelial cells invade the basement membrane through adhesive podosomes, which are similar to the invadopodia of cancerous cells. A parallel cascade of events is set in the associated stromal cells, some of which may eventually differentiate into the pericytes and other mural cells during the growth or stabilization of the sprouts.

Not all the activators of the angiogenic switch are well understood. The best understood is the hypoxia-inducible factor (HIF) pathway, which is one of the angiogenic "master regulator" transcription factors. Endothelial cells carry oxygen sensors, which have prolyl hydroxylase activity that hydroxylates HIF1a and targets it for ubiquitin-mediated degradation. In the hypoxic state, intact HIF1a combines with constitutively produced HIF1b and activates genes with hypoxia response elements. The angiogenic cascade goes through sequential phases, with initiation happening through a tissue- and context-dependent angiogenic switch, for example, suppression of quiescence mediators and upregulation of activation mediators, which likely happens through a cooperation or convergence of ETS transcription factors like ETS1 (originally named "erythroblast transformation specific") and Erg (ETS-related gene), and HIF1 and 2. The initial angiogenic signal is magnified through transcriptional, intracrine, autocrine, and paracrine short- and long-feedback amplification loops, which can be diverse and tissue context dependent.

Compared with the quiescent state, the activated endothelial cells have a different protein expression profile. They synthesize a large gamut of angiogenic soluble factors; adhesion molecules, including integrins $\alpha v\beta 3$ and $\alpha 5\beta 1$; and proteases, including MMP2 and MMP9, in a cascade fashion. The activation state may be context dependent and may have multiple levels of activation or deactivation. Some experimental examples of the angiogenic transcription switch studied relatively more in tumor models include HOX B7, which can upregulate pro-angiogenic mediators VEGF, basic fibroblast growth factor (bFGF) (FGF2), GROα (CXCL1), interleukin (IL) 8 (CXCL8), and MMP9, but downregulate Ang1, and upregulate angiostatic Ang2 in the HOX B7–transfected SKBR3 breast carcinoma cell line which is known to lack HOX B7. While these examples are about transcriptional switch upstream of the factors, even downstream of these growth factors, there is recruitment of secondary activating transcription factors, for example, HOX D3 downstream of FGF2 and AP1 downstream of IL18. HOX D3 in turn mediates $\alpha v\beta 3$ and $\alpha 5\beta 1$ integrins and urokinase-type plasminogen activator (uPA) expression downstream of bFGF. These steps further enhance the expression of mitogens, matrix degradation enzymes, and activated integrins and cause shedding of pro-angiogenic soluble cell adhesion molecules (s-CAMs), like CD146, soluble E-selectin, and soluble vascular cell adhesion molecule (VCAM) 1. Many of these soluble adhesion molecules are capable of supporting angiogenesis. Over the years, a long list of soluble factors, adhesion molecules, and ECM fragments involved in angiogenesis have been discovered. A brief discussion of the relevant ones to this context will follow in a later part of this chapter. These factors feedback amplify the angiogenic response and recruit neighboring cells by autocrine and paracrine mechanisms. The knowledge of various factors, including the newer factors, for example, micro-RNAs (miRNA), which also works in a combinatorial network, has made the field far more complex than what we knew just a few years back.

Many of the so-called pro-angiogenic mediators (e.g., most classically VEGFA) are now known to have multiple atypical isoforms and, for example, alternative start sites, several splice variants, and translational read-through products, at least some of which are clearly antiangiogenic (Qiu et al. 2009; Eswarappa et al. 2014). Transforming growth factor (TGF) β1 is one factor known to be able to switch splicing of VEGFA to antiangiogenic isoforms in podocytes. Diabetic retinopathy, a disease that shares a lot in common with psoriasis, has been suspected to be associated with a switch of the VEGF isoform splicing from the antiangiogenic to the pro-angiogenic type. On the flip side, so-called classic antiangiogenic factors like thrombospondin (TSP) 1 are now known to be even directly pro-angiogenic in some contexts, for example, when working along with syndecan 4, a proteoglycan that is also involved in many other signaling pathways (FGF, DC-HIL, etc.) in endothelial and leukocytes and happens to be one of the candidates genes at a moderately associated psoriasis locus in some genome-wide association studies (GWASs) (Stuart et al. 2010). Pro-angiogenic mediators are kept from too much action by counterbalancing extracellular antiangiogenic factors (like endostatin and angiostatin), some of which are released by longer (or stronger) activation of the same mechanisms that release the pro-angiogenic factors. If angiogenesis is normally regulated, the actions of the endothelial activation steps amplified, for example, by HOX D3 are temporally succeeded by *feed-forward inhibition* by sequential recruitment of reverse acting players, for example, HOX B3, at the transcriptional level that stabilize vessel morphogenesis by inducing ephrin A1 and other vessel maturation factors at the extracellular level, followed finally by factors like HOX D10 (Myers et al. 2002), which reinstalls the quiescent state by bringing back the balance of opposing factors described earlier. A translational implication of a complex network of feedback, as well as feed-forward inhibitions, is that a simple blockade of a random node in these networks can produce paradoxical effects, and exploration of critical "hubs" in the network is important.

5.1.3 Historical Importance of Psoriasis in Early Angiogenesis Research

The term *angiogenesis* was coined in 1787 by John Hunter, a British surgeon, but the field hardly grew for almost two centuries. Only sporadic anatomical observations of tumor neovascularization were performed until the 1960s, when the "father of angiogenesis," Judah Folkman, a professor of pediatric surgery at Harvard University's Boston Children's Hospital, started his seminal work in this field. The first angiogenesis-related publications by Folkman appeared in 1971 in the *Journal of Experimental Medicine* and the *New England Journal of Medicine* (Folkman 1971; Folkman et al. 1971) and were related to "tumor angiogenesis." The very next year, Folkman published a paper titled "Angiogenesis in Psoriasis: Therapeutic Implications" in the *Journal of Investigative Dermatology* (Folkman 1972).

In the abstract of this historic 1972 paper, Folkman wrote,

> In this paper an analogy is drawn between tumor angiogenesis and the angiogenesis which accompanies psoriasis. If the relationship between psoriatic epithelium and its capillary endothelium turns out to be similar to the integration of capillaries by solid tumors then "antiangiogenesis" may eventually become a useful therapeutic approach in psoriasis.

Indeed, now we have some proofs of the principle predicted by Folkman 45 years back.

For example, during this era of a multitude of antiangiogenesis therapies, there are several examples where an antiangiogenic drug was administered for the treatment of cancers in patients who also happened to have psoriasis and the psoriasis underwent remission (Datta-Mitra et al. 2014). However, a lot of opposite examples also exist, where some antiangiogenesis drugs paradoxically precipitated or exacerbated psoriasis-like reactions (Yiu et al. 2016). We further discuss this in

Sections 5.4.7.2 and 5.4.7.3. It does not necessarily mean that the efforts on antiangiogenesis should be abandoned for this disease. Rather, it could possibly mean that the process is multistep and complex, and we need better understanding in order to target the whole process more effectively.

5.1.4 Relationship between Inflammation, Angiogenesis, and Carcinogenesis

Inflammation is the body's nonspecific defense mechanism, usually regarded as part of innate immunity to preserve live tissue from pathogens or injury. Pathogen-associated molecular patterns (PAMPs) and damage-associated molecular patterns (DAMPs), or alarmins, act as "danger signals" (e.g., alarmins) to the body and are identified by pattern recognition receptors (PRRs) of the innate immune system (e.g., Toll-like receptor [TLR] and NOD-like receptor [NLR] families), which mounts a series of inflammatory processes. It starts with acute inflammation, which is generally destructive and, if not resolved within days, changes its nature and evolves into "chronic inflammation" and may either resolve through tissue healing and remodeling or sometimes continue for a long duration and is often pathological. Inflammatory cells from blood are recruited through vessels, and during chronic inflammation, the vessels themselves undergo proliferation through angiogenesis, thus helping the inflammation maintain its "chronicity." So in a simplified sense, chronic inflammation and angiogenesis form a positive feedback loop, feeding back to each other. But as it will be explained later, the story is far more complex. The fact remains that most inflammatory conditions, like inflammatory arthritis, chronic airway inflammation, inflammatory bowel disease (IBD), and atherosclerosis, include angiogenesis-like mechanisms in their core pathology.

Cancers are often considered a "wound that never heals," and many chronic inflammatory conditions are known to be "precancerous" and treatment of inflammation is known to be able to prevent or reduce the chances of progression to cancer. Some have even speculated that angiogenesis might be the link between inflammation and cancer (Kobayashi and Lin 2009); that is, the cancer-preventing actions of the anti-inflammatory drugs, including cyclooxygenase 2 (COX2) inhibitors, might be working through prevention of angiogenesis (Sahin et al. 2009).

5.2 ANGIOGENESIS IN PSORIASIS

5.2.1 Psoriatic Diseases versus Other Inflammatory Skin and Joint Diseases

The term *psoriasis*, from Greek *Psora*, meaning "itch," was known to the Greek and other ancient civilizations. According to a 2016 WHO report on psoriasis, it "is a chronic, noncommunicable, painful, disfiguring and disabling disease for which there is no cure (so far) and with great negative impact on patients' quality of life (QoL)." Contrary to the about 2% prevalence that has often been quoted for psoriasis in the Caucasian population of Europe and North America, the prevalence of psoriasis has been increasing and has almost doubled from what it was in the 1970s, and it also increases almost linearly with aging, is twice as common in Caucasian Americans than in African Americans, and has reached as high as 11.43% in Norway. The most common presentation of the disease is the skin manifestations of psoriasis (psoriasis vulgaris), developing sharply demarcated, scaly, erythematous plaques that wax and wane slowly over time. It might be underdiagnosed, as the majority suffer from a mild form of the disease. Up to 34% of patients also develop a so-called specific comorbid condition, PsA, whereas relatively nonspecific comorbid conditions include metabolic syndrome and nonalcoholic fatty liver disease; colitis similar to IBD, especially Crohn's disease; duodenitis; and uveitis. A new entity, "psoriatic colitis," has also occasionally been proposed. IBD-associated spondyloarthropathy is gradually emerging as an important comorbid spectrum that shares a very similar niche to psoriatic diseases and frequently occurs with uveitis. All these comorbid conditions have a central theme in common: angiogenesis and inflammation. A complex interaction between genetic and environmental factors, potentially including obesity, insulin resistance, stress, infections, smoking, and some medications, has been speculated to trigger the disease.

Differences between psoriasis and atopic dermatitis show that epidermal hyperplasia, chronic inflammation, and vasodilation, although qualitatively different, are common to both. However, one of the major distinguishing pathogenesis factors is that angiogenesis is seen only in psoriasis but not in atopic dermatitis. Also, we will see later that plasmacytoid dendritic cells (pDCs), a transient cell population involved in the initiation of inflammatory cascade psoriasis, may be either absent or questionably present in a late window in atopic dermatitis. However, some of the animal models of atopic dermatitis, for example, K14-IL4 Tg (transgenic mice with IL4 driven by keratin 14 promoter locally overexpressed in basal epidermis) show prominent angiogenesis, thus blurring the boundary between the two diseases.

Although psoriasis is a chronic inflammatory condition, the lesions themselves are known to be relatively spared from predisposition to malignancy, but the same is also true for atopic dermatitis and Darier's disease. When the psoriasis resolve, they are remarkably without scars—a phenomenon that is well known but still not completely understood. One of the hypotheses put forward to explain the paradox is that the lesions themselves may not be transforming into cancerous processes, but the patient as a whole is inflamed and is predisposed to cancers, including lymphoma, and immunosuppressive therapy might add to the risk.

In psoriasis patients who do develop PsA, there is no correlation in severity of the skin and joint problems. Of these, only 15% develop both simultaneously, but the majority (60%–70%) develop the skin condition first, with a mean time of 10–12 years in between, and 10%–30% may develop it in reverse order; in some cases, the specific joint symptoms may even precede the skin manifestation by 10–15 years. The "sine psoriasis" subset of PsA, who might not show detectable dermal psoriasis but might have first- or second-degree relatives with psoriasis, is part of the reason the term *psoriatic disease* has been proposed; it covers the spectrum of diverse conditions. PsA, or at least a subset of it, is also known to be genetically divergent from psoriasis and similar to Crohn's disease (Ho et al. 2005). Until about 10 years ago, PsA, which is now regarded as a distinct entity, was not paid its due respect and diagnostic and treatment strategies were mostly extrapolated from ankylosing spondylitis and rheumatoid arthritis (RA). The musculoskeletal problems of PsA, which belongs to the family of seronegative spondyloarthropathies, include tendonitis, enthesitis, dactylitis, and arthritis, which might be mono-oligo or polyarticular. About 85% of patients with PsA and 40%–50% of patients with psoriasis in general develop nail involvement. In the initial phase of PsA, there may be waxing and waning course, but in contrast to RA, PsA may precipitously progress to joint destruction much faster and continue even after part of the inflammation has subsided (McGonagle et al. 2007).

Subclinical enthesopathy is common in both psoriasis and PsA. Up to 50% of psoriasis patients without arthritis might have asymptomatic enthesopathy and osteitis. However, its degree is much more severe in PsA, as documented by power Doppler studies, which are a noninvasive way of assessing the degree of angiogenesis. The anatomic, functional, and physiologic interdependence between the synovial membrane and the "enthesis organ" has recently given rise to a proposal for the concept of the "synovio-entheseal complex" (SEC) and a belief by some experts that "autoinflammatory" factors, rather than autoimmune factors, might be more important in PsA (McGonagle et al. 2007).

On the background of genetic predisposing factors, covered in prior chapters, environmental factors like trauma and infection can precipitate psoriatic plaque formation. The widely recognized Koebner's isomorphic phenomena, recognized by German dermatologist Heinrich Koebner (1872), that psoriatic plaques can arise at sites of prior trauma (although not specific, the characteristic of psoriasis is seen in about 25%–50% of cases) and a corresponding traumatic factor (deep Koebner phenomenon), has been described for the arthritis. The molecular mimicry of autoimmunity hypothesis for streptococcal M protein and keratin 16 and 17 is now shown to be not as straightforward as thought earlier, and the paradigms have been drifting more toward autoinflammation. However, PsA, like other spondyloarthropathies, has shown some association with gut microbiome dysbiosis that elicits a systemic IL23 response (Ritchlin et al. 2017).

5.2.2 Role of Angiogenesis in Core Pathology of Psoriatic Disease

5.2.2.1 Angiogenesis in Psoriatic Skin Lesions

5.2.2.1.1 Morphology of Normal Microcirculation in Skin

Normal cutaneous microcirculation consists of two horizontal plexuses: (1) an upper (superficial) horizontal network, about 1–1.5 mm below the skin surface, from which nutritive vertical capillary loops project into the dermal papillae, and (2) a lower (deeper) horizontal plexus at the dermal–subcutaneous interface, with additional networks supplying the hair papillae and glands. In the areas of prominent epidermal rete ridges, as found physiologically in the skin overlying the extensor aspects of the joints or pathologically psoriatic plaques, nonbranching vertical capillary loops extend into the elongated dermal papillae, with usually only one loop within each papilla, with a hairpin turn at the top. The loops may be divided into an intrapapillary and an extrapapillary portion by an imaginary plane along the tips of adjacent rete ridges. The deep extrapapillary portion of the descending loop becomes venular with a multilaminated basement membrane, and the rest of the loop is usually arteriolar with a homogenous basement membrane. In normal skin, usually only the capillaries supplying the glands and hair papilla show a venular structure, with bridge fenestrations that allow the rapid exchange of molecules.

5.2.2.1.2 Morphology of Microvasculature in Psoriatic Skin Lesions

The marked dilation of dermal vessels in psoriatic lesions was mentioned at least as early as 1896 by Unna, and some of the capillary morphology work predates Folkman's works on angiogenesis (Telner and Fekete 1961). A detailed description of dermal microvascular growth in psoriasis by Braverman is almost contemporary to the original works of Folkman in the early 1970s. Braverman (1972, 2000) demonstrated very nicely that the dermal vascular loops elongate in psoriatic plaques by venulization, that is, grow exclusively from the venous end and show ultrastructural features of bridge fenestrations and a multilayered basement membrane. But uninvolved skin of psoriasis patients and healed lesions have normal loops, with most of the length of an arteriolar capillary nature. The ultrastructural features of the capillary loops in pustular psoriasis and psoriasis vulgaris are not different according to Braverman. The loops in the psoriatic plaque are more tortuous than normal loops, and the ascending and descending loops are generally twisted one or two turns around each other. The crest, instead of a normal hairpin loop, forms a broad curve, sometimes with sinuous tortuosity in planes at various angles to the loop, and usually shows the highest density of bridge fenestrations. The loops become twice or thrice the normal diameter, with the descending portion sometimes reaching 20–30 μm diameter, compared with the normal 3.5–6 μm throughout the loops, with the crest and descending loop wider by 1–1.5 μm. It is from this very large-diameter part that the diapedesis, especially of neutrophils, lymphocytes, and macrophages, takes place. The neutrophils emigrate into the epidermis to form Munro's microabscess in the stratum corneum and spongiform pustules of Kogoj in the stratum spinosum.

Thus, chronic psoriatic plaque demonstrates several prominent vascular features: elongated, dilated, and thin-walled tortuous venulized capillary loops with large endothelial gaps; increased capillary permeability; increased endothelial cell proliferation; and increased blood flow through the skin (Braverman 1972, 2000). These venules are so thin, with large gaps between the endothelial cells, that Braverman initially wondered at the electron micrographs and whether they could be lymphatics. But he found red blood cells inside them, which ruled out a lymphatic identity.

The angiogenesis in the psoriatic plaque clinically manifests as the Auspitz sign, named after Austrian dermatologist Carl Heinrich Auspitz (1835–1886 AD), who may have noted the sign when he was a medical student; however, some consider it a misnomer, as it may have been discovered even earlier. It is the view of the array of pinpoint capillary bleeding from the tips of psoriatic papillae containing the dilated loops when the silvery scaly parakeratotic epidermal roof is peeled off.

5.2.2.1.3 Resolution of Controversy about Existence of Angiogenesis in Psoriasis

Initial morphometric studies of the psoriatic skin plaques had raised a controversy about whether true angiogenesis involving proliferation of endothelial cells is really increased in psoriasis. Some works had suspected that there is only a "pseudoelongation" of blood vessels in psoriatic skin, and speculated that it was due to inward growth of the epidermis into the dermis, which could possibly cause crowding of the intervening vessels (Bacharach-Buhles et al. 1993). However, works by Creamer et al. (1997a) conclusively showed, using endothelial marker and proliferation marker double immunohistochemistry (JC70A and MIB1), that in active psoriasis, angioproliferation is episodic and intermittent, with endothelial cells in only a few loops actively proliferating, interspersed between quiescent loops, which could be the reason it was missed in some of the earlier studies.

5.2.2.1.4 Uniqueness of Angiogenesis in Psoriatic Skin

Some aspects of elongation, tortuosity, or dilation of the dermal papillary vessels are also seen in a few other skin conditions. For example, in eczema, coiled papillary vessels are present adjacent to or surrounded by normal vessels; in lichen planus and dermatitis, herpetiformis patchy irregular coiling of the dermal papillary vessels is seen; and in port wine stains, the capillary width is increased.

In contrast to the above diseases, however, psoriasis is unique in many ways:

- Papillary vessel changes are dramatic and uniformly distributed throughout clinical lesions.
- In the lesions, the number of loops in the dermal papillae is unchanged, that is, one loop per papilla, similar to normal. Although the sinuous tortuosity (instead of the normal hairpin turn) at the crest sometimes gives an apparent glomeruloid appearance from the top, it is purely through elongation and tortuosity; there are no anastomoses.
- Braverman et al. (1977) classified the loops into different patterns, mainly based on the site of transition from the arteriolar-type capillary to the venular type, but within an individual lesion, the patterns were essentially uniform.
- There is almost a fourfold increase in surface area of the superficial plexus but no significant increase in the deeper plexus (Creamer et al. 1997a).
- Compared with normal skin, the cutaneous blood flow is 9–13 times higher in lesional skin and 2.5–4.5 times greater in perilesional skin, but remotely uninvolved skin had the same blood flow (Hern and Mortimer 2007).
- The added length of the capillary is of the venular type (in contrast to the arteriolar type in a normal capillary loop) and happens at the venular end by endothelial proliferation, and during successful treatment, the resorption also takes place at the same end.
- Fenestration in the intrapapillary capillary allows leakage of various plasma proteins (Parent et al. 1990).
- Psoriatic plaques, as well as guttate psoriasis lesions, show a two- to fourfold increase in the relative microvasculature area in lesional skin with large interindividual differences. The overall change in the vascularity of the lesions is similar to the average extents in volume, as well as the fractal dimension in the two types of patients, and a study that also attempted to show any direct mathematical correlation with the dermoepidermal surface complexity could not find it (Uhoda et al. 2005).

5.2.2.1.5 Lymphangiogenesis in Psoriasis Skin

The lymphatics in the psoriatic skin are also dilated, but the wave of changes in the lymphatics takes place later than the changes in the blood vessels and continues at a slower pace (Henno et al. 2010). The lymphangiogenesis in psoriasis also shows some unique features:

- Lymphangiogenesis in psoriasis may be somewhat unusual, as it shows upregulation of D2-40 (podoplanin) but not lymphatic vessel endothelial hyaluronan receptor (LYVE) 1 by immunohistochemistry (Moustou et al. 2014).

- Lymphatic vessels in psoriasis patients were at a normal distance from the epidermal basement in the nonlesional skin, but in the psoriatic lesions the lymphatic capillaries were significantly closer to the epidermis (Henno et al. 2009, 2010). Lymphatic capillary density increases in the lesional skin; however, it starts late and grows at a much slower rate than the blood vessels. These lesional lymphatic vessels, although more dilated, remain mostly collapsed.
- Another study corroborated the above findings and showed that even after 12 weeks of etanercept treatment, the lymphatics remained collapsed and closer to the epidermis and LYVE1 levels also remained low (Suárez-Fariña et al. 2011).

5.2.2.1.6 Angiogenesis in Nail Fold Psoriasis

The seminal work of Moll and Wright in 1973 highlighted the importance of microvascular changes in the nail bed and cited observations from an earlier New York–based capillaroscopic study of rheumatologic diseases (Redisch et al. 1970).

Wavy undulation is seen in <5% of normal loops, usually in the transitional or efferent limbs, and rarely in afferent limbs. Undulations of one limb crisscrossing the other limb give the appearance of a figure-of-eight and are called "tortuosity" and are considered increased when >10% loops show it. Meandering is the combination of undulation and coiling. Meandering with tight terminal convolutions describes meandering tightly compacted near the transition at the apex of the loop, as opposed to meandering with loose convolutions, which is spread across the length of the loop.

Normal nail fold capillaries show hairpin-like capillary loops with a sharp bend at the top, similar to skin in the ventral forearm and malleoli.

The psoriatic nail bed capillaries show that the capillary loop has meandering with tight terminal convolutions (Redisch et al. 1970; Moll and Wright 1973), as opposed to the meandering with loose convolutions seen in systemic lupus erythematosus (SLE). The tight terminal convolutions might reduce the apparent length of the loop compared with nail folds near RA joints in which loops are long and straight and a number of loops also increased. In psoriatic involvement of the nail (which is often associated with PsA and dactylitis), the number of the loops decrease in number, which might be due to vascular injury from PsA (Bhushan et al. 2000).

5.2.3 Dermal Angiogenesis versus Epidermal Hyperplasia: Cause or Effect? A Series of Chicken-and-Egg-Type Questions

There has been an apparent controversy regarding whether the trigger, as well as initial detectable functional and structural changes, of a newly forming psoriatic lesion starts in the vasculature or the epidermis. In 1924, Civatte et al. wrote,

> Whether the dermatosis originates in the dermis or in the epidermis. The question can be considered from different standpoints, and therefore admits of apparently contradictory opinions. It is in the dermis that the lesion commences, since the exocytosis starts from the papillary body; but it is in the rete that it first becomes characteristic; moreover we are ignorant of the site of the agent which provokes it. Opinions vary according to the manner in which a problem is visualized.

Indeed, as Civatte envisioned, the controversy still continues. Ragaz and Ackerman in 1979 observed the entire spectrum of lesions, including prepinpoint papules and macules, and concluded that the dilation of venules and lymphatics in the upper and mid-dermis, and sometimes in the deep dermal plexus, accompanied by perivascular accumulation of mononuclear cells, followed by intrapapillary capillary dilation and tortuosity and papillary dermal edema, was the initial event.

Kerkhof et al. (1983), as a part of his thesis work in the Netherlands, published in the *British Journal of Dermatology*, showed that "disturbances in the epidermis extend only 2–4 mm into the 'uninvolved' skin, whereas the capillary is metabolically abnormal for a distance of about 2 cm ahead of the advancing edge of the plaque."

On the other side of the controversy, Parent et al. (1990), using immunohistochemistry for filaggrin, involucrin, and epidermal membrane-bound transglutaminase for the epidermis versus albumin, fibrinogen, and immunoglobulin (Ig) G for capillary leakiness, and mapping distances relative to the center of a plaque, concluded the following: "Spreading of Psoriatic Plaques: Alteration of Epidermal Differentiation Precedes Capillary Leakiness and Anomalies in Vascular Morphology," the title of their paper.

Goodfield et al. (1994), using changes in keratin expression profiles, mast cell numbers, and psoriatic morphology of the vasculature, concluded the opposite, again in the title of their paper: "Investigations of the 'Active' Edge of Plaque Psoriasis: Vascular Proliferation Precedes Changes in Epidermal Keratin."

Hern and Mortimer (2007), using video-detailed capillaroscopy studies, concluded that

> prior to the development of clinical lesions there are no significant morphological differences between the dermal microvessels in the clinically uninvolved skin of psoriatic subjects and the dermal microvessels in the normal skin of healthy volunteers. However, during plaque formation, the superficial papillary microvessels in plaque skin undergo a striking, characteristic change, i.e. elongation, widening and tortuosity. These blood vessels must therefore, at least in part, play an important, necessary, but probably secondary role in the pathogenesis of clinical lesions in psoriasis.

The recent literature also echoes that the earliest microscopically discernible features consist of focal spongiotic foci in the lower stratum spinosum of the epidermis at a point in time when vascular changes and mast cell degranulation are detectable ultrastructural or functional events, but are not visible by light microscopy (Menter and Ryan 2017).

The epidermis no doubt is a source of several of the chemoattractant and angiogenic factors and harbors transcriptional and posttranscriptional responsiveness to the predisposing genetic and epigenetic factors; however, it is the immune cells transported through the dermal vessels that seem to be able to transmit the disease. This has accidentally been proven in several instances of allogeneic bone marrow transplants, where bone marrow transplant grafts from donors with psoriasis transmitted it and grafts from normal donors into hosts with psoriasis resolved the disease, whereas in autologous marrow or stem cell transplants, psoriasis temporarily remits but usually recurs after a time lag.

One of the currently upcoming paradigms is that in the "initiation phase" of psoriasis, self-DNA complexed with cathelicidin LL37 activates TLR9 or self-RNA complexed with LL37 activates TLR7 in a transient population of pDCs, which are capable of mounting an interferon α response against self–nucleic acid, and later activates myeloid dendritic cells (mDCs), which themselves can sense self-RNA bound to LL37 through TLR8. Seminal work by Nestle et al. (2005) showed high concentrations of pDCs throughout the T cell–rich infiltrate in the dermis of early primary psoriatic plaque lesions, whereas pDCs were completely absent in the normal skin of healthy donors. Interferon α, which is produced only transiently in the local milieu, leaves a sustained imprint in the form of the persisting expression of a battery of interferon response genes. pDCs, the source of this putative transient interferon burst, are also mostly absent from atopic dermatitis, except their questionable presence in some reports, possibly during an intermediate phase when the acute Th2 shifts toward Th1.

Other than the LL37–nucleic acid complex, several other specific and nonspecific autoantigens have been speculated as the trigger for psoriasis, for example, heat shock proteins, melanocytic antigen ADAMTS-like protein 5 (ADAMTSL5), and possibly also unknown antigens released from entheseal microdamage.

A next chicken-or-egg-type question would be, what places pDCs in that opportune location of the perivascular infiltrate in the dermis? pDCs are attracted to the perivascular dermis in psoriatic plaques probably due to

- Adhesion molecules (homing molecules ligating to addressins)
  - Cutaneous lymphocyte antigen (CLA), an epitope of P-selectin glycoprotein ligand (PSGL) 1 (CD162) on pDC, may help homing through E-selectin (CD62E) in high endothelial venules in the skin. This could partly explain the localization, but it is specific for neither the cell type nor the disease.
- Chemoattractant gradients
  - CXCL3 ligands work on pDCs, but again, they are not specific enough for the cell type, disease, or stage of the disease.
  - Chemerin (CMKLR1 ligand) is an attractive candidate that is secreted as an adipokine and is leaked through plasma in the local milieu and is processed into the highly active form by neutrophil elastase and processed to a less active form by mast cell tryptase and chymase.

Of late, the story has been again starting to swing back toward the epidermis, when the skin barrier function genes identified by GWASs seem to be critical for development of psoriasis susceptibility (Sano 2015).

It is increasingly becoming apparent that the answer to the question (what comes first) may not be a mutually exclusive one but is rather an interaction between the innate and the adaptive immune system on the background of a complex interplay of genetic epigenetic and environmental triggers.

5.2.4 Putative Cellular Players of Angiogenesis in Psoriasis

5.2.4.1 Keratinocytes

Psoriatic epidermal keratinocytes strongly secrete several angiogenic factors, for example, VEGF, IL8, tumor necrosis factor (TNF) α, TGFβ, and TSP1. VEGF and VEGFR2 are expressed by psoriatic keratinocytes and act in an autocrine fashion on keratinocyte proliferation and on endothelial cells causing angiogenesis. Thymidine phosphorylase (TP), an endothelial cell chemotactic factor, is also coexpressed by the keratinocytes, along with VEGF (Creamer et al. 2002a).

Many of the successful animal models of psoriasis are based on keratinocyte-specific promoters. Some examples are discussed here and some in other animal model sections.

The major angiopoietin receptor Tie2, when overexpressed under its own Tie2 promoter, is overexpressed not only in endothelial cells but also unexpectedly in keratinocytes and produces the psoriasis phenotype. But when overexpressed under another Tie1 promoter, it remained restricted to endothelial cells and gave dermal vascular expansion without the epidermal phenotype, whereas overexpression under the K5 basal keratin promoter caused it to reproduce the whole psoriasis phenotype (Wolfram et al. 2009).

Overexpression of VEGF in keratinocytes can produce psoriasis, but either when further triggered by inflammation or injury or when left on for 6 months. K14-driven VEGF can also extend the duration of psoriasis phenotype of the chemical imiquimod-induced psoriasis model, which otherwise wanes in a week. Targeted constitutive expression of the STAT3 transcription factor in basal keratinocytes also produces a psoriasis phenotype, and although it is dependent on mediation by the activity of T cells, unlike NFkB overexpression models, it does not need the NFkB to be overexpressed in both epithelial and T cells.

While keratinocytes are blamed for secreting a huge gamut of pro-inflammatory molecules, for example, TNF, IL1β, IL15, IL36, β-defensins, LL37, and S100 members, their role is not unipolar. Some of the "epidermal stromal cells," that is, keratinocytes, especially those in the dermal epidermal junction, possibly the same cells that under stress release DNA, LL37, and so forth, also dampen inflammation by antagonists like soluble IL15Rα. These counterintuitive processes also affect angiogenesis. IL15, like several of the inflammatory markers, is also directly angiogenic in many different tissues, for example, skin and synovia, and sIL15Rα would probably be an endogenous antagonist for IL15-mediated angiogenesis, whose significance is currently unclear. But antagonists presumably would cause containment of the agonists within the lesion and might explain the sharpness of the lesion boundary.

5.2.4.2 Endothelial Cells

Creamer et al. (1995) noted a significant increase in αvβ3 integrin expression and a significant decrease in β4 integrin expression in psoriatic lesional versus nonlesional skin. There were no significant changes in α2, α5, α6, or β1 integrin expression between these two groups.

Sera from psoriasis patients versus controls have been tested on macrovascular cells (human umbilical vein endothelial cells [HUVECs]) and microvascular endothelial cells (Lowe et al. 1995), which showed increased angiogenesis, thus later leading to finding an increased presence of circulating angiogenic factors. Sera of psoriasis patients were found to have increased VEGF and endothelial cell–stimulating angiogenesis factor (ESAF), and the psoriatic severity is correlated with the VEGF serum levels (Creamer et al. 2002a). Since VEGF induces proliferation of endothelial cells, it would be intuitive to think that endothelial cells in psoriasis would be in a highly proliferative state. However, on the contrary, in psoriasis the proliferation of endothelial cells at any one point in time happens only in some of the venular roots of the hairpin loops, which may not be next to each other, a phenomenon that eluded many investigators before the work by Creamer et al. (1997a).

Several meta-analyses suggests that endothelial function is significantly impaired in patients with psoriasis and PsA, compared with the general population. They have significantly increased arterial stiffness, impaired endothelial-dependent vasodilation as measured by pulse wave velocity, flow-mediated dilation, nitroglycerine-induced vasodilation, carotid intima-media thickness, peripheral arterial tonometry, or aortic stiffness parameters. Circulating endothelial precursors (EPCs) are reduced, another sign of endothelial dysfunction. TNFα inhibitors may potentially improve endothelial function to some extent according to preliminary data.

5.2.4.3 Neutrophils and Myeloid Subpopulations

The history of the role of neutrophils (and mast cells) in psoriasis, especially related to angiogenesis, has come full circle from initial importance to the bottom of importance (there has been a trough in publication for almost 20 years, 1990–2010) and back up into the limelight again. Neutrophils are second only after lymphocytes, among leukocytes, to reach the psoriatic lesions, and they start to be seen when the papules have grown beyond pinhead size (Ragaz and Ackerman 1979). Neutrophil-rich Munro's microabscess (also called Munro–Saboureau microabscess) in the parakeratotic subcorneal layer and spongiform pustules of Kogoj in the stratum spongiosum are pathognomonic of psoriasis lesions at an early stage of the disease. William J. Munro, an Australian dermatologist, described the microabscess in 1898, and Franjo Kogoj, a Slovenian-Viennese dermatologist, described the spongiform pustules in 1927. Psoriatic lesions and, to a greater extent, guttate psoriasis are rich in IL8 (CXCL8), which is a classic neutrophil chemoattractant and possibly contributes toward the maintenance of the neutrophil accumulation.

Adhesion of activated polymorphonuclear cells/neutrophils (PMNs) to endothelial cells can cause angiogenesis in vitro and in vivo. ICAM1 and E-selectin, two adhesion molecules, and neutrophil elastase are essential for this action of PMNs, and ETS1, a transcription factor acting downstream of ICAM1, acts as a common factor downstream of VEGF and bFGF, and is involved in transcriptional activation of proteases like uPA and MMP1, 3, and 9. In a mouse model of multistage carcinogenesis, infiltrating neutrophils, presumably acting through MMP9 rather than MMP9-containing macrophages, were found to mediate the initial angiogenic switch and lead to the VEGF-VEGFR associations.

IL17, which is considered one of the central players in both psoriasis and the angiogenesis of psoriasis, is now known to be secreted to a large extent by neutrophils in the psoriatic epidermis, rather than Th17 cells. Neutrophils can also be associated with RORγt—the transcription factor associated with Th17. The IL17 secretion by neutrophil is possibly secreted along with the neutrophil extracellular trap (NET) (Lin 2011). NETs, discovered in 2004, produced by NETosis or ETosis, are the active cellular process of throwing out DNA, along with specific subsets of primary, secondary, and tertiary granule contents, especially many antimicrobial proteins (Brinkmann et al. 2004). This was originally thought to be a form of cell death but was later found to also be possible without cell death, and mitochondrial DNA, rather than genomic DNA, is thrown out in this "vital" form of NETosis. NETs are rich in many known intracellular self-antigens and are also known to be able to stimulate angiogenesis itself.

The mechanism of NETosis in RA and psoriasis or PsA, although not very well tested, may be speculated to be different. RA has shown circulating anticitrullinated peptide antibodies, which could presumably be against the citrullinated histone-like autoantigens found in the cell death–associated NET. Psoriasis and PsA are both very strongly associated with neutrophilic exudates but not with autoantibodies against citrullinated peptides, thus making it tempting to speculate that the NETosis in psoriasis could be more related to the vital form involving mitochondrial DNA and antimicrobial peptides.

DNA, the major constituent of NET, is also one of the central features of the newer hypotheses of psoriasis pathogenesis. The DNA release from stressed keratinocytes, which is one of the putative candidate initial triggers for psoriasis implicated in the binding to LL37 and transiently stimulating pDCs, could also be potentially complemented by DNA in NETs. Neutrophils link the innate and the adaptive immune system, and antipsoriatic therapies exert their effects, at least in part, through interference with neutrophils. However, initial attempts to block neutrophil, for example, by trying to specifically block IL8 and E-selectin, failed, possibly because the inhibition was too specific in a redundant network setting; for example, neutrophil chemoattraction in psoriasis may be a combination of CXCL1, CXCL2, IL8, IL18, and other factors, and the homing may be through multiple selections and vascular adhesion protein (VAP).

None of the three spontaneous psoriasis-like mouse mutants—(1) Sharpin/cpdm (chronic proliferative dermatitis), (2) Ttc7/Fsn (Flaky skin), and (3) Scd1 (stearoyl CoA desaturase)/Asebia—show any microabscess; however, neutrophil depletion can alleviate psoriasis-like skin disease in the flaky skin mice.

Although normal neutrophils are supposed to be short-lived, neutrophils in psoriatic plaques are relatively longer-lived, partly due to decreased apoptosis, for example, caused by CEACAM1.

Neutrophils might become more and more important in the understanding and treatment of psoriasis—not only in inflammatory aspects but also in angiogenic ones. Neutrophils have multiple subsets, and some not only secrete VEGF and multiple other angiogenic factors (in addition to IL17 and NET, described before) but also have their cognate receptors for autocrine and paracrine amplification. By some yet poorly understood mechanism, neutrophils might be capable of causing elongation-type angiogenesis of psoriasis, whose other parallel is seen in angiogenesis in the female reproductive system, especially the endometrium (Gambino et al. 2002). The endometrium shows very sharp focal expression of VEGF associated with segments of microvessels that have neutrophils marginating or adherent within them.

It must also be noted that neutrophils have a dual potential role in inflammation, as well as angiogenesis. Neutrophils can be polarized like Th1 versus Th2 helper T cells or M1 versus M2 macrophages into N1 versus N2 cells. The so-called inflammatory cell neutrophil is now known to have an anti-inflammatory form, N2, which in the original classification scheme was supposed to be the angiogenic phenotype (Piccard et al. 2012). It is also gradually becoming apparent that the phenotypes of neutrophils are more complex than just the binary N1 or N2 can explain. A convenient way to classify neutrophils based on the Ficoll density gradient shows that low-density neutrophils coisolate with peripheral blood mononuclear cells (PBMCs) and high-density neutrophils have different angiogenic properties. Low-density neutrophils might be a heterogenous population with some immature cells, including myeloid-derived suppressor cells (MDSCs), described later, and some mature neutrophils, under the influence of factors like TGFβ, can become large. It is not only the degree of differentiation or plastic redifferentiation but also the degree of activation that matters, because full activation releases both primary and secondary granules, with angiostatic factors in the primary granule dominative, but partial activation of neutrophils, for example, by CXCR2, can release preferentially secondary granules, which may contain more pro-angiogenic molecules, for example, VEGF, hepatocyte growth factor (HGF), and IL12. Thus, neutrophils have now turned out to be one of the most important cells in angiogenesis.

5.2.4.4 BMDCs, MDSCs, RBCCs, and Vascular Modulatory Cells

MDSCs are relatively recently rediscovered heterogenous immature cells of bone marrow myeloid origin related only by lineage to their corresponding terminal states, like granulocyte, monocyte, or dendritic cells, but functionally immunosuppressive for T cells and NK cells, and were originally dubbed the natural suppressor (NS) cell population in the 1960s. In humans, MDSCs express myeloid cell markers such as CD11b+ and CD33+, and in mice, MDSCs express Gr1+ and CD11b+ myeloid markers. They are more heterogenous than originally thought and may include multipotent progenitor cells. Some studies use the term *bone marrow–derived cells* (BMDCs), which might be a broader population of cells that may include MDSCs, and possibly also bone marrow–derived EPCs or hemangiocytes and PPCs. However, a distinction is made from EPCs and PPCs, and the other circulating cells are sometimes referred to as recruited bone marrow–derived circulating cells (RBCCs) and called *vascular modulatory cells*, not to be confused with vascular mural cells. These cells are summoned to the target organ by VEGF, and retained near the vessels by stromal cell–derived factor, that is, SDF1 (CXCL12), chemokine gradient. These cells rarely incorporate into the endothelium, but rather play diverse paracrine and juxtacrine angiogenic and accessory roles. One example of such a role, discussed earlier, is myeloid bridge cells, which help tip cells find partners and anastomose. According to some studies (Rafii et al. 2008), BMDCs are dependent on platelets for both recruitment and retention to angiogenic compartments. BMDCs and MDSCs may also potentially provide neuropilin coreceptors for VEGF signaling or MMP9 for angiogenesis.

BMDC recruitment and retention may be helped by platelets. Platelet aggregation through glycoprotein (gp) IIb–IIIa (the αIIbβ3 integrin) causes inward receptor signaling and platelet activation and, at hypoxic angiogenic sites, induces accumulation of VEGF (the recruitment factor for BMDCs) and MMP9-mediated release of SDF1 (the retention factor for BMDCs). BMDCs may be unable to adhere directly to the exposed ECM, but tether through PSGL1 on their surface, ligating to P-selectin on platelets. This pro-angiogenic action of platelets on BMDCs may be kept partially in check by antiangiogenic platelet factors, for example, TSP1 and platelet factor 4 (PF4 and CXCL4 chemokine).

The monocytic MDSCs, dubbed Mo-MDSCs, found in psoriasis are reported to produce more IL23, IL1β, and CCL4 cytokines than Mo-MDSCs from healthy controls, and are dysfunctional on their suppressive action on T cells. Circulating MDSC levels are significantly increased in psoriasis than in healthy controls. These cells are also capable of producing MMP9, MMP1, IL8, GROα, and modified citrus pectin (MCP) 1, thus contributing to inflammation and angiogenesis.

5.2.4.5 Mast Cells

Mast cells are long-lived cells strategically placed at immune effector sites and usually next to vessels. They are classically known for vasodilatory action but now are becoming the center of renewed interest for angiogenesis as well. Mast cell degranulation is one of the earliest features of nascent psoriatic lesions (Brody 1984). At immune effector sites, the number of tryptase and chymase-positive mast cells increases rapidly during early stages of psoriasis, for example, seen during the Koebner phenomenon. By degranulation-dependent or independent mechanisms, and in a trigger-dependent rapid or slow pace, mast cells can secrete a number of soluble mediators, such as serine proteinases, histamine, lipid-derived mediators, cytokines, chemokines, and growth factors. Mast cells can express major histocompatibility complex (MHC) class II and costimulatory molecules and present antigens. They avidly interact with other cells, such as endothelial cells, keratinocytes, sensory nerves, neutrophils, T-cell subsets, and antigen- presenting cells, contributing to the development of skin inflammation and angiogenesis in psoriasis.

Mast cells are targets of IL9 and can maintain the production of large amounts of angiogenesis factors, for example, bFGF, VEGF, platelet-derived growth factor (PDGF), IL8, TGFβ, TNFα, IL17, and IL22. Many of these factors, for example, IL17, are present in the granules that need degranulation or ETosis. However, mast cells can secrete some of these factors, for example, VEGF121 and VEGF165, in degranulation-independent ways as well. In the dermis of psoriasis lesions, mast cells, rather than Th17, are the strongest source of IL17 (in contrast to epidermis, where neutrophil is the strongest source). There have been controversies about whether mast cells actually transcribe IL17. Mast cells from the tonsil only endocytose, concentrate, and release IL17 upon trigger. However, mast cells at least from psoriatic skin have been shown to transcribe and sort and pack IL17 in an exocytic compartment.

Similar to neutrophils, mast cells also throw extracellular traps, known as mast cell extracellular traps (MCETs). MCETs are also known to be associated with the release of IL17 and other pro-angiogenic factors. The hypoxia-dependent master regulator of angiogenesis HIF is also involved in the formation of MCET.

It must be remembered that mast cells are also present in many other disease, for example, atopic dermatitis, which does not show much angiogenesis compared with psoriasis. Mast cells also have dual roles with some pro-angiogenic and antiangiogenic mediators, with an example of the latter being prostaglandin D2 (PG-D2).

5.2.4.6 Lymphocyte Populations

Since lymphocytes are part of the first wave of cell recruitment in the initial psoriatic plaque, the angiogenesis was also naturally attributed and tested first on the role of lymphocytes.

The SCID mouse human skin xenograft was historically used to inject various types of manipulated activated lymphocytes, for example, NKT cells that are capable of producing psoriasis phenotypes. The study of lymphocytes in psoriasis has a long history, and studies on the pathogenesis of psoriasis have been published more than 18,000 times in the literature, so it is not possible to cover them in detail here. However, a few interesting cell populations are briefly mentioned.

5.2.4.6.1 T-Cell Subsets

In the older theory of helper T-cell polarization, psoriasis was considered more of a Th1-type disease and atopic dermatitis was considered more of a Th2-type disease. However, in light of the newer immune concepts, more and more Th17, Th22, and Th9 components are being invoked in psoriasis. One of the running paradigms is that Th17 cells are more notorious in causing autoimmunity or autoinflammation, and Tregs are better at suppressing them. TGFβ is necessary for the development of both Tregs and Th17, but a context of IL6 and IL21 can switch off Foxp3—necessary for Treg development—and switch on RORγt via activation of transcription factor STAT3. Th17 cells are now known to be longer-lived than earlier thought. An even longer-lived, difficult-to-regulate (by Treg), and highly proliferative novel subset of cells named ex-Th17, or noncanonical Th1, and their role in psoriasis are gradually coming into light.

The angiogenesis in psoriasis is partly dependent on a Th1/Th17-type response. In early psoriatic lesions, the dermis is mainly infiltrated by CD4+ Th1 and Th17 cells, which produce interferon γ and IL17, but not IL4 or IL10. However, it is increasingly becoming clear that the Th17 cell itself is only a minor source of this inflammatory and angiogenic cytokine. Some of the cells now known to contribute to IL17 in the local milieu of psoriasis are

Neutrophils
Mast cells
Macrophages
Dendritic cells

Th17 cells
  Adaptive Th17 cells
  Natural Th17 cells
Tc17 cells
Innate lymphoid cells (ILCs)
  ILC3 producing IL17
  NKp44+ (NCR+) ILC3 producing IL17 and IL22
γδT cells
(IL17-related discussions are also found in Sections 5.3.3.2 and 5.2.5.16.2.)

5.2.4.6.2 Conventional (Adaptive) Th17 Cells

These are a subset of activated CD4+ T helper cells that produce high levels of IL17A, IL17F, and IL22, and express IL23R. They are CD4+ TCRα/β+, a source of IL17, and have been classically implicated in autoimmune diseases. They are relatively more implicated in RA pathogenesis, but in psoriasis and PsA, the other sources are more important.

5.2.4.6.3 Natural Th17 Cells

These are a subset of thymic Th17 cells that express effector properties before peripheral antigen exposure. They have a TCR gene arrangement and signaling different from that of conventional Th17 cells.

5.2.4.6.4 Tc17 Cells

These are CD8+ cells, as opposed to CD4+ Th17 cells, and are the cytotoxic counterpart of Th17 cells. They use CCR6 to home to CCL20 to home to skin and contribute to the epidermally localized disease memory cells.

5.2.4.6.5 Innate Lymphoid Cells: ILC3 and NKp44+ (NCR+) Cells

Innate is generally used as the opposite of *adaptive*, and for T cells, it generally also means without a functional T-cell receptor and associated CD4 or CD8. The ILC, unlike the other and better-known innate cells, like natural killer (NK) cells, is noncytotoxic. ILCs consist of three distinct groups, of which the third one, that is, ILC3 cells, expresses copious amounts of IL17 and is found in psoriasis lesions. ILC3, in itself a heterogenous group, is primarily classified by chemokine receptor signature. A subset of ILCs expressing activating-type NK receptors termed the natural cytotoxicity receptors (NCRs) also express IL22 and are thought to be important in the pathogenesis of psoriasis (Artis and Spits 2015).

5.2.4.6.6 iNKT Cells

Invariant natural killer T (iNKT) cells are cells with properties of both NK cells and T cells that express a (semi-)invariant, that is, limited-diversity, αβ-T-cell receptor and are restricted to recognizing endogenous lipid antigens presented on CD1d MHC-like molecules.

Stimulated by CD1d-bound endogenous lipid antigens, iNKT cells show a constitutive memory phenotype and are capable of rapidly responding to stimulation, producing a broad range of cytokines. In addition, through direct and indirect interactions, for example, via CD1d and CD40L-CD40 signaling, iNKT cells are capable of maturing dendritic cells and activating B cells, and thus are crucial in enhancing antigen-specific B- and T-cell responses. iNKT cells are an alternative source of IL17 when IL6 stimulation for Th17 cells is not available. IL17+ iNKT cells express IL23R and IL1R1.

5.2.4.6.7 γδT Cells

In mouse imiquimod models of psoriasis, IL17-secreting γδT cells expand in lymph nodes and traffic to skin, where they persist as long-term resident memory-like cells capable of rapid reactivation due to increased IL1R1 expression. In humans, long-term dermal resident γδT cells are also receiving renewed interest.

5.2.4.7 Monocyte, Macrophage, and Dendritic Cell Subpopulations

5.2.4.7.1 Monocytes

These cells are very familiar circulating blood cells that are precursors of tissue macrophages. In human peripheral circulation, three distinct monocyte populations have been phenotyped: classical monocytes (Mon1: CD14++ CD16– CCR2+), intermediate monocytes (Mon2: CD14++ CD16+ CCR2+), and nonclassical monocytes (Mon3: CD14+ CD16++ CCR2–). The classical monocytes have been considered osteoclast progenitor cells, although all three are capable of giving rise to osteoclasts. The intermediate subset has been reported to be pro-angiogenic and the main producers of reactive oxygen species (ROS) during homeostasis. Psoriasis patients, who also exhibit a propensity to cardiovascular disease as a comorbidity, have been reported to have elevated levels of a circulating intermediate monocyte population.

Induction of CD16 on the intermediate monocyte and its adhesion to the vascular endothelium (e.g., through the Mac1 integrin) and transendothelial migration can be facilitated by monocyte–platelet interaction. Circulating monocyte–platelet aggregates (MPAs) are considered a robust marker of platelet activation and an indicator of inflammatory conditions, including coronary artery disease-like states. Keratinocyte–Tie2 transgenic mouse models of psoriasis show an increased number of monocyte–monocyte doublets with upregulation of adhesion molecules, for example, integrins, sarcoglycan, collagen type VI, integrins α1 and α2, disintegrins, and CD56 (NCAM1), compared with plastic adherent monocytes.

Monocytes constitute the dominant population among circulating cells expressing VEGFR2. Some pro-angiogenic monocytes express the angiopoietin receptor Tie2 and are called Tie2-expressing monocytes (TEMs). However, the existence of such specific pro-angiogenic subtypes of monocytes is somewhat controversial. The so-called circulating EPCs, when isolated by older adhesion and culture-based methods, were found to be largely of monocytic origin—a subpopulation of monocytes that, when stimulated by VEGF, produce endothelial cell phenotypes in culture. In such cultures, the "early outgrowth" endothelial progenitors include monocytes and T cells, and their formation is strictly dependent on the presence of monocytes. But the cells are nonetheless strongly supportive of angiogenesis and have been named "circulating angiogenic cells" (CACs) by some authors and are likely to overlap with BMDCs, as described in Section 5.2.4.4.

5.2.4.7.2 Macrophages

In contrast to circulating monocytes, which have been classified into Mon1, 2, and 3, tissue macrophages were originally classified into M1 and M2 subpopulations, similar to T-helper Th1-Th2 polarization. Classically activated, that is, M1, macrophages are stimulated by interferon γ, TNFα, and lipopolysaccharide (LPS), and secrete nitric oxide (NO) and pro-inflammatory cytokines IL1, IL6, IL12, IL23, TNFα, and so forth. Alternatively, activated, that is, M2, macrophages are stimulated by IL4 and IL10 and secrete the growth-promoting molecule ornithine, and anti-inflammatory but pro-angiogenic cytokines, for example, IL10 and TGFβ. But such bipolar classification has shortcomings; for example, sometimes so-called anti-inflammatory M2 macrophages behave in pro-inflammatory ways. Even subdividing M2 macrophages into a, b, c, and d may not always overcome these issues, and several alternative classification schemes have been used. Macrophages may be either "recruited" from monocytes (R-Mac), which are usually short-lived, or "tissue-resident" (TR-Mac) long-lived macrophages. The recruited monocytes and macrophages may undergo "education" (reprogramming) by local factors like VEGF, which can enhance their angiogenic role, making them a part of MDSCs (related to MoMDSCs), discussed earlier in Section 5.2.4.4.

5.2.4.7.3 Dendritic Cells

As described earlier, currently the most dominant paradigm of psoriasis initiation is related to LL37 bound to self-DNA activating pDCs. Normally, self-DNA cannot act as self-antigens, as they are methylated on CpG islands, and also, they cannot cross the membrane barrier topology to be presented to intracellular TLR9-containing compartments. However, LL37 can help circumvent these barriers, and the perivascular cellular infiltrate initially rich in pDCs is stimulated to produce a transient spike of interferon α, which itself does not persist in established psoriasis lesions. The baton is later passed from pDCs to mDCs, which persist in the lesion and amplify the TNF signal. Dendritic cells are also known to directly and indirectly stimulate (or sometimes inhibit) angiogenesis through growth factors and cytokines, but their exact role in this regard is an emerging field of research.

5.2.4.8 Mural Cells

The vessels once formed by neoangiogenesis are invested initially by pericytes, followed by smooth muscles, fibroblasts, and a variety of other mural cells, which also may arguably include an interesting population named the telocytes (described below). Dysregulation of proper mural cell layer formation is the reason for the leakiness of neoangiogenesis seen in cancer and other pathologic conditions. TGFβ, the Ang-Tie system, PDGF, SP1, and so forth, a multitude of signaling cascades, are involved in the angiogenic process related to mural cells and vascular remodeling, many of which have been implicated in psoriasis, for example, Tie2-mediated animal models.

5.2.4.9 Telocytes

These cells are elusive but ubiquitous "interstitial cells of Cajal"-like atypical myofibroblastic cells with very long, moniliform processes (telopods with podoms and podomeres) that form an interconnected network and play diverse roles related to communication, pacemaker activity, stem niche formation, and potentially mesenchymal stem cell function. In dermal perivascular adventitia, they have been described as veiled cells by Braverman et al. (1986). Manole et al. (2015) believe that in psoriatic lesions the telocyte network is disrupted and their number is decreased (but recovers after corticosteroid therapy), and they believe that this might explain the mechanistic basis of the *Auspitz sign*. Telocytes also make contact with endothelial cells, pericytes, smooth muscle cells and play important roles in both vasomotor control and angiogenesis.

5.2.4.10 Platelets

Platelets, the smallest "cells" in circulation, are known classically for hemostasis, but also have many other roles, including roles in angiogenesis (some of which have been discussed above in Section 5.2.4.4). Platelets are anucleate products specially derived from mature bone marrow megakaryocytes that have polyploid nuclei. Platelets circulate for 7–10 days and stay in the outer lamina of blood in vessels (unlike larger and heavier cells, which stay in the center of vessels) in close contact with endothelial cells. Platelets have two main types of secretory granules, with α-granule being the main storage granule (50–80 in number, occupying 10% of cytosolic volume; they contain a diverse load of protein in the lumen as well as on the membrane), and a few δ-granules contain ATP, calcium, polyphosphate, serotonin, and so forth. Platelets can have different degrees of activation, with potentially selective release of some granule contents, along with different degrees of aggregation and αIIb-β3 integrin-mediated retraction of the aggregate. The strongest activation of platelets releases platelet microparticles, which are strongly thrombogenic and angiogenic.

The platelets play a lot of major roles in vasculogenesis and angiogenesis. An example of the role in vasculogenesis involves platelet plugs separating the early lymphatic vasculogenesis from the venous vasculature through interaction of CLEC2, a C-type lectin receptor on platelets, and podoplanin on the lymphatic endothelium. Platelet α-granules literally contain hundreds of proteins, many of which are angiogenesis related, for example, VEGFA and C. VEGF levels increase almost threefold within minutes of platelet clot formation, and serum contains significantly more VEGF than plasma due to the same effect. However platelet α-granules contain a lot of both pro- and antiangiogenic factors. Whether and how platelets selectively sort and secrete a set of one type of agonists or the opposite in a polarized manner has been a matter of marvel and research. In injury or inflammation, protease-activated receptor PAR1 is supposed to preferentially release VEGF and suppress endostatin release, thus promoting angiogenesis and wound healing. In contrast, protease-activated receptor PAR4 is supposed to preferentially do the reverse, that is, release endostatin and suppress release of VEGF, thus inhibiting angiogenesis and wound healing. Platelets also help regulate angiogenesis in many other ways; for example, engagement by pathogens or alarmins of TLRs on platelets can lead to platelet–neutrophil interaction, followed by activation of neutrophils, leading to NETosis and amplification of IL17 and VEGF signals, which can promote angiogenesis (discussed earlier). The platelet–neutrophil interaction was originally thought to happen through P-selectin on platelets and PSGL1 on neutrophils (discussed later in this chapter). However, neutrophil β2 integrins, for example, Mac1 and platelet gpIb, are also important and block Mac1 (CD18/CD11b) but not LFA1 (CD18/CD11a) in mice and humans, significantly reducing NET formation. Platelet gpIb inhibition by gene deletion or blocking antibodies also affects the formation of NETs, suggesting that platelets participate in NETosis. Platelets are sticky cells and help bridge interaction between a lot of cell types, for example, lymphocyte to high endothelial venules, and monocytes and MDSCs to angiogenic compartments (discussed above). While platelets can increase IL17 release through NETosis, IL17 in turn can also stimulate platelet function through the extracellular signal-regulated kinase (ERK) 2 signaling pathway. Not all platelet leukocyte complexes are inflammatory; platelet-bound monocytes formed under low-shear-stress conditions have been claimed to show an anti-inflammatory phenotype, which suppresses production of pro-inflammatory cytokines, for example, IL1β, and augments anti-inflammatory cytokines, for example, IL10.

Psoriasis and PsA patients show increased platelet reactivity (especially to ADP) and increased levels of platelet-derived microparticles and soluble P-selectin, as well as increased numbers of platelet–monocyte complexes.

5.2.5 Angiogenic Molecular Mediators in Psoriasis

VEGF and angiopoietins are so far more well discussed and well researched. So, this chapter focuses relatively more on the lesser-known molecular players that should be better researched in relation to psoriatic diseases.

5.2.5.1 VEGF

VEGF was discovered in 1983 and initially named vascular permeability factor (VPF); it was later independently discovered as VEGF in 1989, and in the same year was found to be the same secreted angiogenic mitogen. VEGF belongs to a family of highly conserved growth factors belonging to the cysteine-knot superfamily. Members of the VEGF family are VEGFA–E and placenta growth factor (PlGF). VEGFA has many splice forms. The commonly observed forms, named after the number of amino acids in mature form, are VEGF121, 145, 148, 165, 183, 189, and 206. These were names of the human isoforms; mouse isoforms are one amino acid shorter. VEGFA, which is often known as just VEGF, and some of its other cofamily members, VEGFA and C and PlGF, work mainly through two receptors: VEGFR2, also known as Flk1 or KDR, the activating receptor, and VEGFR1, also known as Flt1, the receptor that is usually inhibitory. These are both receptor tyrosine kinases. Neuropilins (Nrp1 and 2), originally discovered as receptors for semaphoring-type neuronal pathfinding molecules, were found to be coreceptors for some VEGFs: VEGFA165, PlGF152 can directly bind Nrp1 and 2, VEGFB binds to Nrp1 but not Nrp2, and VEGF145 and VEGFC bind Nrp2 but not Nrp1. VEGFC and D bind to VEGFR3 and 4 and are mostly lymphangiogenic.

VEGF, unlike most other angiogenic growth factors, causes leaks by endothelial caveolae modified into vesiculovacuolar organelles (VVOs) and fenestrations. In addition, it can also loosen up interendothelial junctions, like many inflammatory mediators.

Genetic studies have associated several VEGF single-nucleotide polymorphisms (SNPs) to early-onset psoriasis (−2578[C/A], −460[C/T], and +405[C/G]) (Guérard and Pouliot 2012). In some studies, the production of VEGF by PBMCs depended on the genotype, whereas production by keratinocytes did not.

VEGF and the soluble form of its receptor are found in both the skin lesion and serum of patients. In one study, VEGF and soluble VEGFR1 (sFlt1) in the sera of patients were respectively two and four times higher than in healthy controls and demonstrated significant correlation with the Psoriasis Area and Severity Index (PASI), but not soluble VEGFR2 (sKDR) (Flisiak et al. 2010). The isoform of VEGF that has been most studied in psoriasis is VEGFA, but VEGFC and, to a small extent, VEGFD have also been found in psoriasis. VEGFC can play roles in both angiogenesis and lymphangiogenesis. VEGFD is usually implicated in lymphangiogenesis. Keratinocytes, neutrophils, mast cells, macrophages and possibly fibroblasts, smooth muscle cells, and so forth, express VEGF in psoriasis. Keratinocytes from psoriatic lesions are known to express several VEGFA splice forms, including VEGF121 (the most common), followed by VEGF189, 165, and a little 145 (Man et al. 2008). One of the smallest splice forms of VEGFA, VEGF121 is weakly acidic and non–heparin binding (compared with the larger basic ones), and thus freely diffusible, and forms a wide shallow gradient in contrast with 189, which is strictly localized, and 165, which forms a gradient steep enough to form tip cells. VEGF121 is also the most abundant form in both psoriasis lesions and uninvolved skin in psoriasis patients compared with controls (Henno et al. 2009). This is a potential explanation as to why so much VEGF does not cause an increase in branching angiogenesis.

It is known from general VEGF angiogenesis models that the heparin-dependent extracellular matrix–bound larger isoforms are usually involved in branching angiogenesis with thinner vessels, whereas this small isoform of VEGF is known to cause more dilated leaky angiogenesis with the least vessel density (Yuan et al. 2011). It has been known that VEGF121 and 165 increase, whereas VEGF189 decreases, vessel diameter, and VEGF165 is good at both increasing in diameter and length (similar to 121) and sprouting (unlike 121), and gives rise to mixed densities of vessels, both low density (121) and high density (189). The smaller isoforms, like VEGF121, need to be studied more with respect to elongation-type angiogenesis. Some of the literature that did study this isoform has noted that VEGF121, rather than causing sprouting angiogenesis, caused accumulation of proliferating endothelial cells in vessel lumina, giving a glomeruloid appearance.

Glomeruloid angiogenesis is in itself considered a separate entity among types of angiogenesis (discussed in Section 5.1.1.2.5). However, both the natural and the experimental model noting this action of VEGF121 (and VEGF164 in mice) were usually in the closed space of the skull. One of the two schools of thoughts is that glomeruloid angiogenesis, at least one subtype or the early forms, is merely loops and convolutions that only superficially resemble the glomerular tufts (Döme et al. 2007). It is tempting to speculate that in a nonenclosed space like the loose stroma of the dermis or the endometrium, the same type of agonist action of VEGF might lead to elongation-type angiogenesis. Neutrophils, the cell type coming back to the limelight in psoriatic angiogenesis, are known to express at least two common VEGF splice variants, VEGF121 and 165, making VEGF121 an especially attractive candidate that can explain the elongation-type angiogenesis seen in psoriasis.

The previously mentioned antagonistic atypical isoforms of VEGF, such as the alternatively spliced xxxb forms, for example, VEGF121b, 145b, 165b, 183b, and 189b (Nowak et al. 2008), and antagonistic translational read-through forms (Eswarappa et al. 2014) have not been well studied in psoriasis, even though some of them have been speculated to play a role in diabetic retinopathy, which may be a disorder with a lot in common.

VEGFRs in normal patients versus lesional and nonlesional biopsies from psoriasis have been investigated (Henno et al. 2009, 2010). They showed no difference for VEGFR1 and 2 and soluble VEGFR1 (sFlt1) levels. However, the soluble neuropilin isoform (inhibitor for VEGF165), designated s12Nrp1 (named after the presence of intron 12–derived sequences), was increased in nonlesional skin. Lymphangiogenic receptor VEGFR3 and its coreceptor Nrp2a mRNA were also increased in nonlesional skin. VEGFC and D the ligands for VEGFR3 are increased in both the lymphatics and the fibroblasts in lesional skin. All these together might suggest readiness for lymphangiogenesis in the nonlesional skin, which responds to the ligands in the lesions.

5.2.5.2 Angiopoietins (Ang1, Ang2, and Receptor Tie2)

The main angiogenic angiopoietin is Ang2, which causes vessel destabilization, initiation of angiogenesis, and transformation of capillaries into inflammatory venules, with increased leakiness and stickiness, in synergism with TNFα. Ang2 is expressed by endothelial cells near the VEGF-expressing epidermal keratinocytes in psoriasis lesions, and the vessel-stabilizing angiopoietin Ang1 is expressed by stromal cells in the vascularized papillary dermis of lesional skin. Their receptors Tie2 and Ang2 could also be upregulated in cultured dermal microvascular endothelial cell upon the addition of angiogenic factors like VEGF or FGF2. Successful antipsoriatic treatment was accompanied by a noticeable reduction of Ang2.

In PsA, high Ang2 and Ang1, as well as a high Ang2/Ang1 ratio, and high VEGF and TGFβ1 were seen in PsA, especially enriched in perivascular/endothelial synovia in comparison with RA synovia, and may potentially explain the tortuous elongation-type angiogenesis in PsA (Fearon et al. 2003). In both PsA and RA, Ang2 expression correlates with arthritis severity.

5.2.5.3 FGF2

Discovered by Folkman et al. in 1984, bFGF or FGF2 is so basic, that is, positively charged, that it could be "purified" 200,000-fold by a single passage over a heparin affinity column. However, now FGFs are known to belong to a large family (FGF1–23; with a rodent FGF15 ortholog of human FGF19), with many family members that would copurify by such methods. Not just the heparin-based purification, but also the heparin binding and non-binding-type classification for growth factors in general, is no more common, as many of these factors have isoforms with different sizes and charge densities. For example, bFGF has isoforms of molecular masses commonly ranging from 18 to 24 kDa.

bFGF was discovered as a tumor-derived capillary angiogenic factor half a decade before VEGF was known for its angiogenic role. However, unlike VEGF, bFGF acts as a mitogen for many different cell types. bFGF remains bound to the subendothelial ECM and is released when the matrix is degraded by MMPs. In this chapter, in different sections above, some roles of bFGF have already been described in various stages of angiogenesis, including low-level signaling during quiescence and higher-intensity signaling during endothelial activation through angiogenic switch. However, the role of FGF is somewhat obscured by the facts; for example, FGF2 knockout mice or FGF1/FGF2 double-knockout mice do not show apparent morphologic defects of impaired vasculogenesis or angiogenesis. Transgenic overexpression of FGF2 in vivo also does not show any appreciable vascular change. However, FGF2 is still a critical angiogenic factor, and the above paradox is probably explained by the redundancy of numerous FGFs in the mammals and also by avian embryogenesis quail–chick chimeric studies showing that FGF2 is necessary for vasculogenesis, as well as the fact that adenovirus-mediated gene transfer of dominant-negative truncated FGFR1 or of FGF2 antisense cDNA does cause abnormal vascular development in mouse embryos. On the other hand, although FGF2 or the FGF system in general may not be totally redundant, endothelial cell–derived VEGF is an important autocrine amplifier of FGF2-induced angiogenesis, which can be largely blocked by anti-VEGF antibodies. FGF2-mediated angiogenesis is regulated by many complex local systems; for example, long-pentraxin PTX3, synthesized locally by endothelial cells in response to IL1β and TNFα, can bind FGF2 and inhibit the downstream pro-angiogenic effects.

In psoriasis skin lesions, FGF2/bFGF is expressed mainly by keratinocytes, endothelial cells, and mast cells. It has been known since the mid-1980s that FGF2 stimulates the proliferation of both endothelial cells and keratinocytes through autocrine and paracrine mechanisms.

In the joint, FGF2 is among the most potent angiogenic factors secreted by the arthritic synovium (Goddard et al. 1992). Sendai virus–mediated FGF2 overexpression in rat joints significantly worsened clinical symptoms, as well as inflammation, angiogenesis, pannus formation, and osteocartilaginous destruction, in a rat adjuvant-induced model of arthritis (AIA), but not in non-AIA joints. In humans, both FGF1 and 2 are expressed by macrophages, synovial lining cells, and fibroblasts in the RA synovium in situ, and it may be extrapolated that they should be present in PsA. But little, if any, specific data exist regarding FGF distribution during different stages of PsA, and SNPs in FGF1 or 2 genes have not been associated with psoriasis, unlike VEGF. Serum levels of FGF2 (bFGF) or FGF1 (acidic FGF) have occasionally been tested in some studies, but the results were not encouraging to use them as biomarkers.

5.2.5.4 IGF1 and 2

Insulin-like growth factors (IGFs) 1 and 2, which are growth factors homologous in structure to proinsulin, are paracrine- as well as endocrine-acting mediators originally known for their downstream mediation of growth hormone (somatotrophin) action, and were thus named somatomedins. Although a number of members in this family are not so large, the system is complex with a large number of binding proteins and their cleaving proteases. IGF1 and 2 act through activating receptor tyrosine kinases.

The level of IGF2, but not IGF1, is significantly elevated in serum and blister fluid from psoriatic lesions.

5.2.5.5 Hepatocyte Growth Factor/Scatter Factor

Active HGF/scatter factor (SF) is a disulfide-bound heterodimeric polypeptide that belongs to the plasminogen subfamily of S1 peptidases but has no detectable protease activity.

HGF is found in psoriasis lesions, but its level is not raised in the serum. It is expressed in keratinocytes and leukocytes and secreted around the dermal vasculature. HGF can directly help angiogenesis by a partly understood mechanism, and indirectly through VEGF or platelet-activating factor (PAF) induction. However, it must be noted PAF is intermediate to many different types of signaling, including the migration downstream of VEGF itself.

5.2.5.6 ESAF

Around 1979, Weiss et al. (1979) in the United Kingdom and McAuslan and Hoffman (1979) in Australia isolated a freely dialyzable low-molecular-weight (<600 Da) compound from the so-called tumor angiogenic factor (TAF), a crude extract of both intracellular material and ECM rat Walker tumors. This compound gave a strong positive result on the chick chorioallantoic membrane angiogenesis test and stimulated proliferation in microvascular endothelial cell culture. They named it ESAF. ESAF, at the nanograms per microliter level, was found to be a specific mitogen and chemoattractant only for microvascular endothelial cells and pericytes in vitro, but possesses no mitogenic activity on aortic cells, large vein endothelial cells, fibroblasts, or any other cell type. Its stimulatory effect on endothelial cells is synergistic with bFGF (Bhushan et al. 1999). ESAF activates procollagenase (MMP1), progelatinase A (MMP2), prostromelysin 1 (MMP3), and so forth (a basis for the ESAF functional assay) and reactivates the MMP complexes with TIMP by dissociating the inhibitor.

The molecular nature of ESAF has been elusive. It is nonprotein, nonenzymatic molecule and is relatively heat stable (35°C for 30 min causes only a 10% loss of activity). The molecular weight was estimated to be approximately 200–300 D on gel filtration by some studies, but the same authors later estimated it to possibly have a larger weight, but less than 1 kDa. It either is dialyzable or precipitates from nondialyzable components if trichloroacetic acid is added up to 15%, and is extractable with 20 mM acetic acid, but is labile in 50 mM acetic acid. Initial attempts of mass spectrometry

(MS) and nuclear magnetic resonance (NMR) were not successful in deciphering its structure until the late 1990s. So the molecular nature of ESAF is probably unknown or unpublished.

Tissue levels of ESAF have been found to be in psoriasis lesions but not raised in nonlesional skin, and the high level correlated with PASI scores (Bhushan et al. 1999). In contrast to VEGF, which is produced predominantly by keratinocytes, and to a far lesser extent by fibroblasts, ESAF is produced in approximately equal amounts by both keratinocytes and fibroblasts. ESAF is also produced by growth plate cartilage and chondrocytes. Circulating ESAF is also found to be higher in psoriatic patients than in controls.

ESAF was originally thought to be primarily involved in angiogenic conditions where inflammatory cells are not evident, such as fetal bone growth and electrically stimulated skeletal muscles and proliferative retinopathy. However, high levels of ESAF occur in inflamed psoriatic skin lesions (Bhushan et al. 1999) and are also known to be elevated in inflamed growing intracranial tumors. Paradoxically, according to works done in the early 1980s, the majority of RA knee synovial fluids do not seem to have ESAF, but osteoarthritis (OA) and ankylosing spondylitis involving the knee seemed to have it. Patients with RA who had detectable ESAF in the synovial fluid had osteophytes. Of the rheumatic diseases, ankylosing spondylitis was found to have ESAF at the highest level.

5.2.5.7 PDGF

Discovery of PDGF as an angiogenic mitogen predates the discovery of the angiogenic function of VEGF by almost two decades. One of the original two papers that ascribed the angiogenic function to VEGF is "Vascular Permeability Factor, an Endothelial Cell Mitogen Related to PDGF" (Keck et al. 1989). PDGF was discovered in the early 1970s by Prof. Russell Ross, a pathologist cum biochemist researching atherosclerosis at the University of Washington, who had hypothesized that arterial smooth muscle proliferation is stimulated by growth-promoting substances that leak from the plasma through injured endothelium. He and his students systematically investigated various fractions of blood and honed in on a factor they named PDGF. Although PDGF is so named because it is synthesized, stored, and released by platelets, it is also produced by many types of cells, including smooth muscle cells, activated macrophages, and endothelial cells (tip cells). PDGF is a family of dimeric glycoproteins with A and B subunits that can form homodimers (AA, BB) or heterodimers (AB) and also includes PDGF-CC and PDGF-DD, which are exclusively homodimers. They activate dimeric PDGF receptors (PDGFRs) possessing intrinsic tyrosine kinase activity. PDGF is a potent mitogen, especially for mesodermal cells (e.g., pericytes, fibroblasts, vascular smooth muscle cells, glial cells, and chondrocytes). It induces chemotaxis and activation of neutrophils, monocytes, and fibroblasts. It also increases ECM synthesis. PDGF synergizes with TGFs in accelerating wound healing and angiogenesis. PDGF-BB especially is one of the most important factors in mural cell maturation and remodeling.

Espinoza et al. (1994) found that PDGFβ and its receptors were high in psoriatic fibroblasts; however, TGFβ production was similar in normal and psoriatic fibroblasts. PDGFR expression in psoriasis lesions was found to be strongly increased by Krane et al. (1991), who showed that this increase was comparable to that of chronic wounds.

5.2.5.8 TNFα

TNFα is an inflammatory cytokine whose antagonists are currently being successfully used in psoriasis, PsA, RA, and so forth. It was originally named TNF or lymphotoxin based on experiments in the late 1960s and early 1970s, when this factor was found to induce necrosis of fibrosarcoma cells. However, this factor is a general apoptotic signal to many cells unless rescued by some growth factor or other rescue mechanisms. It is one of the acute phase reactants circulating in blood that goes up during inflammatory conditions. Commonly, it is produced in response to danger signals or alarmins by activated macrophages or dendritic cells, although it can be produced by many other cell types, such as Th1 cells, NK cells, neutrophils, mast cells, keratinocytes, and endothelial cells. Structurally, it is a homotrimer that is formed in a membrane-bound state shed from the membrane by TNFα-converting enzyme (TACE), a "secretase." Originally, TACE was ADAM17, but now the action is known to be possible by ADAM9, 17, and 19 and MMP7 and 17. TNFα is the prototype member of a large superfamily of cytokines that cause receptor-mediated cell death.

TNFα has pleiotropic actions, including upregulation of adhesion molecules in vessels, and at the same time loosens up the junction, thus increasing edema, inflammatory cell recruitment, tip cell formation, sprouting angiogenesis, and expression of MHC molecules and antigen presentation. TNFα may downregulate VEGFR1 and 2 on endothelial cells in vitro, but in vivo, TNFα is often strongly angiogenic, with potency comparable to that of FGFs. Thus, it has a dual role in angiogenesis. TNFα is now considered a powerful and faster-acting upstream activator of VEGF.

Large amounts of TNFα have been found in all the layers of the epidermis and dermal vessels and inflammatory infiltrates, sera of psoriasis patients, the synovial membrane, and synovial fluids of PsA patients. In the arthritic synovial tissue, macrophages and endothelial cells express antigenic TNFα. Originally, TNFα in these diseases was thought to be a part of a Th1-type immune response. But as our understanding keeps increasing, Th17, Th22, and Th9 components have been invoked, and TNFα can collaborate with them.

5.2.5.9 NGF

Nerve growth factor (NGF) is an evolutionarily conserved polypeptide neurotrophin. It is secreted as a precursor complex of about a 130 kDa (7S) ternary complex of α, β, and γ subunits. The β and γ subunits are members of the kallikrein family of serine proteases, causing cleavage of the 7S precursor and generation of the active β-NGF. β-NGF causes promotion of neuronal survival, proliferation, and neurite outgrowth.

NGF receptors are tyrosine kinase A (TrkA), a receptor tyrosine kinase, and p75 neurotrophin receptor (p75NTR) (a neurotrophin receptor), a receptor that belongs to the TNF family. p75NTR is a common receptor for other neurotrophins, such as BDNF and NT3 and 4. TrkA and p75NTR together form the high-affinity receptor complex producing pro-survival and proliferative signaling. When p75NTR is expressed in the absence of TrkA, NGF can induce apoptosis through p75NTR-induced Rac GTPase-dependent activation of the c-Jun N-terminal kinase (JNK), including an injury-specific JNK3. The α9β1 integrin is a third receptor for NGF, which mimics TrkA in activity.

The nervous and vascular development share a lot of guidance and survival signals, and their interactions are bidirectional; that is, NGF can cause growth, survival, and migration of endothelial cells, and VEGF can do the same for neurites. NGF-induced angiogenesis is dependent on the α9β1 integrin, to which NGF can directly bind.

Psoriatic keratinocytes express high levels of NGF, as shown by Raychaudhuri et al. (1998) in the mid-1990s. Skin traumatized by tape stripping (simulated Koebner phenomenon) shows a marked upregulation of NGF in Koebner-positive lesions in 24 h and peaks in the next week. Cultured keratinocytes from nonlesional skin of psoriasis patients produced 10 times higher NGF than keratinocytes from healthy controls. The NGF receptors, p75NTR and TrkA, are upregulated in the terminal cutaneous nerves of psoriatic lesions. Autologous PBMCs activated by NGF and injected into the human skin SCID mouse xenotransplant reproduces psoriasis morphology, including the angiogenesis.

Rapid proliferation of terminal cutaneous nerves in the active psoriatic plaque has been documented. Elevated levels of neuropeptides, such as substance, calcitonin gene-related peptide (CGRP), and vasoactive intestinal peptide (VIP), in psoriatic lesions have been reported by a number of authors. All these together suggest that psoriasis may be considered a neuroimmunologic disease with neurogenic inflammation.

5.2.5.10 TGFβ

TGFβ belongs to the TGF and bone morphogenetic protein (BMP) family, whose founding members are TGFβ isotypes 1–3. TGFβ family members are homodimers, which are secreted in an inactive form. The dimerized proTGFs are cleaved by furin convertase to form a pair of latency-associated peptides (LAPs) derived from the N-terminal pro-domain noncovalently bound to the

TGFβ dimer, forming a small latent complex (SLC). SLC in turn binds to the latent TGFβ binding protein (LTBP), forming a larger complex called large latent complex (LLC), which is secreted, and after which LTBP may further complex with ECM components, for example, fibronectin and fibrillin. Activation or release of TGFβ requires proteolytic cleavage from the latent complex by extracellular proteases like MMPs and elastase.

TGFβ receptors are a superfamily of heterodimeric single-pass membrane serine/threonine kinase receptors (types I and II and type III [β-glycan]), and accessory receptor-like molecules, for example, endoglin, are not core TGFβ receptors. These receptors bind members of the TGFβ superfamily of growth factors, BMPs, growth differentiation factors (GDFs), activins inhibins, and so forth. The ligand-mediated sequential recruitment and phosphorylation of type II and then the type I receptor complex leads to a signaling complex that activates the SMAD family of transcription factors.

TGFβ is one of the most important mediators of wound healing and granuloma formation—a process dominated by angiogenesis. Like TNFα, TGFβ also shows the paradox of the inhibitory effect on endothelial cells in vitro but the stimulating effect in vivo, possibly due to recruitment of angiogenic accessory cells and also through ECM deposition and integrin upregulation. TGFβ has been speculated to stimulate angiogenesis indirectly by recruiting angiogenic macrophages, while it eventually also dampens the angiogenic response and stabilizes vessels by pericyte recruitment. TGFβ has a dual activity in modulating angiogenesis. It can stimulate the secretion of pro-angiogenic uPA receptor and MMPs, and it is also capable of upregulating the so-called "angiostatic" matrix metalloproteinase inhibitors (TIMPs). Thus, TGFβ is likely involved relatively more in later stages of angiogenesis, especially in vessel wall stabilization in collaboration with PDGF-BB and others.

One interesting piece of information about the potential role of TGFβ in psoriasis comes from the animal model–based finding that forced expression of wild-type TGFβ1 in the epidermis using a keratin 5 promoter causes the psoriasis phenotype to develop, and it even responds to drugs that work in psoriasis, for example, etanercept (TNFα blocker) and rosiglitazone (insulin sensitizer acting on PPARγ).

TGFβ1 is barely detectable in normal human skin epidermis because of its short half-life. In psoriasis patients, there is increased TGFβ1 in the epidermis and the serum, which correlates with disease severity. Increased TGFβ1 could possibly come from activated endothelial cells, fibroblasts, or inflammatory cells in psoriasis patients, all of which can produce more TGFβ1. However, whether a TGFβ1 increase in the lesion is a cause or consequence of the disease is not clear. There is a significant decrease of TGFβ receptors in lesional epidermis, which could potentially be a compensatory effect of the increased TGFβ1 ligand. Successful treatment decreases serum levels of TGFβ1 in patients with psoriasis (Flisiak et al. 2008).

Endoglin, a TGFβ accessory receptor, is known to be sharply localized to the margin zone of psoriasis and might be a part of the explanation for sharpness of the margin.

5.2.5.11 ECGF1 or PD-ECGF or TP or Gliostatin

Platelet-derived endothelial cell growth factor (PD-ECGF or ECGF1) is the same as the enzyme thymidine phosphorylase (TP) and is an endothelial-specific mitogen of modest potency (Micali et al. 2010). Extracellular DNA may be hydrolyzed to thymidine, which may act as a substrate for TP, which converts thymidine to 2-deoxy-D-ribose, which is chemotactic for endothelial cells and might be the basis for the angiogenic action of TP.

In psoriasis lesions, it is strongly expressed in epidermis with nuclear localization in basal keratinocytes and cytoplasmic localization in suprabasal layers (Creamer et al. 1997b).

5.2.5.12 Developmental Wingless and Hedgehog Pathways

5.2.5.12.1 Wingless Pathway

Wingless agonist Wnt5a is found to be upregulated, and inhibitors WIF1 (Wnt inhibitory factor 1) and Dkk (Dickkopf) were downregulated in both the dermis and epidermis of psoriasis lesions, suggesting effective activation of the Wnt pathway, which is angiogenic (Gudjonsson et al. 2010).

5.2.5.12.2 Hedgehog Pathway

This is another developmental pathway known to be involved in the regenerative process. One expression study showed increased expression of Shh, Kif7, and Gli1, and decreased SUFU and Gli3 RNA isolated from lesional epidermis, suggesting increased activity of the hedgehog pathway (Man and Zheng 2015).

TSP1 is the founding member of the TSP family. It is a multidomain adhesive matrix glycoprotein that mediates cell–cell and cell–matrix interactions. It can form disulfide-linked homotrimers or heterotrimers with TSP2. It is present in high concentrations in platelet α-granules, where it was discovered by Lawler et al. in 1978. It is also secreted by a wide range of epithelial and mesenchymal cells, including endothelial cells, smooth muscle cells, and fibroblasts.

It plays diverse roles in platelet aggregation, angiogenesis, and tumorigenesis. TSP1 and 2 are secreted into the ECM, but rather than serving structural roles, they have regulatory influence on cellular behavior by interaction with numerous receptors, proteases, cytokines, and so forth, and are thus are termed "matricellular" proteins.

Originally thought of as a natural inhibitor of neovascularization and tumorigenesis, TSP1 is capable of both positive and negative modulation (discussed in the general angiogenesis Section 5.1.2) of endothelial cell adhesion, migration, and proliferation.

The interactome of TSP1 is large. Some important examples include

- Adhesion molecules, for example, fibrinogen, fibronectin, laminin, and type V collagen
- Cell adhesion receptors, for example, CD36, β3 integrins (αvβ3 and αIIbβ3), β1 integrins (e.g., α3β1, α4β1, α6β1, and α9β1), syndecan, and integrin-associated protein (IAP) or CD47
- Proteases involved in angiogenesis, for example, plasminogen, urokinase, MMP, thrombin, cathepsin, and elastase

TSP, a matricellular protein, may regulate angiogenesis in dose-dependent and context-dependent ways and among some of the most pleiotropic regulators of angiogenesis. As early as 1994, Nicosia and Tuszynski (1994) had observed concentration-dependent microvascular outgrowth from aortic ring explants in collagen and fibrin matrices containing TSP1. Wound healing was also paradoxically delayed in TSP1-null and TSP1 and 2 double-null mice and was accompanied by a reduction in blood vessels and inflammatory cells, as opposed to TSP2-null, where wounds heal faster than normal, which was initially thought to be due to reduced macrophage chemotaxis and decreased latent TGFβ activation. TSP1 receptors CD36 and β1 integrin associate with the VEGFR2. The coclustering of receptors that regulate angiogenesis may provide the endothelial cell with a platform for the integration of positive and negative signals. Such clusters have sometimes been considered modular signallosomes called "angosomes." TSP1 can be directly pro-angiogenic in some contexts, for example, when working with syndecan 4.

The TSP level is decreased in psoriasis, which is probably a part of the proof of concept that TSP1 is an angiogenesis inhibitor. Nickoloff et al. (1994) showed a marked reduction in the level of TSP1 (accompanied by an increase in IL8) in conditioned medium of cultured human keratinocytes isolated from psoriasis, as opposed to normal keratinocytes that secrete TSP in abundance. This is in contrast to the increase in TSP1 (and endostatin) found in chronic urticaria.

In contrast to psoriasis, in which the low TSP level fits the age-old paradigm of TSP as an angiogenesis inhibitor, in PsA, TSP1 levels are increased and also raise another well-known inhibitor, endostatin (Sedie et al. 2013).

5.2.5.13 PAF

PAF is 1-O-alkyl-2-acetyl-sn-glycero-3-phosphocholine, a potent biolipid with its own receptor, "PAF receptor," a G-protein-coupled receptor (GPCR), involved in signaling in leukocyte recruitment, antigen presentation, inflammation, and angiogenesis. It is produced by all variety of cells, depending on the balance between its synthesis and degradation. PAF synthesis can happen through several routes. For example, in the case of PAF generation downstream of VEGF, it happens through a "remodeling pathway" of membrane phospholipid conversion into lyso-PAF by phospholipase A2 (sPLA2-V). Lyso-PAF is in turn acetylated into PAF by acetyl CoA:lyso-PAF acetyltransferase (lyso-PAF AT). PAF biological activity is abrogated by its platelet-activating factor acetyl hydrolase (PAF-AH). Autocrine loops of PAF signaling, at least in part, mediate many different angiogenic factors: VEGF, FGF, HGF, angiopoietins, TNFα, and so forth. VEGF signaling might be an intermediate step of amplification upstream of PAF, for example, for HGF and angiopoietins.

In K5.hTGFβ1 transgenic mice, PAF produced psoriasis lesions and its blockade can ameliorate more than the baseline (without exogenous PAF application). PAF blockade is able to block the autocrine upregulation of PAF itself, as well as expression Th17–related cytokines IL17A, IL17F, IL23, IL12A, and IL6 and the level of activated transcription factor STAT3.

5.2.5.14 YKL40

YKL40 is also variously known as chitinase 3–like protein 1 (CHI3L1) or cartilage gp39, breast regression protein 39 (BRP39), the 38 kDa heparin binding glycoprotein (gp38k), and chondrex. It is an enzymatically inactive (pseudochitinase or chitinase-like) member of the glycosyl hydrolase 18 (mammalian chitinase) family. The name YKL40 is derived from the first three amino acids present on the N-terminus of the secreted form and its molecular mass, 40 kDa. Chitin is (β-1-4)-linked N-acetyl-D-glucosamine. Although mammals do not produce chitin, after cellulose, chitin is the second most abundant biopolymer on earth. Chitin is a major component of a variety of environmental allergens, including house dust mites or fungal spores, and can act as a foreign alarmin to which YKL40 acts as the PRR and bridges innate and adaptive immunity. YKL40 has a highly conserved chitin binding domain but is enzymatically inactive due to substitution of an essential glutamic acid with leucine in the chitinase 3–like catalytic active site.

YKL40 is one of the major secreted proteins from many structural cells, for example, human articular chondrocytes, synovial cells, endothelial cells, and vascular smooth muscle cells, as well as inflammatory cells, for example, macrophages and mature neutrophils, and many tumor cells, especially the very aggressive and vascular ones, for example, gliomas. The biological functions of YKL40 are poorly understood, especially if there is any receptor. It seems to participate in many physiological and pathological processes, such as proliferation, inflammation, angiogenesis, mitogenesis, and remodeling. It is implicated in cancers, cardiovascular diseases, infections, and other disorders, for example, atherosclerosis, diabetes, psoriasis, atopic dermatitis, PsA, RA, OA, Crohn's disease, cystic fibrosis, Alzheimer's disease, and schizophrenia. Although no specific receptor is known, its ability to bind both proteins (e.g., type I collagen) and carbohydrates makes it a putative linking factor between proteomics and glycomics.

Circulating YKL40 increases with age, and it also acts as an acute phase reactant. Its level is influenced by IL6 and IL18, but not so much by TNFα. YKL40 in the serum is usually 10% higher than plasma but highly correlated. YKL40 knockout mice suggest that it has potential roles in T-cell, macrophage, and dendritic cell responses (especially Th2), and also apoptosis and tissue repair. However, chitin binding can cause a shift in the response, for example, from M2 to M1 for macrophages. Recently, it was shown that it is produced by human Th17 cells and correlates with inflammation in juvenile idiopathic arthritis.

Works of Rong Shao's group (e.g., Francescone et al. 2011) have shown that YKL40 plays a role in the upregulation of VEGF expression and enhances angiogenesis synergistically with VEGF. YKL40 has been shown to induce interaction of syndecan 1 and integrin αvβ3 in endothelial cells of αvβ5 in tumor cells through binding heparan sulfate chains of syndecan 1 on the cell surface and downstream activation of focal adhesion kinase (FAK) and ERK1 and 2, thus inducing VEGF-mediated further angiogenic cascade. The action of YKL40 on vascular smooth muscle action is supposed to restrict vascular leakage, and stabilizes vascular networks. Vascular sprouting and stability mediated by smooth muscle–like cells are dependent on signaling activation induced by YKL40, including

N-cadherin with β-catenin and smooth muscle α actin in cytoskeleton. The adhesion and permeability of human microvascular endothelial cells (HMVECs) modulated by YKL40 depend on the interaction of VE-cadherin with β-catenin and actin. Neutralizing anti-YKL40 antibodies (e.g., clone "mAY" for mice) have been shown to inhibit migration and tube 12 formation induced by YKL40 in a dose-dependent fashion, and also inhibited the VEGFR2 (Flk1/KDR) induction and mitogen-activated protein kinase (MAPK) ERK1 and 2 activation downstream of YKL40. Thus, targeting YKL40 is an important potential antiangiogenic target.

YKL40 serum levels have been shown to be high in psoriasis and even higher in PsA, but while some studies claimed correlation with disease activities, other studies did not find a direct correlation.

5.2.5.15 OPN

Osteopontin (OPN) is a highly negatively charged (acidic) phosphorylated sialoglycoprotein known by various names like bone sialoprotein (BSP) 1 and early T-lymphocyte activation (ETA) 1. It is produced by various immune cells, epithelial tissue, smooth muscle cells, osteoblasts, and tumors. OPN contains Arg-Gly-Asp (RGD) and other integrin-interacting motifs. Like VEGF, OPN is a hypoxia response protein. OPN is also a pro-inflammatory mediator involved in tissue repair and angiogenesis.

OPN is expressed at a higher level in psoriasis lesional skin than in nonlesional skin or controls, and its serum level has also been found to be high in psoriasis. In psoriasis, it is overexpressed in PBMCs and the skin of psoriatic lesions, but surprisingly, no correlation was found in patients with severity of disease, and PsA. It seems to interact with integrins and CD44 in a way that may aid Th1 and inhibit Th2 response. Thus, it has been suggested that OPN could represent a potential target for therapeutic intervention in psoriatic patients.

The angiogenic effect of OPN was earlier thought to work through IL1 upregulation in human monocytes, as it was supposedly abrogated by IL1 blockade. However, OPN is now known to confer direct as well as indirect endothelial cytoprotection through the activation of PI3K/AKT → Bcl-xL and NFkB, with VEGF acting as an amplifying intermediary. OPN induces VEGF through AKT and ERK. VEGF in a positive-feedback autocrine loop further amplifies PI3K/AKT and the ERK1/2 pathway. Blocking the feedback signal by either anti-VEGF antibody, PI3K inhibitor, or ERK inhibitor can partly block the OPN-induced endothelial cell (HUVEC) motility, proliferation, and tube formation. But blocking by anti-OPN or anti-αv3 integrin antibody completely abrogates the biological effects of OPN on HUVECs. The anti-OPN antibody is better than the anti-VEGF antibody in vivo as well. OPN might be a valuable target (potentially better than VEGF) for developing novel antiangiogenesis therapy.

5.2.5.16 Interleukins

A large number of ILs as a part of a complex cytokine network are involved in psoriatic angiogenesis, which is beyond the scope of this chapter (the roles of some of the integrins are covered in other chapters in this book). Some of the important ILs involved in angiogenesis of psoriasis are

- IL8 (CXCL8)
- IL17/IL23 axis
- IL20
- Some IL1 family members, especially IL18, IL33, and IL36

5.2.5.16.1 IL8

IL8, also called CXCL8, is a CXC family chemokine. IL8 is a chemokine with a defining CXC amino acid motif that was initially characterized for its leukocyte chemotactic activity, and is now known to possess tumorigenic and pro-angiogenic properties. IL8 is synthesized primarily as a 99-amino-acid peptide, processed to yield several active IL8 isoforms, with 72- and

77-amino-acid-long forms being the most common; the 72 variant is the major form secreted by monocytes and macrophages in culture, and the 77 variant is the major secretory product of nonimmune cells. Although originally named neutrophil chemoattractant, IL8 is a very potent chemoattractant for neutrophils, basophils, mast cells, and T lymphocytes, but not monocytes. It is involved in autoimmune, inflammatory, and other innate and adaptive immune responses. Transcriptional regulation by NFkB, AP1, and C-EBP/NF-IL6 and posttranscriptional regulation of mRNA stability by the AU-rich RNA instability element (ARE) regulated by MAPK are the main regulator of IL8 levels.

The IL8 receptors include CXCR1 and CXCR2, both GPCRs, and the Duffy antigen receptor for cytokines (DARC), another GPCR-like 7TM protein that is mostly endocytic for CXC and CC chemokines but is not G-protein coupled at the cytosolic end. The pro-angiogenic activity of IL8 occurs predominantly through CXCR2, which is common to other CXC chemokines, but CXCR1 also has some angiogenic action and is unique to IL8 and possibly GCP2 (CXCL6).

IL8 is directly angiogenic, as it can cause proliferation, survival, protease activation, and capillary tube formation of CXCR1- and CXCR2-expressing endothelial cells and enhances production of MMPs. The pro-angiogenic nature of IL8 is largely related to the Glu-Leu-Arg (ELF) motif immediately proximal to first N-terminal cysteine. ELF-positive CXC chemokines IL8 (CXCL8), ENA78 (CXCL5), GCP2 (CXCL6), and GRO-a, -b, and -c (CXCL1, 2, and 3) are all pro-angiogenic due to ELF. On the other hand, the ELF-negative CXC chemokine platelet factor 4 (CXCL4), Mig (CXCL9), and γ-interferon-inducible protein 10 (CXCL10) are antiangiogenic and block ELF-positive CXC chemokines and related VEGF and FGF actions.

5.2.5.16.2 IL17

In this chapter, IL17 mostly refers to IL17A and IL17F, which can form homo- as well as mutual heterodimers (unlike other members of this family). IL17 is central to the pathogenesis of psoriasis and PsA and all the other comorbidities. Cellular sources of IL17 have already been discussed in detail in Sections 5.2.4.6 and 5.3.3.2. Here it is reemphasized that IL17 is also a direct angiogenic cytokine. It was earlier thought that IL17 in itself probably had no direct mitogenic effect on vascular endothelial cells, and only stimulated migration and cord formation. However, some studies now show that at 20% oxygen, IL17 does stimulate proliferation, migration, and tubulogenesis in vitro. Whereas in a hypoxic environment it did not affect their migration and proliferation, it did increase their survival and tubulogenic properties. IL17 also has synergistic effects on bFGF-, HGF-, and VEGF-mediated angiogenesis through enhancing the respective proliferative rates of vascular endothelial cells compared with the agents used alone on endothelial cells. Using an endothelial cell–specific array, it was found that IL17-treated human and mouse aortic endothelial cells in vitro induced four genes, Cxcl1, Cxcl2, Il6, and Csf2, which are related to endothelial cell activation and are necessary for adhesion of monocytes to endothelial cells (Mai 2014). Activation of HMEC (a human dermal microvascular endothelial cell line procured from Sciencell, Carlsbad, California in Yuan et al. [2015]) with IL17 induced STAT3 phosphorylation and nuclear translocation, which was also associated with the induction of angiogenic cytokines GROα, granulocyte-macrophage colony-stimulating factor (GM-CSF), and IL8, and neutrophil recruitment. IL17 targeting is one of the most promising therapies for psoriasis and is covered in the therapy sections.

5.2.5.17 Antimicrobial Peptides and Alarmins Involved in Angiogenesis

As discussed in Section 5.1.4, pathogens or tissue damage produces PAMP and DAMP or alarmins. Most antimicrobial proteins are potent alarmins that activate PRR TLR or NLR and trigger the innate immune system and prime the adaptive immune system. It is becoming clear that many of the antimicrobial proteins are multifunctional, rather than pleiotropic. Many of these alarmins are charged molecules (usually positive), usually do not have a leader sequence, and thus are secreted by nonclassical secretion pathways, and can cross lipid membrane compartments. A large number of them not only activate the immune system but also modulate angiogenesis. Some examples relevant to psoriasis are briefly described below.

5.2.5.17.1 Cathelicidin Fragment LL37

Human cathelicidin antimicrobial protein hCAP18 is the only human cathelicidin whose mature fragment is LL37, which is a multifunctional polypeptide. LL37 is a basic and hydrophobic amino acid–rich 37-amino-acid peptide that is positively charged (6+) at pH 7.4. It is a naturally disordered peptide that folds upon binding to negatively charged nonself or hidden-self surfaces (e.g., DNA or f-actin). It aids in the development of the danger signal, and thus is a central component of innate immunity. Originally discovered for its microbicidal activity, LL37 transactivates the endothelial growth factor receptor (EGFR), inducing cytokine release and cell migration. It stimulates chemotaxis and angiogenesis through the GPCR, FPR2. LL37 is an inducer of tissue repair and wound healing, as well as tumor growth and progression. It is upregulated in ovarian, breast, and lung tumors. LL37 also recruits multipotent mesenchymal stromal cells into tumors.

In addition to the other important roles discussed above, it also has direct angiogenic action on endothelial cells, possibly through (1) formyl peptide receptor–like 1 and/or (2) LL37 → COX1 → PGE2 → EP3 signaling. In EPCs, through NFkB activation it leads to increased PSGL1 and E-selectin expression, which recruits them to ischemic tissue.

A key role for LL37 has emerged in the pathogenesis of psoriasis, RA, SLE, atherosclerosis, and so forth. Its role in developing the initial trigger of psoriasis by transporting self-DNA or -RNA to TLR9, or TLR7 or 8 in the opportune intracellular compartment has already been described earlier in this chapter.

5.2.5.17.2 S100 Family Members

The S100 proteins are a family of low-molecular-weight (9–13 kDa), ubiquitously expressed vertebrate proteins. They are called S100 because of their solubility in a 100% saturated solution with ammonium sulfate at neutral pH, as discovered by B. W. Moore in 1965. Each of them has two calcium binding EF-hand motifs in the monomer and forms antiparallel homodimers and occasionally heterodimers within themselves (e.g., S100A8/A9) and other proteins. They are not enzymes, but they are calcium-activated molecular switches similar to calmodulin or troponin C. They have pleiotropic intracellular and extracellular functions, for example, proliferation, differentiation, migration, energy metabolism, Ca2+ homeostasis, inflammation, and cell death. There are at least 25 members of S100, and some of their specific functions include scavenging of ROS and NO (i.e., S100A8/A9), cytoskeleton assembly (e.g., S100A1, S100A4, S100A6, and S100A9), membrane protein docking and trafficking (e.g., S100A10 and S100A12), transcription regulation and DNA repair (e.g., S100A4, S100A11, S100A14, and S100B), cell differentiation (e.g., S100A6, S100A8/A9, and S100B), release of cytokines and antimicrobial agents (degranulation) (e.g., S100A8/A9, S100A12, and S100A13), muscle cell contractility (e.g., S100A1), cell growth and migration (e.g., S100A4, S100A8/A9, S100B, and S100P), and apoptosis (e.g., S100A6, S100A9, and S100B). The S100 proteins, once extracellular, are saturated with calcium and do not act as a calcium sensing switch, but can now scavenge other transition metal ions, for example, Zn, Cu, and Mn, which might be part of their antimicrobial action.

Many of the S100 protein genes are clustered in the epidermal differentiation complex in human chromosome 1q21, which includes the PSORS4 locus, and 13 S100 proteins (S100A2, S100A3, S100A4, S100A6, S100A7, S100A8, S100A9, S100A10, S100A11, S100A12, S100A15, S100B, and S100P) are expressed in normal and/or diseased epidermis (Eckert et al. 2004). Of these, the following are overexpressed in psoriasis; some are regulated under the aryl hydrocarbon receptor nuclear translocator (Arnt)/Hif1b and are known to have angiogenic properties:

- S100A7 (psoriasin)
- S100A8 (calgranulin A, myeloid-related protein [MRP] 8)
- S100A9 (calgranulin B, MRP14)
- Calprotectin: Heterodimer of S100A8 and S100A9 (also called leukocyte protein L1 or cystic fibrosis antigen)

- S100A12 (calgranulin C, EN-RAGE)
- S100A15 (koebnerisin)

S100 proteins are involved in angiogenesis and modulate MMPs, TGFβ, FGF, VEGF, and so forth. The S100 proteins that are classically known to affect angiogenesis are S100A4, A7, A10, and A13, of which A7 is mainly increased in psoriatic epidermis and A4 is present in neutrophils. S100A4 dimerized with annexin 2, which enhances plasmin-mediated angiogenesis; also, it transcriptionally activates MMP13 and synergizes with VEGF for HUVEC migration via the receptor for advanced glycation end products (RAGE) receptor. S100A10 is also angiogenic in vivo. S100A13 affects angiogenesis through release of FGF1.

5.2.5.17.2.1 S100A7 S100A7 is also called psoriasin. S100A7 differs from the other S100 proteins of known structure in its lack of calcium binding ability in one EF hand at the N-terminus. The protein (and its close homolog S100A15, or koebnerisin) is overexpressed in the epidermal suprabasal compartment of hyperproliferative skin diseases, including psoriasis, and hence the name. S100A7 is present in the nucleus and cytoplasm in basal cells but is associated with the plasma membrane in spinous cells. Along with S100A10 and A11, S100A7 and A15 are targets for cornification through transglutaminase cross-linking (but not S100A8 or A9). S100A7 is known to strengthen the epithelial tight junction barrier via the GSK-3-β-catenin pathway, as well as MAPK pathways.

S100A7 expression is associated with increased blood vessel density in human breast cancer and acts through a dramatic regulation of MMP13 and VEGF, which shows opposite effects in vitro and in vivo. S100A7 also acts through upregulating pro-inflammatory pathways and recruiting myeloid cells, modulating multifunctional gene and CD74, and so forth. Serum S100A7 levels are increased in psoriasis. An S100A7 SNP has been associated with PsA. S100A7 has been shown to enhance osteoclast formation in vitro. Higher levels of S100A7 in the psoriatic plaques have been associated with PsA.

5.2.5.17.2.2 S100A8 and A9 S100A8 is also called calgranulin A or MRP8. S100A9 is also called calgranulin B or MRP14. At the time of discovery in 1987, they were actually called macrophage migration inhibitory factor (MIF)–related proteins: MRP8 and MRP14 (see Section 5.2.5.20). They preferentially form the S100A8/A9 heterodimer, which is called leukocyte protein L1 or cystic fibrosis antigen or calprotectin. These are abundantly expressed in myeloid cells, for example, neutrophils, monocytes, and early macrophages, and also to some extent in keratinocytes. In inflamed microvasculature, the S100A8/A9 complex is deposited onto the endothelium of venules associated with extravasating leukocytes. Normal tissue macrophages do not express S100A8/A9. Chronic inflammatory macrophages, for example, in RA, sarcoidosis, tuberculosis, or onchocerciasis, express both S100A8 and A9, but macrophages in acute inflammation usually express only S100A9. In neutrophils, the S100A8/A9 complex is the most abundant cytosolic protein and may represent almost 45% (30%–60%) of the soluble cytosolic protein content, and the level is 40-fold less in monocytes. This protein is also present in neutrophil granules, especially secondary granules, but the localization is blurred by the cytosolic abundance. IL10 indirectly and slowly stimulates S100A8/A9 production in a COX2-cAMP-dependent way, whereas Th2 cytokines IL4 and IL13 suppress them. Neutrophilic calprotectin, possibly largely cytosolic, is actively extruded with NETs, and this calprotectin is absolutely necessary for antifungal activity of NET in vitro.

It is present in most inflammatory exudates and is involved in neutrophil migration to the inflammatory sites. Fecal calprotectin has been used as a stool marker for IBD. BMDCs and MDSCs and tumor-associated macrophages secrete S100A8/A9. High levels of S100A9 in turn inhibit the differentiation of dendritic cells and induce accumulation of MDSCs. S100A8/A9 regulates neutrophil survival by the MEK-ERK signaling pathway via TLR4 and αMβ2 (Macl) integrin. In S100A9-deficient mice, the number of bone marrow neutrophils is decreased. Hypercalprotectinemia is a rare hereditary syndrome with extremely elevated serum levels of S100A8/A9 and S100A12 presenting with anemia, frequent infections, arthralgia, hepato- and splenomegaly, and stunted growth.

The autocrine action of S100A8/A9 on MDSCs acts through the RAGE and carboxylated glycans on MDSCs, activates NFkB and MAPK, and helps MDSC migration and sustains their perivascular accumulation. Many cytokines and growth factors, for example, TNFα, TGFβ, and VEGFA, can act upstream and stimulate S100A8/A9 expression, which is involved in the recruitment of BMDCs and MDSCs, helping the angiogenic milieu. The paracrine action of S100A8/A9 secreted by MDSCs acts on the endothelial cells through glycans, and possibly RAGE, and activates Macl and other integrins.

Serum levels of S100A8 and9 increase in psoriasis and correlate with disease activity. PsA synovium shows rich accumulation of S100A8 (calgranulin A, MRP8) and S100A9 (calgranulin B, MRP14) in the sublining regions, especially around the enlarged vessels (Ritchlin et al. 1998). In a transcriptomic microarray study, calprotectin was shown to induce a thrombogenic, inflammatory response in HMVECs by increasing pro-inflammatory chemokine and adhesion molecule mRNA and decreasing junction proteins and monolayer integrity, thus helping leukocyte (especially MDSC) transmigration.

5.2.5.17.2.3 S100A12 S100A12 is a relatively recent member, an additional phagocyte-specific S100 protein that is also called calgranulin C, calcium binding protein in amniotic fluid 1, and the extracellular newly identified receptor for advanced glycation end product binding protein (EN-RAGE). Neutrophils and macrophages bind tightly to S100A12-stimulated endothelium, possibly due to the VCAM1 and ICAM1 increase on endothelial cells. This upregulation is due to a signaling cascade downstream of S100A12 binding to EN-RAGE and heparan proteoglycans, partly mediated by NFkB, as shown by several works from Foell and Roth (2004).

5.2.5.17.2.4 S100A15 S100A15, also known as koebnerisin (named after the Koebner phenomenon of psoriasis), is a newer member of this family. It is highly homologous to psoriasin (S100A7) but has a distinct expression, function, and mechanism of action. It sometimes shows an opposite synergistic action from psoriasin. It has also been shown to enhance angiogenesis in murine breast cancer models, possibly associated with the induction of MMP2 and VEGF.

5.2.5.17.3 Human β-Defensins

β-Defensins directly and indirectly influence angiogenesis. Sometimes considered antiangiogenic, β-defensins do have known documented pro-angiogenic actions. IL17A and IL22 stimulate the expression of human β-defensin (HBD) 2. Human β-defensins are also noncognate ligands for chemokine receptor CCR6 and induce chemotaxis of dendritic cells and T cells, which can induce the angiogenic program. HBD2 stimulates chemotaxis of human endothelial cells to a level comparable to that of VEGF.

5.2.5.17.4 Azurocidin 1 or Cationic Antimicrobial Protein 37 or Heparin Binding Protein

This cationic antimicrobial protein, weighing 37 kDa, deserves special mention. Originally discovered from the azurophilic granule of neutrophil, this nonenzymatic protein structurally belongs to the serprocidin subgroup of the chymotrypsin-like protease superfamily comprising neutrophil elastase, cathepsin G, and proteinase 3, but two of the critical amino acids in the active site are changed. Primarily secreted by neutrophils, it can also be synthesized in endothelial cells. It causes opening up of endothelial junctions, and contraction of fibroblasts and endothelial cells, and specifically attracts, arrests, and recruits monocytes around vessels (remember from Section 5.2.4.4 that monocytes are an important component of both types of BMDCs: EPCs and RBCCs). Interestingly, azurocidin 1 is also taken up by endothelial cells and is targeted to the mitochondrial compartment, and it protects endothelial cells from apoptosis. Its role in atherosclerosis is under investigation by several groups, and its role in angiogenesis in the context of psoriasis is also worth exploring.

5.2.5.17.5 Catestatin

Catestatin (CST) is a 21-amino-acid cationic hydrophobic peptide derived from chromogranin A (CgA) 352–372 released by the autonomic nervous system. It is the major protein costored and coreleased with catecholamines from the storage vesicles in adrenal chromaffin cells and adrenergic neurons. It was originally described as an antihypertensive neuropeptide that inhibits nicotine-induced catecholamine release, acting as a physiological brake, which is behind the meaning of its name: cate-statin. Since metabolic syndrome is a strongly associated comorbidity of psoriasis, it must be noted that the CST plasma level is very tightly linked to hypertension, not only in clinically manifest hypertensive patients but also in their still normotensive offspring. The antiadrenergic action of CST is not yet fully understood. It requires a PI3K-dependent NO release from endothelial cells, and a possible mechanism might be its colocalization with heparan sulfate proteoglycans and their caveola-dependent endocytosis that activates endothelial nitric oxide synthase.

CST not only activates endothelial cells, but also enters and activates neutrophils, mast cells, monocytes, keratinocytes, and so forth. CST has recently also been found to be a cutaneous antimicrobial peptide. Like many of the other cationic antimicrobial proteins, CST also probably enters the cells through plasma membrane by a mechanism similar to the "trojan peptide" penetratin: the amphiphilic antennapedia homeodomain-derived 16-amino-acid peptide.

It can cause smooth muscle cell proliferation, monocyte and human mast cell migration, degranulation, and cytokine and chemokine amplification, especially of GM-CSF, MCP1/CCL2, MIP-1α/CCL3, and MIP-1β/CCL4, at the protein level. CST has been established as a pleiotropic hormone having effects on promoting angiogenesis in a bFGF-dependent mechanism. Thus, catestatin is an attractive candidate mediator for psoriasis-associated angiogenesis. One downside of comparing studies that measure CST is the wide variation between normal ranges, which might be due to the use of different antibodies that additionally detect larger interfering precursor peptides (CgA fragments) to different degrees.

It must also be remembered that CST does not act in isolation. CgA is a glycosylated, sulfated, and phosphorylated protein, 439 residues long, stored in the secretory vesicles of many neuroendocrine cells, neurons, and mast cells. CST is only one of many bioactive CgA fragments. Full-length Cg1–439 is antiangiogenic. Proteolytic cleavage of either Q76-K77 or R373–R374 bonds in CgA trims an antiangiogenic end, and the intermediate fragment is pro-angiogenic. The N-terminal fragments vasostatin 1 (CgA1–76) and vasostatin 2 (CgA1–113) are VEGF and HIF1a antagonists. The distal C-terminal 410–439 is also antiangiogenic and further processed into serpinin 411–436. On the other hand, as already mentioned, the catestatin 352–372 fragment is strongly pro-angiogenic. The mixture of circulating polypeptides forms a balance of anti- and pro-angiogenic factors that can be perturbed by thrombin or plasmin or other endogenous protease systems.

5.2.5.17.6 Lipocalin 2

An adipokine and an antimicrobial protein, this protein is known by several names: lipocalin 2 or siderocalin or neutrophil gelatinase (MMP9)-associated lipocalin (NGAL), human neutrophil lipocalin (HNL), 24p3, super-inducible protein 24 (SIP24), uterocalin, neu-related lipocalin (NRL), α2-microglobulin-related protein, and so forth. This 178-amino-acid-long protein may be found as a 24 kDa monomer, a 46 kDa disulfide-linked homodimer, or a disulfide-linked heterodimer with gelatinase B, that is, MMP9. Its strongest sources are neutrophils and kidney tubular cells when triggered by stress or cytokines. But it is also produced at low baseline levels in neutrophils, adipocytes, chondrocytes, endometrial cells, keratinocytes, macrophages, epithelial and endothelial cells, fibroblasts, vascular smooth muscle cells, hepatocytes, mesangial and microglial cells, pneumocytes, splenocytes, and thymocytes.

This molecule belongs to the lipocalin family of small lipid (and other hydrophobic molecule) binding proteins, which are as ancient as gram-negative bacteria and have only structural conservation but very little sequence homology; thus, it was difficult to discover by genomic searches.

The myriad names of lipocalin 2 testify to its multitude of actions. It was called a siderocalin, as it sequesters bacterial siderophores, thus restricting iron supply to bacteria. In the neutrophil granule, it binds to MPO, MMP9 β-galactosidase, and so forth, and is an important component of neutrophil intracellular traps. NGAL might protect proMMP9 from premature activation. Extracellular NGAL is internalized through several receptors, which also triggers several signaling pathways that are not yet fully elucidated. It may act as an intracellular iron metabolism regulator and also has an effect on subcellular localization of transmembrane proteins, such as cadherins and catenins. Several other lipocalins, for example, retinol binding proteins, are also potentially important for angiogenesis in psoriasis. The mother family "calycin," to which lipocalins belong, also includes fatty acid binding proteins (FABPs), some of which, for example, FABP4 and FABP5, are important in endothelial cell function and psoriasis.

It can also act as a pro-inflammatory cytokine and upregulate IL6, CXCL1, and CXCL8 (IL8). Lipocalin 2 blood and urine levels sharply rise by 1000-fold within 24–48 h in response to acute kidney injury, and it is now the most sensitive (but not so specific) biomarker for acute kidney injury. Lipocalin 2 is also considered a novel regulator of angiogenesis. In breast cancer, it is known to increase invasiveness and angiogenesis, which is ERK → HIF → VEGF dependent. However, in colon, pancreatic, and ovarian cancers, it has conflicting data, and some studies show it to suppress invasiveness and angiogenesis partly by suppressing VEGF and FAK.

High lipocalin 2 might be a marker of psoriasis and associated cardiovascular or metabolic risk, for example, association with high LDL. But if it remains high after treatment, it may not be a reliable indicator of inflammation, severity of psoriasis, or efficacy of antipsoriatic treatment. Lipocalin 2 has been implicated in exacerbating psoriasiform skin inflammation by augmenting IL17 immune cells. Lipocalin 2 is also considered a novel regulator of angiogenesis, an activity that is ERK → HIF → VEGF dependent.

5.2.5.17.7 RNAse 7

This is a lysine-rich cationic antimicrobial peptide of the RNAse A family related to angiogenin (RNAse 5). RNAse 7 so far has not been directly proven to be angiogenic, but it is highly expressed in psoriatic epidermis and is supposed to downregulate Th2.

5.2.5.17.8 Y-P30 and Other Dermicidin Peptides

In contrast to the cationic antimicrobials above, dermicidin (DCD) is an anionic antimicrobial protein secreted by eccrine sweat glands, and it is also a skeletal muscle myokine. It is secreted as a 110-amino-acid precursor whose first 30 amino acids may be cleaved into Y-P30. Although DCD expression is constitutive in eccrine sweat glands and is not supposedly increased in inflammatory conditions like psoriasis, DCD is known to be upregulated in chronic wounds. Y-P30 multimerizes with pleiotrophin and binds to syndecan 2 and 3. The survival-promoting peptide Y-P30 has neurite outgrowth-promoting effects in vitro and is known to also be expressed in placenta—a highly angiogenic organ. DCD and its 526 bp splice variant DCD-SV, coding for a 12.1 kDa protein with a different C-terminus without the hydrophobic coiled-coil structure (amino acids 80–103), are thought to be essential for the antibacterial function, and are involved in the aggressiveness of breast carcinoma through ERB-B signaling. Downregulation of DCD resulted in decreased levels of several genes involved in oxidative stress, hypoxia, and angiogenesis, including disulfide isomerase–associated 3, 4, and 6 (PDIA); the stress 70 kDa protein chaperone (STCH); the heat shock 70 kDa protein 5 (GRP78); hypoxia-inducible gene 2 protein (HIG2), and VEGFA and B.

5.2.5.17.9 Galectin 3

Galectins are a family of at least 15 soluble mammalian β-galactoside binding lectin-type alarmins with pleiotropic intracellular and extracellular functions. Galectin 3 (Gal3) is unique among galectins in that it is the only member of the chimera-type group with a C-terminal carbohydrate recognition domain (CRD) and a large N-terminal protein binding domain, and it can also uniquely form pentamers. Some of the functions of Gal3 include RNA splicing, differentiation, apoptosis, and cell–cell or cell–matrix interactions. Gal3 may be expressed as MMP cleavable and noncleavable forms. Gal3 has complex context-dependent immune functions. It was earlier considered to be a Th2 polarizing factor and is also known to induce monocyte–macrophage differentiation, interfere with dendritic cell fate decision, regulate apoptosis of T lymphocytes, and inhibit B-lymphocyte differentiation into plasma cells. Gal3 is considered an important mediator downstream of VEGF- and bFGF-mediated angiogenic responses. In angiogenic pericyte endothelial cross talk, Gal3-dependent oligomerization is supposed to potentiate NG2-mediated activation of α3β1 integrins. A part of Gal3 action is through blocking VEGFR internalization. MCP is a natural inhibitor of Gal3, which might prevent the last action and is a candidate antiangiogenic drug.

Gal3 is constitutively expressed in normal keratinocytes, upregulated in atopic dermatitis, and downregulated in keratinocytes and dendritic cells of psoriatic epidermis. However, the psoriatic capillaries strongly upregulate Gal3 and Gal3-reactive glycoligands.

A very high level of Gal3 is found in RA fibroblast-like synoviocytes and induces mononuclear cell–recruiting chemokines (especially CCL5) uniquely from synovial fibroblasts, but not matched skin fibroblasts, via a PI3K signaling pathway. Gal3 has been proposed as a serologic signature of pre-RA. Earlier, it was thought that extracellular Gal3 is deleterious for the joint, and Gal3-blocking clinical trials are going on (NCT02800629). However, now it seems that Gal3 reinforces the lubricin boundary layer of synovial fluid, which, in turn, enhances cartilage lubrication and, along with its antiapoptotic properties, likely helps delay the onset and progression of OA. Thus, Gal3 is now suspected to have dual and/or concentration-dependent bimodal functions in synovial joints, with direct mechanical and cytoprotection, but possibly indirect development of arthritis through immune and possibly angiogenic mechanisms.

5.2.5.18 Clusterin or Apolipoprotein J

Clusterin is a 40 kDa glycoprotein that was originally discovered as being responsible for allowing trypsinized Sertoli cells to form clusters. It has multiple functions related to apoptosis, inflammation, complement regulation, proliferation, tissue differentiation, tissue remodeling, membrane recycling, lipid transportation, cell–cell or cell–substratum interaction, and extracellular chaperoning. Also known as apolipoprotein J, it is associated with HDL and can promote cholesterol and phospholipid export from macrophage foam cells, and exhibit cytoprotective and anti-inflammatory actions by interacting with lots of known inflammatory proteins. It also plays important roles in vascular smooth cell migration, adhesion, and proliferation, thus regulating angiogenesis and vascular remodeling. Overexpression of clusterin in ovarian cancer has been associated with increased angiogenesis and partly associated with increased VEGF. In prostate cancer, it was shown that the secreted form of clusterin may have antiapoptotic properties, whereas the nuclear form has proapoptotic properties. Similarly, increased free clusterin or apolipoprotein J in hyperlipidemia serum is paradoxically associated with decreased apolipoprotein J content in lipoproteins. Thus, overall clusterin is a multifunctional protein with pleiotropic regulatory effects on angiogenesis-related diseases.

Clusterin circulating levels are supposed to be low in psoriasis. In the joints, it is predominantly expressed by synoviocytes and is also detected in synovial fluids. It is capable of inducing apoptosis in fibroblast-like synoviocytes, which is thought to be a homeostatic mechanism. It is downregulated in RA compared with OA, possibly consistent with the pannus formation. Clusterin antisense oligonucleotides using a capillary endothelial (HUVEC) viability assay have been studied as a candidate antiangiogenic therapy in inflammatory arthritis.

5.2.5.19 Chemerin

Chemerin belongs to adipokines, that is, adipose tissue–derived cytokines, which also happen to include molecules as famous as TNFα and IL6. As already discussed, chemerin is the strongest candidate for the pDC recruitment chemoattractant in psoriasis, and like many other adipokines, it is also directly pro-angiogenic.

Chemerin levels in psoriasis skin were high compared with those of normal skin and atopic dermatitis, and the timing specifically coincides with early psoriatic skin lesions and especially the time of pDC recruitment (Albanesi et al. 2009). Thus, it supports a role for the chemerin/ChemR23 axis in the early phases of psoriasis.

Several other adipokines, for example, leptin, resistin, visfatin, vaspin, and omentin, are known to be upregulated in both psoriasis and metabolic syndrome—a comorbidity associated with increased but pathological adipose tissue metabolism. On the other hand, some other adipokines, for example, adiponectin, showed conflicting data.

5.2.5.20 Macrophage Migration Inhibitory Factor

MIF was discovered more than a half century ago in the mid-1950s, and it still remains an enigma and has been dubbed the "most interesting factor." It was characterized as one of the first lymphokines or cytokines discovered from activated T-cell products, which halted "random migration" of macrophages in vitro and was thought to be involved in delayed-type hypersensitivity. It had to wait to 1989 to be cloned, and in the 1990s, it was rediscovered several times, for example, as a "pituitary-derived cytokine that potentiates lethal endotoxemia." At first, T cells were thought to be the main cellular source of MIF. However, monocytes, macrophages, blood dendritic cells, B cells, neutrophils, eosinophils, mast cells, basophils, and so forth, were added sources. It can be produced by virtually every cell irrespective of epithelial, mesenchymal, or endothelial lineage, with especially high levels of expression in cells and tissues that are in direct contact with the environment, such as the lung, the epithelial lining of the skin, and the gastrointestinal and genitourinary tracts and parts of the brain that sense blood, for example, the hypothalamopituitary axis, and some neuroendocrine tissue, for example, the adrenal. It has many unique features, and one feature is constitutive production, which makes it unique among all cytokines, with most of the others being induction dependent. Like several other cytokines (e.g., IL1), MIF is secreted by a nonconventional leader-peptide-less pathway, but in this case, it involves an ABC transporter. It also enters target cell cytoplasm by crossing the membrane, somewhat similar to many of the antimicrobial peptides, but after endocytosis in this case.

Despite the narrow sense of its function implied by its name, it is now known as a highly pleiotropic protein. One major function of MIF is to act as a counterregulatory hormone to glucocorticoid and "critical upstream regulator" of innate immunity, likely regulating the baseline set point and magnitude of peak of an immune response. Its plasma levels generally rise along with ACTH or glucocorticoid. In antigen-presenting cells, the invariant (Ii) chain associated with class II MHC necessary for MHC peptide loading happens to come to the cell surface in the name of CD74 and act as one of the receptors for MIF, and CD44 is a coreceptor. MIF is also known as a glycosylation-inhibiting factor (GIF), possibly because it can suppress IgE synthesis and N-glycosylation.

In fibroblasts, MIF is secreted through a PKC-dependent pathway following cell adhesion to the ECM and plays important roles in integrin-mediated signaling and MAPK, cyclin D1 expression, and cell cycle progression. In monocytes and mesenchymal cells, MIF production paradoxically enhanced by glucocorticoids or TLR signaling and in a autocrine loop that activates several pathways, especially sustained ERK1/2 MAPK, is initiated by extracellular action of MIF and is further aided intracellularly by MIF crossing into cytosol and the JAB1-MIF complex, resulting in cytosolic PLA2 that produces arachidonic acid and pJNK and activated AP1, which can lead to the production of TNF and other pro-inflammatory cytokines, inhibit p53, and give survival signals. Upstream MIF signaling is important in maintaining the expression of TLR4 (LPS receptor) through the ETS family of transcription factors, for example, PU.1. In B lymphocytes, CD74, upon binding MIF, undergoes "regulated intramembrane proteolysis" (RIMP), and the intracellular fragment has several transcription activities, including regulating NFkB.

MIF does not belong to any cytokine superfamily, and its only other sequence-based homolog in the human genome is the closely linked L-dopachrome isomerase (D-DT), which also has similar action. MIF itself has at least two enzymatic actions, but their relation to its activity has been drawing controversy. It has a tautomerase action that can be blocked by a large number of drugs that show anti-inflammatory potential. It also has an active thioreductase domain. Drugs that inhibit tautomerase activity protect against death due to sepsis. The mature MIF is 115 amino acids long, of which 12.5 kDa monomers trimerize into a barrel-shaped protein. Its unique structure gives a topological resemblance to IL8 with a pseudo-ELR motif and can also bind CXCR2 and CXCR4, which explains its migration arrest-type chemokine action and also a part of its angiogenic actions. MIF knockout mice were initially thought to be phenotypically normal. However, they show premature birth and subtle defects in lung maturation due to a delay in developmental regulation by VEGF and glucocorticoids. MIF knockout studies also show a regulatory role for MIF in hyperoxia-induced injury in the developing murine lung and angiopoietins 1 and 2, and their receptor Tie2 synergizes with it. Gremlin 1, which is a natural antagonist of BMPs, for example, BMP2, 4, and 7, has also been shown to be an antagonist of MIF.

Several studies have shown that angiogenic and tumor-promoting action of MIF and anti-MIF significantly reduced tumor-induced angiogenesis in in vitro models. MIF is known to promote all aspects of angiogenesis in HUVECs, and possibly through MAPK- and PI3K-dependent ways. SiRNA knockdown of MIF has been shown to reduce the level of VEGFC through MAPK signaling in MCF7 breast cancer cell lines. Some of the enzyme inhibitors, as well as some anti-MIF antibodies, are currently being explored, for example, orally active inhibitors from Avanir AVP-13546 and AVP-13748 as anti-inflammatory drugs, and the anti-MIF antibody studied in tumors in a registered clinical trial (NCT01765790). However, MIF action is not unipolar. MIF is also involved in M2-to-M1 macrophage polarization. MIF downregulation has been recently discovered as a novel mechanism of resistance to antiangiogenic (bevacizumab) therapy, leading to M2 macrophage polarization and compensatory angiogenesis.

When MIF was discovered as macrophage MIF in the 1950s and 1960s, the "random migration" out of capillaries was explored as a random historical technique. However, the concept of BMDCs and MDSCs (see Section 5.2.4.4) was not known at that time. MIF-depleted tumors not only grow slowly and have less angiogenesis, but they also have fewer MDSCs and less metastasis. Thus, the migration halting was no random action, and MIF is now a well-established recruiter of MDSCs. MIF has also been nicknamed metastasis/MDSC-inducing factor. Thus, in addition to SDF1 (CXCL12), MIF plays an important role in "retaining" vascular supportive BMDCs and MDSCs near the vessels.

MIF action has been associated with the mechanism of a lot of inflammatory immune and infectious diseases, including human psoriasis, RA, diabetes, atherosclerosis, cardiovascular disease, SLE, and many animal models, including experimental arthritis. Two polymorphisms in the MIF gene promoter are associated with psoriasis, PsA, RA, and systemic-onset juvenile arthritis (Donn et al. 2004). MIF has already been considered a therapeutic target in RA because MIF stimulates TNFα, IL1, IL6, IL8, and prostaglandin synthesis from macrophages, and IL8, VEGF, RANKL (receptor activator of NFkB ligand), MMP1 and 3, phospholipase A2, COX2 in synovial fibroblasts, and MMP9 and MMP13 osteoblasts, and activates osteoclasts. It should be considered a target in PsA and psoriasis as well. It may potentially be a factor even more upstream of the IL23/IL17 axis, though some studies claim that the IL17 rise in obesity is independent of the high MIF also seen in obesity. The more upstream a factor is, the better is its potential to be a magic bullet target for a pathway.

5.2.5.21 MicroRNAs as Regulators of Angiogenesis in Psoriasis

miRNAs (or miRs) belong to a class of non-protein-coding regulatory RNAs. Since their discovery in 1993, literally thousands of miRNAs have been reported in public repositories and are thought to regulate more than one-third of all protein-coding genes. Thus, miRNAs are probably the most abundant regulators of gene expression in humans. miRNAs have now been associated with almost every physiologic and pathologic process, including chronic inflammatory skin diseases and arthritis.

Specific miRNAs that been shown to regulate angiogenesis in vivo are sometimes dubbed angio miRNAs. Some example angiomiRNAs include the following:

- miR126, an endothelial-restricted miRNA, regulates vessel integrity and development.
- miR378, miR296, and the miR17–92 cluster have roles in tumor angiogenesis.

Micro RNAs that have been found to be differentially expressed in psoriasis (Hawkes et al. 2016) can be further classified into relatively enriched miRs and relatively downregulated miRs.

Micro RNAs known to be relatively enriched in Psoriasis include:

- miR21 (promotes inflammation and inhibits apoptosis)
- miR31 (feedback amplification through NFkB)
- miR221 and 222 (via activated metalloproteases)
- miR146 (SNP predisposition, targets regulators of TNF e.g., IRAK1 & TRAF6)
- miR203 (suppresses SOCS-3 causing sustained activation of STAT3)
- miR184 (affects biogenesis of miRs by by targeting Argonaut in RISC)
- miR210 (regulates Tregs by targeting FoxP3)
- miR31 (regulates NF-kB by STK40, keratinocyte proliferation by protein phosphatase 6)

Micro RNAs reported to be relatively downregulated in Psoriasis include:

- miR125b (targets FGFR2)
- mir99a (targets IGF1R & MEK1, Cyclin E1)
- miR 424 (also targets IGF1R & MEK1, Cyclin E1)

Some of the synthetic miRNA agonists and antagonists are under intense research. Some show preliminary encouraging research. For example, miR21 has been one of the short-listed candidate targets (Huang et al. 2015), as it is upstream of both VEGF and IL6.

5.2.5.22 Regnase 1 or ZC3H12A or MCPIP1

Zinc finger CCCH-type containing 12A (ZC3H12A) or monocyte chemotactic protein–induced protein 1 (MCPIP1), also known as regnase 1, is a 599-amino-acid 66 kDa multifunctional intracellular protein. It contains three functional domains: a PIN domain with endoribonucleolytic activity like RNase-L, a CCCH-type zinc finger domain that mediates AU-rich mRNA binding similar to tristetraprolin (TTP), and a ubiquitin binding domain with deubiquitinase activity. It can act as a rapid-response endoribonuclease antimicrobial protein that is expressed in high levels by psoriatic keratinocytes and reduces to normal levels after clinical treatments with anti-IL17A/IL17R neutralizing antibodies. In monocytes, regnase 1 downregulates IL6 and IL12B mRNAs, thus suppressing inflammation, whereas in T cells, it reduces T-cell activation by targeting c-Rel, Ox40, and IL2 mRNAs.

In an ischemia–reperfusion injury model of angiogenesis, it is upregulated and modulates cell migration and apoptosis of HUVECs through MAPK and PI3K/AKT pathways. It also enhances the angiogenic and cardiomyogenic potential of murine bone marrow–derived mesenchymal stem cells. It is also known to play a role in EndMT.

5.2.5.23 Other Potential Angiogenic Mediators

The list of angiogenic factors (pro, anti, and dual) is very long and not possible to catalog here. Only some were covered above, and just a few more, which were once thought important but are no longer so much favored by evidence from animal experiments, are mentioned just to give some examples.

TGFα is member of the epidermal growth factor (e.g., F) family and binds to the EGFR, which is upregulated in psoriasis lesions and could potentially be an angiogenic mediator. But the animal model of TGFα overexpression does not support its role in causality for psoriasis or associated angiogenesis.

Keratinocyte growth factor (KGF), also known as FGF9, is strongly upregulated in psoriasis epidermis and is capable of stimulating angiogenesis. But its angiogenic role in psoriasis is not supported by animal models.

A very large number of known and unknown angiogenic mediators are potentially involved, and we are just barely starting to understand some of the patterns within such complex phenomena. A lot of neutrophil and mast cell substances may play important roles. For example, molecules as well known as cathepsins and tryptase may play angiogenic roles, as well as immunomodulatory roles.

5.3 ANGIOGENESIS IN PSORIATIC ARTHRITIS

5.3.1 Overview of Angiogenesis in Psoriatic Joints

Rheumatologists and immunologists have had a special interest in angiogenesis. The majority of studies in regard to angiogenesis in inflammatory diseases had been carried out in RA since the early observation of marked prominence of vascular tissue in the pannus of a RA synovium, which grows in an angiogenesis-dependent tumor-like locally invasive fashion. Like RA, psoriasis can also develop pannus of the synovium. However, the synovial thickening itself in psoriasis might not be as remarkable as RA, but the early dilated blood vessels and angiogenesis in PsA are usually more remarkable and start very early compared with the progress of arthritis.

The angiogenic phenotype of PsA is somewhat similar to reactive arthritis, in which eventually the elongated tortuous dilated vessels in irregular bushy shapes can be seen in video arthroscopy (Reece et al. 1999) developing relatively rapidly in contrast to the autoimmune RA, where straight well-remodeled angiogenesis with straight branches develops slowly over time, leading to the thick hyperplastic synovium (McGonagle et al. 2007). PsA has a 20% risk of becoming the mutilating type, and thus early intervention to prevent angiogenesis is a very high-priority research topic.

5.3.1.1 Microcirculation of Normal Synovium

The synovial joints require us to maintain stability despite preserving movement capacity and weight bearing, and have evolved into a structure that normally has a division of labor between the cartilage and the synovium. The articular cartilages are generally smooth avascular hyaline cartilage that constitutes the extremely smooth gliding surfaces, which also bear the weight. They are avascular and yet metabolically active. To compensate for the avascular nature of the cartilage, normal synovium, especially the lining region, has a high density of microvessels very close to the intima, including fenestrated capillaries that both contribute a component of the lubricating synovial fluid and satisfy the oxygenation and metabolic demands of the juxtaposed avascular hyaline cartilage, especially the articulating surfaces of the cartilage. The deepest part of the articular cartilage may be supported by oxygen and metabolites diffusing a short distance from subchondral vessels in the bone that themselves do not cross the osteochondral junction. But this diffusion in adults is limited by calcification of the deepest cartilage layer, leaving the synovium as the major nutrient and oxygen supplier of the cartilage.

The synovial supplying arteries anastomose and branch in a few well-organized layers of arcades that have a higher density of thin-walled vessels toward the synovial lining region, fewer but thicker vessels in deeper synovium, and another layer of thinner vessels feeding the capsule (Walsh and Pearson 2001). The microvasculature also forms a lot of sinuous convolutions to accommodate the joint movements (Levick 1995). The vascular arcades of the synovium, once formed, are generally stable and constitute phenotypically mature vessels with normal innervation and vasoregulatory systems. Angiogenic proliferation is not usual in the normal synovium.

5.3.1.2 Microcirculation of Arthritic Synovium

In chronic arthritis, inflammation increases angiogenesis as well as concurrent regression, leading to destabilization and disorganization. Thus, the hierarchy of the arcades is lost. The synovial lining layer, which needs the most blood supply, may develop relatively less vascularity with somewhat bigger vessels, and in contrast, the deeper layer may now have a higher number of smaller vessels that are immature, unstable, and leaky. The modal depth of capillaries from the intima in normal synovium is about 35 microns in the human knee, but in RA it increases to 75 microns (Levick 1995). On the other edge of the synovium, the very superficial region near the capsule might not always show much vascular change unless the capsule is overstretched. The newer vessels that form in the inflamed synovia may have a different type of innervation, for example, fine unmyelinated pain fibers, that may increase pain sensation and also may not be able to generate the regular vasomotor responses, potentially leading to shunting of more oxygenated blood away from the articular surfaces and toward skin aggravating the local hypoxia.

In classic inflammatory-type arthritis typified by RA, but also to some extent spondyloarthropathies including PsA, the thickened vascularized synovium may form invasive structures called pannus that show a tumor-like invasion into articular cartilage and subchondral bone from the synovial side and may also erode and interpose between the joints aggravating pain on movement. Whereas in degenerative arthritis typified by OA, but also to some extent by aging and a subset of PsA, subchondral vessels may show increased angiogenesis that no longer respects the osteochondral junction, and invades from the bony side both directly and indirectly, through endochondral ossifications and osteophytes, into the cartilage and the synovium.

5.3.1.3 Noninvasive Detection of Angiogenesis and Inflammation in the Joint

Noninvasive detection of angiogenesis and inflammation, for example, by power Doppler ultrasound or MRI, has been employed in patients to detect synovitis at earlier stages (Wakefield et al. 2004) or follow disease progression or treatment response. Dynamic contrast-enhanced (DCE) MRI that involves injection of an IV contrast, followed by detection of time-dependent changes in MRI signal, demonstrates the degree of synovial inflammation, especially vessel permeability, and has been shown to be a sensitive tool to detect changes after treatment, which may cause reduced vascularity and/or reduced inflammation. Labeled cyclic RGD peptides have been used for noninvasive imaging, for example, through positron emission tomography scans, and have been used to measure the angiogenic activity in arthritis.

5.3.2 "Entheseal Organ" in Normal versus PsA versus Aging and Overlap Syndromes

The synovium, as an anatomical rule, attaches to bone at the bone–cartilage interface, rather than encroaching on the surface of the hyaline articular cartilage. This is also the site where the joint capsule and its ligaments insert, that is, the enthesis. *Enthesis* is a general term for insertion sites into bone for a variety of structures, including tendons, ligaments, joint capsules, or fascia. The articular enthesis, like the sublining immediately below the synovium, is also very highly vascular in structure. However, the so-called extra-articular enthesis is also frequently associated with synovium-like structures, for example, the subtendinous bursa, and is the basis of the SEC concept described below (see also Section 5.2.1).

Fibrocartilaginous metaplasia, that is, conversion of tendons or sometimes ligaments into fibrocartilage, is common at compression stress-bearing sites, for example, entheses and wraparound pulleys. Fibrocartilage, unlike hyaline cartilage, develops with hyaline vessels, which also help align collagen bundles.

Enthesitis is observed in 30%–50% of PsA patients and most commonly involves the plantar fascia and Achilles tendon, but may involve the patella, iliac crest, epicondyles, and supraspinatus insertions. McGonagle et al. (1999) proposed that entheseopathy may be the much sought after "common thread" between PsA and the other spondylarthropathies (SpA). The pathology in the SpA, including PsA, is to a large extent centered around enthesiopathies. Although traditionally considered focal, insertional disorders, MRI, and Doppler ultrasound imaging of enthesiopathies suggest the presence of more diffuse changes with involvement of the adjacent bone and soft tissue. McGonagle et al. have been proposing to view these insertion sites not merely as focal attachments, but as parts of an "enthesis organ complex" that may dissipate stress concentration at the bony interface away from the attachment site itself. They have furthered the concept to SEC based on the anatomic, functional, and physiologic interdependence between the synovial membrane and entheses. The stress-bearing nature of SEC makes it prone to microdamage that may produce chronic inflammation and angiogenesis spreading into the associated synovia in SpA. Whether SpA may involve the release of autoantigens from the enthesis organ has been speculated but not yet proved, and unlike RA, where autoantibodies like rheumatoid factor and anti-cyclic citrulinated peptide are rare in Ps or PsA, McGonagle et al. have proposed that rather than autoimmunity, these diseases are autoinflammatory. It is an extension of "Mechnikov's thorn" or Polly Matzinger's "danger signal" hypothesis extrapolated from their demonstration that subclinical enthesitis starts to develop around relatively more mechanically strained joints (McGonagle and McDermott 2006) that get highly vascularized.

This entheseopathy theory of disease also provides an anatomical explanation of why nail involvement in psoriasis predicted both PsA development and distal interphalangeal (DIP) joint involvement in PsA (McGonagle and Tan 2015). DIP joint entheses, including the extensor tendons, collateral ligaments, and dermal ligaments, provide an elaborate anchorage mechanism to the nail.

Power Doppler ultrasound imaging and contrast MRI in PsA can be even more useful than RA because of the prominent angiogenesis and enhanced blood flow in regions of arthritis synovitis, tenosynovitis, enthesophytes, and early erosive disease.

5.3.3 Differences between Angiogenesis in PsA and Other Arthritis

5.3.3.1 Angiogenesis in RA versus PsA/SpA and OA Overlap

One of the upcoming patterns of concepts distinguishing the etiopathogenesis of RA and SpA is that RA is more autoimmune in nature and starts in the synovium, where the angiogenesis may be secondary to the inflammation and hypoxia, whereas SpA is more autoinflammatory in nature and starts from nonhealing microdamages in enthesis organs, which involves angiogenesis at a very early stage. In fact, some of the animal models earlier considered to be models for RA are now being shifted to be more of a model for SpA, for example, the TNFα transgenic model, liver overexpressing IL23 model, and SKG mouse model. This model reclassification was mainly due to early-stage histologic investigations that showed primary enthesitis subsequently spreading to the adjacent tissues, including synovium (McGonagle and Tan 2015).

There are many references that have listed histomorphological differences between PsA and RA and OA, most of which note that the pattern of vascularization is the most reliable feature of PsA (Georg Fassbender 2003; Veale and Fearon 2015). The RA synovium is dominated by lining layer thickening and pannus formation, and so the vascular volume, although increased compared with baseline, is outcompeted by growth of the dense and edematous fibrous stroma of RA, which makes the microvascular arcades somewhat receded from the lining and dysregulated branching sprouting angiogenesis all through the depth of the synovium. In contrast, in early PsA episodes, the lining layer thickening is transient, and dominated by increased length, dilation, and further thinning of the walls of the microvascular arcade loops that grow into the slender synovial villi, possibly by elongation-type angiogenesis similar to that of the psoriatic plaques (Georg Fassbender 2003; Veale and Fearon 2015). However, in late PsA the synovium is dominated by small immature capillaries with swollen endothelium (Espinoza et al. 1982; Veale and Fearon 2015).

5.3.3.2 Possible Mechanistic Explanation for the Different Types of Angiogenesis

One explanation for neovascularization in the early phases of PsA that has been offered is the potentially increased expression of the αvβ3 integrin (Georg Fassbender 2003) or higher levels of TGFβ1 and VEGF in the synovial membrane (Fearon et al. 1998). Lower levels of the leukemia inhibitory factor (LIF) and oncostatin M explain why PsA has less lining layer hyperplasia despite a higher degree of angiogenesis near the lining.

However, the newer literature is gradually zeroing in on the immune pathomechanistic differences between RA and PsA. While RA is driven primarily by B- and T-cell autoreactivity, PsA and SpA are driven by innate immune cells (e.g., macrophages, PMN cells, and mast cells). Seropositive RA was generally supposed to exhibit more profound destruction of trabecular bone architecture than seronegative RA or PsA, suggesting that seropositive RA is a disease entity that is distinct from seronegative RA and PsA. Apparently, many of the same cytokines are present in both RA and SpA, but with dynamic differences that result in substantial differences in characteristic bone changes. In RA, TNFα is the primary pro-inflammatory driver, causing RANKL-driven osteoclast erosion and suppressing osteoblastogenesis. In contrast, in PsA and SpA in general, the IL17A pathway seems to play the driving role for osteoclastogenesis, and local and circulating Th17 and other IL17-producing cells are higher in number, degree of differentiation, and polyfunctionality. For example, Tc17 (also discussed in Section 5.2.4.6.4) has been shown to be a stronger source of IL17 in patients with PsA than RA, where the primary IL17 source is Th17 cells. The bone destruction in SpA and PsA is no less, as exemplified by the mutilans form of PsA. A role of angiogenesis has been implicated in the extra-articular and periarticular pathology. Bone destruction seen in RA and PsA and Tie2 transgenic mice has been putatively explained by the roles of VEGF and Ang1. VEGF upregulates RANKL, and both VEGF and Ang1 induce osteoclast chemotaxis through an ERK1/2 MAPK–dependent mechanism.

Individual molecular players implicated in the pathogenesis of psoriatic angiogenesis have mostly been covered earlier in this chapter, under psoriasis, with a reference to PsA at the end of the description of each player, immediately after its role in psoriasis.

In contrast to RA, which shows bone destruction more often, and OA, which shows bone deposition, for example, osteophytes, more often, PsA can show features of both and excessive bone remodeling. TNFα downstream pathways, for example, the RANK-RANKL pathway, act on osteoclasts, and Dkk1 inhibits the Wnt pathway on osteoblasts in RA. But in PsA, the second pathway shows some aberration, along with BMP dysregulation. Thus, unless SMAD or some of the related signaling is corrected, anti-TNFα treatment might only help stop bone degradation, but might aggravate the bone formation part of PsA (Mensah et al. 2008).

5.4 ADHESION MOLECULES IN ANGIOGENESIS OF PSORIASIS

Cell adhesion is an ancient and basic process of any living system. Even unicellular organisms interact with the extracellular environment (e.g., protozoa invading a host) using CAMs, in addition to receptors for soluble molecules. The term *membrane receptor* usually applies to a cell membrane molecule whose ligand is soluble, whereas when the ligand is large or insoluble or bound to another cell or matrix, then the receptor, and sometimes the ligand as well, may be considered a CAM, although the nomenclature is largely convention based. When the ligand is very similar to the receptor itself and located in another cell, it is called a homotypic adhesion molecule (e.g., cadherin), and when the ligand on the other cell is different, it is called heterotypic CAM. CAMs are involved in the development, differentiation, and function of all cells. We will focus on the role of adhesion molecules in inflammation and angiogenesis.

The origin of metazoan life depends on the formation of supracellular structures, which involve cell–cell and cell–matrix adhesions, which are mediated by CAM. Cell adhesion is such an important process that it has evolved many times independently in the evolution of life and diverged, and metazoan adhesion molecules are mostly different from protozoal and plant CAMs. Among the metazoans, vertebrate circulation has further evolved its unique feature of a continuous endothelial lining layer made of endothelial cells adhering within themselves, and also selectively allowing some blood cells to adhere and be recruited to specific tissues.

5.4.1 Classes of Major Cell Adhesion Molecules

Most of the metazoan CAMs can be classified into five main families:

1. Immunoglobulin superfamily (IgSF)
2. Selectins

3. Integrins
4. Cadherins
5. Mucinous cell adhesion ligands, for example, sialoglycoproteins

5.4.1.1 Immunoglobulin Superfamily

This is the largest and one of the most ancient families of cell surface molecules, only a subset of which are CAMs. CAMs under IgSF include, but are not restricted to,

- ICAM1, 2, 3, 4, 5 (intercellular adhesion molecule)
- VCAM1, 2 (vascular cell adhesion molecule)
- MadCAM1 (mucosal addressin cell adhesion molecule)
- PECAM1 (platelet endothelial cell adhesion molecule)
- CEACAM1 (carcino embryonic antigen-related cell adhesion molecule)
- MCAM (melanoma cell adhesion molecule) or CD146/MUC18
- ALCAM (activated leukocyte cell adhesion molecule) or CD166
- JAM-A, -B, and -C (junctional adhesion molecule)
- CD2 family (CD2, CD48, CD58, CD150, CD229, and CD244)
- CD90 (Thy1)
- Nectin family
- NCAM
- L1 family

Note: It must not be assumed that all names ending in CAM belong to this superfamily; for example, lung endothelial cell adhesion molecule (Lu-ECAM) 1 is a chloride channel, epithelial cell adhesion molecule (EpCAM, once written as ECAM1) does not belong to any of the four major adhesion molecule families, and LECAM1 was the old name for L-selectin.

5.4.1.2 Selectins (CD62)

Selectins are C-type (calcium-dependent) lectins. Leukocytes express L-selectin, activated platelets express P-selectin, and activated endothelial cells express E-selectin as well as P-selectin. The Ca2+-dependent interactions of the lectin domain with sialoglycoprotein ligands. The first leukocyte-endothelial adhesion molecule, L-selectin (erstwhile LECAM1), was discovered in 1983 by Gallatin et al. and named "peripheral lymph node homing receptor." All selectins, with their C-type lectin domain, show calcium-dependent low-affinity binding to glycans with terminal components that include α2-3-linked sialic acid and α1-3-linked fucose, typified by the sialyl Lewis x (sLex).

5.4.1.3 Cadherins

Cadherins are a family of ionic calcium-dependent CAMs with more than 100 members. Almost all cadherins are single-pass transmembrane glycoproteins with repetitive extracellular β-sandwich extracellular cadherin domains that adopt a similar fold to Ig domains. There are only a few exceptions, for example, (1) nonclassical member invertebrate flamingo/starry-night and its vertebrate homolog Celsrl,2,3 (cadherin, EGF laminin-G seven-pass G-type receptor 1), which are seven-transmembrane GPCRs with the N-terminus like a cadherin, and (2) T-cadherin, which instead of a transmembrane tail has a gpI anchor. Large organized clusters of cadherin zip up along zones across the cell membrane, leading to various forms of cell–cell junctions, like zonula adherens (or adherens junctions), for example, in epithelial cells, macula adherens (desmosome), and in keratinocytes, fascia adherens (e.g., part of the intercalated disc in cardiomyocytes).

Classic cadherins are homotypic in nature, that is, bind to cadherins similar to themselves on the extracellular side. On the intracellular side, they may bind to a tissue-dependent cytoskeletal complex, for example, α- and β-catenin–actin complexes and plakophilin/plakoglobin–desmoplakin–intermediate filament complexes. In addition to cell adhesion, these complexes participate in many types of signaling, for example, catenin in Wnt signaling, Rho-Rac-mediated MAPK signaling, and the PI3K/AKT pathway.

Cadherins are also a large family of evolutionarily ancient molecules related to the very root of evolution of metazoa. Cadherins can be broadly divided into three subfamilies: (1) classical cadherins involved primarily in adherens junction formation; (2) protocadherins, which might undergo somatic recombination and create Ig gene-like every large combinatorial diversity; and (3) atypical cadherins, for example, those involved in planar cell polarity (e.g., fat, dachsous, and flamingo). Classic cadherins have five EC repeats, are homotypic, and can be further divided into (1) typical or type I, which have a His-Ala-Val (HAV) motif with a single tryptophan (W) preceding the first calcium binding site in EC1, and (2) atypical or type II, which have a variant HAV motif with two Ws. Vertebrates have 6 type I and 13 type II members. A detailed description of cadherins is beyond the scope of this chapter. Cadherin distribution is tissue dependent. Some example distributions of classical cadherins are E-cadherin present in many epithelial tissues; N-cadherin in nervous, smooth muscle, fibroblast, and endothelial cells; placental (P) cadherin in placenta and mammary glands; R-cadherin in retina; and VE-cadherin (a classic type II cadherin) present only in endothelial cells. Some example diseases related to catenins are some of the blistering diseases, like pemphigus, which are caused by autoantibodies against some of the skin cadherins (desmogleins); some of the cardiomyopathies caused by misexpression of cardiac cadherins; and loss of E-cadherin or switching cadherin type, which may lead to increased severity of some carcinomas (e.g., breast carcinoma) or EMT.

Cadherins in endothelial cells include VE-cadherin, N-cadherin, VE-cadherin 2 (protocadherin 12), T-cadherin (H-cadherin/cadherin 13), and R-cadherin.

5.4.1.4 Sialoglycoprotein Ligands

These include carbohydrate moieties on PSGL1, CD43, CD44 GlyCAM1, VAP1, and so forth. PSGL1, which also binds to E-selectin, is the most studied selectin ligand, which harbors the famous epitope line, CLA, which incorporates a sLex. It is named CLA because almost all T cells in the extravascular compartment at sites of inflammatory skin disease are CLA+, in contrast to noncutaneous inflammatory sites where T cells lack it. Initially described as an epitope PSGL1, CLA epitope and E-selectin binding function are also present in CD43 and CD44. CLA is produced by key glycosyltransferases, including α1,3-fucosyltransferases FucT VII and FucT IV.

5.4.1.5 Integrins

Integrins are activatable adhesion receptors that connect or, to be more specific, bidirectionally integrate cells to ligands in the ECM or to other cells and also transduce signals. Structurally, type I αβ heterodimers, at least 24 distinct integrins generated from 18 α and 8 β subunits, are known among mammals. Integrins may be classified in many different ways. One of the ways to classify them is according to ligands.

All integrins (except β4) have small cytosolic domains, but no intrinsic kinase activity. The α subunits largely determine the ligand specificity, and the β1 subunit is relatively more associated with the cytoskeleton. Integrins undergo large conformational changes (activation) in their extracellular domains in response to signaling events inside cells (inside-out signaling), finally acting by adapter proteins, for example, talin and kindling, repositioning the cytoplasmic tails of the α and β integrin subunits relative to each other and to the plasma membrane. The ligand binding domain in resting integrins is not readily accessible to adhesive ligands until they are activated, which can change the affinity for ligand by 10,000-fold in the case of leukocytes (Ley et al. 2016).

Upon activation, integrins initiate ligand-dependent outside-in signaling that involves, in part, ligand-dependent integrin clustering, which brings the signaling domains of integrin-proximal proteins close enough together to initiate intracellular signals, for example, activation of spleen tyrosine kinase (SYK)3,4 and SRC family protein tyrosine kinases, and NADPH oxidase in leukocytes. For substrate adherent cells, unbinding the integrins may lead to a form of apoptosis known as anoikis.

Integrins are considered functional hubs for angiogenesis pathways and interact with and regulate a diversity of molecules, including growth factor receptors, other cell surface adhesion receptors, ECM components, pro- and anti-angiogenic ECM fragments, cytoplasmic adaptors, signaling molecules, cell surface–acting proteases, and their receptors and inhibitors.

5.4.1.5.1 Integrins That Bind RGD Peptide Sequence–Containing Ligands

The mapping of the minimal cell adhesion site in a prototypic integrin ligand, fibronectin, historically led to the discovery of the amino acid sequence RGD serine in the early 1980s. A slightly shorter sequence, RGD, is common to integrin ligands like vitronectin, fibrinogen, and the LAP complex part of inactive TGFβ, and many other ECM proteins (Humphries et al. 2006).

The RGD binding integrins are

- All five αv-containing integrins: αvβ3, αvβ5, αvβ6, αvβ8, and αvβ1
- Two other β1-containing integrins: α5β1 and α8β1
- αIIbβ3 integrin

5.4.1.5.2 Native Collagen Binding Integrins

Although the RGD sequence is present in collagen, it is not accessible in native collagen; instead, there is a triple helical GFOGER sequence with a critical glutamate (E) providing the critical cation coordination. The collagen binding integrins are

- Four β1 integrins with A (also called αI) domain–containing α chains: α1β1, α2β1, α10β1, and α11β1, of which the first three also bind laminin

5.4.1.5.3 Laminin Binding Integrins

These are integrins that act specifically as a laminin receptor, but the sequence target has not been deciphered.

- Three β1 integrins with non–A domain–containing α subunits: α3β1, α6β1 (usually in focal adhesion), and α7β1
- α6β4 integrin usually in hemidesmosomes

5.4.1.5.4 LDV Binding Integrins

An acidic motif, termed LDV, functionally related to RGD is present in fibronectin, and related sequences are present in VCAM1 and MAdCAM1. An unrelated sequence, but somewhat similar integrin specificity, is seen in OPN. The LDV binding integrins are

- So-called "leukocyte integrins": All four β2 integrins are found predominantly on leukocytes αLβ2 (LFA1), αMβ2 (Mac1), αDβ2, and αXβ2.
- VCAM binding integrins
  - Two β1 integrins: α4β1 and α9β1
  - Both β7 integrins: α4β7 and αEβ7

5.4.2 Role of Adhesion Molecules in Different Stages of Inflammatory Cell Recruitment

The leukocytes unbound to quiescent endothelium generally pass through at a relatively high local speed unless loosely captured to endothelial cells by interactions between the adhesion molecules and their ligands. Leukocyte extravasation has been known for more than a quarter of a century.

It happens through different stages. The multistep paradigm for the recruitment of circulating leukocytes to a tissue-like skin is the following:

Free-flowing leukocytes → tethering → rolling → activation → diapedesis → chemotaxis

The adhesion molecules involved in the skin homing of leukocytes are listed stepwise (Fuhlbrigge and Weishaupt 2007), with the most important adhesion molecules in bold.

(A summary table of the adhesion molecules and their corresponding ligands and function is given in Table 5.1.)

- Step 1: Tethering
  - **Leukocyte cell adhesion molecules**
    - E-selectin ligands
      - **PSGL1**
      - CD43
      - CD44
    - Selectin
      - CD62L
    - Integrin
      - VLA4
  - **Endothelial cell adhesion molecules**
    - Selectins
      - **E-selectin**
    - sLex
      - PNAd (peripheral node addressin)
    - Ig family
      - VCAM1
- Step 2: Rolling
  - **Leukocyte cell adhesion molecules**
    - E-selectin ligands
      - PSGL1
      - CD43
      - CD44
    - Selectin
      - L-selectin (CD62L)
    - Integrin
      - VLA4
    - C-type lectin
      - CD209
  - **Endothelial cell adhesion molecules**
    - Selectins
      - E-selectin
      - P-selectin
    - sLex
      - PNAd
    - Ig family
      - VCAM1
      - ICAM3

TABLE 5.1
Adhesion Molecules Important in Leukocyte Recruitment

Family	Adhesion Molecule	Alternative Names	Distribution	Ligands	Function
Immunoglobulin superfamily (IgSF)	ICAM1 (intercellular cell adhesion molecule 1)	CD54	Activated ECs, monocytes, B and T cells, keratinocytes	LFA1 (integrin αLβ2, CD11a/CD18)	Leukocyte–EC firm adhesion
IgSF	ICAM2 (intercellular cell adhesion molecule 2)	CD102	ECs, monocytes, dendritic cells, lymphocyte subsets	LFA1 (integrin αLβ2, CD11a/CD18)	Leukocyte–EC firm adhesion
IgSF	ICAM1 (intercellular cell adhesion molecule 3)	CD50	Leukocytes, epidermal dendritic Langerhans cells	LFA1 (integrin αLβ2, CD11a/CD18)	Leukocyte–EC adhesion and activation
IgSF	VCAM1 (vascular cell adhesion molecule 1)	INCAM110, CD106	Activated ECs, macrophages, dendritic cells	VLA4 (integrin α4β1, CD49d/CD29)	Leukocyte–EC firm adhesion
IgSF	LFA3 (leukocyte function antigen 3)	CD58	Antigen-presenting cells	CD2	Immunologic synapse (leukocyte–leukocyte adhesion)
IgSF	CD90	Thy1	ECs in high endothelial venules, inflamed and psoriatic dermal vessels	Mac1 (integrin αMβ2, CD11b/CD18)	Monocyte and neutrophil homing
IgSF	Junctional adhesion molecule B (JAM-B)	JAM2, VE-JAM	Leukocytes, platelets, ECs, epithelial cells, germ cells, Schwann cells	Homophilic with JAMs, heterophilic with α4β1 integrin	Leukocyte transendothelial migration, cell polarization, tight junction
Integrin	LFA1 (leukocyte functional antigen 1)	Integrin αLβ2, CD11a/CD18	All leukocytes	ICAM1, 2, 3	Leukocyte–EC adhesion, leukocyte–leukocyte adhesion
Integrin	VLA4 (very late antigen 4)	Integrin α4β1, CD49d/CD29	Many cell types, including most leukocytes	VCAM1, MAdCAM1, fibronectin, OPN, ADAM, ICAM4, TSP	Leukocyte–EC adhesion, cell anchoring to ECM
Integrin	p150, 95	Integrin αXβ2, CD11c/CD18	Leukocyte	Fibrinogen, possibly iC3b complement fragment	Leukocyte–EC/matrix adhesion, phagocytes

(Continued)

TABLE 5.1 (CONTINUED)
Adhesion Molecules Important in Leukocyte Recruitment

Family	Adhesion Molecule	Alternative Names	Distribution	Ligands	Function
Selectin	E-selectin	CD62E, ELAM-1, LECAM2	Constitutively expressed on ECs but further enhanced by shear or TNFα	Sialyl Lewis x/a in PSGL1, ESL1, CD43, CD44	Leukocyte rolling
Selectin	P-selectin	CD62P, granule membrane protein 140, PADGEM	Stored in ECs, translocated to surface on activation by TNF, IL1, or LPS, activated platelets, neutrophils, monocytes	Sulfated sialyl Lewis x/a, sulfated chondroitin	Leukocyte rolling, platelet leukocyte aggregation
Selectin	L-selectin	CD62L, LECAM1, MEL14, Leu8	Lymphocytes, monocytes, neutrophils	Sialyl Lewis x/a structures in GlyCAM1, MadCAM1, PSGL1, CD34	Leukocyte homing, rolling
Sialoglycoprotein	VAP1 (vascular adhesion protein 1)	Amine oxidase, copper containing 3 (AOC3), semicarbazide-sensitive amine oxidase (SSAO)	High endothelial venules, adipocytes, myocytes	Sialic acid binding counterreceptors (independent of L-selectin)	Subtype-specific T lymphocyte binding to high endothelial venules and neutrophil rolling in inflamed endothelium
Cadherin	VE-cadherin (vascular endothelial cadherin)	CD144, cadherin 5 type 2	Endothelial cells	Homophilic with VE-cadherin from another EC	Endothelial adherens junctions, also regulate endothelial proliferative state

Step 3: Activation
- CC chemokines
  - CCL1, 2, 5, 11, 13, 26
  - **CCL17 (TARC)**
  - **CCL27 (CTACK)**

Step 4: Firm adhesion
- **Leukocyte integrins**
  - **LFA1**
  - Mac1
  - VLA4
- **Endothelial IgSF CAMs**
  - **ICAM1**
  - ICAM2
  - VCAM1

Step 5: Diapedesis
- **Leukocyte CAMs**
  - Integrins
    - LFA1
    - Mac1
  - Ig family
    - JAM-C
  - C-type lectin
    - CD209
- **Endothelial CAMs**
  - IgSF
    - PE-CAM1
  - ICAM2, ICAM3
  - JAM-A, -B, -C
  - Cadherins
    - VE-cadherin
  - Type II membrane protein
    - CD-99

Step 6: Chemotaxis
- CC chemokine receptors
  - CCR1, 2, 3, **4**, 5, 6, 8, **10**
- CXC chemokine receptors
  - CXCR3, 4
- CX3C chemokine receptors
  - CX3CR1

The adhesion molecules described above and the interaction with their ligands are not one-on-one-type interactions but most of the time involve clustering and self-organizing microdomain-forming interactions, somewhat similar to immunological "kinapse" (short for "kinetic synapse"; see below) formation.

Leukocytes flowing through microvessels, especially in the postcapillary venules (PCVs), first lightly tether to the endothelial cells, and roll at a reduced velocity along the surface (Fuhlbrigge and Weishaupt 2007). The most important molecules mediating tethering and rolling are E-selectin (CD62E) and P-selectin (CD62P) on endothelial cells. P-selectin is produced in general by all endothelia and stored in Webel–Palade bodies for rapid transport to the luminal surface in response to an inflammatory trigger. E-selectin is expressed constitutively on PCVs, mainly in skin and rarely in other tissues, although it can be induced in other vessels by inflammation.

PSGL1 (CD162) is the main ligand on leukocytes for endothelial P-selectin. The E-selectin functional ligand is a sialylated and fucosylated carbohydrate epitope similar or identical to sLex that may be carried by several distinct glycoproteins, for example, PSGL1, CD43, and CD44, at distinct stages of development in various leukocytes (Fuhlbrigge and Weishaupt 2007). Relatively, the skin specificity of endothelial E-selectin explains why leukocytes expressing these ligands home to skin. A monoclonal antibody called HECA-452, which recognizes this E-selectin functional ligand dubbed cutaneous lymphocyte-associated antigen (CLA) (Fuhlbrigge et al. 1997), has been used as a specific marker for skin homing leukocytes. It is expressed by the majority of T cells in skin. The production of CLA carbohydrate epitopes and their like is regulated by the glycosyltransferases α1,3-fucosyltransferases IV and VII.

The α4β1 (VLA4) and α4β7 integrins are important leukocyte homing (organ "addressin"-specific targeting) receptors. The main ligands of these two integrins are VCAM1 and fibronectin. A4β7 can also bind to MAdCAM1 in high endothelial venules of mucosal lymphoid organs, which cause mucosa-specific homing. Another integrin α6β1 is also important in leukocyte firm adhesion and transmigration in general.

The leukocyte-mediated opening of the endothelial junction needs complex cooperation; for example, in the case of neutrophils, β2 integrin engagement leads to degranulation and secretion of the cationic heparin binding protein (described in Section 5.2.5.17.4). CXCL chemokines (CXCL1, 2, 3, and 8), leukotrienes, and thromboxanes also play a role in increasing the permeability.

5.4.3 Role of Adhesion Molecules in Angiogenesis

Adhesion molecules are as important in angiogenesis as they are in inflammation and leukocyte recruitment. As already discussed, several adhesion molecules, especially integrins, are major hubs in the network of angiogenesis-related signaling.

5.4.3.1 Role of Integrins

A variety of integrin heterodimers containing β1, β3, β4, β5, and β8 subunits have been shown to play roles in angiogenesis. Endothelial cells during quiescence express several β1 integrins (e.g., α1β1, α2β1, α3β1, α5β1, and α6β1), α6β4, and αvβ5 integrins. These integrins are mostly receptors for basement membrane collagen and laminin, with the exception of integrins αvβ5 and α5β1, which tend to bind provisional matrix ligands vitronectin and fibronectin, respectively. When activated, ECs upregulate the α5β1 and switch on expression of the αvβ3 integrin, which is absent in the quiescent state. Although the expression level of other integrins may not change, that does not mean they are not important for angiogenesis. Among them, α1β1 and α2β1 integrins, which can mediate interactions with some forms of digested type IV and type I collagens, when inhibited by function-blocking antibodies, inhibit angiogenesis. In fact, now it is known that VEGFR2-mediated EC activation involves relocalization of α6β1 integrin from focal adhesions bound to laminin α4, to podosome rosettes that are cellular foot processes of ECs that drill through the basement membrane.

Interestingly, while blocking αvβ5 and αvβ3 inhibits angiogenesis, mouse knockout of β3 or both β3 and β5 causes paradoxically increased angiogenesis, with elevated levels of VEGFR2 (also called Flk1) in ECs. The explanation proposed for this paradoxic function is through the context-dependent action of the integrins (Robinson and Hodivala-Dilke 2011):

- When αvβ3 integrins are present in ECs and engaged to their ligand (vitronectin) in the ECM, it is a pro-angiogenic condition leading to EC survival and proliferation or migration.
- When αvβ3 integrins are present in ECs but are not engaged by their appropriate ligand, it is an anti-angiogenic condition and the EC is likely to die by apoptosis. It can happen in multiple subscenarios:
  - When a 3-D matrix of a nonligand molecule, for example, collagen, is used (e.g., Matrigel), the nonligated αvβ3 initiates integrin-induced death by recruiting apoptotic machinery to the cell membrane.
  - When a high dose of a competing RGD-containing soluble inhibitor (e.g., cilengitide) is around, it can almost completely displace the ligand. (However, a low dose of the same inhibitor can cause a pro-angiogenic situation.)
- When αvβ3 integrins are themselves downregulated or absent from ECs (e.g., in some advanced aggressive or metastatic tumors), it is again a pro-angiogenic situation.

While absence of the ligand can cause integrin-mediated apoptosis of delaminating nascent tip cells, high doses of VEGF and FGF can rescue them, albeit through somewhat different mechanisms. VEGF usually activates the MAPK pathway through αvβ5-mediated activation of FAK and SRC and protects ECs from receptor-mediated apoptosis. On the other hand, bFGF acts through αvβ3-mediated activation of PAK (p21-activated kinase), which targets c-Raf (of the MAPK pathway) to mitochondria and protects ECs from stress-induced death. VEGF may partly mediate its angiogenic action via β1 integrin–dependent mechanisms (Senger et al. 1997). VEGFR2 activation also induces β3 integrin tyrosine phosphorylation, which, in turn, is crucial for VEGF-induced tyrosine phosphorylation of VEGFR2 (Somanath et al. 2009).

5.4.3.1.1 α9β1 Integrin in Angiogenesis and Lymphangiogenesis

In addition to traditional adhesion ligands like VCAM1, tenascin C, OPN, coagulation factor XIII, and von Willebrand factor (VWF), the α9β1 integrin has been known to directly bind soluble signaling molecules like VEGFC, VEGFD, and NGF, and is the only integrin that is absolutely essential for embryonic lymphangiogenesis. However, in 2007 it was discovered that it is also necessary for action of VEGFA, for example, both VEGF121 and 165. It is different from integrins α3β1 and αvβ3, whose blocking interferes with VEGF165 binding and response in endothelial cells, but not that of VEGF121. Blocking α9β1 modulates VEGF121 and 165 binding, cell adhesion, and migration response in endothelial cells, but it does not interfere with FGF signaling.

5.4.3.1.2 Role in Regulation of Angiogenesis through VWF

Integrin αvβ3 also happens to be the main endothelial receptor for VWF. VWF is an integral and unique component of the subendothelial basement membrane and is known to be important in angiogenesis. It may modulate angiogenesis partly through interaction with αvβ3 on the activated endothelial cells. In VWF-deficient endothelial cell αvβ3 levels, function and trafficking are known to be decreased, suggesting that VWF may also regulate αvβ3 activity in various ways. Ang2 has been reported to stimulate the internalization and degradation of αvβ3 and may directly or indirectly regulate a VWF effect on angiogenesis.

α1β1 integrin (VLA1) has been found to be a "key checkpoint" for the accumulation of epidermal T cells and the development of psoriasis. This integrin binds collagen and is exclusively expressed by epidermal, but not dermal, T cells. α1β1+ T cells were found to be mostly effector memory cells and contained high levels of interferon γ, but not IL4. Blocking α1β1 integrin inhibited migration of T cells into the epidermis in a xenotransplantation model, paralleled by a complete inhibition of psoriasis development, comparable to TNFα blockers. These results define a crucial role for α1β1 integrin in controlling the accumulation of epidermal type 1 polarized effector memory T cells. Additional receptor–ligand interactions, for example, αEβ7 on lymphocytes versus E-cadherin on keratinocytes, have been speculated to be a key factor for the retention of effector cells in the epidermis.

5.4.3.1.3 Role in TGFβ Activation

Epithelial αvβ6 and αvβ8, by binding RGD in LAP, are the major integrins that activate TGFβ in vivo, either by allosteric changes in TGFβ-LAP (αvβ6) or by inducing MMP14 and causing a proteolytic release of TGFβ. Myofibroblast β1 integrins can also induce a mechanical strain-dependent TGFβ activation.

5.4.3.2 Role of Cadherins

VE-cadherin is unique in distribution to endothelial cells, and it can act as a master regulator in vasculogenesis. N-cadherins may be found in primitive ECs or in EC mural cell junctions. Unlike other cells where N-cadherin is expressed, in endothelial cells, N-cadherin is often found diffusely all over the EC surface, whereas VE-cadherin is usually found in EC-EC junctions, from where it eventually displaces N-cadherin. VE-cadherin homotypic engagement usually stabilizes vessels and decreases permeability or proliferation. In contrast, N-cadherin usually permits endothelial cell proliferation and motility.

Similar to E-cadherins in epithelia interacting in cis with growth factor receptors, for example, EGFR and HGFR/c-Met, and influencing their response, in endothelial cells, N-cadherin can interact in cis with FGFR, and VE-cadherin can interact in cis with VEGFR2 and TGFβ receptors. However, while VE-cadherin usually acts as a negative regulator of VEGF signaling, possibly through junctional phosphatases such as DEP-1, N-cadherin may act as a positive regulator of FGF signaling. However, the VE-cadherin influence on VEGFR2 is not entirely negative, as it helps transduce a basal endothelial cell survival signal mediated by the PI3K/AKT pathway that requires the VE-cadherin and VEGFR2 association. VE-cadherin is also a positive and EC-specific regulator of TGFβ signaling. VE-cadherin can bind in cis to TGFβRII, ALK1, ALK5, and endoglin and help recruit its active receptor complex. It helps maintain the quiescent state of endothelial cells.

VE-cadherin phosphorylation is a necessary step for the endothelial switch from the quiescent to the angiogenic phenotype. Several protein tyrosine phosphatases, for example, VE-PTP and PTP-mu, directly interact with VE-cadherin and help maintain the quiescent phenotype. VE-cadherin phosphorylation might be associated with disruption of EC-EC junctions and endocytosis of VE-cadherin, but that does not mean VE-cadherin levels are downregulated. It not only relocalizes, but in some angiogenic states, VE-cadherin levels are further upregulated. The VE-cadherin gene is one of the targets of ETS transcription factors that are part of the angiogenic switch. VE-cadherin in tip cells is relocalized to the filopodia (where CD34 is also localized), and it can help by partnering with opposing tip cells. In stalk cells, VE-cadherin eventually helps localize CD34 in the process of lumen formation. The role of VE-cadherin in migration and proliferation in angiogenesis deserves further investigation. Since VE-cadherin expression is specific to endothelial cells, its inhibition by antibodies has been attempted to target tumor angiogenesis with some preliminary success.

Soluble VE-cadherin is its extracellular domain shed through a metalloproteinase-dependent mechanism. Soluble VE-cadherin may potentially act as a competitive inhibitor of full-length VE-cadherin, as suggested by its inhibitory effect on tumor angiogenesis and tumor growth. According to one study on inflammatory skin conditions, vasculitis, vascular tumors, and normal controls, only psoriasis and atopic dermatitis were found to have low-serum-soluble VE-cadherin levels. Although VE-cadherin is an interesting candidate, with renewed interest in the angiogenesis field, not much clear data are available on the role of cadherins in angiogenesis associated with Ps or PsA.

5.4.3.3 Role of Selectins and Other Adhesion Molecules in Angiogenesis in Psoriasis

The roles of selectins in angiogenesis have already been covered in bits and pieces earlier, for example, the role in leukocyte recruitment by direct binding to the endothelium (see Section 5.4.2) and in indirect binding through platelets (described in Sections 5.2.4.4 and 5.2.4.10). Resting endothelial cells mainly express P-selectins, but when activated, P-selectin is upregulated and E-selectin is induced, along with leukocyte integrin ligands, for example, ICAM1 and VCAM1.

In psoriasis, both the leukocytes and the endothelium have been found to have increased stickiness, and this has been attributed to increased adhesion molecules (e.g., Thy1, ICAM1, VCAM1, and MHC II) (Schön and Boehncke 2005), some of which are shed in soluble forms as well. Shedding of ectodomains of some of the adhesion molecules is rapid and part of the leukocyte adhesion process, for example, L-selectin, which can be cleaved either by sheddase/secretase enzymes (e.g., TACE and ADAM17) (Lee and Iruela-Arispe 2008) or "mechanically." This may explain why the baseline level of soluble l-selectin in health is high (approximately 1.6 μg/mL of soluble L-selectin). For shedding of other adhesion molecules, for example, ICAM1, the soluble form has two sources. One is direct synthesis of the soluble full-length extracellular domain, and the other is the EC domain fragment shed by various proteolytic enzymes, for example, neutrophil elastase or metalloproteases. Soluble monomeric ICAM1 does not significantly inhibit the cellular ICAM1-LFA1 interactions; however, higher-order multimers might potentially compete.

Some studies claim that the shed adhesion molecules, for example, L-selectin are coming from leukocytes, so some leukocyte subsets have correspondingly reduced levels of l-selectin due to the shedding. One study showed that L-selectin expression levels on CD4+ T cells, B cells, monocytes, and neutrophils from patients with severe psoriasis (PASI ≥15) were significantly decreased (Inaoki et al. 2000).

Soluble adhesion molecules, for example, soluble ICAM1, soluble selectins, and soluble VCAM1, are often increased during inflammatory episodes. Most of the studies done on psoriasis or PsA found increased soluble adhesion molecules, for example, soluble E-selectin and increased ICAM1, and correlation with disease severity has been claimed. However, a more recent study, which looked at ankylosing spondyloarthritis, did not find any significant rise in sE-selectin, sP-selectin, sICAM1, or sVCAM1 (Sari et al. 2010).

One study shows that sICAM1 may promote angiogenesis both in vivo and in vitro. In vitro, it stimulates endothelial cell migration, tube formation, and sprouting from aortic rings. In vivo, it induces neovascularization in chicken eggs and stimulates tumor implant growth in mice.

5.4.4 Role of Adhesion Molecules in Immunological Synapses

Psoriasis is a T-cell-dependent disease. T-cell function is critically dependent on antigen presentation, which happens through a special temporary cell–cell junction that is called "immunological synapse" if static and stable and "immunological kinapse" or "kinapse" if transient or moving across the cell surface.

The efficiency of the immunological synapse can be life or death for T cells, as well as for the organism. The synapse must be specific enough to recognize as few as ~10 activating peptide–MHC complexes (pMHCs) among hundreds of self-pMHCs, and sensitive enough to produce the signals of the right intensity for the right amount of time, which requires the cells to stay in touch (within 13 nm of each other).

Molecules involved in immunologic synapse are listed below.

APC (Antigen Presenting Cell)*	T Cell
LFA1	ICAM1
CD2	LFA3
CD28 (or CTLA4)	CD80/CD86
TCRab (+ CD3 + CD4)	MHC + Ag

Immunological synapse involves formation of a bull's-eye pattern with a central cluster of TCR-pMHC, dubbed cSMAC (central supramolecular activation complex), surrounded by a ring of the integrin LFA1 and its ligand ICAM1, defined as the pSMAC (peripheral SMAC). It has been shown that microclusters of the MHC complex surrounded by microrings of adhesion molecules, especially LFA1, and the focal adhesion complex forming over a timescale of 0.5–1 min are critical for the formation of the immunological synapse or kinapse (Hashimoto-Tane et al. 2016). Thus, it is no surprise that inhibition of LFA1 was very effective in preventing helper T-cell activation by immunological synapse and was effective in psoriasis, which is possibly a T-cell-dependent disease.

5.4.5 Blocking of Leukocyte Extravasation/Trafficking

As already mentioned in Section 5.4.2, blockade of leukocyte extravasation is a very important and relevant topic. Blockade of the initial steps has been already covered in many reviews and books (Zollner et al. 2007). However, scant literature is available on the targeting of the later parts of the process.

All single selectin blockades tested for psoriasis failed, for example, E-selectin blockade (Bhushan et al. 2002). However, pan-selectin antagonists have shown encouraging results in psoriasis, including bimosiamose, TBC1269, and efomycine.

Some integrin blockades were already described in other sections of this chapter. An interesting integrin ligand that may be also relevant in psoriasis is described here: Thy1. Thy1 (CD90) belongs to IgSF. When expressed on ECs, it is an atypical counterreceptor for Mac1 expressed by polymorphonuclear leukocytes (PMNs) (Wetzel et al. 2006). The usual ligand for Mac1 is ICAM1.

* Antigen-presenting cell.

But Thyl is upregulated in dermal vasculature endothelium by IL1β and TNFα, both of which are high in psoriasis. The psoriatic neutrophils adhere to Thyl (but not ICAM1) more strongly than neutrophils from healthy controls. Thus, activated by Thyl, neutrophils secrete IL8 and MMP9, which creates an autocrine–paracrine loop of recruiting more neutrophils and allowing basement membrane degradation to expedite their extravasation. Thyl-Macl interaction is an important blockable target worth exploring in psoriasis. However, Thyl-directed targeting is fraught with the problem of mesangioproliferative glomerulonephritis in animal models because Thyl is also expressed in mesangial cells. This complication will need to be bypassed in order for it to be used in psoriasis models.

5.4.6 Adhesion Molecules as Therapeutic Targets

5.4.6.1 Targeting Integrins

The first integrin-targeted drug, abciximab (antiplatelet integrin), was introduced in 1994. Currently, ClinicalTrials.gov lists 108 search hits with *integrin* as the search word, which may be either the target of therapeutic drugs, imaging agents, or the biomarker. All integrin antagonists currently on the market or in late-stage clinical trials target the ligand binding sites of integrins that are expressed on blood cells: leukocytes or platelets. The affinities of both leukocyte and platelet integrins are highly responsive to inside-out signaling.

Targeting leukocyte integrins has proven applications in diseases such as multiple sclerosis, Crohn's disease, and ulcerative colitis. Four leukocyte integrins, αLβ2, α4β1, α4β7, and αEβ7, have been targeted by monoclonal antibodies that have been investigated in patients.

5.4.6.1.1 Efalizumab

Humanized monoclonal antibody efalizumab (marketed as Raptiva by Genentech) is a full-length IgG1κ against the αL (CD11a) integrin subunit. It was previously on the market for psoriasis but was withdrawn in 2009 because of a rare association of progressive multifocal leukoencephalopathy (PML) due to reactivation of a polyoma virus, John Cunningham virus (JCV). Multicenter randomized controlled trials had shown that efalizumab was effective in psoriasis; for example, subcutaneous efalizumab (1 or 2 mg/kg/week) was significantly superior to placebo. Adverse events, including headache, chills, pain, and fever, were more common in patients receiving efalizumab, but serious adverse events and infections were not statistically more common than in those receiving placebo. One must wonder why this drug was not continued even though the percentage of PML was not more than that of natalizumab, which is continuing for multiple sclerosis.

The risk for developing PML after treatment with natalizumab, an anti-α4 integrin used for multiple sclerosis, has been estimated to be approximately 2 in 1000 for patients treated for more than 2 years. The unexpected development of PML in patients treated with natalizumab triggered its voluntary withdrawal from the market in February 2005, but it returned in July 2006 under Tysabri Outreach: Unified Commitment to Health (TOUCH) monitoring because there were not many effective alternatives for MS. However, in the case of psoriasis, until 2009, four cases were described within a cohort of 6000 patients who had received efalizumab for psoriasis (i.e., incidence less than that for natalizumab), but it lead to voluntary withdrawal of efalizumab in 2009 partly because psoriasis has alternative treatments, unlike MS. A newer α4β7 heterodimer-specific integrin inhibitor, vedolizumab, is under trial for IBD, which has shown promise, as no PML cases have so far been described, although it was predicted to have similar PML frequency as natalizumab. Unfortunately, vedolizumab is so far thought to be useful for gut inflammation but not joint or skin inflammation. Vedolizumab, AMG181, and so forth, target the integrin heterodimer α4β7, thus blocking their interaction with MAdCAM1 in mucosa. Inspired by the success of these molecules, similar heterodimer target approaches are being attempted for other integrins. A synthetic peptide

("peptide 3.1," CKSTHDRLC) with specificity for the human arthritic synovium has been putatively identified in similar ways.

PML seems to be a true drug effect, as neither multiple sclerosis, Crohn's disease, or psoriasis is directly associated with PML. There is no known treatment, prevention, or cure for PML, and the infection usually leads to death or severe disability. The wide future use of anti-integrin monoclonal antibodies for the treatment of IBD, multiple sclerosis, or psoriasis has to circumvent the occurrence of this rare but potentially fatal complication.

5.4.6.1.2 Other Therapeutic Antibodies That Have Been Tested in Related Angiogenic Diseases but Not Yet in Psoriasis or PsA

5.4.6.1.2.1 Etaracizumab The $\alpha v\beta 3$ integrin is preferentially expressed on developing and activated endothelial cells, but not quiescent mature vasculature, and is thus considered the most important integrin for angiogenesis. Its primary ligand is vitronectin, but it also binds fibrinogen, fibronectin, and TSP, and associates in cis with MMP2, PDGF, insulin, and VEGFR2. Etaracizumab specifically blocks the binding of vitronectin and other ligands to the $\alpha v\beta 3$ integrin and can cause inhibition of angiogenesis. However, blocking this integrin will at least have dose-dependent effects, and so it should be used with caution (the four different scenarios were discussed in relation to $\alpha v\beta 3$ integrin inhibition in the earlier section on the introduction to integrins).

5.4.6.1.2.2 Volociximab Volociximab, a IgG4 chimeric humanized monoclonal antibody $\alpha 5\beta 1$ integrin, has been through clinical phase II trials for solid tumors in renal cell carcinoma, metastatic melanoma, pancreatic cancer, ovarian cancer, and non-small-cell lung cancer. It has also completed a phase I trial for age-related macular degeneration.

5.4.7 General Appraisal of Molecular Targeting Approaches

There are many alternative approaches to anti-adhesion-based approaches or inhibitor therapies that aim to suppress a cellular process like angiogenic activation. Some examples include the following:

- Most direct and common approaches: Blockade of receptor–ligand interactions by
  - Steric inhibition by
    - A monoclonal antibody binding near the ligand binding site
    - Antibody binding near other functional or docking sites
  - Soluble receptor (e.g., sFlt1 for VEGF) that decoys or chelates ligand
  - Soluble endogenous inhibitor (e.g., endostatin)
  - Competing nonactivating ligand mimetic
    - Synthetic peptide (e.g., cyclic RGD-containing peptide)
    - Natural inhibitor (e.g., RGD disintegrin for integrins such as echistatin)
    - Small-molecule ligand mimetic
  - Strategies that work in vitro, which are very difficult to implement vivo or in patients (e.g., supraphysiological concentration, calcium chelation, or trypsinization or overexpression of a dominant negative so far only work in vitro or, to some extent, in animal models)
- Modulators that regulate
  - Receptor affinity
    - For example, direct allosteric modulators that affect the conformational changes necessary for activation
  - Expression level and structural integrity of the receptor or ligand
    - Decrease synthesis

    - For example, succinobucol (AGI-1067), an antioxidant compound also capable of inhibiting VCAM1 gene expression
    - Dimethyl fumarate
  - Increased degradation
  - Dysregulation of processing
    - For example, agents that interfere with appropriate glycosylation of ligands for selectin receptors
- Localization (e.g., retargeting to endocytosis or lysosome or proteasome)
- Antagonists of downstream signaling pathways: Usually small molecules that easily enter into cells (e.g., kinase inhibitors)
- Modulators of an accessory process, for example, inhibiting ECM degradation or modulating stiffness to prevent angiogenesis
- Interfering with an important known hub in an interactome connected to the process
  - Antagomirs against a critical miR
  - Inhibiting a transcriptional master regulator
- Inhibition further upstream in a process
  - For example, interfering with transendothelial migration of angiogenic cellular players would inhibit angiogenesis
  - Examples of existing VEGF inhibitors that are being tried in psoriasis
    - Directed against VEGF protein, for example, anti-VEGF monoclonal antibodies
      - Bevacizumab
      - Ranibizumab
      - Newer-generation monoclonal antibodies, for example, G6–31, MF1, and DC101
    - Directed against VEGFR
      - Aflibercept/VEGF-Trap
      - Pegaptanib
    - Inhibition of tyrosine kinase–specific VEGFR2 for or common to multiple receptor tyrosine kinases
      - Sunitinib
      - Sorafenib
      - Vandetanib
      - Pazopanib

5.4.7.1 Why Adhesion Molecules

Adhesion molecule inhibition, the first of the approaches listed above, is the most intuitive straightforward approach to halt a physiologic process right at first contact. However, there are multiple issues with adhesion molecule inhibition in contrast to other types of angiogenesis inhibition. Thus, the development of effective intervention has been frustrating. Despite the frustration, efforts must go on, as this is potentially the most accessible and manipulable target. Some of the points against adhesion therapy include the high level of redundancy and complexity; for example, blocking individual selectins did not work at all, but a pan-selectin antagonist gave some effect.

However, the adhesion molecules are likely to come back as therapeutic targets because targeting other angiogenic processes, for example, kinase signaling, has been fraught with even bigger problems of causing paradoxic exacerbation, compared with the ineffectiveness of adhesion targeting.

5.4.7.2 Issues with Antiadhesion and Antiangiogenic Drugs in Psoriasis

Several antiadhesion and antiangiogenesis drugs have been tried in psoriasis. In addition to anti-integrin, for example, efalizumab and the VEGF or VEGFR-related antibodies and antikinases described above, some other drugs that have inhibited angiogenesis in psoriasis include the Goeckerman (coal tar + UVB) regimen, psoralens, and PUVA; other antikinases, for example,

PKC inhibitor AEB071, Jak inhibitor tofacitinib, and P38 MAPK inhibitors BMS-582949 and doramapimod/BIRB796; IL17 ligand or receptor antagonists (covered elsewhere); anti-TNF drugs; pan-selectin antagonists, for example, bimosiamose; cytotoxic drugs, for example, methotrexate, 6-thioguanine, hydroxyurea, azathioprine, 6-mercaptopurine, and piritrexim; antimetastatic drugs, for example, razoxazone; phosphodiesterase 4 inhibitors, for example, apremilast/CC10004; cyclosporin and other T-cell activation inhibitors; immunologic synapse inhibitors; and natural product–derived VEGF antagonists, for example, shark cartilage extract AE-941/neovastat/benefin. Razoxazone, once considered most effective for psoriasis, until the early 1980s, was later stopped due to secondary carcinogenesis. Antiadhesion molecules have faced either ineffectiveness (e.g., anti-individual selectins) or too much effectiveness against immune function, leading to immunosuppression (e.g., PML seen with efalizumab, natalizumab, etc.). However, other types of angiogenesis blockers have faced a peculiar problem of disease exacerbation or de novo disease precipitation, which deserves special mention.

5.4.7.2.1 Paradoxic Exacerbations (More Common with Other Inhibitors than Antiadhesion Agents)

Paradoxical exacerbation of angiogenesis and the inflammatory disease process in general has been seen in several treatment modalities. It is possibly due to compensatory processes in vivo that offset or reverse the effect of the inhibitor; for example, psoriasis may be aggravated with angiogenesis inhibitors classically exemplified not only by sorafenib but also by many TNF inhibitors and other drugs.

In 90% of patients treated with angiogenesis inhibitors, adverse skin reactions are seen, and in some cases, the severity of the reactions parallels the treatment efficacy and tumor response. But given that these drugs act on critical steps of angiogenesis and that psoriasis is centrally dependent on angiogenesis, it is counterintuitive to use these drugs to aggravate or even cause psoriasis.

The paradoxical effect may not necessarily be about psoriasis, but possibly about angiogenesis in general. Psoriasis is not the only angiogenesis-dependent disease that might be exacerbated with some antiangiogenesis therapy—like sorafenib. Crohn's disease, another angiogenesis-dependent disease and a comorbidity of psoriasis, is also occasionally known to paradoxically exacerbate, for example, with sunitinib (Boers-Sonderen et al. 2014).

5.4.7.2.1.1 Sorafenib Sorafenib is an orally acting small-molecule multikinase inhibitor that blocks the receptor tyrosine kinase activity of VEGFR2 and 3, PDGFR, c-kit, Flt3, RET, and nonreceptor kinases Raf1 and B-Raf. It has antiangiogenic and antiproliferative activity. There are anecdotal reports of sorafenib healing psoriasis when used for causes unrelated to psoriasis (Fournier and Tisman 2010). However, there are many reports where the use of sorafenib has paradoxically led to causation of psoriasis-like lesions without any previous history or, in some cases, aggravation (Hung et al. 2012; Du-Thanh et al. 2013; Yiu et al. 2016).

5.4.7.2.1.2 Sunitinib Sunitinib is another orally acting multikinase inhibitor for tyrosine kinases VEGFR1, 2, and 3; PDGFRα and β; colony-stimulating factor 1 receptor (CSF1R), c-kit, RET, and Flt3. It is Food and Drug Administration (FDA) approved for several cancers. In some cases, psoriasis has improved due to sunitinib use for unrelated causes, for example, renal cell carcinoma. Unlike sorafenib, full-blown psoriasis has not been precipitated by sunitinib. However, psoriasiform rashes have been reported with the use of sunitinib, which become particularly severe when in scrotal and genital or inguinal skin (Diamantis and Chon 2010). Crohn's disease, a comorbidity of psoriasis, is also known to be occasionally paradoxically exacerbated, for example, with sunitinib (Boers-Sonderen et al. 2014).

5.4.7.2.1.3 Bevacizumab Bevacizumab is a recombinant humanized (93% human, 7% murine) anti-VEGF monoclonal antibody that neutralizes all the isoforms of VEGF. It is administered by an intravenous route for treatment (in combination) of colorectal and breast carcinoma, renal cell carcinoma, non-small-cell lung cancer, ovarian and fallopian tube cancer, and so forth. Bevacizumab has led to improvement of psoriasis when administered for unrelated causes in anecdotal cases (Akman et al. 2009). However, there have been cases where bevacizumab was given for unrelated causes in a psoriasis case and the case still progressed on to PsA while on bevacizumab (Graceffa et al. 2012).

5.4.7.2.1.4 Tocilizumab Similar to the above, many cases of paradoxical psoriasis-like reactions have been reported for humanized monoclonal antibody, tocilizumab. It is a IL6 receptor blocker. The phenomenon which happens likely due to shunting of the IL6 to bind to noncognate targets.

5.4.7.2.1.5 Gefitinib Exacerbation of psoriasis is also seen with EGFR tyrosine kinase inhibitor gefitinib (Zorzou et al. 2004).

5.4.7.2.2 Paradox Is More Common with TNF Inhibitors

All three common TNFα antagonists, which have now become first-line agents in the treatment of moderate to severe psoriasis, have been known to have produced new psoriasis-like lesions or exacerbated psoriasis in hundreds of patients (Wollina et al. 2008) and might potentially paradoxically precipitate PsA (Napolitano et al. 2017). Some Crohn's disease patients who developed psoriasis-like lesions under treatment with TNFα inhibitors were known to go into remission when switched to vedolizumab, a new α4β7 heterodimer-specific integrin inhibitor that specifically prevents mucosal homing of leukocytes. All three TNF inhibitors together have an average incidence of about 1.04 in 1000 person-years of de novo precipitation of psoriasis in treated RA patients (Toussirot and Aubin 2016). Adalimumab has 4.6 times more risk than etanercept and 3.5 times more risk than infliximab. Psoriasis, Crohn's disease, and hidradenitis suppurativa are considered paradoxic adverse events (PAEs) but may include borderline PAEs, for example, uveitis, scleritis, sarcoidosis and other granulomatous diseases (granuloma annulare and interstitial granulomatous dermatitis), vasculitis, vitiligo, and alopecia areata, many of which are angiogenesis or immune-related exacerbations.

5.4.7.3 Rise, Fall, and Coming Back of Antiadhesion and Antiangiogenesis Therapies

As explained in much of this chapter, angiogenesis seems to be central to almost all the comorbidities of psoriasis, and the process is complex, with many cellular and molecular players. In contrast to RA, where angiogenesis is possibly secondary to TNFα-mediated inflammation, angiogenesis is itself one of the starting points of psoriasis pathogenesis. Interferon α may be one of the transient initial triggers, and IL17 might be one of the maintaining triggers. Perivascular aggregation of BMDCs, mast cells, and NETs set up signaling gradients and play critical roles in the angiogenesis of psoriasis, which we are merely beginning to understand. Adhesion molecules seem to play bigger roles in many of the steps of angiogenesis than was earlier thought, as almost all the growth factors, including VEGF, extensively cross-talk with adhesion receptors.

It is very important to assess the risk–benefit ratio of the therapeutic agents in a big picture. Just the ineffectiveness of initial attempts of inhibition or the paradoxic worsening or new precipitation of the disease with some of the so-called effective inhibitors does not preclude exploration of variations of these drugs. However, it does elicit a question about the best strategies to solve this problem. The main issue is in understanding the complexity of the network of interactions that involves parallel actions, feedback and feed-forward inhibition loops, and dynamic spatiotemporal oscillations. Parallel actions may lead to redundancy, and circuitous loops may lead to compensatory paradoxical effects if one intermediate step of a process is blocked. Since the mechanisms of angiogenesis are shared between organs, off-target effects also need to be minimized. Thus, targeting and organ or disease specificity of the drugs need to be improved.

It must be noted that not all antibodies or antagonists are created equal. The binding site and interaction of the antagonist with the target may not be very intuitive. The same target might behave differently with different antibodies and differently in animal models and in humans. Thus, if one drug fails against one target, it puts some strain on further studies but does not preclude them. The next drug against the same target might show entirely different pharmacodynamics. A drug might also be reintroduced if the perception of risk is outweighed by the benefit. An example was discussed in the case of natalizumab for multiple sclerosis, in which there were not many effective choices, as opposed to the case of efalizumab for psoriasis.

Damage of psoriatic disease is better intercepted at an earlier stage, as currently there is no "cure." Most of the mechanistic research has indeed so far focused on the initial pathogenesis of psoriatic diseases. Blocking the initiation of inflammation is effective, but little mechanistic insight is available on how to intercept the disease once it has progressed. Thus, disease stage–specific targeting strategies are much awaited.

The temporal progression is not to be confused with downstream signaling. For the purpose of blocking a process, the most upstream triggers are usually better points of intervention; otherwise, signaling intermediates that start to accumulate upstream of a block reroute their path into some in vivo compensatory network, which might lead to paradoxic action. Unlike TNFα in RA, IL17 in psoriasis seems to be either acting upstream of TNFα or involved parallelly, feeding independently into critical steps of inflammatory cascades. Thus, TNFα blocking alone could lead to paradoxic action. Potential other upstream signals could be miRNAs. Some of the synthetic miRNA agonists (e.g., angiomir) and antagonists (e.g., antagomirs) are under intense research. Some are showing preliminary encouraging research. As already mentioned, miR21 has been one of the short-listed candidate targets (Huang et al. 2015), as it is upstream of both VEGF and IL6. Also, MIF (see Section 5.2.5.20), which might be an even more upstream factor than the IL23/IL17 axis, is also worth exploring as a target, as exemplified by AVP-13546, which is an inhibitor of the tautomerase activity of MIF (Garai and Lóránd 2009). Given the complexity of the signaling circuit, it is possible that a large part of the circuit is yet to be discovered. A lot of research should be conducted to understand the circuit, so that it can be better manipulated.

Adhesion molecules, for example, integrin-based interventions, are potentially somewhat downstream from the highest upstream trigger, whose nature may not yet be resolved. However, it is possibly a strong brake jam in the amplification circuit because it might apply to several critical nodes in the network, some of which might have an absolute permissive role for the maintenance cycle of the inflammation to go on. It might be so powerful that the main concern is overshooting rather than ineffectiveness, for example, immunosuppression leading to activation of weak pathogens like the JCV, causing PML. So the final challenge would be to either find antivirals to directly circumvent this side effect or, even better, block the circuit at the right place in the right way so that only the intended effect takes place, that is, curing psoriasis in only the involved organs, for example, the skin joint. The successful mucosal targeting by vedolizumab in IBD has reinvigorated the hopes in the antiadhesion therapeutic field.

There are always many gaps between theory and practice. Predictions may fail in either direction. When TNFα blockade was initially being strategized, there was little theoretical hope because TNFα is such a redundant family. The fact that TNFα blockers worked so well in RA and psoriasis was a surprise. The same goes for the anti-B-cell treatment rituximab in RA, which was originally thought to be T cell dependent. However, in psoriasis anti-B-cell therapy does not work. On the other hand, antiadhesion therapy for psoriasis or angiogenesis did work, as in the case of efalizumab. It did not show paradoxical effects, but rather showed too much immunosuppression. Thus, despite setbacks, antiadhesion therapy for blocking angiogenesis in psoriasis deserves intense reattempts and fine-tuning in the future.

REFERENCES

Akman, A., E. Yilmaz, H. Mutlu, and M. Ozdogan. 2009. Complete remission of psoriasis following bevacizumab therapy for colon cancer. *Clinical and Experimental Dermatology* 34 (5): e202–e204.

Albanesi, C., C. Scarponi, S. Pallotta, R. Daniele, D. Bosisio, S. Madonna, P. Fortugno, S. è Gonzalvo-Feo, J.-D. Franssen, and M. Parmentier. 2009. Chemerin expression marks early psoriatic skin lesions and correlates with plasmacytoid dendritic cell recruitment. *Journal of Experimental Medicine* 206 (1): 249–258.

Artis, D., and H. Spits. 2015. The biology of innate lymphoid cells. *Nature* 517 (7534): 293–301.

Bacharach-Buhles, M., S. El Gammal, B. Panz, and P. Altmeyer. 1993. The pseudo-elongation of capillaries in psoriatic plaques. *Acta Dermato-Venereologica* 186 (Suppl.): 133–137.

Bhushan, M., T. O. Bleiker, A. E. Ballsdon, M. H. Allen, M. Sopwith, M. K. Robinson, C. Clarke et al. 2002. Anti-E-selectin is ineffective in the treatment of psoriasis: A randomized trial. *British Journal of Dermatology* 146 (5): 824–831.

Bhushan, M., B. McLaughlin, J. B. Weiss, and C. E. M. Griffiths. 1999. Levels of endothelial cell stimulating angiogenesis factor and vascular endothelial growth factor are elevated in psoriasis. *British Journal of Dermatology* 141 (6): 1054–1060.

Bhushan, M., T. Moore, A. L. Herrick, and C. E. M. Griffiths. 2000. Nailfold video capillaroscopy in psoriasis. *British Journal of Dermatology* 142 (6): 1171–1176.

Boers-Sonderen, M. J., S. F. Mulder, I. D. Nagtegaal, J. F. M. Jacobs, G. J. Wanten, F. Hoentjen, and C. M. van Herpen. 2014. Severe exacerbation of Crohn's disease during sunitinib treatment. *European Journal of Gastroenterology and Hepatology* 26 (2): 234–236.

Braverman, I. M. 1972. Electron microscopic studies of the microcirculation in psoriasis. *Journal of Investigative Dermatology* 59 (1): 91–98.

Braverman, I. M. 2000. The cutaneous microcirculation. *Journal of Investigative Dermatology* 5: 3–9.

Braverman, I. M., and A. Yen. 1977. Ultrastructure of the capillary loops in the dermal papillae of psoriasis. *Journal of Investigative Dermatology* 68 (1): 53–60.

Braverman, I. M., J. Sibley, and A. Keh-Yen. 1986. A study of the veil cells around normal, diabetic, and aged cutaneous microvessels. *Journal of Investigative Dermatology* 86 (1): 57–62.

Brinkmann, V., U. Reichard, C. Goosmann, B. Fauler, Y. Uhlemann, D. S. Weiss, Y. Weinrauch, and A. Zychlinsky. 2004. Neutrophil extracellular traps kill bacteria. *Science* 303 (5663): 1532–1535.

Brody, I. 1984. Mast cell degranulation in the evolution of acute eruptive guttate psoriasis vulgaris. *Journal of Investigative Dermatology* 82 (5): 460–464.

Civatte, A. 1924. Psoriasis and seborrhoeic eczema: Pathological anatomy and diagnostic histology of the two dermatoses. *British Journal of Dermatology* 36 (11): 461–476.

Creamer, D., M. Allen, R. Jaggar, R. Stevens, R. Bicknell, and J. Barker. 2002a. Mediation of systemic vascular hyperpermeability in severe psoriasis by circulating vascular endothelial growth factor. *Archives of Dermatology* 138 (6): 791–796.

Creamer, D., M. Allen, A. Sousa, R. Poston, and J. Barker. 1995. Altered vascular endothelium integrin expression in psoriasis. *American Journal of Pathology* 147 (6): 1661.

Creamer, D., M. H. Allen, A. Sousa, R. Poston, and J. N. W. N. Barker. 1997a. Localization of endothelial proliferation and microvascular expansion in active plaque psoriasis. *British Journal of Dermatology* 136 (6): 859–865.

Creamer, D., R. Jaggar, M. Allen, R. Bicknell, and J. Barker. 1997b. Overexpression of the angiogenic factor platelet-derived endothelial cell growth factor/thymidine phosphorylase in psoriatic epidermis. *British Journal of Dermatology* 137 (6): 851–855.

Creamer, D., D. Sullivan, R. Bicknell, and J. Barker. 2002b. Angiogenesis in psoriasis. *Angiogenesis* 5 (4): 231–236.

Datta-Mitra, A., N. K. Riar, and S. P. Raychaudhuri. 2014. Remission of psoriasis and psoriatic arthritis during bevacizumab therapy for renal cell cancer. *Indian Journal of Dermatology* 59 (6): 632.

Diamantis, M. L., and S. Y. Chon. 2010. Sorafenib-induced psoriasiform eruption in a patient with metastatic thyroid carcinoma. *Journal of Drugs in Dermatology* 9 (2): 169–171.

Djonov, V., O. Baum, and P. H. Burri. 2003. Vascular remodeling by intussusceptive angiogenesis. *Cell and Tissue Research* 314 (1): 107–117.

Döme, B., M. J. C. Hendrix, S. Paku, J. Tóvári, and J. Tímár. 2007. Alternative vascularization mechanisms in cancer. *American Journal of Pathology* 170 (1): 1–15.

Donn, R. P., D. Plant, F. Jury, H. L. Richards, J. Worthington, D. W. Ray, and C. E. M. Griffiths. 2004. Macrophage migration inhibitory factor gene polymorphism is associated with psoriasis. *Journal of Investigative Dermatology* 123 (3): 484–487.

Du-Thanh, A., C. Girard, G.-P. Pageaux, B. Guillot, and O. Dereure. 2013. Sorafenib-induced annular pustular psoriasis (Milian-Katchoura type). *European Journal of Dermatology* 23 (6): 900–901.

Eckert, R. L., A.-M. Broome, M. Ruse, N. Robinson, D. Ryan, and K. Lee. 2004. S100 proteins in the epidermis. *Journal of Investigative Dermatology* 123 (1): 23–33.

Espinoza, L. R., C. G. Espinoza, M. L. Cuellar, E. Scopelitis, L. H. Silveira, and G. R. Grotendorst. 1994. Fibroblast function in psoriatic arthritis. II. Increased expression of beta platelet derived growth factor receptors and increased production of growth factor and cytokines. *Journal of Rheumatology* 21 (8): 1507–1511.

Espinoza, L. R., F. B. Vasey, C. G. Espinoza, T. S. Bocanegra, and B. F. Germain. 1982. Vascular changes in psoriatic synovium. A light and electron microscopic study. *Arthritis and Rheumatism* 25 (6): 677–684.

Eswarappa, S. M., A. A. Potdar, W. J. Koch, Y. Fan, K. Vasu, D. Lindner, B. Willard, L. M. Graham, P. E. DiCorleto, and P. L. Fox. 2014. Programmed translational readthrough generates anti-angiogenic VEGF-Ax. *Cell* 157 (7): 1605–1618.

Fearon, U., K. Griosios, A. Fraser, R. Reece, P. Emery, P. F. Jones, and D. J. Veale. 2003. Angiopoietins, growth factors, and vascular morphology in early arthritis. *Journal of Rheumatology* 30 (2): 260–268.

Fearon, U., R. Reece, J. Smith, P. Emery, and D. J. Veale. 1998. Differential cytokines and growth factor expression: Basis for different pathogenesis of psoriatic and rheumatoid arthritis. *Arthritis and Rheumatism* 41 (9).

Flisiak, I., P. Zaniewski, and B. Chodynicka. 2008. Plasma TGF-β1, TIMP-1, MMP-1 and IL-18 as a combined biomarker of psoriasis activity. *Biomarkers* 13 (5): 549–556.

Flisiak, I., P. Zaniewski, M. Rogalska, H. Myśliwiec, J. Jaroszewicz, and B. Chodynicka. 2010. Effect of psoriasis activity on VEGF and its soluble receptors concentrations in serum and plaque scales. *Cytokine* 52 (3): 225–229.

Foell, D., and J. Roth. 2004. Proinflammatory S100 proteins in arthritis and autoimmune disease. *Arthritis and Rheumatism* 50 (12): 3762–3771.

Folkman, J. 1971. Tumor angiogenesis: Therapeutic implications. *New England Journal of Medicine* 285 (21): 1182–1186.

Folkman, J. 1972. Angiogenesis in psoriasis: Therapeutic implications. *Journal of Investigative Dermatology* 59 (1): 40–43.

Folkman, J., E. Merler, C. Abernathy, and G. Williams. 1971. Isolation of a tumor factor responsible for angiogenesis. *Journal of Experimental Medicine* 133 (2): 275.

Folkman, J., Y. Shing, R. Sullivan, C. Butterfield, J. Murray, and M. Klagsbrun. 1984. Heparin affinity-purification of a tumor derived capillary endothelial cell growth factor. *Science* 223: 1296–1300.

Fournier, C., and G. Tisman. 2010. Sorafenib-associated remission of psoriasis in hypernephroma: Case report. *Dermatology Online Journal* 16 (2): 17.

Francescone, R. A., S. Scully, M. Faibish, S. L. Taylor, D. Oh, L. Moral, W. Yan, B. Bentley, and R. Shao. 2011. Role of YKL-40 in the angiogenesis, radioresistance, and progression of glioblastoma. *Journal of Biological Chemistry* 286 (17): 15332–15343. doi:10.1074/jbc.M110.212514

Fuhlbrigge, R. C., J. D. Kieffer, D. Armerding, and T. S. Kupper. 1997. Cutaneous lymphocyte antigen is a specialized form of PSGL-1 expressed on skin-homing T cells. *Nature* 389 (6654): 978.

Fuhlbrigge, R. C., and C. Weishaupt. 2007. Adhesion molecules in cutaneous immunity. *Seminars in Immunopathology* 29 (1): 45–57.

Gallatin, W. M., I. L. Weissman, and E. C. Butcher. 1983. A cell-surface molecule involved in organ-specific homing of lymphocytes. *Nature* 304 (5921): 30.

Gambino, L. S., N. G. Wreford, J. F. Bertram, P. Dockery, F. Lederman, and P. A. W. Rogers. 2002. Angiogenesis occurs by vessel elongation in proliferative phase human endometrium. *Human Reproduction* 17 (5): 1199–1206.

Garai, J., and T. Lóránd. 2009. Macrophage migration inhibitory factor (MIF) tautomerase inhibitors as potential novel anti-inflammatory agents: Current developments. *Current Medicinal Chemistry* 16 (9): 1091–1114.

Georg Fassbender, H. 2003. New aspects in joint and bone processes in psoriatic arthritis (PSA). *Acta Clinica Croatica* 42 (2): 133–137.

Goddard, D. H., S. L. Grossman, W. V. Williams, D. B. Weiner, J. L. Gross, K. Eidsvoog, and J. R. Dasch. 1992. Regulation of synovial cell growth: Coexpression of transforming growth factor β and basic fibroblast growth factor by cultured synovial cells. *Arthritis and Rheumatism* 35 (11): 1296–1303.

Goodfield, M., S. Macdonald Hull, D. Holland, G. Roberts, E. Wood, S. Reid, and W. Cunliffe. 1994. Investigations of the 'active' edge of plaque psoriasis: Vascular proliferation precedes changes in epidermal keratin. *British Journal of Dermatology* 131 (6): 808–813.

Graceffa, D., E. Maiani, A. Pace, F. M. Solivetti, F. Elia, C. De Mutiis, and C. Bonifati. 2012. Psoriatic arthritis during treatment with bevacizumab for anaplastic oligodendroglioma. *Case Reports in Rheumatology* 2012: e208606.

Gudjonsson, J. E., A. Johnston, S. W. Stoll, M. Riblett, X. Xing, J. J. Kochkodan, J. Ding et al. 2010. Evidence for altered Wnt signaling in psoriatic skin. *Journal of Investigative Dermatology* 130 (7): 1849–1859.

Guérard, S., and R. Pouliot. 2012. The role of angiogenesis in the pathogenesis of psoriasis: Mechanisms and clinical implications. *Journal of Clinical and Experimental Dermatology Research* S2: 2.

Hashimoto-Tane, A., M. Sakuma, H. Ike, T. Yokosuka, Y. Kimura, O. Ohara, and T. Saito. 2016. Micro-adhesion rings surrounding TCR microclusters are essential for T cell activation. *Journal of Experimental Medicine* 213 (8): 1609–1625.

Hawkes, J. E., G. H. Nguyen, M. Fujita, S. R. Florell, K. C. Duffin, G. G. Krueger, and R. M. O'Connell. 2016. MicroRNAs in psoriasis. *Journal of Investigative Dermatology* 136 (2): 365–371.

Henno, A., S. Blacher, C. Lambert, A. Colige, L. Seidel, A. Noël, C. Lapière, M. De La Brassinne, and B. V. Nusgens. 2009. Altered expression of angiogenesis and lymphangiogenesis markers in the uninvolved skin of plaque-type psoriasis. *British Journal of Dermatology* 160 (3): 581–590.

Henno, A., S. Blacher, C. A. Lambert, C. Deroanne, A. Noël, C. Lapiere, M. de la Brassinne, B. V. Nusgens, and A. Colige. 2010. Histological and transcriptional study of angiogenesis and lymphangiogenesis in uninvolved skin, acute pinpoint lesions and established psoriasis plaques: An approach of vascular development chronology in psoriasis. *Journal of Dermatological Science* 57 (3): 162–169.

Hern, S., and P. S. Mortimer. 2007. In vivo quantification of microvessels in clinically uninvolved psoriatic skin and in normal skin. *British Journal of Dermatology* 156 (6): 1224–1229.

Ho, P., I. N. Bruce, A. Silman, D. Symmons, B. Newman, H. Young, C. E. M. Griffiths, S. John, J. Worthington, and A. Barton. 2005. Evidence for common genetic control in pathways of inflammation for Crohn's disease and psoriatic arthritis. *Arthritis and Rheumatism* 52 (11): 3596–3602.

Huang, R.-Y., L. Li, M.-J. Wang, X.-M. Chen, Q.-C. Huang, and C.-J. Lu. 2015. An exploration of the role of microRNAs in psoriasis. *Medicine* 94 (45).

Humphries, J. D., A. Byron, and M. J. Humphries. 2006. Integrin ligands. *Journal of Cell Science* 119 (Pt. 19): 3901–3903.

Hung, C.-T., C.-P. Chiang, and B.-Y. Wu. 2012. Sorafenib-induced psoriasis and hand–foot skin reaction responded dramatically to systemic narrowband ultraviolet B phototherapy. *Journal of Dermatology* 39 (12): 1076–1077.

Inaoki, M., S. Sato, Y. Shimada, S. Kawara, D. A. Steeber, and T. F. Tedder. 2000. Decreased expression levels of L-selectin on subsets of leucocytes and increased serum L-selectin in severe psoriasis. *Clinical and Experimental Immunology* 122 (3): 484–492.

Keck, P. J., S. D. Hauser, G. Krivi, K. Sanzo, T. Warren, J. Feder, and D. T. Connolly. 1989. Vascular permeability factor, an endothelial cell mitogen related to PDGF. *Science* 246 (4935): 1309.

Kerkhof, P. C. M., H. Rennes, R. Grood, F. W. Bauer, and P. D. Mier. 1983. Metabolic changes at the margin of the spreading psoriatic lesion. *British Journal of Dermatology* 108 (6): 647–652.

KilarsKi, W. W., and P. GerWins. 2009. A new mechanism of blood vessel growth—Hope for new treatment strategies. *Discovery Medicine* 8 (40): 23–27.

Kobayashi, H., and P. C. Lin. 2009. Angiogenesis links chronic inflammation with cancer. In *Inflammation and Cancer: Methods and Protocols*, Vol. 1, *Experimental Models and Practical Approaches*, 185–191. New York: Humana Press.

Krane, J. F., D. P. Murphy, A. B. Gottlieb, D. M. Carter, C. E. Hart, and J. G. Krueger. 1991. Increased dermal expression of platelet-derived growth factor receptors in growth-activated skin wounds and psoriasis. *Journal of Investigative Dermatology* 96 (6): 983–986.

Lawler, J. W., H. S. Slayter, and J. E. Coligan. 1978. Isolation and characterization of a high molecular weight glycoprotein from human blood platelets. *Journal of Biological Chemistry* 253: 8609–8616.

Lee, M. L., S. S. T. To, A. Cooper, M. Jones, and L. Schrieber. 1993. Augmented lymphocyte binding to cultured endothelium in psoriasis. *Clinical and Experimental Immunology* 91 (3): 346–350.

Lee, S., and M. L. Iruela-Arispe. 2008. The extracellular matrix and VEGF processing. *Antiangiogenic Agents in Cancer Therapy*, 85–97.

Levick, J. R. 1995. Microvascular architecture and exchange in synovial joints. *Microcirculation* 2 (3): 217–233.

Ley, K., J. Rivera-Nieves, W. J. Sandborn, and S. Shattil. 2016. Integrin-based therapeutics: Biological basis, clinical use and new drugs. *Nature Reviews Drug Discovery* 15 (3): 173–183.

Lin, A. M., C. J. Rubin, R. Khandpur, J. Y. Wang, M. Riblett, S. Yalavarthi, E. C. Villanueva, P. Shah, M. J. Kaplan, and A. T. Bruce. 2011. Mast cells and neutrophils release IL-17 through extracellular trap formation in psoriasis. *The Journal of Immunology* 187 (1): 490–500.

Lowe, P. M., M.-L. Lee, C. J. Jackson, S. S. T. To, A. J. Cooper, and L. Schrieber. 1995. The endothelium in psoriasis. *British Journal of Dermatology* 132 (4): 497–505.

Mai, J. 2014. Role of Interleukin-17 in Endothelial Cell Activation and Vascular Function. ProQuest Dissertations Publishing, Temple University.

Man, X.-Y., X.-H. Yang, S.-Q. Cai, Z.-Y. Bu, and M. Zheng. 2008. Overexpression of vascular endothelial growth factor (VEGF) receptors on keratinocytes in psoriasis: Regulated by calcium independent of VEGF. *Journal of Cellular and Molecular Medicine* 12 (2): 649–660.

Man, X.-Y., and M. Zheng. 2015. Role of angiogenic and inflammatory signal pathways in psoriasis. *Journal of Investigative Dermatology* 17 (1): 43–45.

Manole, C. G., M. Gherghiceanu, and O. Simionescu. 2015. Telocyte dynamics in psoriasis. *Journal of Cellular and Molecular Medicine* 19 (7): 1504–1519.

McAuslan, B. R., and H. Hoffman. 1979. Endothelial stimulating factor from Walker carcinoma cells. *Experimental Cell Research* 199: 181–190.

McGonagle, D., P. G. Conaghan, and P. Emery. 1999. Psoriatic arthritis: A unified concept twenty years On. *Arthritis and Rheumatism* 42 (6): 1080–1086.

McGonagle, D., R. J. U. Lories, A. L. Tan, and M. Benjamin. 2007. The concept of a "Synovio-Entheseal Complex" and its implications for understanding joint inflammation and damage in psoriatic arthritis and beyond. *Arthritis and Rheumatism* 56 (8): 2482–2491.

McGonagle, D., and M. F. McDermott. 2006. A proposed classification of the immunological diseases. *PLoS Medicine* 3 (8): e297.

McGonagle, D., and A. L. Tan. 2015. The enthesis in psoriatic arthritis. *Clinical and Experimental Rheumatology* 33 (5 Suppl. 93): 36–39.

Mensah, K. A., E. M. Schwarz, and C. T. Ritchlin. 2008. Altered bone remodeling in psoriatic arthritis. *Current Rheumatology Reports* 10 (4): 311–317.

Menter, M. A., and C. Ryan. 2017. *Psoriasis*. 2nd ed. Boca Raton, FL: CRC Press.

Micali, G., F. Lacarrubba, M. L. Musumeci, D. Massimino, and M. R. Nasca. 2010. Cutaneous vascular patterns in psoriasis. *International Journal of Dermatology* 49 (3): 249–256.

Moll, J. M. H., and V. Wright. 1973. Psoriatic arthritis. *Seminars in Arthritis and Rheumatism* 3: 55–78.

Moustou, A. E., P. Alexandrou, A. J. Stratigos, I. Giannopoulou, T. Vergou, A. Katsambas, and C. Antoniou. 2014. Expression of lymphatic markers and lymphatic growth factors in psoriasis before and after anti-TNF treatment. *Anais Brasileiros de Dermatologia* 89 (6): 891–897.

Myers, C., A. Charboneau, I. Cheung, D. Hanks, and N. Boudreau. 2002. Sustained expression of homeobox D10 inhibits angiogenesis. *American Journal of Pathology* 161 (6): 2099–2109.

Napolitano, M., F. Caso, L. Costa, M. Megna, T. Cirillo, A. Balato, and R. Scarpa. 2017. Paradoxical onset of psoriatic arthritis during treatment with biologic agents for plaque psoriasis: A combined dermatology and rheumatology clinical study. *Clinical and Experimental Rheumatology* 35 (1): 137–140.

Nestle, F. O., C. Conrad, A. Tun-Kyi, B. Homey, M. Gombert, O. Boyman, G. Burg, Y.-J. Liu, and M. Gilliet. 2005. Plasmacytoid predendritic cells initiate psoriasis through interferon-α production. *Journal of Experimental Medicine* 202 (1): 135–143.

Nickoloff, B. J., R. S. Mitra, J. Varani, V. M. Dixit, and P. J. Polverini. 1994. Aberrant production of interleukin-8 and thrombospondin-1 by psoriatic keratinocytes mediates angiogenesis. *American Journal of Pathology* 144 (4): 820.

Nicosia, R. F., and G. P. Tuszynski. 1994. Matrix-bound thrombospondin promotes angiogenesis in vitro. *Journal of Cell Biology* 124 (1): 183–193.

Nowak, D. G., J. Woolard, E. M. Amin, O. Konopatskaya, M. A. Saleem, A. J. Churchill, M. R. Ladomery, S. J. Harper, and D. O. Bates. 2008. Expression of pro- and anti-angiogenic isoforms of VEGF is differentially regulated by splicing and growth factors. *Journal of Cell Science* 121 (20): 3487–3495.

Parent, D., B. A. Bernard, C. Desbas, M. Heenen, and M. Y. Darmon. 1990. Spreading of psoriatic plaques: Alteration of epidermal differentiation precedes capillary leakiness and anomalies in vascular morphology. *Journal of Investigative Dermatology* 95 (3): 333–340.

Patan, S. 2013. How Is The Branching of Animal Blood Vessels Implemented? *Madame Curie Bioscience Database*. Austin, TX: Landes Bioscience.

Piccard, H., R. J. Muschel, and G. Opdenakker. 2012. On the dual roles and polarized phenotypes of neutrophils in tumor development and progression. *Critical Reviews in Oncology/Hematology* 82 (3): 296–309.

Qiu, Y., C. Hoareau-Aveilla, S. Oltean, S. J. Harper, and D. O. Bates. 2009. The anti-angiogenic isoforms of VEGF in health and disease. *Biochemical Society Transactions* 37 (Pt. 6): 1207–1213.

Rafii, D. C., B. Psaila, J. Butler, D. K. Jin, and D. Lyden. 2008. Regulation of vasculogenesis by platelet-mediated recruitment of bone marrow–derived cells. *Arteriosclerosis, Thrombosis, and Vascular Biology* 28 (2): 217–222.

Ragaz, A., and A. B. Ackerman. 1979. Evolution, maturation, and regression of lesions of psoriasis: New observations and correlation of clinical and histologic findings. *American Journal of Dermatopathology* 1 (3): 199–214.

Raychaudhuri, S. P., W. Y. Jiang, and E. M. Farber. 1998. Psoriatic keratinocytes express high levels of nerve growth factor. *Acta Dermatovenereologica-Stockholm* 78: 84–86.

Redisch, W., E. J. Messina, G. Hughes, and C. McEwen. 1970. Capillaroscopic observations in rheumatic diseases. *Annals of the Rheumatic Diseases* 29 (3): 244.

Reece, R. J., J. D. Canete, W. J. Parsons, P. Emery, and D. J. Veale. 1999. Distinct vascular patterns of early synovitis in psoriatic, reactive, and rheumatoid arthritis. *Arthritis and Rheumatism* 42 (7): 1481–1484.

Ritchlin, C., S. A. Haas-Smith, D. Hicks, J. Cappuccio, C. K. Osterland, and R. J. Looney. 1998. Patterns of cytokine production in psoriatic synovium. *Journal of Rheumatology* 25 (8): 1544–1552.

Ritchlin, C. T., R. A. Colbert, and D. D. Gladman. 2017. Psoriatic arthritis. *New England Journal of Medicine* 376 (10): 957–970.

Robinson, S. D., and K. M. Hodivala-Dilke. 2011. The role of β3-integrins in tumor angiogenesis: Context is everything. *Current Opinion in Cell Biology* 23 (5): 630–637.

Şahin, M., E. Şahin, and S. Gümüşlü. 2009. Cyclooxygenase-2 in cancer and angiogenesis. *Angiology* 60 (2): 242–253.

Sano, S. 2015. Psoriasis as a barrier disease. *Dermatologica Sinica* 33 (2): 64–69.

Sari, I., A. Alacacioglu, L. Kebapcilar, A. Taylan, O. Bilgir, Y. Yildiz, A. Yuksel, and D. L. Kozaci. 2010. Assessment of soluble cell adhesion molecules and soluble CD40 ligand levels in ankylosing spondylitis. *Joint, Bone, Spine* 77 (1): 85–87.

Schön, M. P., and W.-H. Boehncke. 2005. Psoriasis. *New England Journal of Medicine* 352 (18): 1899–1912.

Sedie, A. D., I. Puxeddu, M. Tronchetti, P. Migliorini, S. Bombardieri, and L. Riente. 2013. AB0075 the endogenous angiostatic mediators endostatin and thrombospondin-1 are increased in psoriatic arthritis. *Annals of the Rheumatic Diseases* 71 (Suppl. 3): 642.

Senger, D. R., K. P. Claffey, J. E. Benes, C. A. Perruzzi, A. P. Sergiou, and M. Detmar. 1997. Angiogenesis promoted by vascular endothelial growth factor: Regulation through α1β1 and α2β1 integrins. *Proceedings of the National Academy of Sciences of the United States of America* 94 (25): 13612–13617.

Somanath, P. R., A. Ciocea, and T. V. Byzova. 2009. Integrin and growth factor receptor alliance in angiogenesis. *Cell Biochemistry and Biophysics* 53 (2): 53–64.

Stuart, P. E., R. P. Nair, E. Ellinghaus, J. Ding, T. Tejasvi, J. E. Gudjonsson, Y. Li et al. 2010. Genome-wide association analysis identifies three psoriasis susceptibility loci. *Nature Genetics* 42 (11): 1000–1004.

Suárez-Fariñas, M., J. Fuentes-Duculan, M. A. Lowes, and J. G. Krueger. 2011. Resolved psoriasis lesions retain expression of a subset of disease-related genes. *Journal of Investigative Dermatology* 131 (2): 391–400.

Telner, P., and Z. Fekete. 1961. The capillary responses in psoriatic skin. *Journal of Investigative Dermatology* 36 (3): 225–230.

Toussirot, É., and F. Aubin. 2016. Paradoxical reactions under TNF-α blocking agents and other biological agents given for chronic immune-mediated diseases: An analytical and comprehensive overview. *RMD Open* 2 (2).

Uhoda, I., G. E. Piérard, C. Pierard-Franchimont, J. E. Arrese, V. Goffin, A. Nikkels, P. Paquet, and P. Quatresooz. 2005. Vascularity and fractal dimension of the dermo-epidermal interface in guttate and plaque-type psoriasis. *Dermatology* 210 (3): 189–193.

Veale, D. J., C. Ritchlin, and O. FitzGerald. 2005. Immunopathology of psoriasis and psoriatic arthritis. *Skin* 27: 28.

Veale, D. J., and U. Fearon. 2015. What makes psoriatic and rheumatoid arthritis so different? *RMD Open* 1 (1): e000025.

Wakefield, R. J., M. J. Green, H. Marzo-Ortega, P. G. Conaghan, W. W. Gibbon, D. McGonagle, S. Proudman, and P. Emery. 2004. Should oligoarthritis be reclassified? Ultrasound reveals a high prevalence of subclinical disease. *Annals of the Rheumatic Diseases* 63 (4): 382–385.

Walsh, D. A., and C. I. Pearson. 2001. Angiogenesis in the pathogenesis of inflammatory joint and lung diseases. *Arthritis Res* 3: 147–153.

Weiss, J. B., R. A. Brown, S. Kumar, and P. Phillips. 1979. An angiogenic factor isolated from tumours: A potent low molecular weight compound. *British Journal of Cancer* 40 (3): 493–496.

Welti, J., S. Loges, S. Dimmeler, and P. Carmeliet. 2013. Recent molecular discoveries in angiogenesis and antiangiogenic therapies in cancer. *Journal of Clinical Investigation* 123 (8): 3190.

Wetzel, A., T. Wetzig, U. F. Haustein, M. Sticherling, U. Anderegg, J. C. Simon, and A. Saalbach. 2006. Increased neutrophil adherence in psoriasis: Role of the human endothelial cell receptor thy-1 (CD90). *Journal of Investigative Dermatology* 126 (2): 441–452.

WHO (World Health Organization). 2016. Global report on psoriasis. Geneva: WHO.

Wolfram, J. A., D. Diaconu, D. A. Hatala, J. Rastegar, D. A. Knutsen, A. Lowther, D. Askew, A. C. Gilliam, T. S. McCormick, and N. L. Ward. 2009. Keratinocyte but not endothelial cell-specific overexpression of Tie2 leads to the development of psoriasis. *American Journal of Pathology* 174 (4): 1443–1458.

Wollina, U., G. Hansel, A. Koch, J. Schönlebe, E. Köstler, and G. Haroske. 2008. Tumor necrosis factor-α inhibitor-induced psoriasis or psoriasiform exanthemata. *American Journal of Clinical Dermatology* 9 (1): 1–14.

Yiu, Z. Z. N., F. R. Ali, and C. E. M. Griffiths. 2016. Paradoxical exacerbation of chronic plaque psoriasis by sorafenib. *Clinical and Experimental Dermatology* 41 (4): 407–409.

Yuan, A., C.-Y. Lin, C.-H. Chou, C.-M. Shih, C.-Y. Chen, H.-W. Cheng, Y.-F. Chen et al. 2011. Functional and structural characteristics of tumor angiogenesis in lung cancers overexpressing different VEGF isoforms assessed by DCE- and SSCE-MRI. *PLoS One* 6 (1): e16062.

Yuan, S., S. Zhang, Y. Zhuang, H. Zhang, J. Bai, and Q. Hou. 2015. Interleukin-17 stimulates STAT3-mediated endothelial cell activation for neutrophil recruitment. *Cellular Physiology and Biochemistry* 36 (6): 2340–2356.

Zollner, T. M., K. Asadullah, and M. P. Schön. 2007. Targeting leukocyte trafficking to inflamed skin—Still an attractive therapeutic approach? *Experimental Dermatology* 16 (1): 1–12.

Zorzou, M.-P., A. Stratigos, E. Efstathiou, and A. Bamias. 2004. Exacerbation of psoriasis after treatment with an EGFR tyrosine kinase inhibitor. *Acta Dermato-Venereologica* 84 (4): 308–309.

6 Multifaceted Role of Th17 Cells in Psoriatic Disease

Soumya D. Chakravarty

CONTENTS

6.1 INTRODUCTION

The recently discovered T-helper 17 (Th17) lymphocytes have transformed our understanding of the pathophysiological mechanisms that contribute to the development of psoriasis and psoriatic arthritis (PsA). Th17 cells represent a subset of CD4+ T cells completely distinct from Th1 and Th2 cells. Historically, the classification of T cells has consisted of two predominant subsets, Th1 and Th2, triggered by antigen presentation to naïve CD4+ T cells and subsequent differentiation into either subclass, depending on the prevailing cytokine signature, namely interleukin 12 (IL-12) for the former and IL-4 for the latter. Classically, Th1 cells have been involved in protection against intracellular organisms through the production of interferon γ (IFNγ). In contrast, Th2 lymphocytes produce cytokines that result in protection against extracellular pathogens, allergic reactions, and humoral immunity. Th17 lymphocytes are characterized in part by their secretion of IL-17, which has been linked in the past to defense mechanisms against protozoa, bacteria, and fungi. However, as will be discussed in this chapter, the role of Th17 cells in the pathogenesis of psoriatic disease also highlights the significance of these cells in mediating autoinflammatory conditions [1].

6.2 OVERVIEW OF PSORIATIC DISEASE

PsA belongs to a group of overlapping, autoinflammatory arthritides, termed the seronegative spondyloarthritides, that commonly affect the joints, entheses, and skin. The disease affects about 2%–3% of the general population and carries a significant health and disability burden to both individuals and society at large [2]. Typically, 6%–42% of patients with preceding psoriasis will go on to develop PsA [2]. Clinical features of PsA typically include psoriasis, enthesitis, dactylitis, nail pitting and/or onycholysis, as well as peripheral and/or axial joint manifestations (Figure 6.1) [3]. It is believed that about 67% of patients with clinical and/or radiological PsA show signs of bone destruction in the form of erosions [2].

The diagnosis of PsA is usually based on clinical presentation and features [3]. Furthermore, the International Classification of Psoriatic Arthritis study proposed the most currently used

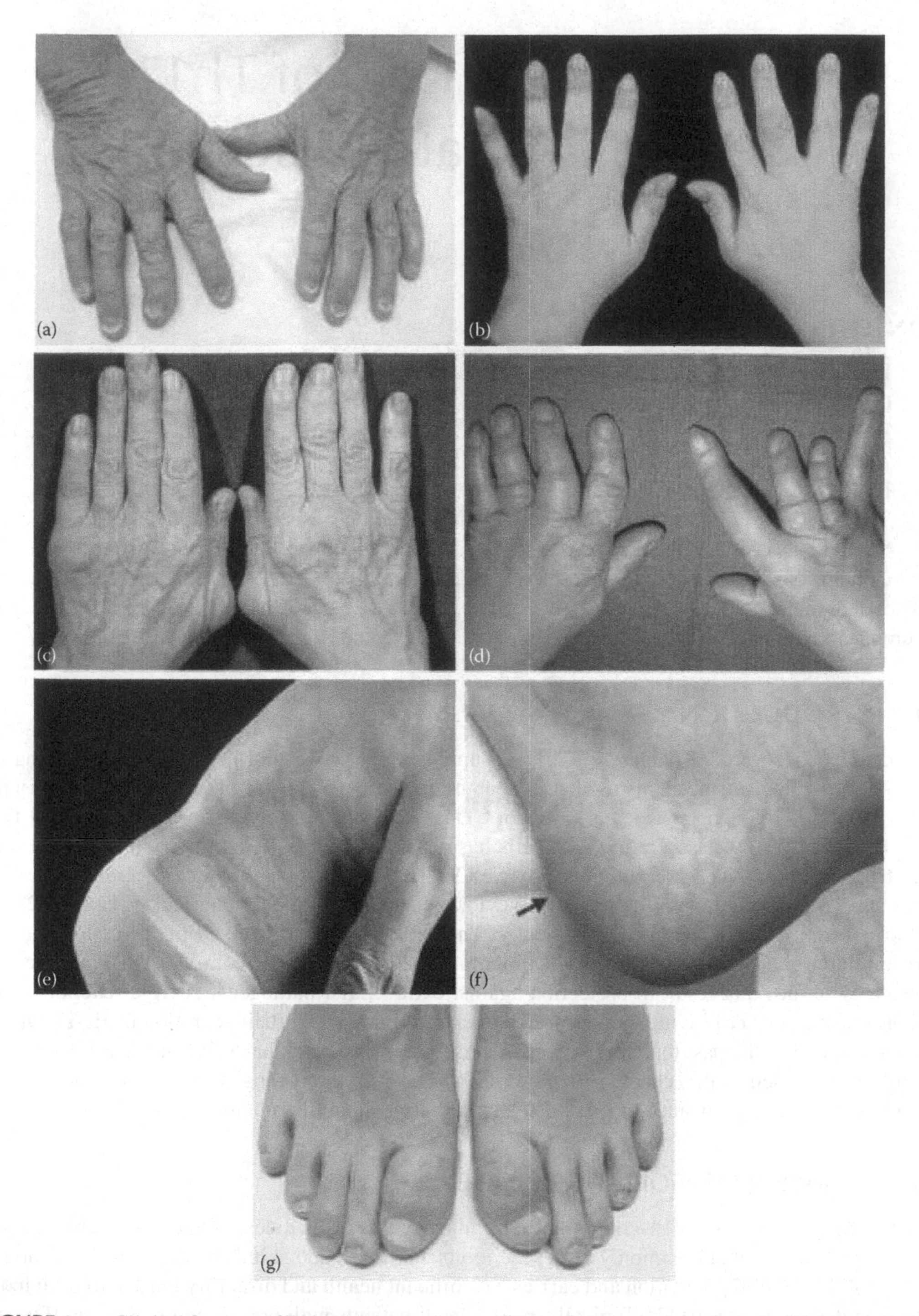

FIGURE 6.1 Clinical features of PsA. (a) Distal subtype of PsA with adjacent onycholysis. (b) Oligoarticular subtype. (c) Polyarticular subtype. (d) Arthritis mutilans, with telescoping of digits and asymmetric and differential involvement of adjacent digits. (e) Spondylitis subtype. (f) Enthesitis of the Achilles tendon (arrow). (g) Dactylitis of the big toes. (From Ritchlin, C.T. et al. *N. Engl. J. Med.*, 376, 957–970, 2017.)

Classification Criteria for Psoriatic Arthritis (CASPAR) utilized for the inclusion and exclusion of patients in clinical research [4]. With validation, their sensitivity has been found to be 91.4%, and specificity 98.7% [4]. A patient is classified as having PsA if he or she has inflammatory articular disease (joint, spine, or entheseal) and at least 3 points from the following [4]:

- Skin psoriasis that is
  - Present—2 points, or
  - Previously present by history—1 point, or
  - A family history of psoriasis, if the patient is not affected—1 point
- Nail lesions (onycholysis, pitting, and hyperkeratosis)—1 point
- Negative rheumatoid factor (RF)—1 point
- Dactylitis (present or past)—1 point
- Juxta-articular bone formation on radiographs (unrelated to osteophytes)—1 point

6.3 PATHOGENESIS OF PSORIATIC DISEASE

The exact etiology of PsA remains unclear. It is believed that PsA results from a complex interaction between a genetically predisposed individual and immune dysregulation as a result of some environmental exposure or trigger. The genetics of PsA are discussed in depth elsewhere in this book.

In 1986, Mossman and Coffman first postulated the Th1/Th2 paradigm when they described two distinct T-helper lymphocyte subsets—Th1 and Th2 cells [5]. It is known that innate immune cells regulate T lymphocytes by secreting specific cytokines and depending on the cytokine milieu, differentiation occurs by either the promotion or inhibition of such cells. IFNγ, produced by Th1 lymphocytes, inhibits the differentiation of IL-4-secreting Th2 cells, whereas IL-4 inhibits the IFNγ-producing Th1 cells [5]. Therefore, IL-12 induces a Th1 response, while IL-4 induces a Th2 response. This proved insufficient when the new IL-23 cytokine was discovered in 2000. The newly discovered IL-23 was found to have a shared p40 subunit with IL-12. IL-12 contains both the p35 and p40 subunits, and its main function is to drive the differentiation of naïve T CD4+ cells to IFNγ-producing Th1 cells [6].

6.4 TH17 CELLS

In 2005, the discovery of CD3+/CD4+ Th17 cells changed the paradigm for understanding autoinflammatory disease processes [7,8]. Th17 cells are a distinct form of CD4+ T cells that by either induction or activation can produce a completely distinct cytokine repertoire. These cells respond to the interleukin 1 receptor 1 (IL-1R1) and interleukin 23 receptor (IL-23R) signaling pathways. It has been postulated that transforming growth factor β (TGFβ), IL-1, IL-6, and IL-23 induce retinoic acid orphan receptors (RORγt and RORα), which result in the upregulation of IL-23R and eventual differentiation of naïve CD4+ T cells into Th17 cells. This has been eloquently summarized in a model for the development of Th17 cells, consisting of three overlapping steps: differentiation, amplification, and stabilization [9]. In particular, TGFβ and IL-6 induce differentiation, IL-21 expressed by developing Th17 cells mediates amplification, and IL-23 expands and stabilizes previously differentiated Th17 cells (also summarized in Table 6.1) [9].

IL-23, consisting of a distinct p19 and shared p40 subunit with IL-12, is considered the critical regulatory cytokine in driving Th17 expansion and survival, whereas IL-12 remains the upstream regulatory cytokine responsible for Th1 differentiation and downstream IFNγ production [1]. Notably, in both humans and mice, naïve CD4+ T cells can also differentiate into Th17 cells in the presence of IL-1, IL-6, and IL-23, without any requirement for TGFβ in the process [10]. The two types of Th17 cells induced by either TGFβ or IL-6, or alternatively, IL-1, IL-6, and IL-23, appear to be functionally and transcriptionally distinct, with potentially different roles in clearing different types of pathogens [9]. In humans, Th17 cells that express IL-17 with IFNγ have specificity for

TABLE 6.1
Th17 Lymphocyte Differentiation

Key Th17 Differentiation Inducers	Key Th17 Differentiation Inhibitors
TGFβ: Essential factor needed for naïve T-cell to Th17 development in concert with IL-6 and IL-23. Il-1β: Involved in early Th17 differentiation. Upregulates RORγt and IRF4. Helps maintain Th17 cytokine profile postpolarization. IL-6: Essential in the activation of IL-17-specific transcription factor RORγt and IL-21 expression, leading to the expression of IL-17A, IL-17F, and IL-23R on Th17 cells. IL-23: Decreases the ability of de-differentiation and plasticity of Th17 cells. Induces expression of the characteristic Th17 cytokines and is essential for their survival and expansion.	IFNγ, IL-2, IL-4, IL-27

Candida albicans, whereas Th17 cells that secrete both IL-17 and IL-10 appear to have specificity for *Staphylococcus aureus* [11]. Hence, Th17 cells clearly demonstrate differing abilities to clear different types of infections, with broader implications as to whether some Th17 cells can be pathogenic versus nonpathogenic in mediating autoimmune disease [9].

Once activated, Th17 cells secrete several cytokines, such as IL-17A, IL-17F, IL-17AF, IL-21, IL-22, IL-26, granulocyte-monocyte colony-stimulating factor (GM-CSF), macrophage inflammatory protein-3α (MIP-3α), and tumor necrosis factor α (TNFα) (Table 6.2).

TABLE 6.2
Th17-Secreted Cytokines

IL-17A

- Regulates local tissue inflammation through coordinated expression of pro-inflammatory and neutrophil-mobilizing cytokines and chemokines
- Secreted as a homodimer and heterodimer

IL-17F

- Involved in neutrophil recruitment and immunity to extracellular pathogens
- Secreted as a homodimer and heterodimer

IL-17AF heterodimer

- Overlaps in function with IL-17A and IL-17F homodimers

IL-21

- Upregulated early in differentiation by IL-6
- Enhances Th17 maintenance by upregulating IL-23R
- Helps promotes/sustain Th17 lineage commitment

IL-22

- Induces antimicrobial peptide and pro-inflammatory cytokine expression on keratinocytes and other nonhematopoietic cells

IL-26

- Enhances Th17 pro-inflammatory response on epithelial cells

GM-CSF

- Critical for the pro-inflammatory functions of Th17 cells
- Promotes M1 macrophage differentiation

MIP-3α

- The ligand for CCR6; blocking delays the onset of arthritis

TNFα

- Pleiotropic immune activator and regulator thought to enhance Th17 pathology

6.5 IL-17

IL-17A (also known as IL-17) is a glycoprotein member of the larger family of IL-17 cytokines, namely IL-17A, IL-17B, IL-17C, IL-17D, IL-17E, and IL-17F. IL-17A most closely relates to IL-17F, with these isoforms resulting in the formation of homodimers or heterodimers. Additionally, IL-17C acts in an autocrine manner and its functions overlap with those of IL-17A [12]. IL-17 is the hallmark cytokine produced by Th17 cells, but notably, αβ CD8+ T cells, innate lymphoid cells type 3 (ILC3s), γδ T cells, NK-T cells, mast cells, and neutrophils can also produce IL-17 as a homodimer or heterodimer with IL-17F. The IL-17 receptor family has five members: IL-17RA, IL-17RB, IL-17RC, IL-17RD, and IL-17RE [9]. IL-17A (in addition to IL-17F) binds its receptor IL-17R (IL-17RA/IL-17RC heterodimer), which is found on the cellular surface of monocytes, keratinocytes, fibroblasts, epithelial cells, and synoviocytes. This triggers the recruitment of nuclear factor κB (NFκB) activator 1 (ACT1) adaptor protein, which in turn activates mitogen-activated protein kinases (MAPKs), such as p38 MAPK. Other signaling pathways, involving c-Jun N-terminal kinase (JNK), extracellular signal-regulated kinase (ERK), Janus kinase (JAK), signal transducer and activator of transcription 3 (STAT3), and phosphoinositol 3 kinase (PI3K), can also be activated [9]. In epithelial and other parenchymal cells, IL-17R activation induces a wide array of pro-inflammatory mediators, such as IL-1, IL-6, IL-8, TNFα, G-CSF, and matrix metalloproteinases (MMPs), thereby causing host tissue to become more pliant to cellular infiltration and tissue inflammation [9]. IL-6 is involved in the development of a febrile response, G-CSF leads to the expansion of neutrophilic lineages, and IL-8 enhances neutrophil migration to the involved tissues [13].

6.6 THE IL-23/IL-17 AXIS AND ITS IMPLICATIONS IN THE PATHOGENESIS OF PSORIATIC DISEASE

Recent studies have repeatedly linked the IL-23/IL-17 axis to the development of several autoinflammatory diseases, including psoriasis, PsA, ankylosing spondylitis (AS), reactive arthritis, and undifferentiated spondyloarthritis (Figure 6.2). Increased expression levels of IL-12, IL-17, IL-22, IL-23, and TNFα have been observed in psoriatic skin lesions [14,15], as well as detection of IL-17/IL-22-producing ILC3s and IL-17-producing CD8+ T cells [16,17]. In addition to psoriatic dermal dendritic cells inducing T cell proliferation and polarization toward Th1 and Th17 cells after antigenic stimulation [18], γδ T cells were also increased in psoriatic skin lesions and ~15% of γδ T cells from psoriatic skin lesions produced IL-17 upon IL-23 stimulation [19]. Previous work has demonstrated how IL-17/IL-17RA are functionally active in PsA synovial fluid and tissues, since Th17 cells, IL-17, and IL-17R are significantly increased [20] and have been colocalized with CD4+ T cells, CD8+ T cells, and macrophages, among other cell types [21]. Interestingly, mast cells have also been identified as a source of IL-17 production in PsA synovial tissue [22]. Furthermore, elevated levels of IL-23 have been found in PsA synovial fluid and are thought to correlate with disease severity [13]. Similarly, IL-17 and IL-23 serum concentration levels have been found to be elevated in AS [23,24]. The proportion of IL-23R-expressing T cells in the periphery was found to be twofold higher in AS patients than in healthy controls, specifically due to a threefold increase in IL-23R-positive γδ T cells in AS patients [25]. Increased IL-23R expression on γδ T cells was associated with enhanced IL-17 secretion and was skewed toward IL-17 production in response to stimulation with IL-23 and/or anti-CD3/CD28 [25]. Moreover, an increased number of IL-17+ cells have been reported in facet joints of postsurgical specimens from patients with AS [26]. More recently, seminal work done examining human entheseal tissue (from individuals with no systemic inflammatory burden) found the presence of ILC3s, with expression of RORγt, STAT3, and IL-23R validating their phenotype [27]. Additionally, normal entheseal digests stimulated with IL-23/IL-1β-upregulated IL-17A expression and histological examination of injured or damaged entheses revealed the presence of RORγt-expressing cells [27].

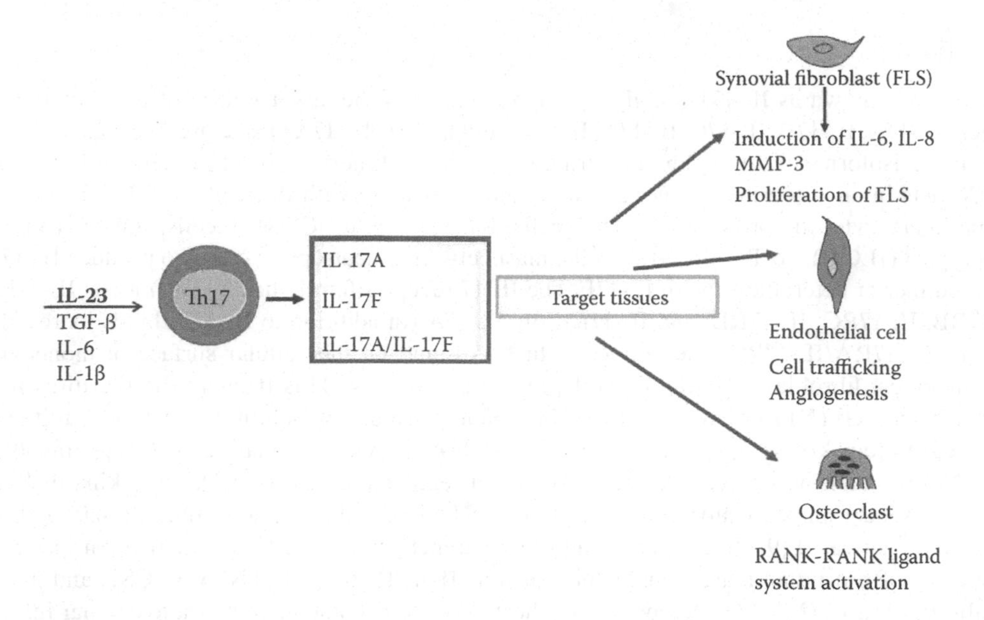

FIGURE 6.2 Regulatory role of IL-23/IL-17 cytokine axis on synovial tissue inflammation, pannus formation, and osteoclast activation. (From Raychaudhuri, S.P., and Raychaudhuri, S.K., *Clin. Rheumatol.*, 35, 1437–1441, 2016.)

Several animal studies, such as in the experimental autoimmune encephalitis (EAE) and collagen-induced arthritis (CIA) mouse models of autoimmunity, have shown how development of the condition depends on IL-23 but not IL-12. Mice lacking IL-23 (IL-23p19–/–) and both IL-23 and IL-12 (IL-23p40–/–) did not develop the disease after antigenic exposure, while IL-12 (IL-12p35–/–)-lacking mice progressed to have severe disease [28]. In addition, recent evidence has demonstrated that IL-23 and resident T cells producing IL-23 and IL-22 lead to enthesitis, synovitis, bone proliferation (nonosteophytic), and bone erosions in autoimmune arthritis mouse models [29].

Specifically, for psoriasis and PsA, animal models have provided critical evidence for the role of the IL-23/IL-17 axis. IL-23-induced psoriasis from lesions in mice was found to be dependent on both IL-17 and IL-22 [30], and furthermore, γδ T cells were determined to be the major producers of these cytokines [31]. Interestingly, the dermal hyperplasia and inflammation induced by IL-23 was significantly decreased when using TCR δ knockout and IL-17 receptor knockout mice [19]. Additional evidence was provided by studying an animal model of psoriasis induced by a TLR7/8 ligand, imiquimod, which triggers dendritic cell IL-23-mediated activation of innate IL-17/IL-22-producing lymphocytes [32]. However, when using IL-23 or IL-17 receptor knockout mice, disease development was shown to be completely inhibited [33]. Another mouse model, a cross between a gp130 knock-in strain that develops chronic arthritis and a transgenic strain overexpressing STAT3 in keratinocytes that develops psoriasis, developed both a severe form of psoriasis and acute inflammatory arthritis, with affected joints showing upregulation of the Th17 pathway [34].

Notably, another critical cytokine in the IL-23/IL-17 axis is IL-22, which is produced by Th17 cells, NK cells, γδ T cells, and Th22 cells [35]. In psoriasis, mast cells appear to be the primary source of IL-22 production [36], which in turn partly drives its pathogenesis. Ex vivo IL-22-induced keratinocyte hyperplasia and upregulation of pro-inflammatory mediators in keratinocytes in vivo have been previously demonstrated [37]. In a mouse model, dermal inflammation and epidermal hyperplasia induced by IL-23 were found to be mediated by IL-22 [38]. Finally, in a separate mouse model of psoriasis, in which transfer of CD4+ CD45RB^{hi}+ cells to severe combined immunodeficiency mice induced disease, IL-22 neutralization prevented progression of disease, partly by reducing skin thickening and pro-inflammatory infiltrates [39].

Of note, IL-17 is involved in the regulation and proliferation of fibroblast-like synovial (FLS) cells and angiogenesis [40,41]. By inducing the release of synoviolin (an antiapoptotic protein) from FLS cells, IL-17 stimulates the survival and proliferation of such cells [42]. Exposure to IL-17 by FLS cells in PsA leads to increased release of pro-inflammatory cytokines, such as IL-6, IL-8, and MMP-3 [13]. In addition, it has been shown that the function of TNFα is enhanced by the synergistic effects of IL-17 on upregulating TNFR2 production and TNFα stabilizing IL-17 mRNA [43].

In addition to psoriasis, the IL-23/IL-17 axis has been implicated in PsA, with prior evidence suggesting that both IL-23 and IL-17A play significant, and perhaps somewhat independent, roles in contributing to bony erosive disease [44]. In vivo systemic expression of IL-23 in a mouse model was shown to result in inflammatory arthritis and severe bone loss partly dependent on CD4+ T cells and IL-17A, but not reproducible with overexpression of IL-17A [45]. In a separate study, in vivo gene transfer of IL-17A and its overexpression in a mouse model mediated bony erosions and induced osteoclast precursor expansion, despite the absence of histological or clinical joint inflammation [46]. Additionally, when IL-17A gene transfer in a CIA mouse model occurred, the inflammatory arthritis was worsened with pannus formation, increased immune cell infiltration, and bony erosions [46]. Interestingly, IL-17A was shown to inhibit bone formation through its negative effects on Wnt signaling in osteoblasts and osteocytes in a mouse model of chronic skin inflammation [47].

These findings aligned with similar observations in which IL-17A-deficient mice induced with inflammatory arthritis exhibited greater periosteal bone formation than wild-type mice, while in vitro IL-17A inhibited osteoblast differentiation by upregulating the expression of secreted frizzled-related protein, a Wnt antagonist [48]. These data illustrate that overabundance of IL-17A favors bony erosions and is consistent with observations that IL-17A can drive parathyroid-induced RANKL expression by osteoblasts and osteocytes, with resultant bone loss [49]. In contrast, IL-22 overexpression is associated with bone formation. In vivo expression of IL-23 in mice was demonstrated to result in enthesitis, with CD3+ CD4– CD8– entheseal resident T cells identified that expressed the IL-23 receptor and, upon stimulation, produced IL-22, IL-6, and IL-17 [29]. IL-22 production by these cells drove both entheseal and periosteal bone formation through the activation of osteoblast STAT3, thereby providing a plausible mechanism for enthesophyte and juxta-articular bone formation observed in PsA [29].

6.7 SHOULD PSORIASIS AND PSORIATIC ARTHRITIS BE CONSIDERED A SPECTRUM OF ONE DISEASE?

A recent study provided the first comprehensive genomic and molecular comparison of matched psoriatic skin lesions and affected synovium in PsA in 12 patients who fulfilled the Moll and Wright criteria for PsA [50]. Samples of tissue from psoriatic skin lesions and synovial tissue from inflamed joints were obtained from the same patient on the same day and subsequently underwent gene expression studies using Affymetrix arrays with confirmatory quantitative real-time polymerase chain reaction (PCR) performed [50]. Their global gene expression analysis indicated that synovial tissue in PsA was much more similar to tissue in psoriatic skin lesions than synovial tissue in other forms of arthritis, such as rheumatoid arthritis, osteoarthritis, or systemic lupus erythematosus [50]. However, it is important to note that their study also showed clear differential inflammatory gene expression between synovial tissue and skin. They found a strong IL-17-related gene signature in skin relative to synovium, with many upregulated genes in skin being IL-17 signature genes [50]. In contrast, TNF appeared to have a more similar gene expression profile in skin and synovium and serves as an upstream regulator in both. Nevertheless, by highlighting the shared gene expression profiles of psoriasis and PsA, this study raises the intriguing possibility that the two disease states may be part of a larger single continuum.

Additionally, the recent development of a mouse model provided novel insights into the pathogenesis of psoriasis and PsA, with a single agent able to induce both. Exposure to mannan from

Saccharomyces cerevisiae was found to induce an acute inflammatory response in inbred mouse strains that resembled clinical psoriasis and PsA [51]. Disease severity was worsened in those mice deficient for generation of reactive oxygen species (ROS), which upon restoration, specifically in macrophages, ameliorated both skin and joint disease [51]. IL-17A neutralization, found to be mainly produced by γδ T cells in this model, prevented the occurrence of disease symptoms, with mice depleted of granulocytes resistant to disease development as well [51]. Intriguingly, this study suggests a shared mechanism of disease triggered by exposure to exogenous microbial antigen that can induce and exacerbate both psoriasis and PsA.

6.8 CONCLUSIONS

In this chapter, the crucial role of Th17 cells in the pathogenesis of psoriatic disease has been discussed. The discovery of this pathway has transformed our understanding of the immunomolecular mechanisms that result in the clinically evident signs and symptoms of psoriatic disease. Cumulative and strong scientific evidence has led to the development of several therapeutic targets within this autoinflammatory pathway, which is covered in Section IV-A of this book.

ACKNOWLEDGMENTS

The author wishes to thank Ronald Yglesias, MD, for initial assistance provided in the drafting of this chapter.

REFERENCES

1. Fragoulis GE, Siebert S, McInnes IB. Therapeutic targeting of IL-17 and IL-23 cytokines in immune-mediated diseases. *Annu Rev Med* 2016, 67:337–353.
2. Gladman DD, Antoni C, Mease P, Clegg DO, Nash P. Psoriatic arthritis: Epidemiology, clinical features, course, and outcome. *Ann Rheum Dis* 2005, 64(Suppl 2):ii14–ii17.
3. Ritchlin CT, Colbert RA, Gladman DD. Psoriatic arthritis. *N Engl J Med* 2017, 376:957–970.
4. Taylor W, Gladman D, Helliwell P, Marchesoni A, Mease P, Mielants H, CASPAR Study Group. Classification criteria for psoriatic arthritis: Development of new criteria from a large international study. *Arthritis Rheum* 2006, 54:2665–2673.
5. Mosmann TR, Cherwinski H, Bond MW, Giedlin MA, Coffman RL. Two types of murine helper T cell clone. I. Definition according to profiles of lymphokine activities and secreted proteins. *J Immunol* 1986, 136:2348–2357.
6. Barnas JL, Ritchlin CT. Etiology and pathogenesis of psoriatic arthritis. *Rheum Dis Clin North Am* 2015, 41:643–663.
7. Harrington LE, Hatton RD, Mangan PR, Turner H, Murphy TL, Murphy KM, Weaver CT. Interleukin 17-producing CD4+ effector T cells develop via a lineage distinct from the T helper type 1 and 2 lineages. *Nat Immunol* 2005, 6:1123–1132.
8. Park H, Li Z, Yang XO, Chang SH, Nurieva R, Wang YH, Wang Y et al. A distinct lineage of CD4 T cells regulates tissue inflammation by producing interleukin 17. *Nat Immunol* 2005, 6:1133–1141.
9. Patel DD, Kuchroo VK. Th17 cell pathway in human immunity: Lessons from genetics and therapeutic interventions. *Immunity* 2015, 43:1040–1051.
10. Ghoreschi K, Laurence A, Yang XP, Tato CM, McGeachy MJ, Konkel JE, Ramos HL et al. Generation of pathogenic T(H)17 cells in the absence of TGF-beta signalling. *Nature* 2010, 467:967–971.
11. Zielinski CE, Mele F, Aschenbrenner D, Jarrossay D, Ronchi F, Gattorno M, Monticelli S, Lanzavecchia A, Sallusto F. Pathogen-induced human TH17 cells produce IFN-gamma or IL-10 and are regulated by IL-1beta. *Nature* 2012, 484:514–518.
12. Singh RP, Hasan S, Sharma S, Nagra S, Yamaguchi DT, Wong DT, Hahn BH, Hossain A. Th17 cells in inflammation and autoimmunity. *Autoimmun Rev* 2014, 13:1174–1181.
13. Raychaudhuri SP, Raychaudhuri SK. IL-23/IL-17 axis in spondyloarthritis—Bench to bedside. *Clin Rheumatol* 2016, 35:1437–1441.

14. Di Cesare A, Di Meglio P, Nestle FO. The IL-23/Th17 axis in the immunopathogenesis of psoriasis. *J Invest Dermatol* 2009, 129:1339–1350.
15. Lee E, Trepicchio WL, Oestreicher JL, Pittman D, Wang F, Chamian F, Dhodapkar M, Krueger JG. Increased expression of interleukin 23 p19 and p40 in lesional skin of patients with psoriasis vulgaris. *J Exp Med* 2004, 199:125–130.
16. Teunissen MB, Yeremenko NG, Baeten DL, Chielie S, Spuls PI, de Rie MA, Lantz O, Res PC. The IL-17A-producing CD8+ T-cell population in psoriatic lesional skin comprises mucosa-associated invariant T cells and conventional T cells. *J Invest Dermatol* 2014, 134:2898–2907.
17. Ward NL, Umetsu DT. A new player on the psoriasis block: IL-17A- and IL-22-producing innate lymphoid cells. *J Invest Dermatol* 2014, 134:2305–2307.
18. Zaba LC, Fuentes-Duculan J, Eungdamrong NJ, Abello MV, Novitskaya I, Pierson KC, Gonzalez J, Krueger JG, Lowes MA. Psoriasis is characterized by accumulation of immunostimulatory and Th1/Th17 cell-polarizing myeloid dendritic cells. *J Invest Dermatol* 2009, 129:79–88.
19. Cai Y, Shen X, Ding C, Qi C, Li K, Li X, Jala VR et al. Pivotal role of dermal IL-17-producing gammadelta T cells in skin inflammation. *Immunity* 2011, 35:596–610.
20. Raychaudhuri SP, Raychaudhuri SK, Genovese MC. IL-17 receptor and its functional significance in psoriatic arthritis. *Mol Cell Biochem* 2012, 359:419–429.
21. van Baarsen LG, Lebre MC, van der Coelen D, Aarrass S, Tang MW, Ramwadhdoebe TH, Gerlag DM, Tak PP. Heterogeneous expression pattern of interleukin 17A (IL-17A), IL-17F and their receptors in synovium of rheumatoid arthritis, psoriatic arthritis and osteoarthritis: Possible explanation for nonresponse to anti-IL-17 therapy? *Arthritis Res Ther* 2014, 16:426.
22. Noordenbos T, Yeremenko N, Gofita I, van de Sande M, Tak PP, Canete JD, Baeten D. Interleukin-17-positive mast cells contribute to synovial inflammation in spondylarthritis. *Arthritis Rheum* 2012, 64:99–109.
23. Mei Y, Pan F, Gao J, Ge R, Duan Z, Zeng Z, Liao F et al. Increased serum IL-17 and IL-23 in the patient with ankylosing spondylitis. *Clin Rheumatol* 2011, 30:269–273.
24. Zeng L, Lindstrom MJ, Smith JA. Ankylosing spondylitis macrophage production of higher levels of interleukin-23 in response to lipopolysaccharide without induction of a significant unfolded protein response. *Arthritis Rheum* 2011, 63:3807–3817.
25. Kenna TJ, Davidson SI, Duan R, Bradbury LA, McFarlane J, Smith M, Weedon H et al. Enrichment of circulating interleukin-17-secreting interleukin-23 receptor-positive gamma/delta T cells in patients with active ankylosing spondylitis. *Arthritis Rheum* 2012, 64:1420–1429.
26. Appel H, Maier R, Wu P, Scheer R, Hempfing A, Kayser R, Thiel A, Radbruch A, Loddenkemper C, Sieper J. Analysis of IL-17(+) cells in facet joints of patients with spondyloarthritis suggests that the innate immune pathway might be of greater relevance than the Th17-mediated adaptive immune response. *Arthritis Res Ther* 2011, 13:R95.
27. Cuthbert RJ, Fragkakis EM, Dunsmuir R, Li Z, Coles M, Marzo-Ortega H, Giannoudis P, Jones E, El-Sherbiny YM, McGonagle D. Brief report: Group 3 innate lymphoid cells in human enthesis. *Arthritis Rheumatol* 2017, 69:1816–1822.
28. Cua DJ, Sherlock J, Chen Y, Murphy CA, Joyce B, Seymour B, Lucian L et al. Interleukin-23 rather than interleukin-12 is the critical cytokine for autoimmune inflammation of the brain. *Nature* 2003, 421:744–748.
29. Sherlock JP, Joyce-Shaikh B, Turner SP, Chao CC, Sathe M, Grein J, Gorman DM et al. IL-23 induces spondyloarthropathy by acting on ROR-gammat+ CD3+CD4–CD8– entheseal resident T cells. *Nat Med* 2012, 18:1069–1076.
30. Rizzo HL, Kagami S, Phillips KG, Kurtz SE, Jacques SL, Blauvelt A. IL-23-mediated psoriasis-like epidermal hyperplasia is dependent on IL-17A. *J Immunol* 2011, 186:1495–1502.
31. Mabuchi T, Takekoshi T, Hwang ST. Epidermal CCR6+ gammadelta T cells are major producers of IL-22 and IL-17 in a murine model of psoriasiform dermatitis. *J Immunol* 2011, 187:5026–5031.
32. Wohn C, Ober-Blobaum JL, Haak S, Pantelyushin S, Cheong C, Zahner SP, Onderwater S et al. Langerin(neg) conventional dendritic cells produce IL-23 to drive psoriatic plaque formation in mice. *Proc Natl Acad Sci U S A* 2013, 110:10723–10728.
33. van der Fits L, Mourits S, Voerman JS, Kant M, Boon L, Laman JD, Cornelissen F et al. Imiquimod-induced psoriasis-like skin inflammation in mice is mediated via the IL-23/IL-17 axis. *J Immunol* 2009, 182:5836–5845.
34. Yamamoto M, Nakajima K, Takaishi M, Kitaba S, Magata Y, Kataoka S, Sano S. Psoriatic inflammation facilitates the onset of arthritis in a mouse model. *J Invest Dermatol* 2015, 135:445–453.

35. Zenewicz LA, Flavell RA. Recent advances in IL-22 biology. *Int Immunol* 2011, 23:159–163.
36. Mashiko S, Bouguermouh S, Rubio M, Baba N, Bissonnette R, Sarfati M. Human mast cells are major IL-22 producers in patients with psoriasis and atopic dermatitis. *J Allergy Clin Immunol* 2015, 136:351–359.e351.
37. Boniface K, Bernard FX, Garcia M, Gurney AL, Lecron JC, Morel F. IL-22 inhibits epidermal differentiation and induces proinflammatory gene expression and migration of human keratinocytes. *J Immunol* 2005, 174:3695–3702.
38. Zheng Y, Danilenko DM, Valdez P, Kasman I, Eastham-Anderson J, Wu J, Ouyang W. Interleukin-22, a T(H)17 cytokine, mediates IL-23-induced dermal inflammation and acanthosis. *Nature* 2007, 445:648–651.
39. Ma HL, Liang S, Li J, Napierata L, Brown T, Benoit S, Senices M et al. IL-22 is required for Th17 cell-mediated pathology in a mouse model of psoriasis-like skin inflammation. *J Clin Invest* 2008, 118:597–607.
40. Numasaki M, Fukushi J, Ono M, Narula SK, Zavodny PJ, Kudo T, Robbins PD, Tahara H, Lotze MT. Interleukin-17 promotes angiogenesis and tumor growth. *Blood* 2003, 101:2620–2627.
41. Saxena A, Raychaudhuri SK, Raychaudhuri SP. Interleukin-17-induced proliferation of fibroblast-like synovial cells is mTOR dependent. *Arthritis Rheum* 2011, 63:1465–1466.
42. Toh ML, Gonzales G, Koenders MI, Tournadre A, Boyle D, Lubberts E, Zhou Y, Firestein GS, van den Berg WB, Miossec P. Role of interleukin 17 in arthritis chronicity through survival of synoviocytes via regulation of synoviolin expression. *PLoS One* 2010, 5:e13416.
43. Hartupee J, Liu C, Novotny M, Li X, Hamilton T. IL-17 enhances chemokine gene expression through mRNA stabilization. *J Immunol* 2007, 179:4135–4141.
44. Suzuki E, Mellins ED, Gershwin ME, Nestle FO, Adamopoulos IE. The IL-23/IL-17 axis in psoriatic arthritis. *Autoimmun Rev* 2014, 13:496–502.
45. Adamopoulos IE, Tessmer M, Chao CC, Adda S, Gorman D, Petro M, Chou CC et al. IL-23 is critical for induction of arthritis, osteoclast formation, and maintenance of bone mass. *J Immunol* 2011, 187:951–959.
46. Adamopoulos IE, Suzuki E, Chao CC, Gorman D, Adda S, Maverakis E, Zarbalis K et al. IL-17A gene transfer induces bone loss and epidermal hyperplasia associated with psoriatic arthritis. *Ann Rheum Dis* 2015, 74:1284–1292.
47. Uluckan O, Jimenez M, Karbach S, Jeschke A, Grana O, Keller J, Busse B et al. Chronic skin inflammation leads to bone loss by IL-17-mediated inhibition of Wnt signaling in osteoblasts. *Sci Transl Med* 2016, 8:330ra337.
48. Shaw AT, Maeda Y, Gravallese EM. IL-17A deficiency promotes periosteal bone formation in a model of inflammatory arthritis. *Arthritis Res Ther* 2016, 18:104.
49. Pacifici R. The role of IL-17 and TH17 cells in the bone catabolic activity of PTH. *Front Immunol* 2016, 7:57.
50. Belasco J, Louie JS, Gulati N, Wei N, Nograles K, Fuentes-Duculan J, Mitsui H, Suarez-Farinas M, Krueger JG. Comparative genomic profiling of synovium versus skin lesions in psoriatic arthritis. *Arthritis Rheumatol* 2015, 67:934–944.
51. Khmaladze I, Kelkka T, Guerard S, Wing K, Pizzolla A, Saxena A, Lundqvist K, Holmdahl M, Nandakumar KS, Holmdahl R. Mannan induces ROS-regulated, IL-17A-dependent psoriasis arthritis-like disease in mice. *Proc Natl Acad Sci U S A* 2014, 111:E3669–E3678.

7 Nerve Growth Factor and Its Receptor System in Rheumatologic Diseases and Pain Management

A New Dimension in Pathogenesis and Novel Drugs in the Pipeline

Smriti K. Raychaudhuri and Siba P. Raychaudhuri

CONTENTS

7.1 INTRODUCTION

Nerve growth factor (NGF), a neurotrophic factor, is expressed in most of the organs, although initially NGF was identified in the nervous system. NGF acts on its two well-recognized receptors (NGF-R): tyrosine receptor kinase A (TrkA), its high-affinity receptor, and p75, the low-affinity receptor. Several studies suggest that an inflammatory state (chronic or acute) is characterized by marked upregulation of NGF at the site of inflammation [1,2]. Cytokines such as interleukin (IL) 1β, tumor necrosis factor (TNF) α, and IL-6 can induce the synthesis of NGF in endothelial cells, fibroblasts, keratinocytes, and glial cells [1–4]. In addition, immune cells involved in innate and acquired immunity show a basal expression of NGF, and its synthesis is enhanced after stimulation with specific antigens and cytokines [1–5]. Also, immune cells and other nonneuronal cells that produce NGF express TrkA, the high-affinity receptor, which, on binding to its ligand, activates the intracellular signaling system and the transcription factors in a similar manner to what happens in neuronal cells [1–5]. In vitro, NGF also influences multiple functions of the purified myeloid or lymphoid cell population, such as proliferation and survival, production of cytokines and immunoglobulins, release of inflammatory mediators, chemotaxis, and proliferation and survival of an array of immune cells [1,2,5]. Thus, NGF has the potential to influence the inflammatory and proliferative cascades directly by regulating the immune cell functions, or indirectly by inducing neuropeptide synthesis or activating the mast cells, which in turn affects an immune-mediated inflammatory reaction. These observations justify a relatively new concept that de novo synthesis of NGF or local induction of NGF by pro-inflammatory cytokines (TNF-α, IL-1α, and IL-6) plays a critical role in the initiation or perpetuation of an inflammatory process, in addition to its role in the pathophysiology of "pain processing" [1–5].

The regulatory role of the NGF/NGF-R system in inflammatory and rheumatologic diseases is an active and a novel research field. Initial evidence for a role of the NGF/NGF-R system in inflammatory disease has been documented in psoriasis [2]. However, with time a contributing role of the NGF/NGF-R system in the inflammatory cascades of multiple inflammatory diseases has been documented, such as in inflammatory bowel disease, inflammatory airway disease, atopic dermatitis, psoriatic arthritis (PsA), and rheumatoid arthritis [1–5]. In addition, because of its regulatory role on the pain pathway, the NGF/TrkA system is under intense research in chronic painful conditions, including degenerative disease of the spine and osteoarthritis (OA) of the peripheral joints. A new discipline is emerging in clinical pharmacology focusing on the development of drugs targeting the neuropeptides, NGF, and TrkA. In this chapter, we describe the role of the NGF and its receptor system in inflammatory diseases, such as in psoriasis, PsA, adjuvant-induced rat arthritis, and arthritic pain of OA.

7.2 ROLE OF THE NGF AND ITS RECEPTOR SYSTEM IN THE INFLAMMATORY AND PROLIFERATIVE CASCADES OF PSORIASIS AND PSORIATIC ARTHRITIS

7.2.1 Psoriasis and Psoriatic Arthritis

Psoriasis is a common skin disease, the most frequent human autoimmune disease. It affects around 2% of the world population. Psoriasis can bring significant morbidity. Extensive pustular lesions, generalized involvement of the body (erythroderma), and PsA, an associated inflammatory arthritis, are severe complications of psoriasis.

Complaints of joint pain, swelling, morning stiffness, and fatigue in a patient with skin psoriasis raise a suspicion for concurrent PsA. PsA is a distinct clinical entity [6]. It is a seronegative inflammatory arthritis associated with psoriasis. PsA involves small joints of the hands, other peripheral joints, and spondyloarthropathy, including both sacroiliitis and spondylitis. Other common rheumatic features of PsA include soft tissue inflammation similar to that seen in seronegative arthritides, enthesitis (inflammation at the site of tendon insertion into bone), tenosynovitis, and dactylitis, which is characterized by diffuse swelling of a whole digit (called "sausage finger"). The most striking radiologic feature of PsA is the coexistence of erosive changes and new bone formation in the distal joints.

7.2.2 Pathogenesis of Psoriasis and Psoriatic Arthritis

To understand the role of NGF/NGF-R in the pathogenesis of psoriasis and PsA, it is essential to know how NGF and its receptor system can influence the critical biological events associated with the disease process of psoriasis and PsA. So in this section, we first briefly narrate the current state of knowledge of pathogenesis of psoriasis and PsA. The exact cause of psoriasis and its associated arthritis has yet to be identified. Genetic, immunologic, and environmental factors all contribute to its pathogenesis [7,8]. PsA is a systemic inflammatory disease mainly involving the skin and the joints. Psoriasis and PsA have similarities in human leukocyte antigen (HLA) phenotyping, cell trafficking mechanisms, nature of T-cell phenotypes, cytokine profiles, and angiogenesis. It is reasonable to postulate that the skin and joint involvement share common pathophysioiogic processes. However, there are also several differences in genetic predisposition such as HLA phenotypes, clinical presentation, therapeutic response, and pathophysiologic events in patients with psoriasis and PsA.

Severity of the skin disease and arthritis often does not correlate. Patients with severe PsA may not have extensive skin lesion, and patients with extensive psoriasis may or may not have arthritis.

Psoriasis has long been known to occur in families. Approximately 40% of patients with psoriasis or PsA have a family history of these disorders in first-degree relatives [7]. The HLA antigens B13, B17, B39, and Cw6 occur with increased frequency in both psoriasis and PsA when compared with the general population [8]. In PsA, additional associations have been found with HLA-B27, chiefly in patients with predominant spinal disease, HLA-B38, HLA-B39, and the class II antigen HLA-DR4 [8].

Inflammatory infiltrates in the skin and joints have been studied extensively. In both tissues, there is a prominent lymphocytic infiltrate, localized to the dermal papillae in the skin and to the sublining layer stroma in the joint. T cells are the most significant lymphocytes in the tissues, with a predominance of CD4+ lymphocytes; in contrast, this ratio is reversed in the epidermis, in the synovial fluid compartment, and at the enthesis, where CD8+ T cells are more common [9–11]. Localization of enriched CD8+ T-cell infiltrates suggests that these cells may be driving the immune response in the joint and skin. This is supported by an association with HLA class I [8]. The cytokine network in the psoriatic skin and synovium is dominated by monocyte and T-cell-derived cytokines: IL-1β, IL-2, IL-10, IL-17, IFN-γ, and TNF-α [12]. In PsA synovium, higher levels of IFN-γ, IL-2, and IL-10 have been detected than in psoriatic skin. An analysis of T-cell receptor β chain variable (TCRβV) gene repertoires revealed common expansions in both skin and synovial inflammatory sites, suggesting an important role for cognate T-cell responses in the pathogenesis of PsA, and that the inciting antigen may be identical or homologous between afflicted skin and synovium [13].

In PsA, involvement of bones and synovium provides another dimension to the pathogenesis of PsA. Until recently, the molecular events underlying osteoclast differentiation (osteoclastogenesis) and activation were not well understood. Elucidation of the receptor activator of nuclear factor κB ligand (RANKL)–RANK signaling pathway, however, revealed the pivotal steps required for osteoclast formation and activation [14]. Specifically, RANKL, expressed on the surface of osteoblasts and stromal cells in the bone marrow and infiltrating T lymphocytes and synoviocytes in the inflamed joint, binds to RANK, a cell-associated TNF receptor–related protein [15]. RANK is expressed on a variety of cell types, including osteoclast precursors and osteoclasts. The interaction between RANKL and its receptor RANK, in the presence of macrophage colony-stimulating factor (M-CSF), is necessary and sufficient for osteoclastogenesis and subsequent bone resorption. In addition, a decoy receptor for RANKL, osteoprotegerin, a molecule released by a wide array of cells, can bind to RANKL and neutralize bioactivity, thus inhibiting osteolysis [16]. Thus, the ratio of RANKL to osteoprotegerin in the pathologic tissue may be a deciding factor for bone resorption and osteolysis.

These observations encouraged study of the significance of RANKL-RANK signaling in the pathogenesis of PsA [17]. Study of the joint and bone tissues obtained from surgical samples of inflamed psoriatic joint has demonstrated abundant osteoclasts at the pannus and bone junction. Immunohistochemical staining of adjacent inflamed PsA synovium with antibodies to RANKL revealed intense expression by the synovial lining cells, while osteoprotegerin staining was relatively faint and limited to the endothelium. Also, staining of tissues with anti-RANK antibodies showed a gradient of RANK+ cells (presumably osteoclast precursors) increasing in number from the blood vessels in the subsynovium to the pannus–bone junction, where osteoclasts were prominently located. Bone from patients with OA contained few osteoclasts, and the synovial tissue did not express RANKL or osteoprotegerin.

Like in other inflammatory diseases, adhesion molecules play a critical role in the pathogenesis of both psoriasis and PsA. Upregulation of intercellular cell adhesion molecule 1 (ICAM-1) and vascular cell adhesion molecule 1 (VCAM-1) is pronounced in the skin and synovial membrane; however, E-selectin appears to be upregulated in the skin more than in the PsA synovial membrane [18]. A very critical observation has been made that cutaneous lymphocyte–associated antigen (CLA) is preferentially expressed on leukocytes "homing" to lesional psoriatic skin but not to the PsA synovial membrane [19]. Recent evidence suggests that local expression of myeloid-related protein also plays a central role in the transendothelial migration of leukocytes in PsA [20]. These observations provide a partial explanation for the preference of homing of pathologic T cells in joints and skin in PsA.

Specific vascular morphological changes have been described in the psoriasis skin, nail fold capillaries, and more recently, PsA synovial membrane, suggesting a common link [21,22]. Angiogenesis is a prominent early event in psoriasis and PsA; elongated and tortuous vessels in skin and joint suggest dysregulated angiogenesis resulting in immature vessels [23,24]. Angiogenic growth factors, including transforming growth factor (TGF) β), platelet-derived growth factor (PDGF), and vascular endothelial growth factor (VEGF), are markedly increased in psoriasis [25]. VEGF and TGF-β levels are high in the joint fluid in early PsA, and expression of angiopoietins, a novel family of vascular growth factors, colocalizes with the VEGF protein and mRNA in PsA synovial membrane perivascular areas [26]. Angiopoietin expression is upregulated in perivascular regions in lesional psoriasis skin [27].

In addition, various multiple factors, such as stress, temperature, humidity, neuroimmunologic mechanisms, and the role of growth factors, such as insulin-like growth factor (IGF) and NGF, have a contributing role in the pathogenesis of psoriasis and PsA. Koebner's phenomenon is the development of psoriasis in areas of traumatized skin. Koebner's reaction may result from upregulation of NGF and release of pro-inflammatory neuropeptides and from nerve endings [28,29]. Very limited information is available about the role of neurogenic inflammation in PsA. Veale et al. reported that substance P (SP) release from the synovial membrane into joint fluid is blocked by nerve damage and can ameliorate PsA [30]. In a second case, sparing of distal interphalangeal (DIP) joint disease and nail dystrophy in a partially denervated digit was reported in a patient with chronic PsA [31]. These common features of vascular morphology and angiogenic growth factors in the skin and joints, in addition to similarity in expression of neuropeptides, reflects a neurovascular pathologic process, which we address in the following sections.

The underlying pathophysiology for the cause of psoriasis and PsA is unfolding. In the last two decades, extensive work has been done to identify the immunological mechanisms involved in psoriatic disease. At the disease sites (both skin and joints) in patients with PsA and/or psoriasis, enrichment of activated T cells has been identified. An active role of T cells in the pathogenesis of psoriatic disease is strongly substantiated by the following observations: (1) immunotherapy targeted specifically against T cells, such as cyclosporine or T-cell-specific cytokines, is therapeutically effective in psoriasis [32], and (2) in severe combined immunodeficient (SCID) mice, transplanted nonlesional psoriatic skin converts to a psoriatic plaque subsequent to intradermal administration of T cells activated with an antigen cocktail [33]. However, it is also true that calcipotriol (Dovonex) and etritinate (Tegison), which affect the differentiation process of keratinocytes, are also very effective in psoriasis. Dovonex and Tegison are not effective in other T-cell-mediated skin diseases, such as in lichen planus or contact dermatitis. No antigen has been identified for psoriasis. In the SCID mouse model, it has been demonstrated that SP or NGF-activated lymphocytes, which are not conventional antigens, can also convert nonlesional psoriatic skin transplants to psoriasis.

These observations suggest that there are regulatory systems other than T cells that also contribute to the inflammatory and proliferative processes of psoriasis. It is likely that cytokines, adhesion molecules, chemokines, neuropeptides, NGF and other growth factors, and T-cell receptors act in an integrated way and contribute to the unique inflammatory and proliferative processes required for psoriasis and PsA.

7.2.3 Neurogenic Inflammation in Psoriasis

A role of neurogenic inflammation in the pathogenesis of psoriasis is considered because of several critical observations: (1) exacerbation of psoriasis during periods of emotional stress; (2) marked proliferation of lesional terminal cutaneous nerves, along with upregulation of neuropeptides (SP, calcitonin gene-related peptide [CGRP], and vasoactive intestinal peptide [VIP]) [34–37]; (3) therapeutic response to neuropeptide-modulating agents with capsaicin, peptide T, and somatostatin; and (4) following traumatic denervation of cutaneous nerve clearance of active plaques of psoriasis at the sites of anesthesia [38–42]. These key observations in psoriasis cannot be explained as a part of an autoimmune process. An antigen-induced T-cell activation process alone fails to clarify several other well-known features of psoriasis. For example, it does not explain the Koebner phenomenon. The T-cell activation process cannot explain the symmetrical distribution of psoriasis, the upregulation of neuropeptides in psoriatic tissue, and the proliferation of lesional cutaneous nerves in psoriatic plaques. Also, the current autoimmune theory for psoriasis cannot explain why a psoriasis plaque would resolve at sites of anesthesia.

7.2.4 Role of Nerve Growth Factor and Its Receptor System in the Pathogenesis of Psoriasis

The following unique features encouraged us and other investigators to search for the mechanism of neural influence in psoriasis: (1) resolution of psoriasis at sites of anesthesia, (2) marked proliferation of terminal cutaneous nerves, and (3) upregulation of neuropeptides in psoriatic plaques. As NGF augments nerve sprouting and thus tissue innervation [43], and also plays a critical role for the secretion of certain neuropeptides (SP and CGRP) [44,45], we investigated the role of NGF in the pathogenesis of psoriasis. We and other investigators have independently reported that keratinocytes from lesional and nonlesional psoriatic tissue express higher levels of NGF than the controls [46,47]. Further, we have reported that there is a marked upregulation of NGF-R in the terminal cutaneous nerves of psoriatic plaques [48].

NGF can influence many pathologic events observed in psoriasis, including keratinocyte proliferation, angiogenesis, T-cell activation, adhesion molecule expression, cutaneous nerve proliferation, and neuropeptide upregulation [1–5,29]. It has been reported that NGF is mitogenic to keratinocytes [29,49]. NGF recruits mast cells and promotes their degranulation [50,51], both of which are early events in a developing lesion of psoriasis. In addition, NGF activates T lymphocytes, recruits inflammatory cellular infiltrates [5,52–54], is mitogenic to endothelial cells, and induces ICAM on endothelial cells [55]. NGF is also known to upregulate the expression of SP [44].

NGF is known to stimulate neural outgrowth in cultured PC12 cells in vitro [56]. Since psoriatic keratinocytes produce very high levels of NGF, it is likely that keratinocyte-derived NGF induces proliferation of nerve fibers in psoriatic lesions in vivo. To test this hypothesis, we transplanted psoriatic plaques and normal skin to the SCID mouse skin. As mouse and human NGF are 90% homologous, we expected that mouse nerves will promptly proliferate into the transplanted plaques on a SCID mouse. Upregulation of the NGF p75 receptor is a unique in vivo effect of NGF [57]. Accordingly, we observed a marked proliferation of NGF-R (p75)-positive nerve fibers in the transplanted psoriatic plaque compared with a few nerves in the transplanted normal human skin. By immunofluoresence and immunoperoxidase staining, we have demonstrated that in these terminal cutaneous nerves there is a marked upregulation of SP. These observations substantiate the in vivo effect of NGF released from the keratinocytes of psoriatic plaques [58]. We have also observed that within 3 weeks in the SCID mouse–psoriasis skin xenograft model, injection of autologous immunocytes activated with NGF can convert a nonlesional psoriatic skin to a psoriatic plaque [59].

These clinical and laboratory studies suggest a critical role of NGF and its receptor system in the inflammatory process of psoriasis; however, direct evidence has been lacking. To determine the significance of the NGF/NGF-R system in the inflammatory process of psoriasis, we evaluated the effects of K252a, a high-affinity NGF-R inhibitor [58]. The transplanted psoriatic plaques on the SCID mice (n = 12) were treated with K252a, a high-affinity NGF-R blocker. Psoriasis significantly improved after 2 weeks of therapy. The control group, treated with normal saline, did not improve. A similar improvement of psoriasis was observed by directly antagonizing NGF with a NGF-neutralizing antibody.

7.2.5 Role of NGF and Its Receptor System in the Pathogenesis of Psoriatic Arthritis

The NGF/TrkA system influences the inflammatory and proliferative mechanisms in psoriasis. As psoriasis and PsA are parts of the same disease spectrum, it is expected that NGF and its receptor system likely play a critical role in the pathogenesis of PsA. Table 7.1 enlists the functions of NGF that are relevant for the pathomechanisms of the inflammatory and proliferative cascades associated with PsA.

There is no animal model for PsA. Transgenic mice expressing the human TNF gene (Tg197) demonstrate increased levels of NGF in the synovium of inflamed joints; further treatment with subcutaneous injection of NGF antibody has demonstrated a reduction of joint inflammation in this mouse model [60]. Both TNF-α and IL-1β promote the synthesis of NGF in the cultured fibroblast-like synovium (FLS) [61]. In patients with PsA and other forms of inflammatory arthritis, no comprehensive work has been carried out to address the role of NGF and its receptor system. Nonetheless, there are reports indicating that SP release from the synovial membrane into joint fluid is blocked by nerve damage and digital denervation prevented the development of arthritis in the interphalangeal joints [30,31]. Kane et al. have also reported on a patient of PsA who developed arthritis mutilans in all digits of both hands with the exception of the left fourth finger, which had prior sensory denervation following traumatic nerve dissection [62]. There are reports that NGF and SP levels in the synovial fluid may be elevated in HLA-B27-associated arthritis [63]. Based on our research work on psoriasis and these case reports suggesting a possible role of neurogenic inflammation in the inflammatory cascades of PsA, we initiated studies to elucidate the role of NGF/NGF-R in PsA.

We observed a marked elevation of NGF in the synovial fluid of PsA compared with patients with OA [4]. The total NGF level was significantly higher in the PsA group (46.5–418.5 pg/mL, median 365.5 pg/mL, standard error of the mean [SEM] 85.2) than in OA patients (median <40 pg/mL). In immunohistochemical staining, we found that psoriatic synovium is enriched with NGF-R-positive proliferating nerves compared with rheumatoid arthritis and OA. Marked proliferation of terminal nerves with expression of NGF-R further substantiates the in vivo effect of NGF in the synovium of PsA. These observations are a replication of our studies in psoriasis plaques and indicate that NGF and its receptor system have a regulatory role in the inflammatory cascades of PsA [64].

TABLE 7.1
Regulatory Role of NGF in Inflammatory Cascades

1. Cell trafficking
   - Induces adhesion molecule
   - Upregulates chemokine
2. Activates T cells and promotes pro-inflammatory cytokine
3. Degranulates mast cells
4. Upregulates expression of neuropeptides
5. Mitogenic to FLS
6. Promotes angiogenesis

7.3 NGF/NGF-R SYSTEM IN THE PATHOPHYSIOLOGY OF PAIN, ITCHING, AND HYPERALGESIA

NGF and its receptor system have a significant contribution to the survival factor for sensory and sympathetic neurons in the developing nervous system. In adults, NGF is not required for survival, although it helps wound healing, including regeneration of terminal nerve endings. It is also currently believed that NGF sensitizes nociceptive neurons and regulates the processing and transmission of pain signals. As these observations are relatively new in the pathophysiology of processing and perception of pain, we provide details of certain experimental and clinical studies explaining the role of NGF in a wide variety of acute and chronic painful conditions.

1. Mutations in the genes that encode TrkA and NGF result in congenital insensitivity to pain. Congenital insensitivity to pain and the inability to sweat (anhidrosis) is an autosomal recessive disease that is caused by null mutations of the gene encoding TrkA (NTRK1) [65]. Subsets of sensory and sympathetic neurons do not develop adequately in this condition, which makes affected individuals unresponsive to pain and unable to sweat. There is also mild cognitive impairment that is believed to reflect dysfunction of NGF-responsive acetylcholine-containing neurons in the basal forebrain. A recently discovered mutation in the gene that encodes human NGF is also associated with diminished pain perception [66].
2. Administration of NGF provokes pain and hyperalgesia. In rodents, NGF causes robust, long-lasting mechanical and thermal hyperalgesia (an increased response to a stimulus that is normally painful) following either local or systemic administration [67,68]. In humans, the ability of NGF to provoke pain came to light in clinical studies to explore its potential in the treatment of polyneuropathies. Subcutaneous injection of NGF into the forearm of healthy volunteers produced allodynia (pain as a result of a stimulus that does not normally cause pain) and hypersensitivity in the surrounding skin that lasted for up to 3 weeks [69], and generalized muscle pain occurred more frequently in subjects who received NGF compared with those who received placebo [70,71]. In a controlled trial of the effects of NGF injection into the masseter muscle of healthy volunteers, local mechanical allodynia and hyperalgesia were observed for at least a week, and pain was observed during strenuous jaw movement [72]. Direct administration of NGF into the sciatic nerve also produces hyperalgesia [73].
3. NGF triggers changes in gene expression in nociceptors. TRPV1 is a cation channel that was identified originally as the capsaicin receptor. It is expressed on polymodal nociceptors and serves as a molecular detector for noxious heat and extracellular acidification, which occurs in tissue inflammation. When activated, TRPV1 enables the influx of monovalent and divalent cations, predominantly Ca2C, which results in membrane depolarization and the generation of action potentials [74]. In culture, NGF rapidly potentiates the activity of TRPV1 channels in dorsal root ganglion (DRG) neurons treated with capsaicin [75,76]. Studies using pharmacological inhibitors in these neurons indicate that the phosphatidylinositol 3-kinase (PI3K) pathway is crucial for mediating sensitization to NGF, with both Ca2C–calmodulin-dependent kinase II and protein kinase C (PKC) acting downstream of PI3K [76,77]. PKC-3 sensitizes TRPV1 by direct phosphorylation, which leads to increased channel activity [78–80] and translocation of the channel to the cell surface [81]. Accordingly, NGF-induced hyperalgesia is inhibited by a PKC-3-selective peptide inhibitor [82]. Retrograde NGF signaling from the peripheral terminals to the cell bodies of nociceptive neurons [83] enhances the expression of several proteins that further sensitize these neurons and facilitate activation of second-order neurons in the central nervous system. This includes SP, which acts at central synapses to increase the activity of second-order nociceptive neurons [84].

4. NGF activates mast cells, upregulates adhesion molecules, induces chemokines, and promotes cell trafficking. Exposure of isolated mast cells to NGF and lysophosphatidylserine (a molecule on the surface of activated platelets), but not to either factor alone, induces the release of 5-hydroxytryptamine (5-HT) [85]. This indicates that NGF sensitizes mast cells under conditions of tissue injury and inflammation. In addition to 5-HT, activated mast cells release other pain mediators, such as prostaglandins, bradykinin, histamine, ATP, and NGF itself, which stimulate nociceptor terminals and potentiate the pain response [85].

Induction of the expression of NGF is an early event in injured and inflamed tissues, and elevated levels of NGF are sustained in chronic inflammation. These changes in the synthesis of NGF appear to be caused, in part at least, by the action of pro-inflammatory cytokines, many of which induce the synthesis of NGF in several cell types in vitro and in vivo [86]. Earlier, we reported that NGF promotes inflammation by inducing adhesion molecules, upregulating chemokines such as RANTES, and activating lymphocytes [2,5,55,87]. In vivo studies have also provided similar observations. Using transplanted human skin on SCID mouse, recently we have observed that within 2 hours intradermal injection of NGF induces extravasations of lymphomononuclear cells and upregulation of ICAM. These positive-feedback loops of inflammatory cascades are also likely to contribute to the pain associated with acute and chronic inflammatory processes.

Thus, NGF/NGF-R influences the generation and processing of pain signals in several ways. It is likely that upregulation of NGF occurs as a part of the tissue response to injury or inflammation. NGF activates TrkA receptors on sensory neurons and modifies the function of the TRPV1 channel and axonal sodium channel to enhance pain signal transmission. The NGF/TrkA interaction on sensory neurons initiates retrograde signaling to the cell body of the neurons and induces expression of genes that encode precursors of neuropeptides, which contribute to the long-term sensitization for the pain response. NGF also can degranulate mast cells, and thus has the potential to initiate the inflammatory machinery by upregulating adhesion molecules (ICAM-1), chemokines (RANTES), and cytokines (IL-1 and TNF-α). An inflammatory reaction will induce the release of many other pain mediators to enhance the pain response.

7.4 DRUG DISCOVERY: NGF/TRKA SIGNALING PATHWAY IS A UNIQUE TARGET TO MANIPULATE THE INFLAMMATORY PROLIFERATIVE CASCADES OF PSORIATIC DISEASE AND OTHER AUTOIMMUNE DISEASES

The recognition that NGF/TrkA signaling pathways have a regulatory role in the pathogenesis of inflammation, inflammatory disease, and pain mechanisms has generated immense initiatives to develop NGF/TrkA-targeted therapies for systemic and localized inflammatory diseases and to develop new therapies for chronic pain conditions. The NGF/TrkA system and its downstream signaling cascades offer multiple drug targets, such as (1) NGF-neutralizing agents, (2) TrkA-blocking agents, and (3) molecules that prevent NGF/TrkA signaling cascades.

We have demonstrated that in a developing psoriasis lesion following cutaneous trauma, keratinocyte proliferation and upregulation of NGF in basal keratinocytes are earlier events and precede epidermotropism of T lymphocytes [29]. Further, we have demonstrated that keratinocytes of psoriatic patients produce a higher level of NGF than those of normal individuals and are functionally active to regulate key pathologic events for the genesis of psoriasis, such as keratinocyte proliferation, angiogenesis, influx of cellular infiltrates, and growth and survival of T cells [2,5,29,55,87]. In view of the indisputable evidence suggesting a key role of NGF in the pathogenesis of psoriasis and PsA, we and others have been working to develop NGF/TrkA-targeted novel therapies for psoriasis and other autoimmune rheumatologic diseases. We have evaluated therapeutic efficacies of K252a, a TrkA inhibitor, and have also used a NGF-neutralizing antibody [58]. In this study, we

TABLE 7.2
Effect of K252a Treatment on the Rete Peg Length (μm) of the Transplanted Psoriatic Plaques (*n* = 20)

Group	Before Treatment	After Treatment
K252a treatment: 50 μg BID for 14 days (*n* = 12)	308.57 ± 98.72	164.64 ± 46.78
Control: Normal saline (*n* = 8)	269.37 ± 57.78	209.37 ± 74.00

used the SCID mouse model of psoriasis—the SCID mouse–psoriasis plaque xenograft model. In this study, we demonstrated that K252a, which blocks signal transductions induced by NGF/TrkA interaction, is therapeutically effective for psoriasis. Compared with the control group treated with normal saline, we observed significant reduction in thickness of the rete pegs and lesional cellular infiltrates (Table 7.2), and also normalization of the stratum corneum in the plaques treated with K252a. The therapeutic success of K252a and NGF-neutralizing antibody proves the regulatory role of NGF and its functional receptor TrkA in psoriasis and has provided a new dimension in understanding of the pathogenesis of psoriasis [58]. This study (Table 7.2) provides direct evidence that NGF/TrkA therapeutic manipulation of the NGF/TrkA interaction and its downstream signal cascades is plausible for the treatment of psoriasis.

Systemic use of K252a has been restricted due to its toxicities. Pincelli and Pignattim have extended our observations and are currently developing a topical preparation of K252a for psoriasis [88]. Many pharmaceutical companies are also in search of an anti-NGF therapy for psoriasis, autoimmune arthritis, and pain control. Shelton et al. from Rinat Neuroscience Corp. have observed the efficacy of anti-NGF antibody in a rat model of autoimmune arthritis [89]. Rats, after development of severe arthritis, received either of these two types of anti-NGF antibody: muMab 911 (a mouse antibody to NGF, i.v., days 14 and 19) or RI 624 (a humanized version of this antibody, i.v., days 14 and 19). Saline and indomethacin (3 mg/kg, p.o.) were the control groups. Treatment with anti-NGF had significant improvement of pain, and the analgesic effect was achieved within 24 h of therapy. Pain relief from anti-NGF therapy was comparable to or better than that of indomethacin.

These in vivo and in vitro studies have provided a clear direction for anti-NGF therapy not only for psoriatic disease but also for chronic pain, OA, and other types of autoimmune arthritis. For autoimmune arthritis, it will serve a dual effect as both an antipain and a disease-modifying anti-inflammatory agent. These results have encouraged the development of human monoclonal anti-NGF/anti-TrkA antibodies, and impressive preliminary results have been reported in OA patients.

The NGF monoclonal antibody tanezumab has been reported to have an excellent therapeutic agent; a patient with knee OA had significant pain reduction in phase I, phase II, and phase III trials [90–92]. Fasinumab, a newly developed anti-NGF agent and a high-affinity NGF-R inhibitor, is also demonstrating a significant analgesic effect in knee and hip OA arthritis, and initial results suggest that it is so far well tolerated [93]. However, there are also certain concerns; osteonecrosis and worsening of OA of the hip, knee, and shoulder were observed more in the study group than in the patients who did not receive tanezumab. It is important to address and overcome these two concerns: osteonecrosis and rapid progress of OA. The Food and Drug Administration (FDA) has concerns about these safety issues and is closely monitoring these aspects of anti-NGF preparations.

7.5 CONCLUSION

The role of NGF and its receptor system has provided a new dimension into the understanding of inflammatory diseases and the pathophysiology of acute and chronic pain conditions. It is likely that NGF-based therapy will be used in various disciplines of medicine, more so by rheumatologists for the treatment of autoimmune arthritis, OA, and chronic musculoskeletal pain syndromes. Currently, there are some concerns that include osteonecrosis of bones. It is important to understand the mechanisms for osteonecrosis. Extensive in vivo and in vitro studies are needed to make anti-NGF therapy totally safe for human use.

REFERENCES

1. Aloe L. Nerve growth factor and neuroimmune responses: Basic and clinical observations. *Arch Physiol Biochem* 2001;109(4):354–6.
2. Raychaudhuri SK, Raychaudhuri SP. NGF and its receptor system: A new dimension in the pathogenesis of psoriasis and psoriatic arthritis. *Arthritis. Ann NY Acad Sci* 2009;1173:470–7.
3. Hattor IA et al. Tumor necrosis factor is markedly synergistic with interleukin 1 and interferon gamma in stimulating the production of nerve growth factor in fibroblasts. *FEBS Lett* 1994;340:177–80.
4. Raychaudhuri SP, Raychaudhuri SK. The regulatory role of nerve growth factor and its receptor system in fibroblast-like synovial cells. *Scand J Rheumatol* 2009;38(3):207–15.
5. Raychaudhuri SP, Raychaudhuri SK, Atkuri KR, Herzenberg LA, Herzenberg LA. Nerve growth factor: A key local regulator in the pathogenesis of inflammatory arthritis. *Arthritis Rheum* 2011;63(11): 3243–52.
6. Moll JMH, Wright V. Psoriatic arthritis. *Semin Arthritis Rheum* 1973;3:55–78.
7. Elder JT et al. The genetics of psoriasis 2001: The odyssey continues. *Arch Dermatol* 2001;137:1447.
8. Gladman DD, Anhorn KAB, Schachter RK, Mervart H. HLA antigens in psoriatic arthritis. *J Rheumatol* 1986;13:586–92.
9. Austin LM, Coven TR, Bhardwaj N, Steinman R, Krueger JG. Intraepidermal lymphocytes in psoriatic lesions are activated GMP-17(TIA-1)+CD8+CD3+ CTLs as determined by phenotypic analysis. *J Cutan Pathol* 1998;25(2):79–88.
10. Costello P, Bresnihan B, O'Farrelly C, FitzGerald O. Predominance of CD8+ T lymphocytes in psoriatic arthritis. *J Rheumatol* 1999;26:1117–24.
11. Laloux L, Voisin MC, Allain J, Martin N, Kerboull L, Chevalier X, Claudepierre P. Immunohistological study of entheses in spondyloarthropathies: Comparison in rheumatoid arthritis and osteoarthritis. *Ann Rheum Dis* 2001;60:316–21.
12. Saxena A, Raychaudhuri SK, Raychaudhuri SP. Cytokine pathways in psoriasis and psoriatic arthritis. In *Psoriatic Arthritis and Psoriasis: Pathology and Clinical Aspects*, ed. A Adebajo, W-H Boehncke, DD Gladman, PJ Mease (pp. 73–82). Berlin: Springer International, 2016.
13. Tassiulas I, Duncan SR, Centola M, Theofilopoulos AN, Boumpas DT. Clonal characteristics of T cell infiltrates in skin and synovium of patients with psoriatic arthritis. *Hum Immunol* 1999;60:479–91.
14. Boyle WJ, Simonet WS, Lacey DL. Osteoclast differentiation and activation. *Nature* 2003;423:337–42.
15. Gravallese EM, Manning C, Tsay A, Naito A, Pan C, Amento E, Goldring SR. Synovial tissue in rheumatoid arthritis is a source of osteoclast differentiation factor. *Arthritis Rheum* 2000;43:250–8.
16. Bengtsson AK, Ryan EJ. Immune function of the decoy receptor osteoprotegerin. *Crit Rev Immunol* 2002;22:201–15.
17. Ritchlin CT, Haas-Smith SA, Li P, Hicks DG, Schwarz EM. Mechanisms of TNF-alpha- and RANKL-mediated osteoclastogenesis and bone resorption in psoriatic arthritis. *J Clin Invest* 2003;111:821–31.
18. Veale D, Rogers S, Fitzgerald O. Immunolocalization of adhesion molecules in psoriatic arthritis, psoriatic and normal skin. *Br J Dermatol* 1995;132:32–8.
19. Pitzalis C, Cauli A, Pipitone N, Smith C, Barker J, Marchesoni A, Yanni G, Panayi GS. Cutaneous lymphocyte antigen-positive T lymphocytes preferentially migrate to the skin but not to the joint in psoriatic arthritis. *Arthritis Rheum* 1996;39:137–45.
20. Kane D, Roth J, Frosch M, Vogl T, Bresnihan B, FitzGerald O. Increased perivascular synovial membrane expression of myeloid-related proteins in psoriatic arthritis. *Arthritis Rheum* 2003;48:1676–85.
21. Braverman IM, Yen A. Ultrastructure of the capillary loops in the dermal papillae of psoriasis. *J Invest Dermatol* 1977;68:53–60.
22. Reece RJ, Canete JD, Parsons WJ, Emery P, Veale DJ. Distinct vascular patterns of early synovitis in psoriatic, reactive, and rheumatoid arthritis. *Arthritis Rheum* 1999;42:1481–4.
23. Creamer D, Sullivan D, Bicknell R, Barker J. Angiogenesis in psoriasis. *Angiogenesis* 2002;5:231–6.
24. Fearon U et al. Angiopoietins, growth factors, and vascular morphology in early arthritis. *J Rheumatol* 2003;30:260–8.

25. Creamer D, Jaggar R, Allen M, Bicknell R, Barker J. Overexpression of the angiogenic factor platelet-derived endothelial cell growth factor/thymidine phosphorylase in psoriatic epidermis. *Br J Dermatol* 1997;137:851–5.
26. Fearon U et al. Synovial cytokine and growth factor regulation of MMPs/TIMPs: Implications for erosions and angiogenesis in early rheumatoid and psoriatic arthritis patients. *Ann NY Acad Sci* 1999;878:619–21.
27. Kuroda K, Sapadin A, Shoji T, Fleischmajer R, Lebwohl M. Altered expression of angiopoietins and Tie2 endothelium receptor in psoriasis. *J Invest Dermatol* 2001;116:713–20.
28. Raychaudhuri SP, Farber EM. Neuroimmunologic aspects of psoriasis. *Cutis* 2000;66(5):357–62.
29. Raychaudhuri SP, Jiang WY, Raychaudhuri SK. Revisiting the Koebner phenomenon: Role of NGF and its receptor system in the pathogenesis of psoriasis. *Am J Pathol* 2008;172(4):961–71.
30. Veale D, Farrell M, Fitzgerald O. Mechanism of joint sparing in a patient with unilateral psoriatic arthritis and a longstanding hemiplegia. *Br J Rheumatol* 1993;32:413–6.
31. Mulherin D, Bresnihan B, FitzGerald O. Digital denervation associated with absence of nail and distal interphalangeal joint involvement in psoriatic arthritis. *J Rheumatol* 1995;22:1211–2.
32. Raychaudhuri SP, Wilken R, Sukhov AC, Raychaudhuri SK, Maverakis E. Management of psoriatic arthritis: Early diagnosis, monitoring of disease severity and cutting edge therapies. *J Autoimmun* 2017;76:21–37.
33. Wrone-Smith T, Nickoloff BJ. Dermal injection of immunocytes induces psoriasis. *J Clin Invest* 1996;98(8):1878–87.
34. Farber EM, Nickoloff BJ, Recht B, Fraki JE. Stress, symmetry, and psoriasis: Possible role of neuropeptides. *J Am Acad Dermatol* 1986;14:305–11.
35. Raychaudhuri SP, Farber EM. Are sensory nerves essential for the development of psoriasis lesions? *J Am Acad Dermatol* 1993;28:488–9.
36. Naukkarinen A, Nickoloff BJ, Farber EM. Quantification of cutaneous sensory nerves and their substance P content in psoriasis. *J Invest Dermatol* 1989;92:126–9.
37. Al'Abadie MS, Senior HJ, Bleehen SS, Gawkrodger DJ. Neuropeptides and general neuronal marker in psoriasis—An immunohistochemical study. *Clin Exp Dermatol* 1995;20(5):384–9.
38. Wallengren J, Ekman R, Sunder F. Occurrence and distribution of neuropeptides in human skin. An immunocytochemical and immunohistochemical study on normal skin and blister fluid from inflamed skin. *Acta Derm Venereol (Stockh)* 1987;67:185–92.
39. Bernstein JE, Parish LC, Rapaport M, Rosenbaum MM, Roenigk HH. Effects of topically applied capsaicin on moderate and severe psoriasis vulgaris. *J Am Acad Dermatol* 1986;15:504–7.
40. Leeman SE, Krause JE, Lembeck F. Substance P and related peptides: Cellular and molecular physiology. *Ann NY Acad Sci* 1991;632:1–58, 263–71.
41. Camisa C, O'Dorisio TM, Maceyko RF, Schacht GE, Mekhjian HS, Howe BA. Treatment of psoriasis with chronic subcutaneous administration of somatostatin analog 201–295 (sandostatin). An open-label pilot study. *Clev Clin J Med* 1990;57:71–6.
42. Farber EM, Cohen EN, Trozak DJ, Wilkinson DI. Peptide T improves psoriasis when infused into lesions in nanogram amounts. *J Am Acad Dermatol* 1991;25:658–64.
43. Wyatt S, Shooeter EM, Davies AM. Expression of the NGF receptor gene in sensory neurons and their cutaneous targets prior to and during innervation. *Neuron* 1990;2:421–7.
44. Lindsay RM, Harmar AJ. Nerve growth factor regulates expression of neuropeptides genes in adult sensory neurons. *Nature* 1989;337:362–4.
45. Schwartz J, Pearson J, Johnson E. Effect of exposure to anti-NGF on sensory neurons of adult rats and guinea pigs. *Brain Res* 1982;244:378–81.
46. Fantini F, Magnoni C, Brauci-Laudeis L, Pincelli C. Nerve growth factor is increased in psoriatic skin. *J Invest Dermatol* 1995;105:854–5.
47. Raychaudhuri SP, Jiang W-Y, Farber EM. Psoriatic keratinocytes express high levels of nerve growth factor. *Acta Derm Venereol* 1998;78:84–6.
48. Raychaudhuri SP, Jiang W-Y, Smoller BR, Farber EM. Nerve growth factor and its receptor system in psoriasis. *Br J Dermatol* 2000;143:198–200.
49. Wilkinson DI, Theeuwes MI, Farber EM. Nerve growth factor increases the mitogenicity of certain growth factors for cultured human keratinocytes: A comparison with epidermal growth factor. *Exp Dermatol* 1994;3:239–45.
50. Aloe L, Levi-Mantalcini R. Mast cells increase in tissues of neonatal rats injected with the nerve growth factor. *Brain Res* 1977;133:358–66.
51. Pearce FL, Thompson HL. Some characteristics of histamine secretion from rat peritoneal mast cells stimulated with nerve growth factor. *J Physiol* 1986;372:379–93.

52. Thorpe LW, Werrbach-Perez K, Perez-Polo JR. Effects of nerve growth factor on the expression of IL-2 receptors on cultured human lymphocytes. *Ann NY Acad Sci* 1987;496:310–1.
53. Bischoff SC, Dahinden CA. Effect of nerve growth factor on the release of inflammatory mediators by mature human basophils. *Blood* 1992;79:2662–9.
54. Lambiase A, Bracci-Laudiero L, Bonini S, Bonini S, Starace G, D'Elios MM, De Carli M, Aloe L. Human CD4+ T cell clones produce and release nerve growth factor and express high-affinity nerve growth factor receptors. *J Allerg Clin Immunol* 1997;100(3):408–14.
55. Raychaudhuri SK, Raychaudhuri SP, Weltman H, Farber EM. Effect of nerve growth factor on endothelial cell biology: Proliferation and adherence molecule expression on human dermal microvascular endothelial cells. *Arch Dermatol Res* 2001;293:291–5.
56. Peunova N, Enicolopov G. Nitric oxide triggers a switch to growth arrest during differentiation of neuronal cells. *Nature* 1995;375:68–73.
57. Wyatt S, Davies AM. Regulation of expression of mRNAs encoding the nerve growth factor receptors p75 and trkA in developing sensory neurons *Development* 1993;119(3):635–48.
58. Raychaudhuri SP, Sanyal M, Weltman H, Raychaudhuri SK. K252a, a high affinity NGF receptor blocker improves psoriasis: An in vivo study using the SCID mouse-human skin model. *J Invest Dermatol* 2004;122(3):812–9.
59. Raychaudhuri SP, Dutt S, Raychaudhuri SK, Sanyal M, Farber EM. Severe combined immunodeficiency mouse-human skin chimeras: A unique animal model for the study of psoriasis and cutaneous inflammation. *Br J Dermatol* 2001;144(5):931–9.
60. Aloe L et al. The synovium of transgenic arthritic mice expressing human tumor necrosis factor contains a high level of nerve growth factor. *Growth Factors* 1993;9(2):149–55.
61. Manni L, Lundeberg T, Fiorito S, Bonini S, Vigneti E, Aloe L. Nerve growth factor release by human synovial fibroblasts prior to and following exposure to tumor necrosis factor-alpha, interleukin-1 beta and cholecystokinin-8: The possible role of NGF in the inflammatory response. *Clin Exp Rheumatol* 2003;21(5):617–24.
62. Kane D, Lockhart JC, Balint PV, Mann C, Ferrell WR, McInnes IB. Protective effect of sensory denervation in inflammatory arthritis (evidence of regulatory neuroimmune pathways in the arthritic joint). *Ann Rheum Dis* 2005;64(2):325–7.
63. Halliday DA, Zettler C, Rush RA, Scicchitano R, McNeil JD. Elevated nerve growth factor levels in the synovial fluid of patients with inflammatory joint disease. *Neurochem Res* 1998;23(6):919–22.
64. Raychaudhuri SP, Raychaudhuri SK. Role of NGF and neurogenic inflammation in the pathogenesis of psoriasis. *Prog Brain Res* 2004;146:433–7.
65. Indo Y. Genetics of congenital insensitivity to pain with anhidrosis (CIPA) or hereditary sensory and autonomic neuropathy type IV. Clinical, biological and molecular aspects of mutations in TRKA(NTRK1) gene encoding the receptor tyrosine kinase for nerve growth factor. *Clin Auton Res* 2002;12(Suppl. 1): I20–32.
66. Einarsdottir E et al. A mutation in the nerve growth factor beta gene (NGFB) causes loss of pain perception. *Hum Mol Genet* 2004;13:799–805.
67. Lewin GR et al. Peripheral and central mechanisms of NGF-induced hyperalgesia. *Eur J Neurosci* 1994;6:1903–12.
68. Della Seta D et al. NGF effects on hot plate behaviors in mice. *Pharmacol Biochem Behav* 1994;49:701–5.
69. Dyck PJ et al. Intradermal recombinant human nerve growth factor induces pressure allodynia and lowered heat-pain threshold in humans. *Neurology* 1997;48:501–5.
70. McArthur JC et al. A phase II trial of nerve growth factor for sensory neuropathy associated with HIV infection. AIDS Clinical Trials Group Team 291. *Neurology* 2000;54:1080–8.
71. Apfel SC. Nerve growth factor for the treatment of diabetic neuropathy: What went wrong, what went right, and what does the future hold? *Int Rev Neurobiol* 2002;50:393–413.
72. Svensson P et al. Injection of nerve growth factor into human masseter muscle evokes long-lasting mechanical allodynia and hyperalgesia. *Pain* 2003;104:241–7.
73. Ruiz G et al. Behavioral and histological effects of endoneurial administration of nerve growth factor: Possible implications in neuropathic pain. *Brain Res* 2004;1011:1–6.
74. Szallasi A, Blumberg PM. Vanilloid (capsaicin) receptors and mechanisms. *Pharmacol Rev* 1999;51: 159–212.
75. Shu X, Mendell LM. Nerve growth factor acutely sensitizes the response of adult rat sensory neurons to capsaicin. *Neurosci Lett* 1999;274:159–62.
76. Bonnington JK, McNaughton PA. Signalling pathways involved in the sensitisation of mouse nociceptive neurones by nerve growth factor. *J Physiol* 2003;551:433–46.

77. Zhuang ZY et al. Phosphatidylinositol 3-kinase activates ERK in primary sensory neurons and mediates inflammatory heat hyperalgesia through TRPV1 sensitization. *J Neurosci* 2004;24:8300–9.
78. Cesare P et al. Specific involvement of PKC-epsilon in sensitization of the neuronal response to painful heat. *Neuron* 1999;23:617–24.
79. Premkumar LS, Ahern GP. Induction of vanilloid receptor channel activity by protein kinase C. *Nature* 2000;408:985–90.
80. Numazaki M et al. Direct phosphorylation of capsaicin receptor VR1 by protein kinase C epsilon and identification of two target serine residues. *J Biol Chem* 2002;277:13375–8.
81. Morenilla-Palao C et al. Regulated exocytosis contributes to protein kinase C potentiation of vanilloid receptor activity. *J Biol Chem* 2004;279:25665–72.
82. Khasar SG et al. A novel nociceptor signaling pathway revealed in protein kinase C epsilon mutant mice. *Neuron* 1999;24:253–60.
83. Delcroix JD et al. NGF signaling in sensory neurons: Evidence that early endosomes carry NGF retrograde signals. *Neuron* 2003;39:69–84.
84. Lindsay RM et al. Nerve growth factor regulates expression of the nerve growth factor receptor gene in adult sensory neurons. *Eur J Neurosci* 1990;2:389–96.
85. Kawamoto K et al. Nerve growth factor activates mast cells through the collaborative interaction with lysophosphatidylserine expressed on the membrane surface of activated platelets. *J Immunol* 2002;168:6412–9.
86. Bennett DLH et al. Nerve growth factor and sensory nerve function. In *Pain and Neurogenic Inflammation*, ed. SD Brain, PK Moore (pp. 167–193). Berlin: Birkhauser, 1999.
87. Raychaudhuri SP, Farber EM, Raychaudhuri SK. Role of nerve growth factor in RANTES expression by keratinocytes. *Acta Derm Venereol* 2000;80(4):247–50.
88. Pincelli C, Pignattim M. Keratinocyte-based mechanisms are trendy again in psoriasis—The role of a k252a derivative as a novel topical treatment. *Eur Dermatol Rev* 2006;3:13–16.
89. Shelton DL, Zeller J, Ho WH, Pons J, Rosenthal A. Nerve growth factor mediates hyperalgesia and cachexia in auto-immune arthritis. *Pain* 2005;116(1–2):8–16.
90. Schnitzer TJ, Marks JA. A systematic review of the efficacy and general safety of antibodies to NGF in the treatment of OA of the hip and knee. *Osteoarthr Cartil* 2015;23(Suppl. 1):S8–17.
91. Lane NE et al. Tanezumab for the treatment of pain from osteoarthritis of the knee. *N Engl J Med* 2010;363:1521–31.
92. Hochberg MC et al. When is osteonecrosis not osteonecrosis? Adjudication of reported serious adverse joint events in the tanezumab clinical development program. *Arthritis Rheumatol* 2016;68:382–91.
93. Maloney J et al. Efficacy and safety of fasinumab for osteoarthritic pain in patients with moderate to severe osteoarthritis of the knees or hips [abstract]. *Arthritis Rheumatol* 2016;68(Suppl. 10):295.

Section III

Psoriatic Disease: Clinical Profiles

8 Psoriasis: Clinical Spectrum

Chelsea Ma, Smriti K. Raychaudhuri, Emanual Maverakis, and Siba P. Raychaudhuri

CONTENTS

8.1 INTRODUCTION

Psoriasis is a chronic skin disease that is considered to be the most prevalent autoimmune disease [1], affecting approximately 2%–5% of the world's population [1,2]. In the United States, as many as 7.5 million individuals have psoriasis [1]. The exact etiology of psoriasis is not well understood, but is thought to involve a complex interplay among the environment, genetics, immune dysfunction, and skin barrier disruption [1–4].

There is currently no cure for the various different subtypes of psoriasis or for psoriatic arthritis. Psoriasis is associated with increased morbidity, and medications currently used can have severe side effects. Several clinical studies have found strong associations between psoriasis and type 2 diabetes, atherosclerosis, and metabolic syndrome, which in the Western world are the leading causes of mortality [5]. In addition, psoriasis patients have decreased quality of life and lower levels of employment and income [6,7]. The cost of long-term therapy combined with the social costs of the disease have had great impacts on the health care system and society. Data from the National Psoriasis Foundation show that the direct and indirect cost of psoriasis in the United States is more than $11 billion annually, with missed workdays comprising 40% of the cost burden [1].

This chapter reviews the clinical spectrum of psoriasis and ways to diagnose the varying manifestations of it. An expert dermatologist will typically use morphologic appearance to diagnose plaque psoriasis and other clinical variants. Histopathology and laboratory tests are not recommended as diagnostic tools for psoriasis. However, psoriasis does have unique histopathological and immunohistochemical features, and on rare occasions, clinicopathological correlations may aid in diagnosis.

8.2 PATHOGENESIS AND THE PATHOLOGY OF PSORIASIS

Here we briefly review the following aspects of psoriasis: immunogenetics, immunopathogenesis, and the histopathological features of psoriasis. This genetic basis of psoriasis is supported by evidence from population-based association studies, linkage studies, and family and twin studies. These studies found keratinocytes and the immune system to be important in the pathophysiology of psoriasis. NF-κB-mediated responses in the skin have been reported to be directed by CARD14, a rare subset of which may lead to psoriasis and psoriatic arthritis—the inflammatory arthritis associated with psoriasis [8,9]. Elder et al. reviewed single-nucleotide polymorphism (SNP) analyses of multiple major studies in this area to corroborate data on the association between psoriasis and numerous loci of the immune system; this included the TH17 pathway (*IL23A*, *IL23R*, *IL12B*, *TRAF3IP2*, and *TYK2*), the TH2 pathway (*IL4* and *IL13*), innate immunity [interferon and NF-κB], signaling pathways (*IL23RA*, *TNFAIP3*, *TNIP1*, *REL*, *NFKBIA*, *TYK2*, and *IFIH1*), and β-defensin, as well as adaptive immunity involving CD8 T cells (*ZAP70* and *ERAP1*) [10].

The underlying pathophysiologic dysregulation in psoriasis results in increased proliferation and abnormal differentiation of keratinocytes. On histology, there is marked epidermal thickening due to keratinocyte hyperproliferation in the interfollicular epidermis, and elongated epidermal rete peg [11–15]. Keratinocyte differentiation is also greatly altered in psoriasis, paralleling "regenerative maturation," which is an alternative cell differentiation program transiently expressed during wound repair. The epidermal granular layer, in which terminal differentiation occurs, is also markedly reduced or absent in psoriatic lesions [12–15]. Consequently, the stratum corneum forms from keratinocytes that are incompletely differentiated and aberrantly retain a cell nucleus (parakeratosis).

The critical role of T cells in psoriasis pathophysiology is strongly substantiated by the following observations: (1) immunotherapy targeting T cells or T-cell cytokines (i.e., IL-17) clears active psoriasis plaques [16–20], and (2) in mice with severe combined immunodeficiency (SCID), transplantation of nonlesional psoriatic skin converts to a plaque after intradermal administration of antigen-activated T cells [21]. SCID mice studies have also found that in addition to traditional inflammatory mediators, nerve growth factor (NGF) and substance P (SP)–activated lymphocytes mediate conversion of nonlesional psoriatic skin transplants to psoriasis [22]. Thus, cytokines (i.e., Th1, Th17, and Th22), chemokines, growth factors, neuropeptides, adhesion molecules, and specific T-cell subpopulations, plus their receptors, all contribute to the unique inflammatory and proliferative processes characteristic for psoriasis.

The inflammatory infiltrates found in the skin and joints of psoriasis patients have been studied extensively. Prominent lymphocytic infiltrates are localized in the dermal papillae of the skin, as well as the sublining layer in the joint. T cells, predominantly CD4+ lymphocytes, are the dominant lymphocytes found in these tissues; in contrast, CD8+ T cells are predominant in the epidermis, synovial fluid compartment, and enthesis [23–25]. These findings suggest that CD8+ T cells may be the driving force behind the immune response in the skin and joints. This is further supported by evidence demonstrating an association between psoriasis and human leukocyte antigen (HLA) class I [10].

In summary, the immunopathologic features in a psoriasis plaque are unique [26]. Histological features of plaque psoriasis include marked epidermal thickening, elongated epidermal rete pegs, parakeratosis, decrease of loss of the granular layer, microabscess of Munro (a collection of neutrophils seen in the stratum corneum), suprapapillary thinning, spongiform pustule of Kojog (an epidermal spongiotic pustule with neutrophilic infiltration), and epidermal or dermal CD3+ T-cell infiltrates with CD8+ T-cell epidermotropism. While psoriatic subtypes may share classic histologic dermal and epidermal features seen in plaque psoriasis, they may also have their own distinct histopathologic characteristics [26,27].

8.3 DIAGNOSIS OF PSORIASIS: CLINICAL SPECTRUM, CLASSIFICATION, AND DIAGNOSIS

8.3.1 Clinical Spectrum

The clinical manifestations of psoriasis are variable. Primary skin lesions may appear as macules, papules, plaques, and pustules (Figure 8.1a–c). The disease is not necessarily restricted to the skin and nails. Around 30% of patients may develop an inflammatory arthritis, which is known as psoriatic arthritis. Psoriasis may also be rarely associated with inflammatory bowel disease and uveitis. Furthermore, the presentation can vary widely from patient to patient. Skin manifestations may be limited or widespread, monomorphic or polymorphic, and can develop at any age. Thus, psoriasis may be viewed as a spectrum; as such, there is currently no definitive diagnostic criteria for the disease.

8.3.2 Disease Classification

The clinical phenotypes of psoriasis have been classified according to various features, including age of onset, morphologic pattern, degree of skin involvement, and body sites of predilection [28–31]. Table 8.1 summarizes the various clinical phenotypes that are observed [28–31].

8.3.3 Diagnosis

Because there is no currently accepted diagnostic criteria for psoriasis, diagnosis is based largely on morphologic evaluation of a skin lesion. Morphology and site of involvement may further be used

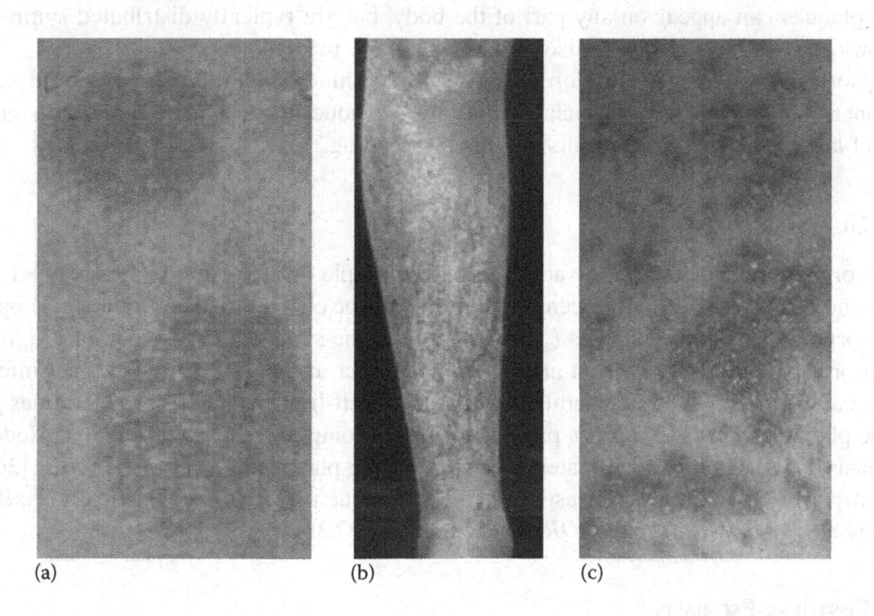

FIGURE 8.1 **(See color insert.)** Morphology of certain psoriasis lesions. (a) Erythematous macular lesions of psoriasis. (b) Stable chronic plaques; some are lichenified. (c) Discrete pustular lesions on an erythematous base.

TABLE 8.1
Psoriasis Can Be Classified in Various Ways Based on Certain Clinical Aspects

Clinical Parameter	Various Clinical Phenotypes
1. Age of onset	Type I psoriasis: Before 40 years of age Type II psoriasis: After 40 years of age
2. Distribution pattern	Seborrheic, inverse, flexor
3. Severity based on body surface area (BSA) involvement	Mild: <5% BSA Moderate: 5%–10% BSA Severe: >10% BSA
4. Location	Localized psoriasis/widespread psoriasis Scalp psoriasis, nail psoriasis, genital psoriasis, palmoplantar psoriasis, inverse psoriasis, anal psoriasis
5. Morphology	Plaque, guttate, pustular (generalized/localized), erythrodermic, elephantine, rupioid
6. Stage of development	Stable plaque psoriasis Unstable eruptive psoriasis

to categorize psoriasis into its various clinical phenotypes (Table 8.1). Clinical features of these subtypes are described in detail by Farber and Nall [32]. In the next section, we describe the telltale diagnostic signs of these phenotypes.

8.4 CLINICAL PHENOTYPES OF PSORIASIS

8.4.1 Plaque Psoriasis

Plaque psoriasis, also known as psoriasis vulgaris, is the most common form of psoriasis, representing almost 90% of psoriatic patients [33]. The lesions typically begin as erythematous macules or papules that extend peripherally and coalesce into plaques. The lesions are characterized by well-defined round or oval erythematous plaques with loosely adherent silvery white scales (Figure 8.1b). Psoriasis plaques can appear on any part of the body, but are typically distributed symmetrically over elbows and knees; the scalp is also a common area of involvement [31].

New psoriasis lesions may develop following direct cutaneous trauma, a response known as the Koebner phenomenon. Another classic feature of plaque psoriasis is the Auspitz sign, where removal of layers of lesion scale results in pinpoint bleeding.

8.4.2 Guttate Psoriasis

Guttate psoriasis is characterized by acute onset of multiple discrete small papules of <1 cm over the trunk and extremities, often in a centripetal fashion. The characteristic morphologic appearance is monomorphic droplet-like papules (gutta) that are at the same stage of evolution (Figure 8.2a). Guttate psoriasis can affect children and adolescents after an upper respiratory tract infection or streptococcal infection [34,35]. Generally, the disease is self-limiting, but it can sometimes progress to chronic plaque psoriasis [34]. Even patients who have complete recovery from an episode of guttate psoriasis have a significantly greater risk of developing plaque psoriasis in the future [36]. Thus, it is not surprising that guttate psoriasis and chronic plaque psoriasis are genetically similar, both with strong associations with the *PSORS1* genetic locus [37,38].

8.4.3 Pustular Psoriasis

Pustular psoriasis presents as multiple tender sterile pustules on an underlying, blotchy, erythematous base (Figure 8.1c). Histology shows diffuse dermal neutrophilic infiltration, as well as

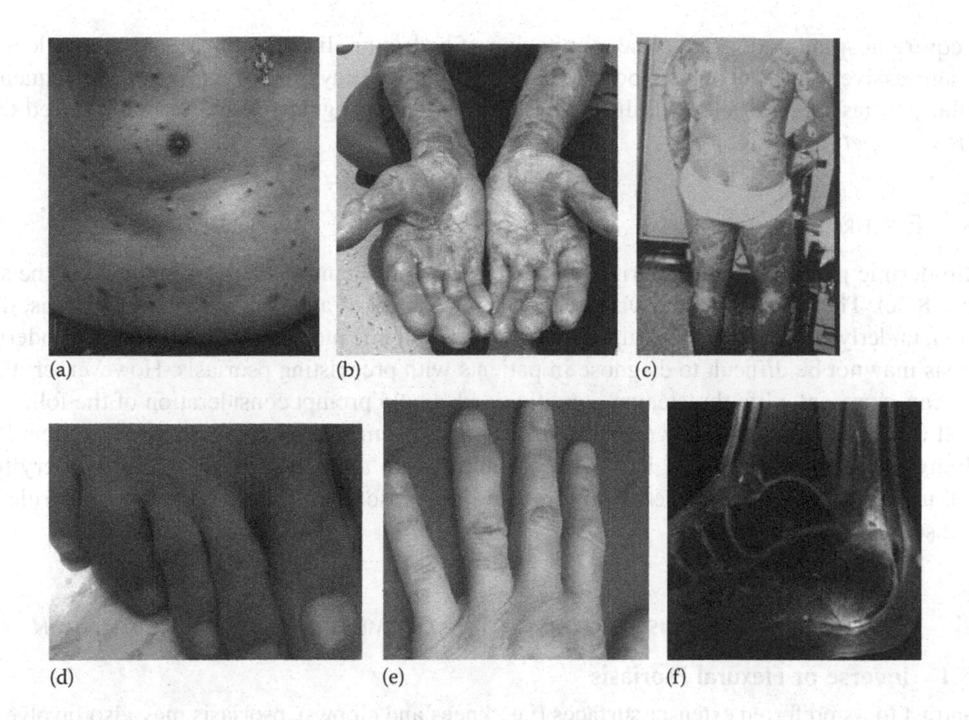

FIGURE 8.2 **(See color insert.)** Many faces of psoriasis. (a) Guttate psoriasis—monomorphic psoriasis lesions at the same stage of evolution. (b) Unstable widespread psoriasis—actively spreading within a few weeks. (c) Erythrodermic psoriasis. (d) Dactylitis—on the fourth toe (sausage digit); indicates inflammation of an entire digit. (e) DIP-predominant variant of psoriatic arthritis involving the DIP joint of the ring finger. (f) MRI demonstrating enthesitis of the right Achilles tendon. There is also thickening of the right plantar fascia at its calcaneal attachment, surrounding soft tissue edema and associated marrow edema involving the plantar aspect of the calcaneal tuberosity, and thickening of the right plantar fascia at its calcaneal attachment.

intraepidermal micropustules. Variations of pustular psoriasis have been described; among these, localized pustular psoriasis and generalized pustular psoriasis (von Zumbusch) are most well recognized [39,40].

Palmoplantar pustulosis and acrodermatitis continua of Hallopeau are distinctive forms of localized pustular psoriasis. Palmoplantar pustular psoriasis is characterized by pustules on the palms and soles with an erythematous base and scale. It is often associated with psoriatic nail involvement. While plaque formation is not normally seen in palmoplantar pustulosis, this variant may be associated with plaque psoriasis. Acrodermatitis continua presents as a pustular eruption on the fingers and toes [41]. The pustules subsequently become confluent and can spread proximally to the dorsal hands and feet. Pustules may become generalized; if left untreated, the disease may lead to osteolysis of the distal phalanx.

Generalized pustular psoriasis is a rare, active, unstable disease. A reported 20% of chronic plaque psoriasis patients may develop pustular lesions during their disease course [42]. Acute generalized pustular psoriasis may be triggered by an infection, drugs, hypocalcemia, pregnancy, topical therapy of plaque psoriasis (i.e., from an irritant in a topical vehicle), or abrupt corticosteroid withdrawal [39,40,42,43]. Onset is often accompanied by fever, nausea, myalgias, and leukocytosis, and patients may have erythematous tender skin [39,40]. Within hours, numerous pustules appear on an erythematous base, which may later become confluent, creating sheets of superficial pus. Eventually, the pustules desiccate and slough off, resulting in a shiny erythematous surface where new pustules may develop. Geographic tongue, cholestasis, and polyarthritis are associated with generalized pustular psoriasis [44]. Patients are often quite sick and require hospitalization and close monitoring of hydration, liver function, and hypocalcemia. With aggressive treatment and supportive care, the disease may go into remission. Infrequently, pustular psoriasis can develop within the first 6 months of pregnancy, a condition referred to as *impetigo herpetiformis* [45].

8.4.4 Erythrodermic Psoriasis

Erythrodermic psoriasis is characterized by generalized erythema affecting a majority of the skin (Figure 8.2c). The condition can develop due to poor control of a patient's existing psoriasis, drug reaction, underlying infection, or abrupt withdrawal of systemic medications [46,47]. Erythrodermic psoriasis may not be difficult to diagnose in patients with preexisting psoriasis. However, erythroderma can represent a life-threatening condition and should prompt consideration of the following in the differential diagnosis: drug rash, airborne contact dermatitis, atopic dermatitis (especially in children), pityriasis rubra pilaris, and Sezary syndrome. In an undiagnosed patient with erythroderma, nail changes can be suggestive of erythrodermic psoriasis. Skin biopsy may help rule out other diseases, as noted above.

8.4.5 Phenotypes of Psoriasis according to Involvement of Anatomical Location

8.4.5.1 Inverse or Flexural Psoriasis

In contrast to its preferred extensor surfaces (i.e., knees and elbows), psoriasis may also involve the flexor surfaces and skinfolds, such as the axillary, inframammary, perineal, intergluteal, and inguinal areas. As these areas are moist, psoriatic lesions are less scaly than in plaque psoriasis.

8.4.5.2 Scalp Psoriasis

The scalp is a common area of involvement in psoriasis [31]. When located around the hairline, the disease can significantly lower quality of life due to its visibility. Particular challenges in the management of scalp psoriasis include difficulties of applying topical therapies and effectively treating severe disease [48,49].

8.4.5.3 Palmoplantar Psoriasis

The thick scales and painful fissures seen in nonpustular palmoplantar psoriasis make it a disabling condition [50]. Treatment of recalcitrant disease is challenging. Symptoms can be reduced with preventive measures, such as avoiding friction and irritants and applying emollients at night.

8.4.5.4 Nail Psoriasis

Psoriasis commonly affects the nails, and occasionally their characteristic changes can fetch a diagnosis [51]. Nail pitting is most characteristic, but onycholysis or detachment of the proximal nail from the nail bed is most commonly seen. Current therapies available for nail psoriasis are limited and often have poor response [52]. Involvement of the nail bed is often indicated by the appearance of orange-yellow areas or "oil spots" beneath the nail plate. The nail plate may also become dystrophic, discolored (often yellow), and thickened; keratinous material may accumulate under the nail plate, a condition called subungual hyperkeratosis.

8.4.5.5 Genital Psoriasis

Psoriasis involving the genitalia occurs in nearly one-third of psoriasis patients and can be observed in all age groups [53,54]. Special attention to this form is important, as quality of life is significantly decreased in both men and women.

8.4.6 Psoriatic Arthritis

Psoriatic arthritis is described in other sections of this book. Evaluation of a psoriasis patient without musculoskeletal examination is considered an incomplete task. Psoriatic arthritis has been classified into five subtypes: DIP-predominant arthritis (Figure 8.2e), asymmetrical oligoarthritis and monoarthritis, symmetrical polyarthritis, predominant spondylitis, and arthritis mutilans. Dactylitis (Figure 8.2d) and enthesopathy (Figure 8.2f) are other major features seen in patients with psoriatic arthritis. In every patient of psoriasis, it is essential to look for evidence of an inflammatory arthritis, the extent or severity of arthritis, the presence of dactylitis or enthesitis, and the degree of nail involvement.

8.5 CONCLUSION

Psoriasis is a multifactorial disease involving various forms and sometimes including extracutaneous manifestations. There are currently no established diagnostic criteria for psoriasis [28]. Classification schemes are organized according to clinical phenotype, age of onset, disease morphology, and disease severity. Despite this broad clinical spectrum, a trained clinician is able to diagnosis psoriasis and its various phenotypes based primarily on clinical presentation. However, this does not mean that psoriasis does not need diagnostic criteria. As Naldi and Gambini suggested, the field will benefit from an internationally coordinated approach to develop standardized, universally accepted diagnostic criteria for psoriasis [28].

CONTRIBUTIONS

S.K.R. and S.P.R. designed the papers. S.P.R. provided the figures from his research work and his clinic patients. All authors together wrote the chapter.

REFERENCES

1. https://www.aad.org/media/stats/conditions/psoriasis.
2. Raychaudhuri SP, Farber EM. The prevalence of psoriasis in the world. *J Eur Acad Dermatol Venereol* 2001;15(1):16–7.
3. Tsoi LC, Stuart PE, Tian C, Gudjonsson JE, Das S, Zawistowski M, Ellinghaus E et al. Large scale meta-analysis characterizes genetic architecture for common psoriasis associated variants. *Nat Commun* 2017;8:15382.
4. Chandran V, Raychaudhuri SP. Geoepidemiology and environmental factors of psoriasis and psoriatic arthritis. *J Autoimmun* 2010;34(3):J314–21.
5. Gelfand JM, Neimann AL, Shin DB, Wang X, Margolis DJ, Troxel AB. Risk of myocardial infarction in patients with psoriasis. *JAMA* 2006;296:1735–41.
6. Raychaudhuri SP, Gross J. Psoriasis risk factors: Role of lifestyle practices. *Cutis* 2000;66(5):348–52.
7. Gelfand JM, Feldman SR, Stern RS, Thomas J, Rolstad T, Margolis DJ. Determinants of quality of life in patients with psoriasis: A study from the US population. *J Am Acad Dermatol* 2004;51(5):704–8.
8. Jordan CT, Cao L, Roberson ED, Duan S, Helms CA, Nair RP, Duffin KC et al. Rare and common variants in CARD14, encoding an epidermal regulator of NF-kappaB, in psoriasis. *Am J Hum Genet* 2012;90(5):796–808.
9. Jordan CT, Cao L, Roberson ED, Pierson KC, Yang CF, Joyce CE, Ryan C et al. PSORS2 is due to mutations in CARD14. *Am J Hum Genet* 2012;90(5):784–95.
10. Elder JT, Bruce AT, Gudjonsson JE, Johnston A, Stuart PE, Tejasvi T, Voorhees JJ, Abecasis GR, Nair RP. Molecular dissection of psoriasis: Integrating genetics and biology. *J Invest Dermatol* 2010;130(5):1213–26.
11. Tonel G, Conrad C. Interplay between keratinocytes and immune cells—Recent insights into psoriasis pathogenesis. *Int J Biochem Cell Biol* 2009;41(5):963–8.
12. Nickoloff BJ. Keratinocytes regain momentum as instigators of cutaneous inflammation. *Trends Mol Med* 2006;12:102–6.

13. Griffiths CE, Barker JN. Pathogenesis and clinical features of psoriasis. *Lancet* 2007;370:263–71.
14. Hertle MD, Kubler MD, Leigh IM, Watt FM. Aberrant integrin expression during epidermal wound healing and in psoriatic epidermis. *J Clin Invest* 1992;89(6):1892–901.
15. Iizuka H, Ishida-Yamamoto A, Honda H. Epidermal remodelling in psoriasis. *Br J Dermatol* 1996;135(3): 433–8.
16. Gottlieb AB, Lebwohl M, Shirin S, Sherr A, Gilleaudeau RN, Singer G, Solodkina G et al. Anti-CD4 monoclonal antibody treatment of moderate to severe psoriasis vulgaris: Results of a pilot, multicenter, multiple-dose, placebo-controlled study. *J Am Acad Dermatol* 2000;43(4):595–604.
17. Raychaudhuri SP, Raychaudhuri SK, Tamura K, Masunaga T, Kubo K, Hanaoka K, Jiang WY, Herzenberg LA, Herzenberg LA. FR255734, a humanized, Fc-silent, anti-CD28 antibody improves psoriasis in the SCID mouse-psoriasis xenograft model. *J Invest Dermatol* 2008;128(8):1969–76.
18. Papp KA, Reich K, Paul C, Blauvelt A, Baran W, Bolduc C, Toth D et al. A prospective phase III, randomized, double-blind, placebo-controlled study of brodalumab in patients with moderate-to-severe plaque psoriasis. *Br J Dermatol* 2016;175(2):273–86.
19. Gordon KB, Blauvelt A, Papp KA, Langley RG, Luger T, Ohtsuki M, Reich K et al. Phase 3 Trials of ixekizumab in moderate-to-severe plaque psoriasis. *N Engl J Med* 2016;375(4):345–56.
20. McInnes IB, Mease PJ, Kirkham B, Kavanaugh A, Ritchlin CT, Rahman P, van der Heijde D et al. Secukinumab, a human anti-interleukin-17A monoclonal antibody, in patients with psoriatic arthritis (FUTURE 2): A randomised, double-blind, placebo-controlled, phase 3 trial. *Lancet* 2015;386(9999): 1137–46.
21. Wrone-Smith T, Nickoloff BJ. Dermal injection of immunocytes induces psoriasis. *J Clin Invest* 1996;98(8):1878–87.
22. Raychaudhuri SP, Jiang WY, Raychaudhuri SK. Revisiting the Koebner phenomenon: Role of NGF and its receptor system in the pathogenesis of psoriasis. *Am J Pathol* 2008;172(4):961–71.
23. Austin LM, Coven TR, Bhardwaj N, Steinman R, Krueger JG. Intraepidermal lymphocytes in psoriatic lesions are activated GMP-17 (TIA-1)+ CD8+ CD3+ CTLs as determined by phenotypic analysis. *J Cutan Pathol* 1998;25(2):79–88.
24. Costello P, FitzGerald O. Disease mechanisms in psoriasis and psoriatic arthritis. *Curr Rheumatol Rep* 2001;3(5):419–27.
25. Laloux L, Voisin MC, Allain J, Martin N, Kerboull L, Chevalier X, Claudepierre P. Immunohistological study of entheses in spondyloarthropathies: Comparison in rheumatoid arthritis and osteoarthritis. *Ann Rheum Dis* 2001;60:316–21.
26. Murphy M, Kerr P, Grant-Kels JM. The histopathologic spectrum of psoriasis. *Clin Dermatol* 2007;25(6): 524–8.
27. Balato N, Di Costanzo L, Balato A. Differential diagnosis of psoriasis. *J Rheumatol Suppl* 2009;83:24–5.
28. Naldi L, Gambini D. The clinical spectrum of psoriasis. *Clin Dermatol* 2007;25(6):510–8.
29. Henseler T, Christophers E. Psoriasis of early and late onset: Characterization of two types of psoriasis vulgaris. *J Am Acad Dermatol* 1985;13:450–6.
30. Pariser DM, Bagel J, Gelfand JM, Korman NJ, Ritchlin CT, Strober BE, Van Voorhees AS et al. National Psoriasis Foundation clinical consensus on disease severity. *Arch Dermatol* 2007;143(2):239–42.
31. Raychaudhuri SP, Gross J. A comparative study of pediatric onset psoriasis with adult onset psoriasis. *Pediatr Dermatol* 2000;17(3):174–8.
32. Farber EM, Nall L. Epidemiology: Natural history and genetics. In HH Roenigk Jr, HI Maibach (eds.), *Psoriasis*. New York: Dekker, 1998, pp. 107–57.
33. Levine D, Gottlieb A. Evaluation and management of psoriasis: An internist's guide. *Med Clin North Am* 2009;93(6):1291–303.
34. Krishnamurthy K, Walker A, Gropper CA, Hoffman C. To treat or not to treat? Management of guttate psoriasis and pityriasis rosea in patients with evidence of group A streptococcal infection. *J Drugs Dermatol* 2010;9(3);241–50.
35. Naldi L, Peli L, Parazzini F, Carrel CF. Family history of psoriasis, stressful life events, and recent infectious disease are risk factors for a first episode of acute guttate psoriasis: Results of a case-control study. *J Am Acad Dermatol* 2001;44(3):433–8.
36. Martin BA, Chalmers RJ, Telfer NR. How great is the risk of further psoriasis following a single episode of acute guttate psoriasis? *Arch Dermatol* 1996;132(6):717–8.
37. Sagoo GS, Tazi-Ahnini R, Barker JW, Elder JT, Nair RP, Samuelsson L, Traupe H, Trembath RC, Robinson DA, Iles MM. Meta-analysis of genome-wide studies of psoriasis susceptibility reveals linkage to chromosomes 6p21 and 4q28-q31 in Caucasian and Chinese Hans population. *J Invest Dermatol* 2004;122(6):1401–5.

38. Asumalahti K, Ameen M, Suomela S, Hagforsen E, Michaelsson G, Evans J, Munro M et al. Genetic analysis of PSORS1 distinguishes guttate psoriasis and palmoplantar pustulosis. *J Invest Dermatol* 2003;120(4):627–32.
39. Baker H, Ryan TJ. Generalized pustular psoriasis. A clinical and epidemiological study of 104 cases. *Br J Dermatol* 1968;80(12):771–93.
40. Kawada A, Tezuka T, Nakamizo Y, Kimura H, Nakagawa H, Ohkido M, Ozawa A et al. A survey of psoriasis patients in Japan from 1982 to 2001. *J Dermatol Sci* 2003;31(1):59–64.
41. Rosenberg BE, Strober BE. Acrodermatitis continua. *Dermatol Online J* 2004;10(3):9.
42. Naldi L, Colombo P, Placchesi EB, Piccitto R, Chatenoud L, La Vecchia C, PraKtis Study Centers. Study design and preliminary results from the pilot phase of the PraKtis study: Self-reported diagnoses of selected skin diseases in a representative sample of the Italian population. *Dermatology* 2004;208:38–42.
43. Ohkawara A, Yasuda H, Kobayashi H, Inaba Y, Ogawa H, Hashimoto I, Imamura S. Generalized pustular psoriasis in Japan: Two distinct groups formed by differences in symptoms and genetic background. *Acta Derm Venereol* 1996;76(1):68–71.
44. Viguier M, Allez M, Zagdanski AM, Bertheau P, de Kerviler E, Rybojad M, Morel P, Dubertret L, Lemann M, Bachelez H. High frequency of cholestasis in generalized pustular psoriasis: Evidence for neutrophilic involvement of the biliary tract. *Hepatology* 2004;40(2):452–8.
45. Oumeish OY, Parish JL. Impetigo herpetiformis. *Clin Dermatol* 2006;24(2):101–4.
46. Farber EM, Nall L. Erythrodermic (exfoliative) psoriasis. *Cutis* 1993;51(2):79–82.
47. Balasubramaniam P, Berth-Jones J. Erythroderma: 90% skin failure. *Hosp Med* 2004;65(2):100–2.
48. Papp K, Berth-Jones J, Kragballe K, Wozel G, de la Brassinne M. Scalp psoriasis: A review of current topical treatment options. *J Eur Acad Dermatol Venereol* 2007;21:1151–60.
49. Schlager JG, Rosumeck S, Werner RN, Jacobs A, Schmitt J, Schlager C, Nast A. Topical treatments for scalp psoriasis. *Cochrane Database Syst Rev* 2016;2:CD009687.
50. Janagond AB, Kanwar AJ, Handa S. Efficacy and safety of systemic methotrexate vs. acitretin in psoriasis patients with significant palmoplantar involvement: A prospective, randomized study. *J Eur Acad Dermatol Venereol* 2013;27(3):e384–9.
51. Salomon J, Szepietowski JC, Proniewicz A. Psoriatic nails: A prospective clinical study. *J Cutan Med Surg* 2003;7(4):317–21.
52. Wozel G. Psoriasis treatment in difficult locations: Scalp, nails, and intertriginous areas. *Clin Dermatol* 2008;26(5):448–59.
53. Meeuwis KA, de Hullu JA, de Jager ME, Massuger LF, van de Kerkhof PC, van Rossum MM. Genital psoriasis: A questionnaire-based survey on a concealed skin disease in the Netherlands. *J Eur Acad Dermatol Venereol* 2010;24(12):1425–30.
54. Meeuwis KA, de Hullu JA, IntHout J, Hendriks IM, Sparreboom EE, Massuger LF, van de Kerkhof PC, van Rossum MM. Genital psoriasis awareness program: Physical and psychological care for patients with genital psoriasis. *Acta Derm Venereol* 2015;95(2):211–6.

38. [illegible] Kr[illegible] M, [illegible] S, [illegible] Evans [illegible] Murray [illegible] [illegible] analysis of [illegible] distinguishes [illegible] and [illegible] pustulosis. [illegible]

39. [illegible] Generalized pustular psoriasis [illegible]

40. [illegible]

41. [illegible]

42. Naldi L, Colombo P, [illegible] Study Centers. Study design [illegible] Development [illegible]

43. Ohkawara A, [illegible] Generalized pustular psoriasis [illegible] Acta Derm [illegible]

44. Viguier M, [illegible] de [illegible] M, Morel P, [illegible] Dubertret L, Bachelez H. [illegible]

45. [illegible]

46. [illegible]

47. [illegible]

48. [illegible] A review of current [illegible]

49. [illegible] A. [illegible] treatments for [illegible]

50. [illegible]

51. [illegible]

52. [illegible]

53. [illegible] von Kossow [illegible]

54. Meadows KA, [illegible] Hendriks [illegible] Smith [illegible] Maddox [illegible] Physical and psychological [illegible] Br J Dermatol [illegible]

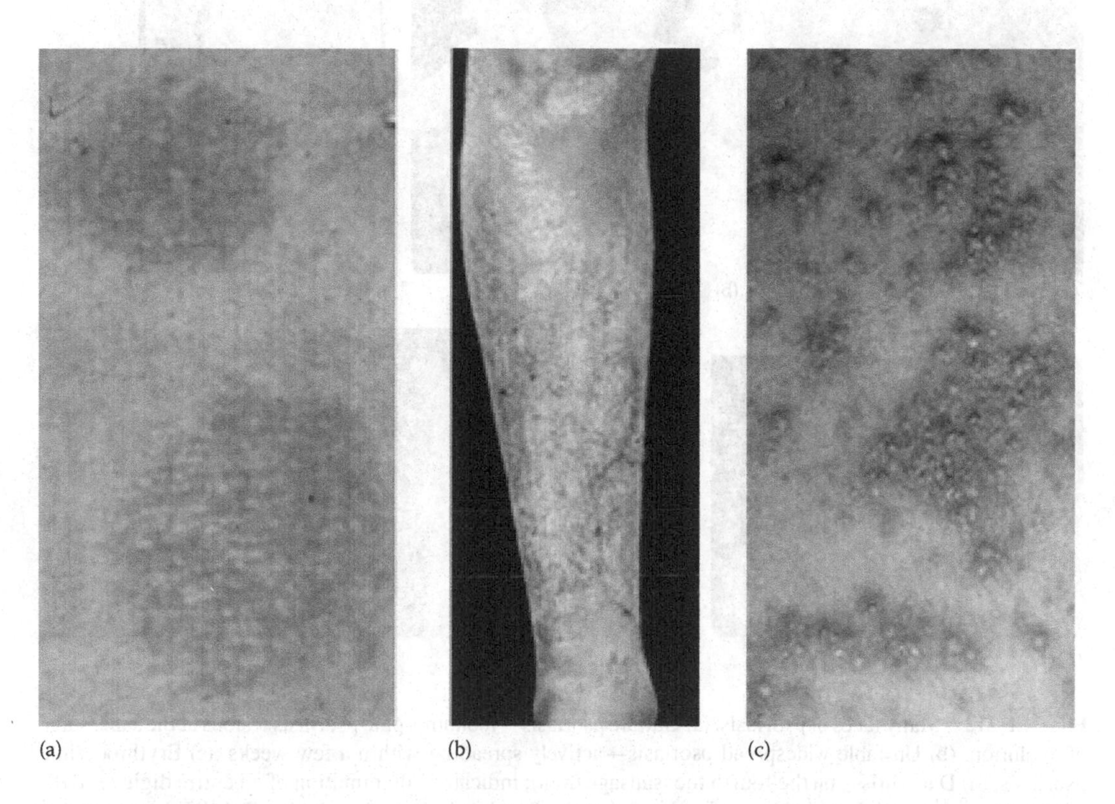

FIGURE 8.1 Morphology of certain psoriasis lesions. (a) Erythematous macular lesions of psoriasis. (b) Stable chronic plaques; some are lichenified. (c) Discrete pustular lesions on an erythematous base.

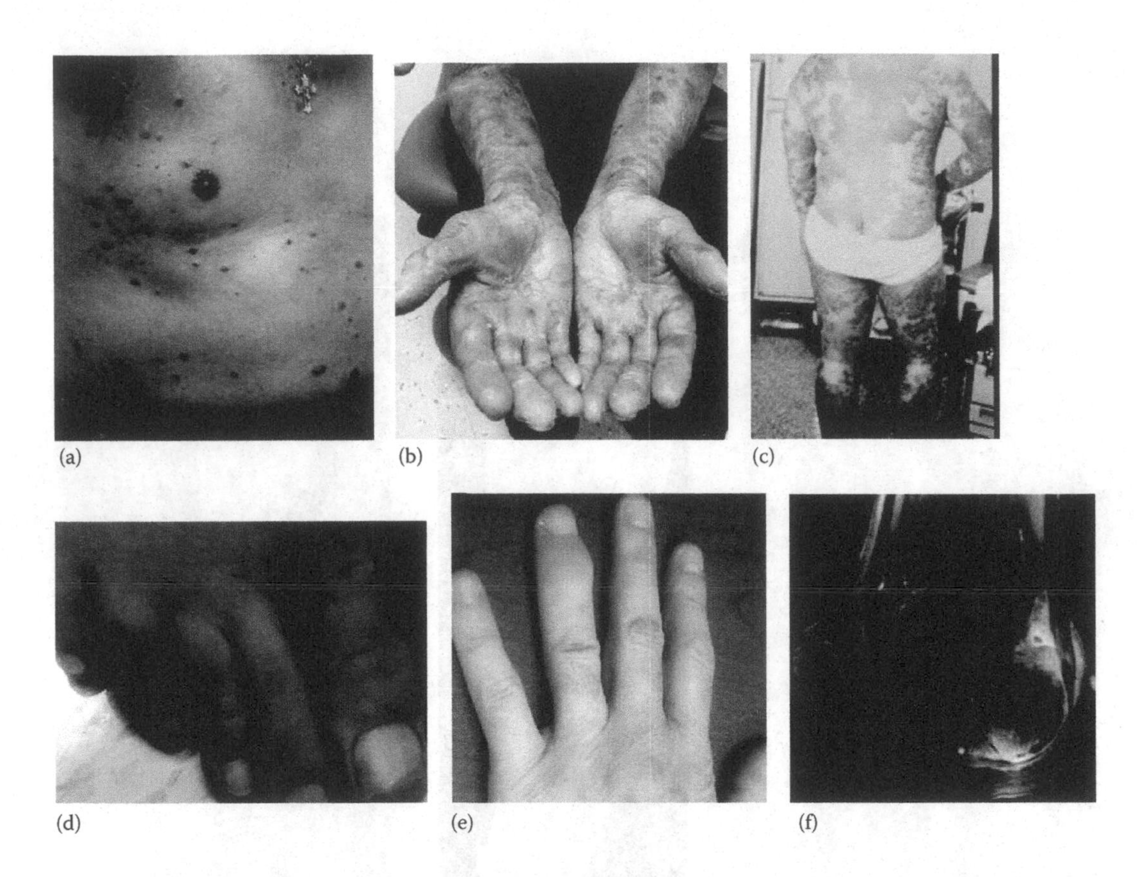

FIGURE 8.2 Many faces of psoriasis. (a) Guttate psoriasis—monomorphic psoriasis lesions at the same stage of evolution. (b) Unstable widespread psoriasis—actively spreading within a few weeks. (c) Erythrodermic psoriasis. (d) Dactylitis—on the fourth toe (sausage digit); indicates inflammation of an entire digit. (e) DIP-predominant variant of psoriatic arthritis involving the DIP joint of the ring finger. (f) MRI demonstrating enthesitis of the right Achilles tendon. There is also thickening of the right plantar fascia at its calcaneal attachment, surrounding soft tissue edema and associated marrow edema involving the plantar aspect of the calcaneal tuberosity, and thickening of the right plantar fascia at its calcaneal attachment.

9 Clinical Spectrum of Spondyloarthritis

Joerg Ermann

CONTENTS

9.1 SPONDYLOARTHRITIS CONCEPT

Spondyloarthritis (SpA) is a family of diseases with overlapping clinical features that include ankylosing spondylitis (AS), psoriatic arthritis (PsA), reactive arthritis, SpA associated with inflammatory bowel disease (IBD), and undifferentiated SpA (Figure 9.1) [1]. HLA-B27-associated uveitis, psoriasis, and IBD (Crohn's disease and ulcerative colitis) are closely related disorders.

As the name suggests, the common denominator of the spondyloarthritides is inflammation in the spine (*spondylos* = vertebra, *arthros* = joint, *itis* = inflammation, Greek). The terms *spondyloarthritis* and *spondyloarthropathy* are often used interchangeably, although it has been argued that spondyloarthritis should be preferred, as this term highlights the inflammatory nature of the underlying disease process [2].

The SpA concept began to emerge in the 1950s. Shortly after the discovery of rheumatoid factor, it was recognized that there was a group of inflammatory arthropathies that were seronegative and clinically distinct from rheumatoid arthritis. This group included AS, PsA, the arthritis of ulcerative colitis, and Reiter's syndrome [3]. The concept was reinforced in the 1970s with the discovery that these diseases were all associated with HLA-B27 [4–8], and the name *seronegative spondarthritis* was introduced in 1974 [9]. *Seronegative* was later dropped to avoid confusion with seronegative rheumatoid arthritis. The terms *reactive arthritis* [7] and *Reiter's disease* [10] were used synonymously in the United States for a long time to describe an inflammatory arthropathy that followed an infection in the intestinal or urinary tract. However, the use of the eponym Reiter's syndrome has been discouraged because of Julius Reiter's involvement in war crimes in Nazi Germany [11].

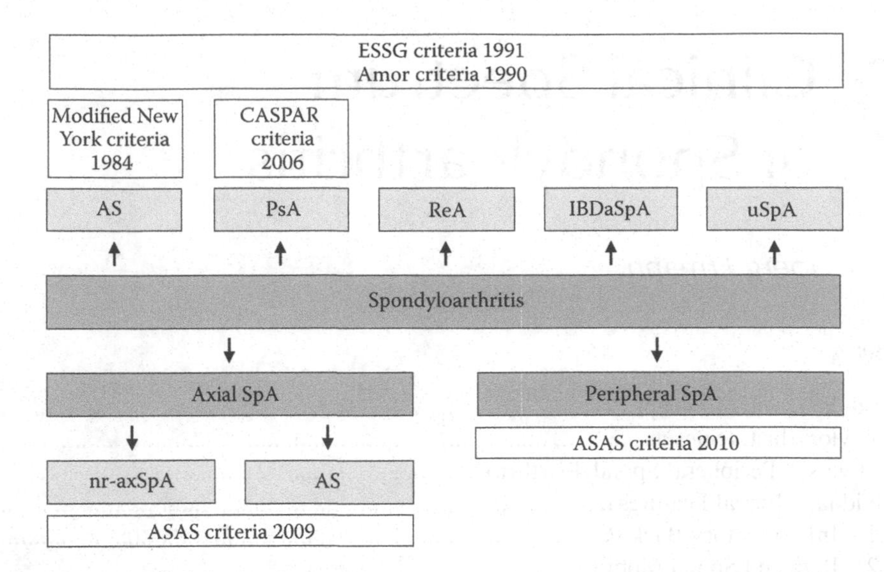

FIGURE 9.1 SpA classification schemes. SpA comprises AS, PsA, reactive arthritis (ReA), IBD–associated spondyloarthritis (IBDaSpA), and undifferentiated SpA. Alternatively, SpA can be distinguished into axial and peripheral SpA, the former including patients with AS [26] and nonradiographic axial SpA. Validated classification criteria exist for AS (modified New York criteria) [26], PsA (Classification Criteria for Psoriatic Arthritis [CASPAR]) [31], axial and peripheral SpA (ASAS criteria) [16,18], and SpA globally [20,21].

9.2 SPONDYLOARTHRITIS SUBSETS

AS is often considered to be the prototypic SpA. AS is characterized by inflammation in the axial skeleton involving the sacroiliac (SI) joints, vertebrae, and facet joints. Axial inflammation manifests clinically as back pain and stiffness. Pathological new bone formation results in fusion of SI and facet joints, the development of syndesmophytes at the edges of vertebral bodies, and fusion of vertebral bodies. The spine becomes stiff (*ankylos* = stiff, Greek), giving rise to the classical and easily recognizable clinical appearance of the AS patient with long-standing disease.

A diagnosis of *PsA* requires evidence for psoriasis at some point in the patient's lifetime. Psoriasis typically precedes or starts at the onset of musculoskeletal symptoms, but may follow the development of arthritis in some patients. Peripheral joints and the spine are variably affected and several subsets of PsA have been described; rheumatoid factor is negative [12]. Dactylitis and enthesis (see below) are typical features of PsA.

Reactive arthritis is defined by inflammation in peripheral joints or spine that develops within 4 weeks of a urinary tract infection or diarrheal illness caused by infection with gram-negative bacteria (*Chlamydia, Yersinia, Salmonella, Shigella, Campylobacter*). Aspirated joint fluid is by definition culture negative [13].

SpA associated with IBD is seen in patients with Crohn's disease or ulcerative colitis. Similar to other SpA variants, patients may have axial disease or peripheral arthritis. In some patients, the arthritis may flare when their IBD is active, while in other patients, the activity of arthritis and intestinal inflammation is uncoupled [14].

Undifferentiated SpA includes disease presentations that do not fit into one of the more defined categories at the time of assessment. Undifferentiated SpA may evolve into a more specific diagnosis, most commonly AS [1].

9.3 AXIAL VERSUS PERIPHERAL SPONDYLOARTHRITIS

A substantial delay between symptom onset and diagnosis is a well-described phenomenon in AS [15]. Attempts to identify patients with axial inflammation earlier led to the development of the axial SpA concept by the Assessment of SpondyloArthritis international Society (ASAS) [16]. Axial SpA includes patients with classical AS but also patients with similar symptoms but lacking unequivocal evidence for sacroiliitis on pelvic radiographs. The latter patients are thought to have nonradiographic axial SpA. Many patients with nonradiographic axial SpA will over time progress to AS, but a substantial fraction of patients may not [17]. Interestingly, nonradiographic axial SpA is somewhat of a misnomer, as these patients may have mild radiographic abnormalities but do not fulfill criteria according to the modified New York criteria.

Shortly after the definition of axial SpA, ASAS also published criteria for peripheral SpA [18]. All patients with SpA should therefore be classifiable as having either axial or peripheral SpA. This classification scheme (Figure 9.1) makes sense, as there is evidence that axial and peripheral disease respond differently to a variety of therapies. However, individual patients may have both axial and peripheral disease, and the severity of axial and peripheral symptoms may change over time, making the unequivocal classification as either axial or peripheral SpA challenging [19]. The complete spectrum of axial and peripheral SpA is embraced by the European Spondyloarthropathy Study Group (ESSG) and the Amor criteria from the early 1990s [20,21].

9.4 INDIVIDUAL CLINICAL FEATURES

9.4.1 Inflammatory Back Pain

Patients with axial SpA typically present with chronic back pain of insidious onset that starts in the second to fourth decade of life. The pain is worse in the morning, associated with morning stiffness, and improves with exercise but not rest. Patients may wake up because of pain and may describe alternating buttock pain. Together, these features constitute inflammatory back pain (IBP), a concept that was inaugurated by Calin et al. in 1977 [22]. Subsequent studies have tried to improve the sensitivity and specificity of the IBP criteria [23,24]. IBP differs qualitatively from mechanical back pain caused by degenerative disease of the spine or other more sinister back pain etiologies, including fracture, malignancy, or infection. NSAIDs are typically beneficial. However, the sensitivity of IBP criteria for a diagnosis of axial SpA is only ~70%; the absence of typical IBP features therefore does not rule out a diagnosis of axial SpA.

9.4.2 Reduced Spinal Mobility

Loss of spinal mobility can be the presenting complaint in some patients with AS. Reduced spinal mobility is irreversible if it is the result of bony fusion of spinal elements. However, inflammation contributes to reduced mobility, and some degree of movement may be recoverable with potent anti-inflammatory therapy [25]. Functionally important are reduced rotation in the cervical spine (impairing the ability to drive) and fixed kyphotic curvature of the spine (negatively affecting forward gaze when standing).

9.4.3 Sacroiliitis

Symmetric inflammation in the SI joints resulting in erosions, subchondral sclerosis, and ultimately fusion of the joints is the defining feature of AS [26]. The clinical correlate of sacroiliitis is pain in the low back and buttocks that is associated with morning stiffness. Magnetic resonance imaging (MRI) is more sensitive to detect SI joint inflammation than plain radiography, which can only detect the sequelae of sacroiliitis. Sacroiliitis may also be encountered in patients with PsA or IBD-associated SpA and then is often asymmetric. Patients with peripheral SpA may have subclinical sacroiliitis [18].

9.4.4 Spondylitis

Inflammation of vertebrae (*spondylos* = vertebra, Greek) is typically seen at the edges of vertebral bodies but may also involve the posterior and lateral vertebral elements, that is, the facet joints, pedicles, transverse and spinous processes. Similar to sacroiliitis, spondylitis manifests as IBP. The earliest detectable lesions are inflammatory vertebral corner lesions on fluid-sensitive MRI sequences. These lesions are thought to progress to fatty corner lesions and ultimately bony syndesmophytes. The radiographic correlate of early inflammation at vertebral edges is the shiny corner or Romanus lesion. Syndesmophyte formation ultimately results in the bridging of vertebral bodies, giving rise to the radiographic finding of the bamboo spine.

9.4.5 Peripheral Arthritis

The peripheral arthritis in SpA is typically an asymmetric oligoarthritis affecting the lower extremities [20,21]. Patients with PsA may have additional patterns: A predominantly distal arthritis involving the distal interphalangeal (DIP) joints of the hands and feet is associated with psoriatic nail disease. Arthritis mutilans is a disabling destructive arthritis of digits that results in bone resorption and telescoping of fingers and toes [12]. Patients with AS frequently have arthritis of the shoulder and hip joints.

9.4.6 Psoriasis

Psoriasis affects 2%–3% of the population. Variants include classical plaque psoriasis, inverse psoriasis, isolated nail psoriasis, and guttate psoriasis. Up to 30% of patients with psoriasis may develop an inflammatory arthropathy [27]. Nail psoriasis is associated with arthritis in the distal interphalangeal (DIP) joints. In the vast majority of patients with PsA, the skin disease is present first or arises at the same time as the joint disease [12]. Patients with bona fide AS may also have psoriasis and may thus fulfill classification criteria for PsA.

9.4.7 Dactylitis

Inflammation of digits results in the sausage appearance of fingers or toes. Dactylitis (dactylos = finger or toe, Greek) may or may not be painful. Imaging studies have demonstrated that the inflammatory process in dactylitis involves multiple structures, including entheses, joints, tendon sheaths, and subcutaneous tissues. Within the SpA spectrum, dactylitis is most commonly seen in PsA and reactive arthritis. It is important to note that the dactylitic appearance of digits, while characteristic of SpA, can also be seen in other circumstances, including sarcoidosis, tuberculosis, cellulitis, and gout [28].

9.4.8 Enthesitis

Entheses are attachment sites of tendons and ligaments to bone. Enthesitis is commonly seen in SpA, and it has been argued that enthesitis (in contrast to the synovitis in rheumatoid arthritis) is the pathological substrate underlying joint inflammation in SpA [29]. Enthesitis manifests as pain and tenderness ± swelling on physical examination. The Achilles tendon and plantar fascia insertions at the calcaneus and the attachment sites of the quadriceps and patellar tendons at the patella and tibia are frequently affected. However, entheses are ubiquitous and enthesitis anywhere may cause local symptoms. In fact, inflammation at vertebral edges may be considered to represent enthesitis.

9.4.9 Uveitis

The uvea is the medial layer of the eye between the retina on the inside and the sclera on the outside. Anterior uveitis involves the iris and ciliary body and may also be called iritis or iridocyclitis. Choroiditis is a synonymous term for posterior uveitis. Uveitis manifests variably as eye pain, redness, and visual disturbances. Anterior uveitis is common in AS and can be unilateral or bilateral. Posterior uveitis is more common in PsA.

9.4.10 Intestinal Inflammation

SpA is strongly associated with intestinal inflammation. Reactive arthritis follows an episode of infectious diarrhea [13]. Two-thirds of patients with AS have subclinical inflammation in their intestine [30]. Patients with clinical IBD may also develop axial or peripheral SpA. Intestinal disease manifestations may therefore vary from asymptomatic to an acute diarrheal illness to the full clinical spectrum of IBD, including abdominal pain, weight loss, bloody diarrhea, fistula formation, and colorectal cancer.

9.5 CONCLUSION

SpA is characterized by inflammation in the spine and/or peripheral joints combined with additional clinical features, including psoriatic skin or nail disease, enthesitis, dactylitis, uveitis, or intestinal inflammation. This spectrum of clinical presentations distinguishes SpA from other inflammatory arthropathies, such as rheumatoid arthritis or gout. There is substantial overlap in clinical presentation between the different SpA entities, reflecting commonalities in genetics and pathophysiology. Moreover, disease phenotypes are not static and may evolve over time. What determines the spectrum of disease manifestations in the individual patient is still largely unknown.

REFERENCES

1. Zochling J, Brandt J, Braun J. The current concept of spondyloarthritis with special emphasis on undifferentiated spondyloarthritis. *Rheumatology (Oxford)* 2005;44:1483–91.
2. François RJ, Eulderink F, Bywaters EG. Commented glossary for rheumatic spinal diseases, based on pathology. *Ann Rheum Dis* 1995;54:615–25.
3. McEwen C, Ziff M, Carmel P, Ditata D, Tanner M. The relationship to rheumatoid arthritis of its so-called variants. *Arthritis Rheum* 1958;1:481–96.
4. Schlosstein L, Terasaki PI, Bluestone R, Pearson CM. High association of an HL-A antigen, W27, with ankylosing spondylitis. *N Engl J Med* 1973;288:704–6.
5. Brewerton DA, Hart FD, Nicholls A, Caffrey M, James DC, Sturrock RD. Ankylosing spondylitis and HL-A 27. *Lancet* 1973;1:904–7.
6. Brewerton DA, Caffrey M, Nicholls A, Walters D, Oates JK, James DC. Reiter's disease and HL-A 27. *Lancet* 1973;302:996–8.
7. Aho K, Ahvonen P, Lassus A, Sievers K, Tilikainen A. HL-A antigen 27 and reactive arthritis. *Lancet* 1973;2:157.
8. Brewerton DA, Caffrey M, Nicholls A, Walters D, James DC. HL-A 27 and arthropathies associated with ulcerative colitis and psoriasis. *Lancet* 1974;1:956–8.
9. Moll JM, Haslock I, Macrae IF, Wright V. Associations between ankylosing spondylitis, psoriatic arthritis, Reiter's disease, the intestinal arthropathies, and Behcet's syndrome. *Medicine (Baltimore)* 1974;53:343–64.
10. Jackson WP. The syndrome known as Reiter's disease (a triad of polyarthritis, urethritis, and conjunctivitis). *Br Med J* 1946;2:197–9.
11. Panush RS, Wallace DJ, Dorff RE, Engleman EP. Retraction of the suggestion to use the term "Reiter's syndrome" sixty-five years later: The legacy of Reiter, a war criminal, should not be eponymic honor but rather condemnation. *Arthritis Rheum* 2007;56:693–4.
12. Moll JM, Wright V. Psoriatic arthritis. *Semin Arthritis Rheum* 1973;3:55–78.

13. Carter JD. Reactive arthritis: Defined etiologies, emerging pathophysiology, and unresolved treatment. *Infect Dis Clin North Am* 2006;20:827–47.
14. Orchard TR, Wordsworth BP, Jewell DP. Peripheral arthropathies in inflammatory bowel disease: Their articular distribution and natural history. *Gut* 1998;42:387–91.
15. Feldtkeller E, Khan MA, van der Heijde D, van der Linden S, Braun J. Age at disease onset and diagnosis delay in HLA-B27 negative vs. positive patients with ankylosing spondylitis. *Rheumatol Int* 2003;23:61–6.
16. Rudwaleit M, van der Heijde D, Landewé R, Listing J, Akkoc N, Brandt J et al. The development of Assessment of SpondyloArthritis international Society classification criteria for axial spondyloarthritis (part II): Validation and final selection. *Ann Rheum Dis* 2009;68:777–83.
17. Sieper J, van der Heijde D. Review: Nonradiographic axial spondyloarthritis: New definition of an old disease? *Arthritis Rheum* 2013;65:543–51.
18. Rudwaleit M, van der Heijde D, Landewé R, Akkoc N, Brandt J, Chou CT et al. The Assessment of SpondyloArthritis international Society classification criteria for peripheral spondyloarthritis and for spondyloarthritis in general. *Ann Rheum Dis* 2011;70:25–31.
19. Zeidler H, Amor B. The Assessment in Spondyloarthritis International Society (ASAS) classification criteria for peripheral spondyloarthritis and for spondyloarthritis in general: The spondyloarthritis concept in progress. *Ann Rheum Dis* 2011;70:1–3.
20. Dougados M, van der Linden S, Juhlin R, Huitfeldt B, Amor B, Calin A et al. The European Spondylarthropathy Study Group preliminary criteria for the classification of spondylarthropathy. *Arthritis Rheum* 1991;34:1218–27.
21. Amor B, Dougados M, Mijiyawa M. Criteria of the classification of spondylarthropathies [in French]. *Rev Rhum Mal Osteoartic* 1990;57:85–9.
22. Calin A, Porta J, Fries JF, Schurman DJ. Clinical history as a screening test for ankylosing spondylitis. *JAMA* 1977;237:2613–4.
23. Rudwaleit M, Metter A, Listing J, Sieper J, Braun J. Inflammatory back pain in ankylosing spondylitis: A reassessment of the clinical history for application as classification and diagnostic criteria. *Arthritis Rheum* 2006;54:569–78.
24. Sieper J, van der Heijde D, Landewé R, Brandt J, Burgos-Vagas R, Collantes-Estevez E et al. New criteria for inflammatory back pain in patients with chronic back pain: A real patient exercise by experts from the Assessment of SpondyloArthritis international Society (ASAS). *Ann Rheum Dis* 2009;68:784–8.
25. Braun J, Sieper J, Breban M, Collantes-Estevez E, Davis J, Inman R et al. Anti-tumour necrosis factor alpha therapy for ankylosing spondylitis: International experience. *Ann Rheum Dis* 2002;61(Suppl 3):iii51–60.
26. van der Linden S, Valkenburg HA, Cats A. Evaluation of diagnostic criteria for ankylosing spondylitis. A proposal for modification of the New York criteria. *Arthritis Rheum* 1984;27:361–8.
27. Greb JE, Goldminz AM, Elder JT, Lebwohl MG, Gladman DD, Wu JJ et al. Psoriasis. *Nat Rev Dis Primers* 2016;2:16082.
28. Healy PJ, Helliwell PS. Dactylitis: Pathogenesis and clinical considerations. *Curr Rheumatol* Rep 2006;8:338–41.
29. McGonagle D, Lories RJ, Tan AL, Benjamin M. The concept of a "synovio-entheseal complex" and its implications for understanding joint inflammation and damage in psoriatic arthritis and beyond. *Arthritis Rheum* 2007;56:2482–91.
30. Van Praet L, Jacques P, Van den Bosch F, Elewaut D. The transition of acute to chronic bowel inflammation in spondyloarthritis. *Nat Rev Rheumatol* 2012;8:288–95.
31. Taylor W, Gladman D, Helliwell P, Marchesoni A, Mease P, Mielants H, CASPAR Study Group. Classification criteria for psoriatic arthritis: Development of new criteria from a large international study. *Arthritis Rheum* 2006;54:2665–73.

10 Comorbidities in Psoriatic Arthritis

Maria J. Antonelli and Marina Magrey

CONTENTS

10.1 INTRODUCTION

Psoriatic arthritis (PsA) is a chronic inflammatory arthritis characterized predominantly by skin and joint inflammation. In addition to skin and joint involvement, other comorbidities are often seen in patients with PsA. Nearly half of patients with PsA have more than one comorbidity, and nearly a fifth have three or more (Salaffi et al. 2009). Studies that have compared patients with PsA-related spondyloarthritis (SpA) with patients with non-psoriatic SpA have reported significantly more and multiple comorbidities in PsA (Hague et al. 2016). It is imperative for a rheumatologist to remain aware of these comorbidities not only for their optimal management but also to improve patient function and quality of life. This chapter outlines common comorbidities seen in PsA patients, as well as their influence on disease activity, presence in light of some treatments, and impact on patient function and outcomes.

10.2 CARDIOVASCULAR DISEASE

The risk of developing cardiovascular disease (CVD) in PsA is high (Kondratiouk et al. 2008; Li et al. 2015; Ogdie et al. 2015). A recent meta-analysis of 11 observational studies revealed that there was a 43% increased risk of CVDs in patients with PsA compared with the general population (pooled odds ratio [OR] 1.43, 95% confidence interval [CI] 1.24–1.66) [Eder et al. 2016]).

Over the years, the understanding of pathogenesis of CVD has evolved to a complex process; it has been linked to low-grade inflammation and the metabolic processes of the blood vessel wall. Studies in patients with PsA have also found abnormalities in endothelial dysfunction, arterial wall stiffness, and plaque formation, resulting in CVD (Gonzalez-Juanatey et al. 2007; Rose et al. 2014).

This so-called "psoriatic march" results in coronary, carotid, and cerebral artery occlusion with resultant myocardial infarction or cerebral vascular disease (Boehncke et al. 2011). Studies evaluating the carotid plaque burden over time suggest disease length may play a role (Eder et al. 2015a). Other studies indicate no association between disease duration and atherosclerosis (Eder et al. 2015a). High psoriatic skin involvement (Psoriasis Area and Severity Index [PASI] scores) is also associated with CVD (Gladman et al. 2009). PsA may be an independent risk factor for CVD.

It has been demonstrated using a large claims database that patients with moderate–severe psoriasis (PsO) and those with PsA also have increased risk for hypertension, hyperlipidemia, diabetes, obesity, and coronary heart disease compared with controls (Feldman et al. 2015). A recent population-based study examined the prevalence and incidence of cardiovascular risk factors, including hypertension, hyperlipidemia, diabetes mellitus (DM), and obesity among patients with PsA and rheumatoid arthritis compared with the general population. The study revealed a high prevalence of hypertension, 33.6% (OR = 1.31, 95% CI 1.26–1.37), hyperlipidemia 17.5% (OR = 1.23, 95% CI 1.18–1.29); DM, 13.5% (OR = 1.38, 95% CI 1.31–1.45); and obesity, 32.7% (OR = 1.69, 95% CI 1.62–1.75) in PsA patients (Jafri et al. 2016). However, between 30% and 50% of PsA patients are noted to have atherosclerosis without traditional risk factors (Gelfand et al. 2006; Gladman et al. 2009). The traditional risk stratification models for CVD, the Framingham risk score, and the Systematic Coronary Risk Evaluation algorithm generally underestimate the risk for cardiovascular events in these patients (Ogdie et al. 2015). There is lack of evidence indicating that treating traditional CVD risk factors will lower risk for cardiovascular events; however, there is the inferred benefit from general population studies (Ogdie et al. 2015).

The incidence of hypertension in PsA patients varies in studies anywhere from 33% (Jafri et al. 2016) to as high as 95% (Favarato et al. 2014). The presence of hypertension is noted to be higher in those PsA patients with known CVD compared with those without CVD (95% vs. 45%, $p < 0.001$), conferring an OR of 21.0 for CVD (Favarato et al. 2014). This is an important comorbidity that perhaps is influenced by the presence and use of chronic nonsteroidal anti-inflammatory drugs (NSAIDs). Although not used commonly for the treatment of PsA, cyclosporine can also contribute to the risk of hypertension.

PsA patients have a notably high incidence of diabetes: studies vary, but most report an incidence of 11.4%–15.9% (Labitigan et al. 2014), and some as high as 20% (Favarato and Goldenstein-Schainberg 2014). Also, glucocorticoid use in these patients increases the risk of developing diabetes; in studies of PsA and rheumatoid arthritis patients, use of topical and oral steroids was associated with a 30% increased risk for developing diabetes (Solomon et al. 2010). Tumor necrosis factor (TNF) antagonist therapy has been associated with a lower risk of developing diabetes than other nonmethotrexate disease-modifying antirheumatic drug (DMARD) therapy (Solomon et al. 2011). Diabetes prevalence in PsA patients with known CVD is noted to be higher than that in those without known CVD (60% vs. 19%, $p < 0.001$), conferring an OR of 5.4 for CVD (Favarato et al. 2014).

Given the concern for increased cardiovascular events with the use of NSAIDs, it is recommended that NSAIDs be used for the shortest time at the lowest possible dose in patients with PsA and known CVD or multiple known risk factors (Ogdie et al. 2015). Similarly, both NSAIDs and glucocorticoids should be limited in patients with known congestive heart failure (CHF), as they may increase the risk of CHF exacerbations (Ogdie et al. 2015). Likewise, glucocorticoids should be avoided in patients with diabetes given their hyperglycemic effects. Methotrexate should be used with caution in patients with obesity and/or diabetes, as there may be an increased risk of elevated liver function test abnormalities and liver fibrosis (Ogdie et al. 2015). For patients with known CHF New York Heart Association (NYHA) class III or IV, TNF antagonists should be avoided due to limited data (Ogdie et al. 2015). Observational data do not suggest a risk of new-onset CHF in patients being treated with TNF antagonist (Ogdie et al. 2015). Although initial studies with interleukin (IL) 12/23 antagonist therapy, briakinumab and ustekinumab, raised interest in a possible increased risk for cardiovascular events, extended studies with ustekinumab have not demonstrated substantial cardiovascular risk in PsO patients and rare events in PsA clinical trials (McKeage 2014).

Studies measuring substitute outcomes (including carotid intima-media thickness, aortic stiffness, platelet reactivity, and postocclusion flow-mediated vasodilatation) suggest favorable outcomes with TNF antagonist therapy and possibly methotrexate (Ogdie et al. 2015). Some data indicate a cardioprotective effect of methotrexate in rheumatoid arthritis patients, but data are inconclusive in PsA and PsO populations (Armstrong et al. 2014). Some preliminary data on the use of TNF antagonists indicate that there may be a reduced risk of cardiovascular events (Armstrong et al. 2014).

10.3 METABOLIC SYNDROME AND OBESITY

Metabolic syndrome is a combination of insulin resistance with two or more CVD risk factor abnormalities (low HDL, high triglycerides, obesity or increased waist/hip ratio, and hypertension). Studies indicate between a quarter (27%) (Labitigan et al. 2014) and more than half (58%) (Raychaudhuri 2012) of PsA patients are found to have metabolic syndrome. It is thought that metabolic syndrome factors play a role in making the normally quiescent endothelial cells of arterial walls highly irritable and active; obesity, insulin resistance, and inflammation induce changes in the endothelial cell adhesion molecule expression, recruiting various classes of leukocytes (Raychaudhuri 2012).

A large portion of PsA patients are noted to be obese (between 30% and 60%), and obesity is associated with a lower probability of achieving sustained minimal disease activity irrespective of therapy (Eder et al. 2015b). Interestingly, in one study over 6 months, increasing weight loss (≥5% total body weight) was associated with increased achievement of minimal disease activity (OR = 4.20, 95% CI 1.82–9.66); the higher the fraction of weight loss, the more patients were able to achieve minimal disease activity (Di Minno et al. 2014). Methotrexate should be used with caution in patients with obesity and PsA, as these patients taking methotrexate were found to be at high risk of cirrhosis (Schmajuk et al. 2014).

10.4 OPHTHALMIC DISEASE

The incidence of comorbid eye disease in PsA patients is not clearly defined; however, one study observes that 16% of PsA patients have ocular involvement (Peluso et al. 2015). Inflammatory eye involvement in PsA can involve uveitis, keratitis, blepharitis, conjunctivitis, episcleritis, and scleritis (Altan-Yaycioglu et al. 2003; Lima et al. 2012). The most serious condition and strongest association is uveitis (Ogdie et al. 2015). Uveitis has been noted in 25.1% (Zeboulon et al. 2008) to 35.48% (Peluso et al. 2015) of PsA patients. This condition has been strongly linked to human leukocyte antigen (HLA) B27 positivity. Of those patients who develop uveitis, approximately half are HLA-B27 positive (Rosenbaum 2015). Uveitis in PsA patients is most likely to be insidious in onset, bilateral, chronic, and posterior (Paiva et al. 2000). Inflammatory eye disease is more common in PsA patients who are male (OR = 1.89, 95% CI 1.09–3.30, $p = 0.023$) (Peluso et al. 2015). In addition, ocular involvement was more common with patients with axial involvement than with peripheral articular manifestations (Peluso et al. 2015). However, another study indicates that uveitis is predominant in males if there is axial involvement, but in females if there is peripheral arthritis (Paiva et al. 2000). Conjunctivitis has been reported to be the most common ocular involvement (64%) in a small retrospective analysis (Peluso et al. 2015), although prior reports indicate it is less common, 20% (Lambert and Wright 1976). These lesions are generally described as demarcated, yellowish-red plaques with xerotic appearance, suggesting "ocular psoriasis" (Rehal et al. 2011).

Although no trials have been done specifically in inflammatory eye disease in PsA, there is evidence and guidelines for the use of oral and topical corticosteroids; traditional DMARDs, including azathioprine, cyclosporine, sulfasalazine, and methotrexate; and other immunosuppressants, including mycophenolate mofetil, tacrolimus, and cyclophosphamide (Jabs et al. 2000; Rosenbaum 2015). More recently, biological use has been demonstrated in uveitis (Servat et al. 2012). Although adalimumab is the only biologic drug approved for use in uveitis, both adalimumab and infliximab have been regularly used for uveitis treatment in PsA patients (Martel et al. 2012). Etanercept is not recommended in uveitis treatment because of concerns that it either causes more flares or is less effective in preventing new flares (Brito-Zeron et al. 2015).

10.5 INFLAMMATORY BOWEL DISEASE

The relationship between the gut and SpA has long been recognized. Subclinical inflammation in the gut has been recognized in two-thirds of SpA patients (Fries 2009). A small study indicated microscopic gut inflammation in all 15 PsA and PsO patients included in the study (Scarpa et al. 2000).

The reported incidence of gastrointestinal involvement in PsA varies between 1.3% and 5.9% (Husni 2015). A small retrospective analysis indicates Crohn disease in 3.9% of PsA patients and ulcerative colitis in 2.6% of PsA patients (Peluso et al. 2015). This study indicated that bowel involvement was more common in patients with established PsA (nearly 20%), as well as patients with axial involvement, than in those with peripheral joint involvement (Peluso et al. 2015). A study from the Nurses' Health Studies indicated a similar increased risk for Crohn disease in patients with PsO, but no associated increased risk of ulcerative colitis; there was an especially high risk of Crohn disease in PsA patients compared with controls (relative risk [RR] = 6.43, 95% CI 2.04–20.32) (Li et al. 2013).

Patients with comorbid inflammatory bowel disease (IBD) and PsA should generally avoid NSAIDs or be monitored carefully given the possibility of exacerbating IBD symptoms. TNF inhibitors are used in both IBD and PsA, with the exception of certolizumab (for Crohn disease only) and golimumab (for ulcerative colitis only) (Ogdie et al. 2015). However, etanercept is not used in IBD given the lack of effectiveness in clinical trials (Ogdie et al. 2015).

10.6 LIVER DISEASE AND NONALCOHOLIC FATTY LIVER DISEASE

Although there are limited studies on the association of fatty liver disease in PsA, an increased prevalence has been noted in PsA patients. The incidence of liver disease has been reported in 2.4% of PsA patients (Husted et al. 2013). Similarly, using a claims database, 3.4% of a large cohort of moderate–severe PsO and PsA patients were noted to have liver disease (Feldman et al. 2015). Among patients with psoriatic skin disease, patients with PsA are among the highest at risk to have nonalcoholic fatty liver disease (NAFLD) (Miele et al. 2009). In addition, compared with patients without PsO, psoriatic-related NAFLD is more likely to cause severe liver fibrosis (Miele et al. 2009).

One prospective study exhibited hepatic steatosis as an independent predictor of not achieving minimal disease activity (hazard ratio [HR] 1.91, 95% CI 1.04–3.38), suggesting that fatty liver disease may influence disease prognosis or therapy response (Di Minno et al. 2012). Additionally, the presence of liver disease limits the choice of therapies, which in turn may influence the ability to attain minimal disease activity.

Patients should be screened for hepatitis B and C prior to initiation of DMARD and biologic therapy with the following laboratory investigations: hepatitis C viral antibody level, hepatitis B core antibody, surface antibody, and surface antigen. DMARDs often typically used in PsA, methotrexate and leflunomide, can affect liver function tests and, in some cases, cause permanent liver damage (Ogdie et al. 2015). Methotrexate and leflunomide should be avoided in patients with known chronic hepatitis B or C infections (Ogdie et al. 2015). Patients with obesity and diabetes, as well as preexisting liver disease, are at increased risk of liver toxicity from methotrexate (Ogdie et al. 2015). NSAIDs, too, can cause liver function test abnormalities and hepatotoxicity (Ogdie et al. 2015). Although TNF inhibitors have been known to also cause liver function test abnormalities in rheumatoid arthritis patients, their combined use with methotrexate seems to have a protective effect from liver fibrosis (Ogdie et al. 2015). TNF antagonist drugs are generally considered to be safe in the setting of chronic hepatitis C infection with careful monitoring; although scant, the most data exist for the safety of etanercept and adalimumab in hepatitis C (Caso et al. 2015). Little has been studied on the safety of IL-12/23 blockade in liver disease, but a small study specifies that ustekinumab is safe in patients with preexisting liver disease (Llamas-Velasco et al. 2015).

10.7 GOUT

Patients with PsA have an associated increased risk of gout (HR = 4.95, 95% CI 2.72–9.01) when compared with persons without PsO (Merola et al. 2015). Physicians should be aware of this important comorbidity, as a gouty flare may be mistaken for a PsA flare. Treatment acutely may not differ drastically, but long-term prevention of gout with urate-lowering therapy would be indicated and change the disease course.

10.8 OSTEOPOROSIS

Osteoporosis has not been well studied in PsA (Del Puente et al. 2012). The prevalence of this comorbidity in PsA patients has been controversial; some studies indicate a prevalence higher than that of the general population, whereas others indicate a normal or no increase in prevalence of osteoporosis (Chandran et al. 2016). The prevalence of osteoporosis among studies varies widely from 1.4% to 68.8% (Chandran et al. 2016). Traditional risk factors (age, female sex, postmenopausal status, and cumulative steroid dose), as well as PsA duration and the presence of erosions, are associated with lower bone mineral density (BMD) (Chandran et al. 2016).

General screening and management of osteoporosis should be done in PsA patients per guidelines for the general population (Ogdie et al. 2015). There are limited data on the effect of PsA treatments and bone quality. However, it has been noted that there is no evidence of an increased fracture risk in PsA patients in whom TNF inhibitor therapy was initiated (Kawai et al. 2013). In PsA patients who are on long-term glucocorticoids, physicians should be mindful of considering the American College of Rheumatology (ACR) recommendations for the prevention and treatment of glucocorticoid-induced osteoporosis (Grossman et al. 2010).

10.9 DEPRESSION AND ANXIETY

Depression and anxiety have a high reported incidence in PsA patients: between 15% and nearly 30% (Husni 2015). The prevalence of both anxiety and depression is noted to be higher in PsA patients than in patients without joint disease (36.6% and 22.2% vs. 24.4% and 9.6%, respectively; $p = 0.12$ and 0.002, respectively) (McDonough et al. 2014). It has been suggested that skin involvement highly influences patients' quality of life, as indicated by studies that compare the health-related quality of life between psoriatic and rheumatoid arthritis patients (Husted et al. 2001). It is important to identify depression and anxiety not only so that they can treated effectively, but also to increase the adherence of treatment for PsA. It has been noted that there is strong evidence for nonadherence to medical treatment related to psychosocial factors (Vangeli et al. 2015). It appears that depression, but not anxiety, may be a risk factor for nonadherence to treatment in inflammatory conditions (Vangeli et al. 2015); this important comorbidity is modifiable and may easily influence treatment outcomes if ignored.

Apremilast, a small-molecule treatment for PsO and PsA, has been known to worsen depression and should be avoided in patients with preexisting depression (Celgene 2016).

10.10 FIBROMYALGIA

It is well known that many autoimmune and chronic inflammatory arthritis patients have comorbid centralized pain syndromes. The overall prevalence of fibromyalgia in PsA patients varies in studies from 17% (Brikman et al. 2016) to 53% (Magrey et al. 2013). The importance of identifying comorbid fibromyalgia is an important aspect of treatment, as PsA-specific disease activity measures are generally worse in patients with comorbid fibromyalgia (Brikman et al. 2016). Manifestations of fatigue, widespread body pain, and sleep disturbance may overlap in those with PsA and fibromyalgia. When physicians are deciding whether a patient has attained minimal disease activity, it is imperative to define if fibromyalgia is present.

10.11 CHRONIC KIDNEY DISEASE

There are limited data on the prevalence of chronic kidney disease (CKD) in PsA patients. One study investigating the prevalence of CKD among seronegative inflammatory arthritis (including PsA patients) and rheumatoid arthritis patients indicates approximately 16% of patients with reduced glomerular filtration rate (GFR) (<60 mL/min), which was comparable between rheumatoid and seronegative patients (Haroon et al. 2011). Renal dysfunction is an important consideration in therapy selection. Renal function should be regularly monitored in patients on chronic DMARD therapy. NSAIDs should generally be avoided in patients with CKD, as there is increased risk for acute renal injury; similarly, methotrexate and leflunomide may have toxicity with decreased renal clearance, resulting in potential pancytopenia and increased liver toxicity.

10.12 MALIGNANCY

Very few studies have evaluated the risk of malignancy in PsA patients compared with the general population. Despite variable rates and controversy, malignancy incidence in PsA patients is noted to be 6.5%–8.9% (Husni 2015). Similar rates of malignancy between rheumatoid arthritis and PsA were indicated in a study of the Consortium of Rheumatology Researchers of North America (CORRONA) registry (Gross et al. 2014). In a study comparing PsA with non-PsA SpA patients, there was an increased incidence of malignancy in the PsA group ($p < 0.05$) (Hague et al. 2016).

Nonmelanomatous skin cancers were the most common malignancy noted among PsA patients (Gross et al. 2014). Specifically, skin cancers are more common in moderate–severe PsO and PsA patients than in controls (not statistically significant) (Feldman et al. 2015); another study indicates comparable rates of nonmelanomatous skin cancer between PsA and non-PsA cohorts (incident rate ratio [IRR] 1.01, 95% CI 0.90–1.13) (Hagberg et al. 2016).

A retrospective database review shows a slightly higher rate of hematologic cancer in a PsA patient cohort than in a non-PsA cohort of a total of 8493 patients (IRR 1.52, 95% CI, 1.10–2.10) (Hagberg et al. 2016). The IRR for solid cancers in PsA cohorts compared with non-PsA cohorts was similar (IRR = 0.97, 97% CI 0.82–1.14) (Hagberg et al. 2016). One study summarizes that overall there is no consistent association that has been demonstrated between PsA and cancer (Feldman et al. 2015).

There are no specific screening guidelines for malignancy in PsA patients; it is recommended that general population screening recommendations be followed. In patients who have been treated with ultraviolet (UV) light therapy, a yearly or periodic skin check should be considered in concern for elevated risk of skin cancers. Studies focusing on malignancy rates in patients treated with anti-TNF drugs show mixed results. Few studies focus on PsA, while most include rheumatoid and PsO patients. One meta-analysis of PsA patients being treated with anti-TNF medications in the short term (12–30 weeks) indicated no increased risk of malignancy (Dommasch et al. 2011). One ACR recommendation suggests that TNF antagonist medication should generally be avoided in the 5 years after cancer remission (Mercer et al. 2013); however, newer rheumatoid guidelines do not include this generalization (Singh et al. 2016).

10.13 INFECTION

The incidence rate of infection has been shown to be higher in patients with PsA than in patients with just PsO. Also, the rate is higher among patients treated with biologics (Haddad et al. 2016).

One meta-analysis of PsA patients treated in the short term with anti-TNF medications indicated an OR for any infectious event of 1.09 (95% CI 0.87–1.37), although 97.6% of these infections were nonserious (not recorded as a serious adverse event) (Dommasch et al. 2011). In that study, 0.61% of PsA and PsO patients treated were affected with a serious infection at some point (Dommasch et al. 2011). Another study found that the IRR for infections was higher in those patients treated for PsA using prescription medications than in those who were not (IRR = 1.71, 95% CI 1.52–1.91) (Hagberg et al. 2016).

10.14 CONCLUSION

Numerous comorbidities that affect many organ systems are associated with PsA; it is not clear if appropriate treatment in the early stage could have an effect on not only the cutaneous and articular manifestations, but also the other features of this complex disease. Although specialists are often focused on their own "system," this pleiotropic disease can affect nearly every organ system. Physicians should be aware and considerate of the many facets that can be affected. Screening, recognizing, and addressing morbidities is key to effectively treating PsA patients.

REFERENCES

Altan-Yaycioglu, R., Y. A. Akova, H. Kart, A. Cetinkaya, G. Yilmaz, and P. Aydin. 2003. Posterior scleritis in psoriatic arthritis. *Retina* 23 (5):717–9.

Armstrong, A. W., E. A. Brezinski, M. R. Follansbee, and E. J. Armstrong. 2014. Effects of biologic agents and other disease-modifying antirheumatic drugs on cardiovascular outcomes in psoriasis and psoriatic arthritis: A systematic review. *Curr Pharm Des* 20 (4):500–12.

Boehncke, W. H., S. Boehncke, A. M. Tobin, and B. Kirby. 2011. The 'psoriatic march': A concept of how severe psoriasis may drive cardiovascular comorbidity. *Exp Dermatol* 20 (4):303–7.

Brikman, S., V. Furer, J. Wollman, S. Borok, H. Matz, A. Polachek, O. Elalouf, A. Sharabi, I. Kaufman, D. Paran, and O. Elkayam. 2016. The effect of the presence of fibromyalgia on common clinical disease activity indices in patients with psoriatic arthritis: A cross-sectional study. *J Rheumatol* 43 (9):1749–54.

Brito-Zeron, P., R. Perez-Alvarez, M. Ramos-Casals, and Biogeas Study Group. 2015. Etanercept and uveitis: Friends or foes? *Curr Med Res Opin* 31 (2):251–2.

Caso, F., L. Cantarini, F. Morisco, A. Del Puente, R. Ramonda, U. Fiocco, E. Lubrano et al. 2015. Current evidence in the field of the management with TNF-alpha inhibitors in psoriatic arthritis and concomitant hepatitis C virus infection. *Expert Opin Biol Ther* 15 (5):641–50.

Celgene. 2016. Otezla [package insert]. http://www.otezlapro.com/content/uploads/2016/08/otezla-pi.pdf (accessed December 22).

Chandran, S., A. Aldei, S. R. Johnson, A. M. Cheung, D. Salonen, and D. D. Gladman. 2016. Prevalence and risk factors of low bone mineral density in psoriatic arthritis: A systematic review. *Semin Arthritis Rheum* 46 (2):174–82.

Del Puente, A., A. Esposito, A. Parisi, M. Atteno, S. Montalbano, M. Vitiello, C. Esposito, N. Bertolini, F. Foglia, L. Costa, and R. Scarpa. 2012. Osteoporosis and psoriatic arthritis. *J Rheumatol Suppl* 89:36–8.

Di Minno, M. N., S. Iervolino, R. Peluso, A. Russolillo, R. Lupoli, R. Scarpa, G. Di Minno, G. Tarantino, and CaRRDS Study Group. 2012. Hepatic steatosis and disease activity in subjects with psoriatic arthritis receiving tumor necrosis factor-alpha blockers. *J Rheumatol* 39 (5):1042–6.

Di Minno, M. N., R. Peluso, S. Iervolino, A. Russolillo, R. Lupoli, R. Scarpa, and CaRRDs Study Group. 2014. Weight loss and achievement of minimal disease activity in patients with psoriatic arthritis starting treatment with tumour necrosis factor alpha blockers. *Ann Rheum Dis* 73 (6):1157–62.

Dommasch, E. D., K. Abuabara, D. B. Shin, J. Nguyen, A. B. Troxel, and J. M. Gelfand. 2011. The risk of infection and malignancy with tumor necrosis factor antagonists in adults with psoriatic disease: A systematic review and meta-analysis of randomized controlled trials. *J Am Acad Dermatol* 64 (6): 1035–50.

Eder, L., A. Polachek, C. F. Rosen, V. Chandran, R. Cook, and D. D. Gladman. 2016. The development of PsA in patients with psoriasis is preceded by a period of non-specific musculoskeletal symptoms: A prospective cohort study. *Arthritis Rheumatol* 69 (3):622–9.

Eder, L., A. Thavaneswaran, V. Chandran, R. Cook, and D. D. Gladman. 2015a. Increased burden of inflammation over time is associated with the extent of atherosclerotic plaques in patients with psoriatic arthritis. *Ann Rheum Dis* 74 (10):1830–5.

Eder, L., A. Thavaneswaran, V. Chandran, R. J. Cook, and D. D. Gladman. 2015b. Obesity is associated with a lower probability of achieving sustained minimal disease activity state among patients with psoriatic arthritis. *Ann Rheum Dis* 74 (5):813–7.

Favarato, M. H., and C. Goldenstein-Schainberg. 2014. Reply to: Cardiovascular risk in psoriatic arthritis; should we focus on hypertension and diabetes only? Gkaliagkousi et al. *Clin Exp Rheumatol* 32 (6):996.

Favarato, M. H., P. Mease, C. R. Goncalves, C. Goncalves Saad, P. D. Sampaio-Barros, and C. Goldenstein-Schainberg. 2014. Hypertension and diabetes significantly enhance the risk of cardiovascular disease in patients with psoriatic arthritis. *Clin Exp Rheumatol* 32 (2):182–7.

Feldman, S. R., Y. Zhao, L. Shi, and M. H. Tran. 2015. Economic and comorbidity burden among patients with moderate-to-severe psoriasis. *J Manag Care Spec Pharm* 21 (10):874–88.

Fries, W. 2009. Inflammatory bowel disease-associated spondyloarthropathies. *World J Gastroenterol* 15 (20):2441–2.

Gelfand, J. M., A. L. Neimann, D. B. Shin, X. Wang, D. J. Margolis, and A. B. Troxel. 2006. Risk of myocardial infarction in patients with psoriasis. *JAMA* 296 (14):1735–41.

Gladman, D. D., M. Ang, L. Su, B. D. Tom, C. T. Schentag, and V. T. Farewell. 2009. Cardiovascular morbidity in psoriatic arthritis. *Ann Rheum Dis* 68 (7):1131–5.

Gonzalez-Juanatey, C., J. Llorca, E. Amigo-Diaz, T. Dierssen, J. Martin, and M. A. Gonzalez-Gay. 2007. High prevalence of subclinical atherosclerosis in psoriatic arthritis patients without clinically evident cardiovascular disease or classic atherosclerosis risk factors. *Arthritis Rheum* 57 (6):1074–80.

Gross, R. L., J. S. Schwartzman-Morris, M. Krathen, G. Reed, H. Chang, K. C. Saunders, M. C. Fisher et al. 2014. A comparison of the malignancy incidence among patients with psoriatic arthritis and patients with rheumatoid arthritis in a large US cohort. *Arthritis Rheumatol* 66 (6):1472–81.

Grossman, J. M., R. Gordon, V. K. Ranganath, C. Deal, L. Caplan, W. Chen, J. R. Curtis et al. 2010. American College of Rheumatology 2010 recommendations for the prevention and treatment of glucocorticoid-induced osteoporosis. *Arthritis Care Res (Hoboken)* 62 (11):1515–26.

Haddad, A., S. Li, A. Thavaneswaran, R. J. Cook, V. Chandran, and D. D. Gladman. 2016. The incidence and predictors of infection in psoriasis and psoriatic arthritis: Results from longitudinal observational cohorts. *J Rheumatol* 43 (2):362–6.

Hagberg, K. W., L. Li, M. Peng, M. Paris, K. Shah, and S. S. Jick. 2016. Rates of cancers and opportunistic infections in patients with psoriatic arthritis compared with patients without psoriatic arthritis. *J Clin Rheumatol* 22 (5):241–7.

Hague, N., R. J. Lories, and K. de Vlam. 2016. Comorbidities associated with psoriatic arthritis compared with non-psoriatic spondyloarthritis: A cross-sectional study. *J Rheumatol* 43 (2):376–82.

Haroon, M., F. Adeeb, J. Devlin, D. O'Gradaigh, and F. Walker. 2011. A comparative study of renal dysfunction in patients with inflammatory arthropathies: Strong association with cardiovascular diseases and not with anti-rheumatic therapies, inflammatory markers or duration of arthritis. *Int J Rheum Dis* 14 (3):255–60.

Husni, M. E. 2015. Comorbidities in psoriatic arthritis. *Rheum Dis Clin North Am* 41 (4):677–98.

Husted, J. A., D. D. Gladman, V. T. Farewell, and R. J. Cook. 2001. Health-related quality of life of patients with psoriatic arthritis: A comparison with patients with rheumatoid arthritis. *Arthritis Rheum* 45 (2):151–8.

Husted, J. A., A. Thavaneswaran, V. Chandran, and D. D. Gladman. 2013. Incremental effects of comorbidity on quality of life in patients with psoriatic arthritis. *J Rheumatol* 40 (8):1349–56.

Jabs, D. A., J. T. Rosenbaum, C. S. Foster, G. N. Holland, G. J. Jaffe, J. S. Louie, R. B. Nussenblatt et al. 2000. Guidelines for the use of immunosuppressive drugs in patients with ocular inflammatory disorders: Recommendations of an expert panel. *Am J Ophthalmol* 130 (4):492–513.

Jafri, K., C. M. Bartels, D. Shin, J. M. Gelfand, and A. Ogdie. 2016. Incidence and management of cardiovascular risk factors in psoriatic arthritis and rheumatoid arthritis: A population-based study. *Arthritis Care Res (Hoboken)* 69 (1):51–7.

Kawai, V. K., C. G. Grijalva, P. G. Arbogast, J. R. Curtis, D. H. Solomon, E. Delzell, L. Chen et al. 2013. Initiation of tumor necrosis factor alpha antagonists and risk of fractures in patients with selected rheumatic and autoimmune diseases. *Arthritis Care Res (Hoboken)* 65 (7):1085–94.

Kondratiouk, S., N. Udaltsova, and A. L. Klatsky. 2008. Associations of psoriatic arthritis and cardiovascular conditions in a large population. *Perm J* 12 (4):4–8.

Labitigan, M., A. Bahce-Altuntas, J. M. Kremer, G. Reed, J. D. Greenberg, N. Jordan, C. Putterman, and A. Broder. 2014. Higher rates and clustering of abnormal lipids, obesity, and diabetes mellitus in psoriatic arthritis compared with rheumatoid arthritis. *Arthritis Care Res (Hoboken)* 66 (4):600–7.

Lambert, J. R., and V. Wright. 1976. Eye inflammation in psoriatic arthritis. *Ann Rheum Dis* 35 (4):354–6.

Li, L., K. W. Hagberg, M. Peng, K. Shah, M. Paris, and S. Jick. 2015. Rates of cardiovascular disease and major adverse cardiovascular events in patients with psoriatic arthritis compared to patients without psoriatic arthritis. *J Clin Rheumatol* 21 (8):405–10.

Li, W. Q., J. L. Han, A. T. Chan, and A. A. Qureshi. 2013. Psoriasis, psoriatic arthritis and increased risk of incident Crohn's disease in US women. *Ann Rheum Dis* 72 (7):1200–5.

Lima, F. B., M. F. Abalem, D. G. Ruiz, A. Gomes Bde, M. N. Azevedo, H. V. Moraes Jr., A. S. Yeskel, and N. Kara-Junior. 2012. Prevalence of eye disease in Brazilian patients with psoriatic arthritis. *Clinics (Sao Paulo)* 67 (3):249–53.

Llamas-Velasco, M., M. J. Concha-Garzon, A. Garcia-Diez, and E. Dauden. 2015. Liver injury in psoriasis patients receiving ustekinumab: A retrospective study of 44 patients treated in the clinical practice setting. *Actas Dermosifiliogr* 106 (6):470–6.

Magrey, M. N., M. Antonelli, N. James, and M. A. Khan. 2013. High frequency of fibromyalgia in patients with psoriatic arthritis: A pilot study. *Arthritis* 2013:762921.

Martel, J. N., E. Esterberg, A. Nagpal, and N. R. Acharya. 2012. Infliximab and adalimumab for uveitis. *Ocul Immunol Inflamm* 20 (1):18–26.

McDonough, E., R. Ayearst, L. Eder, V. Chandran, C. F. Rosen, A. Thavaneswaran, and D. D. Gladman. 2014. Depression and anxiety in psoriatic disease: Prevalence and associated factors. *J Rheumatol* 41 (5):887–96.

McKeage, K. 2014. Ustekinumab: A review of its use in psoriatic arthritis. *Drugs* 74 (9):1029–39.

Mercer, L. K., A. S. Low, J. B. Galloway, K. D. Watson, M. Lunt, D. P. Symmons, K. L. Hyrich, and BSRBR Control Centre Consortium. 2013. Anti-TNF therapy in women with rheumatoid arthritis with a history of carcinoma in situ of the cervix. *Ann Rheum Dis* 72 (1):143–4.

Merola, J. F., S. Wu, J. Han, H. K. Choi, and A. A. Qureshi. 2015. Psoriasis, psoriatic arthritis and risk of gout in US men and women. *Ann Rheum Dis* 74 (8):1495–500.

Miele, L., S. Vallone, C. Cefalo, G. La Torre, C. Di Stasi, F. M. Vecchio, M. D'Agostino et al. 2009. Prevalence, characteristics and severity of non-alcoholic fatty liver disease in patients with chronic plaque psoriasis. *J Hepatol* 51 (4):778–86.

Ogdie, A., S. Schwartzman, and M. E. Husni. 2015. Recognizing and managing comorbidities in psoriatic arthritis. *Curr Opin Rheumatol* 27 (2):118–26.

Paiva, E. S., D. C. Macaluso, A. Edwards, and J. T. Rosenbaum. 2000. Characterisation of uveitis in patients with psoriatic arthritis. *Ann Rheum Dis* 59 (1):67–70.

Peluso, R., S. Iervolino, M. Vitiello, V. Bruner, G. Lupoli, and M. N. Di Minno. 2015. Extra-articular manifestations in psoriatic arthritis patients. *Clin Rheumatol* 34 (4):745–53.

Raychaudhuri, S. P. 2012. Comorbidities of psoriatic arthritis—Metabolic syndrome and prevention: A report from the GRAPPA 2010 annual meeting. *J Rheumatol* 39 (2):437–40.

Rehal, B., B. S. Modjtahedi, L. S. Morse, I. R. Schwab, and H. I. Maibach. 2011. Ocular psoriasis. *J Am Acad Dermatol* 65 (6):1202–12.

Rose, S., J. Dave, C. Millo, H. B. Naik, E. L. Siegel, and N. N. Mehta. 2014. Psoriatic arthritis and sacroiliitis are associated with increased vascular inflammation by 18-fluorodeoxyglucose positron emission tomography computed tomography: Baseline report from the Psoriasis Atherosclerosis and Cardiometabolic Disease Initiative. *Arthritis Res Ther* 16 (4):R161.

Rosenbaum, J. T. 2015. Uveitis in spondyloarthritis including psoriatic arthritis, ankylosing spondylitis, and inflammatory bowel disease. *Clin Rheumatol* 34 (6):999–1002.

Salaffi, F., M. Carotti, S. Gasparini, M. Intorcia, and W. Grassi. 2009. The health-related quality of life in rheumatoid arthritis, ankylosing spondylitis, and psoriatic arthritis: A comparison with a selected sample of healthy people. *Health Qual Life Outcomes* 7:25.

Scarpa, R., F. Manguso, A. D'Arienzo, F. P. D'Armiento, C. Astarita, G. Mazzacca, and F. Ayala. 2000. Microscopic inflammatory changes in colon of patients with both active psoriasis and psoriatic arthritis without bowel symptoms. *J Rheumatol* 27 (5):1241–6.

Schmajuk, G., Y. Miao, J. Yazdany, W. J. Boscardin, D. I. Daikh, and M. A. Steinman. 2014. Identification of risk factors for elevated transaminases in methotrexate users through an electronic health record. *Arthritis Care Res (Hoboken)* 66 (8):1159–66.

Servat, J. J., K. A. Mears, E. H. Black, and J. J. Huang. 2012. Biological agents for the treatment of uveitis. *Expert Opin Biol Ther* 12 (3):311–28.

Singh, J. A., K. G. Saag, S. L. Bridges Jr., E. A. Akl, R. R. Bannuru, M. C. Sullivan, E. Vaysbrot et al. 2016. 2015 American College of Rheumatology Guideline for the Treatment of Rheumatoid Arthritis. *Arthritis Rheumatol* 68 (1):1–26.

Solomon, D. H., T. J. Love, C. Canning, and S. Schneeweiss. 2010. Risk of diabetes among patients with rheumatoid arthritis, psoriatic arthritis and psoriasis. *Ann Rheum Dis* 69 (12):2114–7.

Solomon, D. H., E. Massarotti, R. Garg, J. Liu, C. Canning, and S. Schneeweiss. 2011. Association between disease-modifying antirheumatic drugs and diabetes risk in patients with rheumatoid arthritis and psoriasis. *JAMA* 305 (24):2525–31.

Vangeli, E., S. Bakhshi, A. Baker, A. Fisher, D. Bucknor, U. Mrowietz, A. J. Ostor, L. Peyrin-Biroulet, A. P. Lacerda, and J. Weinman. 2015. A systematic review of factors associated with non-adherence to treatment for immune-mediated inflammatory diseases. *Adv Ther* 32 (11):983–1028.

Zeboulon, N., M. Dougados, and L. Gossec. 2008. Prevalence and characteristics of uveitis in the spondyloarthropathies: A systematic literature review. *Ann Rheum Dis* 67 (7):955–9.

Section IV-A

Treatment Regimen

Pharmaceuticals and Treatment

11 Current Recommendations for the Treatment of Psoriasis

Chelsea Ma and Emanual Maverakis

CONTENTS

11.1 INTRODUCTION

The history of psoriasis treatment spans over a century, with the first modern treatment consisting of anthralin in the late 1800s. In 1925, dermatologist William H. Goeckerman discovered an adjunctive effect of coal tar and ultraviolet radiation on psoriasis plaques.[1] In terms of effectiveness, Goeckerman therapy was the gold standard treatment regimen for several decades, although therapy sessions are time-consuming and require patients to attend day centers. In 1952, 2 years after the Nobel Prize was awarded for the development of cortisone, topical hydrocortisone was found to successfully treat inflammatory skin conditions. This revolutionized the treatment of psoriasis and remains the mainstay of topical treatments today. Other topical therapies, including retinoids and vitamin D, were later developed in the 1980s.

The Food and Drug Administration (FDA) approved methotrexate as the first systemic treatment for psoriasis in 1972, followed by cyclosporine in 1997. However, these immunosuppressive agents are sometimes poorly tolerated and/or are associated with significant adverse events, such as organ toxicities. The 1990s also saw the innovation of biologic agents, which are injectables with specificities for unique aspects of the immune system, mainly soluble mediators of inflammation. However, the first biologic developed for psoriasis, alefacept, blocked CD2 on T cells from interacting with the lymphocyte function–associated antigen (LFA) 3 on antigen-presenting cells. This agent was approved by the FDA for psoriasis in 2003.[2] The next wave of biologic agents targeted tumor necrosis factor (TNF). Most recently, interleukin (IL)-targeting biologics have become more widely used, but all of these agents have made a substantial impact on psoriasis treatment given their favorable tolerability and short- and long-term efficacies. Even in the setting of this treatment revolution, therapeutic discovery in psoriasis remains an active and dynamic area, with newer agents striving to achieve enhanced safety, efficacy, convenience, and immunological selectivity.

Ironically, Goeckerman therapy remains a gold standard for therapeutic efficacy, but today only a few treatment centers remain.

This chapter reviews the multiple psoriasis treatment options that are currently available, including traditional topical therapies, phototherapy, systemic therapies, and the latest addition of biological therapies. These various modalities are designed to target the different components of the diverse pathways involved in the pathophysiology of psoriasis. Treatment is guided by severity of disease, type of psoriasis, treatment response, patient comorbidities, and patient preference. Oftentimes, the physician will combine therapeutics to achieve optimal outcomes.

11.2 TOPICAL THERAPIES

Topical corticosteroids remain the mainstay treatment for psoriasis, and are effective as monotherapy for mild disease or combined with other topicals or systemic therapies for moderate to severe disease. They exert their effects by binding to the glucocorticoid receptor, affecting gene transcription that results in anti-inflammatory, antiproliferative, immunosuppressive, and vasoconstrictive effects.[3,4] They come in various strengths (Table 11.1) and are available in a wide array of vehicles, including creams, lotions, ointments, gels, oils, shampoos, and sprays. Ointment formulations traditionally provided higher drug penetration, but newer formulations, such as sprays, have been shown to be very potent and allow access to areas that are difficult to reach.[5,6]

Limitations of topical corticosteroids include skin atrophy and suppression of the pituitary–adrenal axis with higher-potency topicals and increased body surface area (BSA) involvement. It is therefore recommended that only low-potency corticosteroids be used in areas such as the face, flexural sites, and genitalia; high-potency corticosteroid application should be limited to 2–4 weeks,[7] although most psoriasis clinicians will allow prolonged use of high-potency corticosteroid topicals in patients who have refractory disease or who cannot be started on systemic agents. Due to the possibility of tachyphylaxis, intermittent application or rotation of the topical agents is sometimes advised for longer treatment courses.

Topical vitamin D analogs used in psoriasis treatment include calcitriol, calcipotriene, and tacalcitol. These analogs all act by binding to the vitamin D receptor, which then binds to a region of DNA called the vitamin D response element. Its downstream effects result in inhibition of keratinocyte proliferation and stimulation of keratinocyte differentiation.[8–10] Calcitriol has also been shown to be immunomodulatory by inhibiting T-cell activity and decreasing the production of TNF-alpha, interferon-gamma, IL-4, IL-6, and IL-12, all of which are implicated in psoriasis.[11–13] Although vitamin D analogs alone have been shown to be less effective than high-potency corticosteroids, their use in combination with corticosteroids has an additive effect.[14–16] The addition of vitamin D analogs may also reduce the frequency of corticosteroid use, thereby decreasing the risk of skin atrophy.[17] The combination of calcipotriol and betamethasone dipropionate ointment was approved by the FDA for plaque psoriasis in 2004. A foam formulation of the drug was approved by the FDA in 2015, and was shown in clinical trials to have significantly greater efficacy than the ointment formulation.[18]

Contraindications to the use of vitamin D analogs include kidney dysfunction, abnormalities of bone or calcium metabolism, pregnancy, and lactation. Excessive application can result in hypervitaminosis; it is therefore recommended that use of calcitriol, calcipotriene, and tacalcitol not exceed 200, 100, and 70 g per week, respectively.

Tazarotene is the only topical retinoid that has been shown to be effective in treating psoriasis plaques.[19,20] It binds selectively to retinoic acid receptor beta and gamma. Studies have shown that tazarotene application can downregulate markers of keratinocyte proliferation and upregulate the tazarotene-induced genes TIG-1, TIG-2, and TIG-3 thought to be involved in antiproliferation.[21,22] Tazarotene was shown to be as effective as fluocinonide in reducing plaque elevation in one study.[23] Irritation in up to 23% of patients limits its use; it is therefore often combined with a topical corticosteroid to enhance efficacy and reduce irritation.[24,25]

TABLE 11.1
Topical Corticosteroids and Considerations for Use in Psoriasis

Potency (Class)	Generic Names	Indications for Use	Duration of Use	Other Considerations
Superpotent (I)	Betamethasone dipropionate Clobetasol propionate Diflorasone diacetate Desoximetasone Fluocinonide Halobetasol propionate	• Severe disease resistant to high-potency corticosteroids	• Short-term use, preferably no longer than 4 weeks at a time • Prolonged use may be needed for refractory disease or patients who cannot be started on systemic agents	• Avoid on thin skin, face, and intertriginous areas • Avoid in patients under 12 years of age • Avoid use on large surface areas
High (II and III)	Betamethasone dipropionate[a] Betamethasone valerate Diflorasone diacetate Desoximetasone Fluocinonide Fluticasone propionate Halcinonide Mometasone furoate	• Severe disease • Effective for thick, hypertrophied, or lichenified skin	• Short-term use, preferably no longer than 4 weeks at a time • Prolonged use may be needed for refractory disease or patients who cannot be started on systemic agents	• Avoid on thin skin, face, and intertriginous areas • Avoid in patients under 12 years of age • Avoid use on large surface areas
Intermediate (IV and V)	Desonide Desoximetasone Fluocinolone acetonide Flurandrenolide Fluticasone propionate Hydrocortisone valerate Mometasone furoate Prednicarbate Triamcinolone acetonide	• Moderate disease • Thin skin • Preferred use on trunk and extremities	• Avoid using beyond 1–2 weeks in infants and children	• Not as effective on thick, hypertrophied, or lichenified skin
Low (VI and VII)	Aclometasone dipropionate Desonide Fluocinolone acetonide Hydrocortisone acetate Hydrocortisone hydrochloride	• Mild disease • Thin skin • Treatment of large areas • Best choice for face and intertriginous areas	• Best choice for long-term treatment	• Not effective on thick, hypertrophied, or lichenified skin • May be used in infants and children

[a] Overlap in potencies for generic names may exist based on concentration, vehicle, and brand name.

Calcineurin inhibitors in psoriasis treatment include tacrolimus and pimecrolimus. These drugs inhibit the phosphorylase enzyme calcineurin, preventing translocation of the nuclear factor of activated T cells, and thereby blocking transcription of cytokines involved in inflammation.[26,27] Calcineurin inhibitors have been shown in studies to be safe and efficacious for the treatment of facial and intertriginous psoriasis.[28,29] In 2006, the FDA placed a black box warning on tacrolimus and pimecrolimus due to their possible link with cases of lymphoma and skin cancer; this association, however, was not shown in subsequent studies.[30,31]

Coal tar, *anthralin*, and *emollients* are other topical modalities that have long been used in psoriasis care and are available without a prescription. Although not first-line therapies, these topicals are typically used as adjunctive therapy. Coal tar and anthralin are the earliest recognized treatments for psoriasis. Tar has additional antipruritic properties and exerts its effect via activation of the aryl hydrocarbon receptor, which stimulates keratinocyte differentiation and restores expression of skin barrier proteins.[32] Its use is contraindicated in pregnancy and lactation due to its mutagenic potential. Anthralin exerts its anti-inflammatory effect via generation of oxygen free radicals and by inhibiting monocyte pro-inflammatory activity.[33,34] It is contraindicated in unstable plaque psoriasis, pustular psoriasis, and erythrodermic psoriasis. Coal tar and anthralin are applied before and after ultraviolet B (UVB) radiation, respectively, in Goeckerman therapy.

Emollients have minimal efficacy in the treatment of psoriasis plaques, but maintain skin hydration and restore barrier function at the epidermal layer.[35] They are often used as part of routine skin care in psoriasis patients.

11.2.1 In the Pipeline

Current research in topical psoriasis therapies focuses on developing more sophisticated and elegant vehicles to enhance drug penetration and increase patient compliance. Also under investigation is the therapeutic potential of topical formulations of small molecules, which are small-molecular-weight inhibitors that can enter cells and inhibit selective signaling pathways. Topical small molecules under phase II clinical trials target Janus-associated kinase (JAK) and phosphodiesterase-4 (PDE4).

Topical tofacitinib and topical ruxolitinib inhibit JAK, a tyrosine kinase that initiates an inflammatory signaling pathway activated by cytokines. Topical tofacitinib, which selectively inhibits JAK1 and JAK3, showed a statistically significant reduction in target plaque severity score at week 4 compared with placebo.[36] Topical ruxolitinib, which selectively inhibits JAK1 and JAK2, was shown to improve lesion thickness, erythema, scaling, and area compared with placebo with good tolerability.[37] Crisaborole is a boron-based molecule that inhibits PDE4, resulting in inhibition of the nuclear factor kappa-B (NF-kB) pathway and decreased pro-inflammatory cytokines. Phase II clinical trials on crisaborole have shown significant reductions in target plaque severity score compared with placebo with no treatment-related adverse events.[38] Larger trials are underway to establish safety and efficacy of these small molecules.

11.3 PHOTOTHERAPY

The formal use of UV exposure for psoriasis treatment began in 1925 after Goeckerman discovered the benefit of treating psoriasis with UV radiation in combination with coal tar, but the use of sunlight to treat skin disease is an ancient concept. The absorption of UV rays by DNA is thought to activate multiple biochemical pathways, resulting in induction of T-cell apoptosis, immunosuppression, alteration of cytokine expression, alterations in antigen-presenting cell activity, inhibition of DNA synthesis, and inhibition of epidermal hyperproliferation.[39] Phototherapy is an option for patients who have moderate to severe disease affecting greater than 5% BSA. Forms of phototherapy for psoriasis include broadband (BB)-UVB, narrowband (NB)-UVB, psoralen with ultraviolet A (PUVA) photochemotherapy, and excimer laser.

BB-UVB (290–320 nm) works best for guttate and seborrheic forms of psoriasis, but is inferior to NB-UVB and PUVA in clearance efficiency and duration of remission.[40] It is typically administered three times weekly until remission, followed by a maintenance regimen to prolong remission.

NB-UVB (311 nm) has largely replaced BB-UVB due to superior clearance and remission times, especially on plaque-type psoriasis.[41] It is also superior to PUVA in terms of photocarcinogenic risk and safety in pregnancy.[42] NB-UVB has been used in combination with multiple topical psoriasis treatments to enhance efficacy and reduce the cumulative UVB dose. Home phototherapy with NB-UVB is an option that has been shown to be as effective as outpatient NB-UVB treatment in one study.[43]

Treatment with PUVA involves oral, topical, or bath psoralen, followed by UVA radiation (320–400 nm). Psoralen is a natural phototoxic compound that penetrates cells and intercalates into DNA. Upon exposure to UVA radiation, the psoralen molecules become activated and bind with DNA base pairs, resulting in DNA cross-linking and apoptosis. PUVA therapy was shown to achieve clearance of psoriasis lesions in 70%–100% of patients in two large systemic reviews.[44,45] Studies comparing clearance with PUVA versus NB-UVB therapy are mixed, but one study showed longer remission times in PUVA therapy.[46] A pitfall to PUVA therapy is its association with skin cancer. Studies have shown an increased risk of cutaneous squamous cell carcinoma in PUVA-treated patients; risk was also increased with high-dose compared with low-dose PUVA, and in patients being treated with PUVA while on cyclosporine.[47–50] The association between PUVA treatment and melanoma is unclear, with multiple large studies demonstrating contradictory results.[51–54] Other adverse effects associated with PUVA treatment include accelerated photoaging, phototoxicity, and gastrointestinal symptoms from psoralen.

Excimer laser is a newer high-energy 308 nm ultraviolet therapy that localizes treatment to involved skin only. This targeted therapy allows higher doses of UVB and has been shown to require fewer treatments than conventional phototherapy.[55,56] The main side effects include erythema, blistering, and hyperpigmentation of treated areas, which resolved with discontinuation of treatment.

11.4 NONBIOLOGIC SYSTEMIC THERAPY

Before the advent of biologic therapies, other systemic therapies, such as methotrexate, cyclosporine, and oral retinoids, were commonly used for psoriasis therapy. While these agents are inferior to biologics in safety, they remain an option for patients with more extensive disease.

Methotrexate was approved by the FDA for psoriasis treatment in 1971 and continues to be a commonly used systemic agent. It is a folic acid antagonist that inhibits DNA synthesis in immunologically active cells by competitively binding to dihydrofolate reductase; this prevents the conversion of dihydrofolate to tetrahydrofolate, a cofactor required in DNA/RNA synthesis. Methotrexate is also thought to exert immunosuppressive effects by blocking migration of activated T cells to tissues and by inhibiting cytokine secretion.[57,58]

Methotrexate is highly efficacious and may be used for all clinical variants of psoriasis. Studies have shown that 50%–60% of patients reached 75% reduction in the Psoriasis Area Severity Index (PASI 75) score at doses of 15–20 mg weekly.[59,60] An initial response is typically seen at 1–4 weeks, with a maximal response at 2–3 months. It is typically administered in once-weekly doses and may be used as long-term therapy. A major adverse effect of methotrexate is hepatotoxicity. Liver biopsy after every 1–1.5 g of cumulative methotrexate was previously recommended for all psoriasis patients.[61] This recommendation has since been revised based on patient-specific risk factors and serologic markers. Other major adverse effects of methotrexate include bone marrow suppression, acute pneumonitis, pulmonary fibrosis, and gastrointestinal symptoms. Methotrexate also increases the risk of cancer, including lymphoma. Folic acid supplementation may reduce hematologic and hepatic adverse effects, but there is concern that coadministration may reduce methotrexate efficacy. Methotrexate is contraindicated in pregnancy and lactation.

Cyclosporine is a calcineurin inhibitor that was approved by the FDA for the treatment of psoriasis in 1997. Due to its rapid onset of action, it is an effective treatment for acute flares, as a bridge to other maintenance therapies, or when rapid clearance is needed. Studies demonstrate statistically significant dose-dependent efficacy and faster remission at higher doses.[62,63] Its maximum dose is 5 mg/kg/day; once a good response has been achieved, the dose may be weaned by 0.5–1 mg/kg/day at 2-week intervals.

A major adverse effect of cyclosporine treatment is hypertension secondary to renal vasoconstriction, which occurs in about 25% of patients.[64] This effect is both time and dose dependent. Patients should be routinely monitored for the development of hypertension and nephrotoxicity. Serum creatinine elevations of greater than 25% above baseline warrant discontinuation by taper until creatinine is within 10% of baseline. Cyclosporine is contraindicated in significant renal impairment and uncontrolled hypertension.

Acitretin is the only systemic retinoid currently approved by the FDA for the treatment of psoriasis. Although less efficacious than other systemic treatments in plaque psoriasis, it has been shown to be more efficacious than methotrexate or cyclosporine in generalized pustular psoriasis, and is effective in palmoplantar and erythrodermic psoriasis.[65–67] Because acitretin lacks immunosuppressive effects, it may be used in patients with active cancer, infection, or HIV. The maximum dosage is 1 mg/kg/day, which may be necessary for pustular psoriasis. Due to its teratogenicity, acitretin is contraindicated during pregnancy and should be avoided up to 3 years prior to pregnancy. Patients on acitretin therapy should have routine monitoring for hypertriglyceridemia and hepatotoxicity.

Apremilast is a relatively new oral small-molecule PDE4 inhibitor that was approved by the FDA in 2014 for the treatment of psoriasis. Large randomized trials demonstrate achievement of PASI 75 in roughly 30% of patients. Its efficacy appears to be dose dependent and is inferior to that of cyclosporine, ustekinumab, and anti-TNF biologic agents.[68,69] Its main advantage is its relative safety, precluding the need for routine lab monitoring. The most common side effect is diarrhea when treatment is initiated; tolerability may be improved by uptitrating the dose by 10 mg/day over 1 week. Other adverse effects include upper respiratory infection, headache, weight loss, and depression. The associated weight loss may be one reason for this drug's popularity.

11.4.1 In the Pipeline

Three oral small-molecule agents that target specific inflammatory signaling pathways are in phase III clinical trials. CF101 (Can-Fite BioPharma Ltd.) is an oral small-molecule agent that binds to the adenosine A3 receptor, which is overexpressed in inflammatory cells.[70–72] This agonism leads to downregulation of inflammatory signaling pathways, including the NF-kB pathway, resulting in decreased levels of inflammatory cytokines and promotion of inflammatory cell apoptosis.[73,74] In a phase II randomized double-blind clinical trial, 35.3% of patients treated with CF101 achieved PASI 50, which is significantly greater clearance than that of placebo.[75]

FP187 (Forward-Pharma) is a dimethyl fumarate currently undergoing phase III clinical trials for its treatment in both psoriasis and multiple sclerosis. Data from phase II clinical studies have not yet been published. Fumaric acid esters have been used to treat psoriasis for decades in northern Europe but are not yet available in the United States. Its mechanism is not entirely understood, but one commonly proposed theory involves decreased translocation of NF-kB, leading to the decreased expression of pro-inflammatory cytokines.[76,77] Progressive multifocal leukoencephalopathy has been reported in case reports of patients who received long-term fumaric acid therapy.[78,79]

Pooled data from two phase III clinical trials showed that oral tofacitinib, which inhibits JAK, achieved PASI 75 in 55.6% and 68.8% of patients with 5 and 10 mg twice-daily dosing, respectively. Efficacy was sustained for 24 months in most patients.[80]

11.5 BIOLOGICAL THERAPIES

Biological therapies are the latest addition to the treatment of moderate to severe psoriasis and have become increasingly utilized due to their high short- and long-term efficacy and good safety profile.

Alefacept was the first biologic approved by the FDA for psoriasis treatment in 2003. It bound to CD2 on T cells, preventing its interaction with the LFA-3 on antigen-presenting cells, thereby preventing T-cell activation. Alefacept's manufacturer discontinued production in 2011. *Efalizumab*, also approved by the FDA in 2003, targeted the CD11a subunit of LFA-1. It was voluntarily withdrawn from the market in 2009 due to reports of progressive multifocal leukoencephalopathy in patients undergoing long-term treatment. Currently available biologics exert their therapeutic effects through inhibition of TNF, IL-12 and IL-23, or IL-17A (Table 11.2). The downstream effects involve reduction of inflammatory cytokines and elimination of pathogenic T cells.

11.5.1 TNF-Targeting Therapeutics

TNF antagonists include *etanercept*, *infliximab*, *adalimumab*, *golimumab*, and *certolizumab*. These agents bind to TNF and prevent its interaction with TNF receptors, thus leading to inhibition of the NF-kB pathway involved in cell proliferation, cell survival, and cytokine production. Infliximab, adalimumab, and golimumab are monoclonal antibodies; etanercept is a dimeric fusion protein composed of two TNF receptors fused to the Fc portion of immunoglobulin (Ig) G1; and certolizumab is a PEGylated Fab′ fragment of a humanized TNF-specific monoclonal antibody. The structural differences among the TNF-targeting therapeutics are thought to explain their differences in efficacy and timing of therapeutic response seen clinically. For example, etanercept can only bind to a single trimer of TNF to form complexes of etanercept and TNF in a 1:1 ratio, but in contrast to the other agents, etanercept can also bind to lymphotoxin, a TNF-related molecule that is also a soluble mediator of inflammation. Infliximab may bind to both TNF monomers and trimers. Infliximab can also cross-link separate TNF molecules, resulting in the formation of larger and more stable complexes. The varying half-lives of these complexes and rates of TNF release affect the efficacy of each drug.[81,82] Furthermore, monoclonal antibodies have the additional benefit of inducing complement-mediated cytotoxicity and antibody-dependent cell-mediated cytotoxicity, leading to cellular apoptosis.[83,84]

Etanercept has demonstrated efficacy in achieving PASI 75 after 12 weeks of treatment compared with placebo.[85–87] Efficacy and safety have also been shown in the pediatric population, although the drug is not FDA approved for patients under the age of 18.[88] Studies have also shown enhanced efficacy when combined with methotrexate.[89,90] Onset of action is slower compared with that of other TNF antagonists, but continued improvement may be seen for up to 6 months. Etanercept is typically administered as a 50 mg subcutaneous injection twice weekly for 3 months, followed by 50 mg once weekly for maintenance therapy. Although the formation of antidrug antibodies may occur, they are not neutralizing and do not seem to have a strong effect on treatment efficacy.[91]

Infliximab, a chimeric (human–mouse) IgG1 monoclonal antibody, has been shown to have higher efficacy and faster onset of action than other TNF antagonists.[92–94] Studies have shown that treatment at 3 or 5 mg/kg achieved PASI 75 at 10 weeks, with efficacy maintained over placebo for 46–50 weeks.[95–97] Duration of response was longer at higher doses. One randomized trial comparing infliximab with methotrexate found that patients treated with infliximab showed greater improvement at 16 weeks (78% vs. 42% achieving PASI 75) and were less likely to switch to an alternative therapy.[98]

Infliximab is typically dosed at 5 mg/kg via intravenous infusion at 0, 2, and 6 weeks, and then every 8 weeks. The formation of neutralizing antidrug antibodies may lead to loss of efficacy over time, as well as greater risk of infusion reactions. These may be prevented with concurrent administration of methotrexate.[99–102]

Adalimumab, a human recombinant IgG1 monoclonal antibody, has been shown to achieve PASI 75 in up to 80% of patients, with response maintained up to 60 weeks.[92,103,104] In one randomized study, adalimumab demonstrated significantly superior efficacy in achieving PASI 75 compared with methotrexate.[105] A multicenter study showed clearance or near clearance at 12 weeks in 34% of patients who had failed etanercept, with treatment success near 50% when adalimumab was given

TABLE 11.2
Current Biological Therapies in Psoriasis Management

Biologic	Structure	Target	Route	Most Common Adverse Effects	Contraindications
Etanercept	Dimeric fusion protein composed of two TNF-alpha receptors fused to the Fc portion of IgG1	TNF	SC	Upper respiratory tract infection, sinusitis, headache, injection site reaction	Active infection, hypersensitivity to etanercept
Infliximab	Chimeric (human–mouse) IgG1 monoclonal antibody	TNF	IV	Rhinitis, sinusitis, transaminitis, headache	Active infection, congestive heart failure, hypersensitivity to murine proteins
Adalimumab	Human recombinant IgG1 monoclonal antibody	TNF	SC	Upper respiratory tract infection, urinary tract infection, nasopharyngitis, headache, cellulitis	Hypersensitivity to adalimumab
Golimumab	Human recombinant IgG1 monoclonal antibody	TNF	SC	Upper respiratory tract infection, nasopharyngitis, injection site reaction	None
Certolizumab	Pegylated Fab fragment of a humanized monoclonal antibody	TNF	SC	Upper respiratory tract infection, urinary tract infection, rash	None
Ustekinumab	Human IgG1 monoclonal antibody	p40 subunit shared by IL-12 and IL-23	SC	Upper respiratory tract infection, nasopharyngitis, headache, fatigue, injection site reaction	Hypersensitivity to ustekinumab
Secukinumab	Human IgG1 monoclonal antibody	IL-17A	IV	Upper respiratory tract infection, nasopharyngitis, diarrhea	Hypersensitivity to secukinumab
Ixekizumab	Human IgG1 monoclonal antibody	IL-17A	SC	Upper respiratory tract infection, tinea infection, nausea, injection site reaction	Hypersensitivity to ixekizumab

Note: SC, subcutaneously.

for an additional 12 weeks.[106] It has quick onset of action, with initial improvement seen within 2 weeks and maximal responses seen at 12–16 weeks. Treatment typically begins with a loading dose of 80 mg subcutaneously, followed by 40 mg every other week beginning 1 week after the initial dose. Treatment response may decrease with the formation of antidrug antibodies.

Golimumab, a human recombinant IgG1 monoclonal antibody, is FDA approved for the treatment of psoriatic arthritis. One study showed significant improvement in psoriatic arthritis and associated skin and nail psoriasis, with efficacy maintained through 24 weeks.[107] It is dosed at 50 mg subcutaneously monthly. Antidrug antibodies have not been shown to affect treatment response.

Certolizumab, a pegylated Fab fragment of a humanized monoclonal antibody, was approved by the FDA for psoriatic arthritis in 2013. It is currently in phase III clinical trials for the treatment of plaque psoriasis.

11.5.2 Important Considerations

Patients treated with TNF antagonists are at increased risk of developing opportunistic infections, such as mycobacterial infections, *Pneumocystis jiroveci* pneumonia, coccidioidomycosis, histoplasmosis, and listeriosis.[108–115] Of these, there is a clear link between TNF-targeting agents and reactivation of latent tuberculosis (TB) or development of new-onset TB.[116–119] This is supported by mouse models showing that TNF plays a critical role in the protective immune response against TB, and prevents disseminated disease.[120–122] Of the TNF-targeting agents, adalimumab and infliximab appear to have a greater risk of TB reactivation than etanercept, but all patients initiating biologic therapy need to be screened for TB with either the tuberculin skin test or interferon-gamma release assay (IGRA) with continued annual TB screening.[82] Patients testing positive for TB must show response to TB treatment prior to initiating biologic therapy.

11.6 INHIBITION OF IL-12 AND IL-23

Ustekinumab is a human IgG1 monoclonal antibody that inhibits IL-12 and IL-23 by binding to the p40 subunit that is shared by both cytokines. This inhibits NK cell activation and the development and survival of Th1 and Th17 cells, which are implicated in psoriasis pathogenesis. Studies show achievement of PASI 75 in 65%–80% of patients treated with ustekinumab after 12 weeks.[123,124] One study showed superior efficacy of ustekinumab at 45 and 90 mg compared with high-dose etanercept at achieving PASI 75.[125] Another study showed efficacy and tolerability of ustekinumab in patients with inadequate response to methotrexate, with 62% of patients achieving PASI 75 at 12 weeks.[126]

Ustekinumab is dosed at 45 mg (if weight <100 kg) or 90 mg (if weight >100 kg) subcutaneously at weeks 0 and 4, and then every 12 weeks. Antidrug antibodies have been reported in 4%–6% of patients, but their effect on efficacy is undetermined.[91] Given its immunomodulatory mechanism, there was concern that ustekinumab placed patients at risk for infection and malignancy. However, safety data collected over 5 years showed no increased risk of infection or malignancy.[127] Data from phase II and III clinical trials led to concern about possible increased risk of major adverse cardiovascular events, which was not observed to be significant in a subsequent meta-analysis.[128]

11.7 INHIBITION OF IL-17A

Secukinumab and *ixekizumab*, approved by the FDA for psoriasis in 2015 and 2016, respectively, are the latest additions to the biologic class of psoriatic therapeutics. They are human IgG1 monoclonal antibodies that target IL-17A, a pro-inflammatory cytokine produced by Th17 cells found at increased levels in psoriatic lesions.[129,130]

Secukinumab is approved for both plaque psoriasis and psoriatic arthritis. In a phase III clinical trial, secukinumab achieved PASI 75 at 12 weeks in 82% of patients in the 300 mg group and

72% of patients in the 150 mg group, compared with 5% of controls. Secukinumab was found to be superior to etanercept in another phase III clinical trial, with PASI 75 achieved in 77% of patients in the 300 mg secukinumab group, 67% of patients in the 150 mg secukinumab group, and 44% of patients in the etanercept group.[131] A randomized double-blind study comparing secukinumab with ustekinumab showed a significantly greater PASI 90 response at week 16 and PASI 75 response at week 4.[132] Dosing is typically 300 mg subcutaneously once weekly for the first 5 weeks, followed by once every 4 weeks thereafter.

Ixekizumab was approved by the FDA for moderate to severe plaque psoriasis in March 2016. In a phase III clinical trial, PASI 75 was achieved in 90% of patients treated with ixekizumab once every 2 weeks compared with 42% of patients treated with etanercept; similar results were reported in a second phase III study.[133] Rates of adverse effects were similar between treatment and placebo groups, with the most common being transient neutropenia in 12% of patients. Dosing for ixekizumab is 160 mg at week 0, followed by 80 mg at weeks 2, 4, 6, 8, 10, and 12, spaced out to 80 mg every 4 weeks.

11.8 IN THE PIPELINE

There are additional investigational drugs with promising therapeutic potential in phase III clinical trials. *Abatacept* is a fusion protein composed of the extracellular domain of CTLA-4 linked to a modified Fc portion of human IgG1. It blocks T-cell activation by binding to the B7 protein on antigen-presenting cells, preventing its interaction with the costimulatory CD28 molecule, which is important for T-cell activation. Abatacept was approved by the FDA in 2005 for rheumatoid arthritis and is currently in phase III clinical trials for the treatment of psoriatic arthritis. In a phase II clinical trial, patients treated with abatacept at 10 mg/kg showed significant improvement in arthritis symptoms compared with placebo.[134]

Brodalumab is an anti-IL-17A monoclonal antibody that has been under consideration for FDA approval for moderate to severe psoriasis as of January 2016. Two phase III randomized trials demonstrate superior efficacy compared with placebo, with about 85% of patients achieving PASI 75 at 12 weeks in both studies. Compared with ustekinumab, brodalumab achieved a higher rate of complete clearance (PASI 100). Adverse effects occurring more frequently than in placebo groups were mild to moderate *Candida* infections and neutropenia.[135] There have been reports of suicidal ideation and two suicides in patients treated with brodalumab, which prompted Amgen to drop brodalumab, leaving AstraZeneca without an additional corporate partner. It is now being developed in conjunction with Valeant Pharmaceuticals.

Tildrakizumab, *guselkumab*, and *BI 655066* (Boehringer-Ingelheim and AbbVie) are human monoclonal antibodies designed to target the p19 subunit of IL-23, blocking IL-23 without blocking IL-12. The reasoning behind this selectivity is the thought that the Th17 pathway mediated by IL-23 may be more important in the pathogenesis of psoriasis than the Th1 pathway mediated by IL-12.

Tildrakizumab was found to be significantly superior to placebo at achieving PASI 75 at 16 weeks, with 74.4% of patients showing response at the highest dose of 200 mg.[136] Efficacy was maintained for 52 weeks of treatment and continued 20 weeks after cessation. The most serious adverse effects included drug-related melanoma, stroke, epiglottitis, bacterial arthritis, and lymphedema, although these were uncommon. Thirteen percent of study participants developed antidrug antibodies, of which 3% were neutralizing.

Guselkumab was shown to be significantly superior to placebo in achieving a Physician's Global Assessment (PGA) score of 0 (cleared psoriasis) or 1 (minimal psoriasis) at 16 weeks.[137] Guselkumab at higher doses was also superior to adalimumab with regards to PGA at 16 and 40 weeks. Up to week 16, infections were observed in 20% of patients in the guselkumab group compared with 12% in the adalimumab group and 14% in the placebo group. Anti-guselkumab antibodies developed in 6% of patients treated with guselkumab, but these were in low titers and nonneutralizing.

A small phase I trial conducted on BI 655066 showed achievement of PASI 75, 90, and 100 in 87%, 58%, and 16% of patients in the treatment group compared with none in the placebo group.[138] Clinical improvement was seen at week 2 and maintained for up to 66 weeks after treatment. No differences in adverse events were noted. Two of 31 patients receiving BI 655066 developed anti-drug antibodies, but these were not associated with loss of efficacy or hypersensitivity reactions. Results of phase II clinical trials have not been formally published.

11.9 CONCLUSION

Treatment options for psoriasis have expanded considerably since the discovery of anthralin one century ago, with accelerated development in the past few decades. Vehicles for topical therapies have become more elegant, enhancing drug penetration and increasing patient adherence. The advent of biologic agents was a critical addition to systemic therapy in their high efficacy and superior safety profile. Ongoing investigations in psoriasis treatment focus on small molecules that target selective signaling pathways important in the inflammatory response. As novel molecular targets in psoriasis are discovered, future therapies will aim to enhance efficacy while reducing toxicity and administration burden.

REFERENCES

1. Goeckerman WH. The treatment of psoriasis. *Northwest Medicine* 1925;24:229–31.
2. Rich SJ, Bello-Quintero CE. Advancements in the treatment of psoriasis: Role of biologic agents. *Journal of Managed Care Pharmacy* 2004;10:318–25.
3. Uva L, Miguel D, Pinheiro C et al. Mechanisms of action of topical corticosteroids in psoriasis. *International Journal of Endocrinology* 2012;2012:561018.
4. Barnes PJ. Anti-inflammatory actions of glucocorticoids: Molecular mechanisms. *Clinical Science* 1998;94:557–72.
5. Menter A. Topical monotherapy with clobetasol propionate spray 0.05% in the COBRA trial. *Cutis* 2007;80:12–9.
6. Bhutani T, Koo J, Maibach HI. Efficacy of clobetasol spray: Factors beyond patient compliance. *Journal of Dermatological Treatment* 2012;23:11–5.
7. Menter A, Korman NJ, Elmets CA et al. Guidelines of care for the management of psoriasis and psoriatic arthritis. Section 3. Guidelines of care for the management and treatment of psoriasis with topical therapies. *Journal of the American Academy of Dermatology* 2009;60:643–59.
8. Rizova E, Corroller M. Topical calcitriol—Studies on local tolerance and systemic safety. *British Journal of Dermatology* 2001;144 (Suppl. 58):3–10.
9. Yamanaka KI, Kakeda M, Kitagawa H et al. 1,24-Dihydroxyvitamin D(3) (tacalcitol) prevents skin T-cell infiltration. *British Journal of Dermatology* 2010;162:1206–15.
10. Jensen AM, Llado MB, Skov L, Hansen ER, Larsen JK, Baadsgaard O. Calcipotriol inhibits the proliferation of hyperproliferative CD29 positive keratinocytes in psoriatic epidermis in the absence of an effect on the function and number of antigen-presenting cells. *British Journal of Dermatology* 1998;139:984–91.
11. Matsumoto K, Hashimoto K, Nishida Y, Hashiro M, Yoshikawa K. Growth-inhibitory effects of 1,25-dihydroxyvitamin D3 on normal human keratinocytes cultured in serum-free medium. *Biochemical and Biophysical Research Communications* 1990;166:916–23.
12. Koeffler HP, Amatruda T, Ikekawa N, Kobayashi Y, DeLuca HF. Induction of macrophage differentiation of human normal and leukemic myeloid stem cells by 1,25-dihydroxyvitamin D3 and its fluorinated analogues. *Cancer Research* 1984;44:5624–8.
13. Staeva-Vieira TP, Freedman LP. 1,25-Dihydroxyvitamin D3 inhibits IFN-gamma and IL-4 levels during in vitro polarization of primary murine CD4+ T cells. *Journal of Immunology* 2002;168:1181–9.
14. Kaufmann R, Bibby AJ, Bissonnette R et al. A new calcipotriol/betamethasone dipropionate formulation (Daivobet) is an effective once-daily treatment for psoriasis vulgaris. *Dermatology* 2002;205:389–93.
15. Vissers WH, Berends M, Muys L, van Erp PE, de Jong EM, van de Kerkhof PC. The effect of the combination of calcipotriol and betamethasone dipropionate versus both monotherapies on epidermal proliferation, keratinization and T-cell subsets in chronic plaque psoriasis. *Experimental Dermatology* 2004;13:106–12.

16. Anstey AV, Kragballe K. Retrospective assessment of PASI 50 and PASI 75 attainment with a calcipotriol/betamethasone dipropionate ointment. *International Journal of Dermatology* 2006;45:970–5.
17. American Academy of Dermatology Work Group, Menter A, Korman NJ et al. Guidelines of care for the management of psoriasis and psoriatic arthritis: Section 6. Guidelines of care for the treatment of psoriasis and psoriatic arthritis: Case-based presentations and evidence-based conclusions. *Journal of the American Academy of Dermatology* 2011;65:137–74.
18. Koo J, Tyring S, Werschler WP et al. Superior efficacy of calcipotriene and betamethasone dipropionate aerosol foam versus ointment in patients with psoriasis vulgaris—A randomized phase II study. *Journal of Dermatological Treatment* 2016;27:120–7.
19. Weinstein GD, Krueger GG, Lowe NJ et al. Tazarotene gel, a new retinoid, for topical therapy of psoriasis: Vehicle-controlled study of safety, efficacy, and duration of therapeutic effect. *Journal of the American Academy of Dermatology* 1997;37:85–92.
20. Weinstein GD, Koo JY, Krueger GG et al. Tazarotene cream in the treatment of psoriasis: Two multicenter, double-blind, randomized, vehicle-controlled studies of the safety and efficacy of tazarotene creams 0.05% and 0.1% applied once daily for 12 weeks. *Journal of the American Academy of Dermatology* 2003;48:760–7.
21. Nagpal S, Thacher SM, Patel S et al. Negative regulation of two hyperproliferative keratinocyte differentiation markers by a retinoic acid receptor-specific retinoid: Insight into the mechanism of retinoid action in psoriasis. *Cell Growth and Differentiation* 1996;7:1783–91.
22. Duvic M, Nagpal S, Asano AT, Chandraratna RA. Molecular mechanisms of tazarotene action in psoriasis. *Journal of the American Academy of Dermatology* 1997;37:S18–24.
23. Lebwohl M, Ast E, Callen JP et al. Once-daily tazarotene gel versus twice-daily fluocinonide cream in the treatment of plaque psoriasis. *Journal of the American Academy of Dermatology* 1998;38:705–11.
24. van de Kerkhof PC. An update on topical therapies for mild-moderate psoriasis. *Dermatologic Clinics* 2015;33:73–7.
25. Gollnick H, Menter A. Combination therapy with tazarotene plus a topical corticosteroid for the treatment of plaque psoriasis. *British Journal of Dermatology* 1999;140 (Suppl. 54):18–23.
26. Reynolds NJ, Al-Daraji WI. Calcineurin inhibitors and sirolimus: Mechanisms of action and applications in dermatology. *Clinical and Experimental Dermatology* 2002;27:555–61.
27. Clipstone NA, Crabtree GR. Identification of calcineurin as a key signalling enzyme in T-lymphocyte activation. *Nature* 1992;357:695–7.
28. Gribetz C, Ling M, Lebwohl M et al. Pimecrolimus cream 1% in the treatment of intertriginous psoriasis: A double-blind, randomized study. *Journal of the American Academy of Dermatology* 2004; 51:731–8.
29. Lebwohl M, Freeman AK, Chapman MS et al. Tacrolimus ointment is effective for facial and intertriginous psoriasis. *Journal of the American Academy of Dermatology* 2004;51:723–30.
30. Tennis P, Gelfand JM, Rothman KJ. Evaluation of cancer risk related to atopic dermatitis and use of topical calcineurin inhibitors. *British Journal of Dermatology* 2011;165:465–73.
31. Siegfried EC, Jaworski JC, Hebert AA. Topical calcineurin inhibitors and lymphoma risk: Evidence update with implications for daily practice. *American Journal of Clinical Dermatology* 2013;14:163–78.
32. van den Bogaard EH, Bergboer JG, Vonk-Bergers M et al. Coal tar induces AHR-dependent skin barrier repair in atopic dermatitis. *Journal of Clinical Investigation* 2013;123:917–27.
33. Kemeny L, Ruzicka T, Braun-Falco O. Dithranol: A review of the mechanism of action in the treatment of psoriasis vulgaris. *Skin Pharmacology* 1990;3:1–20.
34. Mrowietz U, Falsafi M, Schroder JM, Christophers E. Inhibition of human monocyte functions by anthralin. *British Journal of Dermatology* 1992;127:382–6.
35. Rim JH, Jo SJ, Park JY, Park BD, Youn JI. Electrical measurement of moisturizing effect on skin hydration and barrier function in psoriasis patients. *Clinical and Experimental Dermatology* 2005;30: 409–13.
36. Ports WC, Khan S, Lan S et al. A randomized phase 2a efficacy and safety trial of the topical Janus kinase inhibitor tofacitinib in the treatment of chronic plaque psoriasis. *British Journal of Dermatology* 2013;169:137–45.
37. Punwani N, Scherle P, Flores R et al. Preliminary clinical activity of a topical JAK1/2 inhibitor in the treatment of psoriasis. *Journal of the American Academy of Dermatology* 2012;67:658–64.
38. Nazarian R, Weinberg JM. AN-2728, a PDE4 inhibitor for the potential topical treatment of psoriasis and atopic dermatitis. *Current Opinion in Investigational Drugs* 2009;10:1236–42.
39. Wong T, Hsu L, Liao W. Phototherapy in psoriasis: A review of mechanisms of action. *Journal of Cutaneous Medicine and Surgery* 2013;17:6–12.

40. Walters IB, Burack LH, Coven TR, Gilleaudeau P, Krueger JG. Suberythemogenic narrow-band UVB is markedly more effective than conventional UVB in treatment of psoriasis vulgaris. *Journal of the American Academy of Dermatology* 1999;40:893–900.
41. Dawe RS. A quantitative review of studies comparing the efficacy of narrow-band and broad-band ultraviolet B for psoriasis. *British Journal of Dermatology* 2003;149:669–72.
42. Menter A, Korman NJ, Elmets CA et al. Guidelines of care for the management of psoriasis and psoriatic arthritis: Section 5. Guidelines of care for the treatment of psoriasis with phototherapy and photochemotherapy. *Journal of the American Academy of Dermatology* 2010;62:114–35.
43. Koek MB, Buskens E, van Weelden H, Steegmans PH, Bruijnzeel-Koomen CA, Sigurdsson V. Home versus outpatient ultraviolet B phototherapy for mild to severe psoriasis: Pragmatic multicentre randomised controlled non-inferiority trial (PLUTO study). *BMJ* 2009;338:b1542.
44. Spuls PI, Witkamp L, Bossuyt PM, Bos JD. A systematic review of five systemic treatments for severe psoriasis. *British Journal of Dermatology* 1997;137:943–9.
45. Griffiths CE, Clark CM, Chalmers RJ, Li Wan Po A, Williams HC. A systematic review of treatments for severe psoriasis. *Health Technology Assessment* 2000;4:1–125.
46. Yones SS, Palmer RA, Garibaldinos TT, Hawk JL. Randomized double-blind trial of the treatment of chronic plaque psoriasis: Efficacy of psoralen-UV-A therapy vs narrowband UV-B therapy. *Archives of Dermatology* 2006;142:836–42.
47. Forman AB, Roenigk HH Jr., Caro WA, Magid ML. Long-term follow-up of skin cancer in the PUVA-48 cooperative study. *Archives of Dermatology* 1989;125:515–9.
48. Cole C, VanFossen R. Measurement of sunscreen UVA protection: An unsensitized human model. *Journal of the American Academy of Dermatology* 1992;26:178–84.
49. Stern RS, Lunder EJ. Risk of squamous cell carcinoma and methoxsalen (psoralen) and UV-A radiation (PUVA). A meta-analysis. *Archives of Dermatology* 1998;134:1582–5.
50. Nijsten TE, Stern RS. The increased risk of skin cancer is persistent after discontinuation of psoralen+ultraviolet A: A cohort study. *Journal of Investigative Dermatology* 2003;121:252–8.
51. Stern RS, Nichols KT, Vakeva LH. Malignant melanoma in patients treated for psoriasis with methoxsalen (psoralen) and ultraviolet A radiation (PUVA). The PUVA Follow-Up Study. *New England Journal of Medicine* 1997;336:1041–5.
52. Chuang TY, Heinrich LA, Schultz MD, Reizner GT, Kumm RC, Cripps DJ. PUVA and skin cancer. A historical cohort study on 492 patients. *Journal of the American Academy of Dermatology* 1992;26:173–7.
53. Hannuksela-Svahn A, Pukkala E, Koulu L, Jansen CT, Karvonen J. Cancer incidence among Finnish psoriasis patients treated with 8-methoxypsoralen bath PUVA. *Journal of the American Academy of Dermatology* 1999;40:694–6.
54. Hannuksela A, Pukkala E, Hannuksela M, Karvonen J. Cancer incidence among Finnish patients with psoriasis treated with trioxsalen bath PUVA. *Journal of the American Academy of Dermatology* 1996;35:685–9.
55. Gerber W, Arheilger B, Ha TA, Hermann J, Ockenfels HM. Ultraviolet B 308-nm excimer laser treatment of psoriasis: A new phototherapeutic approach. *British Journal of Dermatology* 2003;149:1250–8.
56. Feldman SR, Mellen BG, Housman TS et al. Efficacy of the 308-nm excimer laser for treatment of psoriasis: Results of a multicenter study. *Journal of the American Academy of Dermatology* 2002;46:900–6.
57. Sigmundsdottir H, Johnston A, Gudjonsson JE, Bjarnason B, Valdimarsson H. Methotrexate markedly reduces the expression of vascular E-selectin, cutaneous lymphocyte-associated antigen and the numbers of mononuclear leucocytes in psoriatic skin. *Experimental Dermatology* 2004;13:426–34.
58. Gottlieb SL, Gilleaudeau P, Johnson R et al. Response of psoriasis to a lymphocyte-selective toxin (DAB389IL-2) suggests a primary immune, but not keratinocyte, pathogenic basis. *Nature Medicine* 1995;1:442–7.
59. Van Dooren-Greebe RJ, Kuijpers AL, Mulder J, De Boo T, Van de Kerkhof PC. Methotrexate revisited: Effects of long-term treatment in psoriasis. *British Journal of Dermatology* 1994;130:204–10.
60. Heydendael VM, Spuls PI, Opmeer BC et al. Methotrexate versus cyclosporine in moderate-to-severe chronic plaque psoriasis. *New England Journal of Medicine* 2003;349:658–65.
61. Roenigk HH Jr., Auerbach R, Maibach H, Weinstein G, Lebwohl M. Methotrexate in psoriasis: Consensus conference. *Journal of the American Academy of Dermatology* 1998;38:478–85.
62. Timonen P, Friend D, Abeywickrama K, Laburte C, von Graffenried B, Feutren G. Efficacy of low-dose cyclosporin A in psoriasis: Results of dose-finding studies. *British Journal of Dermatology* 1990;122 (Suppl. 36):33–9.
63. Ellis CN, Fradin MS, Messana JM et al. Cyclosporine for plaque-type psoriasis. Results of a multidose, double-blind trial. *New England Journal of Medicine* 1991;324:277–84.

64. Grossman RM, Chevret S, Abi-Rached J, Blanchet F, Dubertret L. Long-term safety of cyclosporine in the treatment of psoriasis. *Archives of Dermatology* 1996;132:623–9.
65. Ozawa A, Ohkido M, Haruki Y et al. Treatments of generalized pustular psoriasis: A multicenter study in Japan. *Journal of Dermatology* 1999;26:141–9.
66. Janagond AB, Kanwar AJ, Handa S. Efficacy and safety of systemic methotrexate vs. acitretin in psoriasis patients with significant palmoplantar involvement: A prospective, randomized study. *Journal of the European Academy of Dermatology and Venereology* 2013;27:e384–9.
67. Lassus A, Geiger JM. Acitretin and etretinate in the treatment of palmoplantar pustulosis: A double-blind comparative trial. *British Journal of Dermatology* 1988;119:755–9.
68. Schmitt J, Rosumeck S, Thomaschewski G, Sporbeck B, Haufe E, Nast A. Efficacy and safety of systemic treatments for moderate-to-severe psoriasis: Meta-analysis of randomized controlled trials. *British Journal of Dermatology* 2014;170:274–303.
69. Papp K, Cather JC, Rosoph L et al. Efficacy of apremilast in the treatment of moderate to severe psoriasis: A randomised controlled trial. *Lancet* 2012;380:738–46.
70. Ochaion A, Bar-Yehuda S, Cohen S et al. The anti-inflammatory target A(3) adenosine receptor is over-expressed in rheumatoid arthritis, psoriasis and Crohn's disease. *Cellular Immunology* 2009;258:115–22.
71. Fishman P, Bar-Yehuda S, Madi L et al. The PI3K-NF-kappaB signal transduction pathway is involved in mediating the anti-inflammatory effect of IB-MECA in adjuvant-induced arthritis. *Arthritis Research and Therapy* 2006;8:R33.
72. Madi L, Cohen S, Ochayin A, Bar-Yehuda S, Barer F, Fishman P. Overexpression of A3 adenosine receptor in peripheral blood mononuclear cells in rheumatoid arthritis: Involvement of nuclear factor-kappaB in mediating receptor level. *Journal of Rheumatology* 2007;34:20–6.
73. Szabo C, Scott GS, Virag L et al. Suppression of macrophage inflammatory protein (MIP)-1alpha production and collagen-induced arthritis by adenosine receptor agonists. *British Journal of Pharmacology* 1998;125:379–87.
74. Fishman P, Cohen S. The A3 adenosine receptor (A3AR): Therapeutic target and predictive biological marker in rheumatoid arthritis. *Clinical Rheumatology* 2016;35:2359–62.
75. David M, Akerman L, Ziv M et al. Treatment of plaque-type psoriasis with oral CF101: Data from an exploratory randomized phase 2 clinical trial. *Journal of the European Academy of Dermatology and Venereology* 2012;26:361–7.
76. Gold R, Linker RA, Stangel M. Fumaric acid and its esters: An emerging treatment for multiple sclerosis with antioxidative mechanism of action. *Clinical Immunology* 2012;142:44–8.
77. Roll A, Reich K, Boer A. Use of fumaric acid esters in psoriasis. *Indian Journal of Dermatology, Venereology and Leprology* 2007;73:133–7.
78. van Oosten BW, Killestein J, Barkhof F, Polman CH, Wattjes MP. PML in a patient treated with dimethyl fumarate from a compounding pharmacy. *New England Journal of Medicine* 2013;368:1658–9.
79. Ermis U, Weis J, Schulz JB. PML in a patient treated with fumaric acid. *New England Journal of Medicine* 2013;368:1657–8.
80. Papp KA, Krueger JG, Feldman SR et al. Tofacitinib, an oral Janus kinase inhibitor, for the treatment of chronic plaque psoriasis: Long-term efficacy and safety results from 2 randomized phase-III studies and 1 open-label long-term extension study. *Journal of the American Academy of Dermatology* 2016;74:841–50.
81. Scallon B, Cai A, Solowski N et al. Binding and functional comparisons of two types of tumor necrosis factor antagonists. *Journal of Pharmacology and Experimental Therapeutics* 2002;301:418–26.
82. Sivamani RK, Goodarzi H, Garcia MS et al. Biologic therapies in the treatment of psoriasis: A comprehensive evidence-based basic science and clinical review and a practical guide to tuberculosis monitoring. *Clinical Reviews in Allergy and Immunology* 2013;44:121–40.
83. Mitoma H, Horiuchi T, Tsukamoto H et al. Mechanisms for cytotoxic effects of anti-tumor necrosis factor agents on transmembrane tumor necrosis factor alpha-expressing cells: Comparison among infliximab, etanercept, and adalimumab. *Arthritis and Rheumatism* 2008;58:1248–57.
84. Van den Brande JM, Braat H, van den Brink GR et al. Infliximab but not etanercept induces apoptosis in lamina propria T-lymphocytes from patients with Crohn's disease. *Gastroenterology* 2003;124:1774–85.
85. Papp KA, Tyring S, Lahfa M et al. A global phase III randomized controlled trial of etanercept in psoriasis: Safety, efficacy, and effect of dose reduction. *British Journal of Dermatology* 2005;152:1304–12.
86. Leonardi CL, Powers JL, Matheson RT et al. Etanercept as monotherapy in patients with psoriasis. *New England Journal of Medicine* 2003;349:2014–22.
87. Tyring S, Gordon KB, Poulin Y et al. Long-term safety and efficacy of 50 mg of etanercept twice weekly in patients with psoriasis. *Archives of Dermatology* 2007;143:719–26.

88. Paller AS, Siegfried EC, Langley RG et al. Etanercept treatment for children and adolescents with plaque psoriasis. *New England Journal of Medicine* 2008;358:241–51.
89. Zachariae C, Mork NJ, Reunala T et al. The combination of etanercept and methotrexate increases the effectiveness of treatment in active psoriasis despite inadequate effect of methotrexate therapy. *Acta Dermato-Venereologica* 2008;88:495–501.
90. Gottlieb AB, Langley RG, Strober BE et al. A randomized, double-blind, placebo-controlled study to evaluate the addition of methotrexate to etanercept in patients with moderate to severe plaque psoriasis. *British Journal of Dermatology* 2012;167:649–57.
91. Hsu L, Snodgrass BT, Armstrong AW. Antidrug antibodies in psoriasis: A systematic review. *British Journal of Dermatology* 2014;170:261–73.
92. Brimhall AK, King LN, Licciardone JC, Jacobe H, Menter A. Safety and efficacy of alefacept, efalizumab, etanercept and infliximab in treating moderate to severe plaque psoriasis: A meta-analysis of randomized controlled trials. *British Journal of Dermatology* 2008;159:274–85.
93. Nast A, Sporbeck B, Rosumeck S et al. Which antipsoriatic drug has the fastest onset of action? Systematic review on the rapidity of the onset of action. *Journal of Investigative Dermatology* 2013;133:1963–70.
94. Reich K, Burden AD, Eaton JN, Hawkins NS. Efficacy of biologics in the treatment of moderate to severe psoriasis: A network meta-analysis of randomized controlled trials. *British Journal of Dermatology* 012;166:179–88.
95. Gottlieb AB, Evans R, Li S et al. Infliximab induction therapy for patients with severe plaque-type psoriasis: A randomized, double-blind, placebo-controlled trial. *Journal of the American Academy of Dermatology* 2004;51:534–42.
96. Menter A, Feldman SR, Weinstein GD et al. A randomized comparison of continuous vs. intermittent infliximab maintenance regimens over 1 year in the treatment of moderate-to-severe plaque psoriasis. *Journal of the American Academy of Dermatology* 2007;56:31.e1–15.
97. Reich K, Nestle FO, Papp K et al. Infliximab induction and maintenance therapy for moderate-to-severe psoriasis: A phase III, multicentre, double-blind trial. *Lancet* 2005;366:1367–74.
98. Barker J, Hoffmann M, Wozel G et al. Efficacy and safety of infliximab vs. methotrexate in patients with moderate-to-severe plaque psoriasis: Results of an open-label, active-controlled, randomized trial (RESTORE1). *British Journal of Dermatology* 2011;165:1109–17.
99. Maini RN, Breedveld FC, Kalden JR et al. Therapeutic efficacy of multiple intravenous infusions of anti-tumor necrosis factor alpha monoclonal antibody combined with low-dose weekly methotrexate in rheumatoid arthritis. *Arthritis and Rheumatism* 1998;41:1552–63.
100. Hsu L, Armstrong AW. Anti-drug antibodies in psoriasis: A critical evaluation of clinical significance and impact on treatment response. *Expert Review of Clinical Immunology* 2013;9:949–58.
101. Anderson PJ. Tumor necrosis factor inhibitors: Clinical implications of their different immunogenicity profiles. *Seminars in Arthritis and Rheumatism* 2005;34:19–22.
102. Baert F, Noman M, Vermeire S et al. Influence of immunogenicity on the long-term efficacy of infliximab in Crohn's disease. *New England Journal of Medicine* 2003;348:601–8.
103. Gordon KB, Langley RG, Leonardi C et al. Clinical response to adalimumab treatment in patients with moderate to severe psoriasis: Double-blind, randomized controlled trial and open-label extension study. *Journal of the American Academy of Dermatology* 2006;55:598–606.
104. Menter A, Tyring SK, Gordon K et al. Adalimumab therapy for moderate to severe psoriasis: A randomized, controlled phase III trial. *Journal of the American Academy of Dermatology* 2008;58:106–15.
105. Saurat JH, Stingl G, Dubertret L et al. Efficacy and safety results from the randomized controlled comparative study of adalimumab vs. methotrexate vs. placebo in patients with psoriasis (CHAMPION). *British Journal of Dermatology* 2008;158:558–66.
106. Bissonnette R, Bolduc C, Poulin Y, Guenther L, Lynde CW, Maari C. Efficacy and safety of adalimumab in patients with plaque psoriasis who have shown an unsatisfactory response to etanercept. *Journal of the American Academy of Dermatology* 2010;63:228–34.
107. Kavanaugh A, McInnes I, Mease P et al. Golimumab, a new human tumor necrosis factor alpha antibody, administered every four weeks as a subcutaneous injection in psoriatic arthritis: Twenty-four-week efficacy and safety results of a randomized, placebo-controlled study. *Arthritis and Rheumatism* 2009;60:976–86.
108. Tsiodras S, Samonis G, Boumpas DT, Kontoyiannis DP. Fungal infections complicating tumor necrosis factor alpha blockade therapy. *Mayo Clinic Proceedings* 2008;83:181–94.
109. Bergstrom L, Yocum DE, Ampel NM et al. Increased risk of coccidioidomycosis in patients treated with tumor necrosis factor alpha antagonists. *Arthritis and Rheumatism* 2004;50:1959–66.

110. Komano Y, Harigai M, Koike R et al. *Pneumocystis jiroveci* pneumonia in patients with rheumatoid arthritis treated with infliximab: A retrospective review and case-control study of 21 patients. *Arthritis and Rheumatism* 2009;61:305–12.
111. Wissmann G, Morilla R, Martin-Garrido I et al. *Pneumocystis jirovecii* colonization in patients treated with infliximab. *European Journal of Clinical Investigation* 2011;41:343–8.
112. Kaur N, Mahl TC. *Pneumocystis jiroveci* (*carinii*) pneumonia after infliximab therapy: A review of 84 cases. *Digestive Diseases and Sciences* 2007;52:1481–4.
113. Mertz LE, Blair JE. Coccidioidomycosis in rheumatology patients: Incidence and potential risk factors. *Annals of the New York Academy of Sciences* 2007;1111:343–57.
114. Bodro M, Paterson DL. Listeriosis in patients receiving biologic therapies. *European Journal of Clinical Microbiology and Infectious Diseases* 2013;32:1225–30.
115. Slifman NR, Gershon SK, Lee JH, Edwards ET, Braun MM. *Listeria monocytogenes* infection as a complication of treatment with tumor necrosis factor alpha-neutralizing agents. *Arthritis and Rheumatism* 2003;48:319–24.
116. Gomez-Reino JJ, Carmona L, Valverde VR, Mola EM, Montero MD, BIOBADASER Group. Treatment of rheumatoid arthritis with tumor necrosis factor inhibitors may predispose to significant increase in tuberculosis risk: A multicenter active-surveillance report. *Arthritis and Rheumatism* 2003;48:2122–7.
117. Keane J, Gershon S, Wise RP et al. Tuberculosis associated with infliximab, a tumor necrosis factor alpha-neutralizing agent. *New England Journal of Medicine* 2001;345:1098–104.
118. Centers for Disease Control and Prevention. Tuberculosis associated with blocking agents against tumor necrosis factor-alpha—California, 2002–2003. *Morbidity and Mortality Weekly Report* 2004;53:683–6.
119. Wallis RS. Tumour necrosis factor antagonists: Structure, function, and tuberculosis risks. *Lancet Infectious Diseases* 2008;8:601–11.
120. Lukacs NW, Chensue SW, Strieter RM, Warmington K, Kunkel SL. Inflammatory granuloma formation is mediated by TNF-alpha-inducible intercellular adhesion molecule-1. *Journal of Immunology* 1994;152:5883–9.
121. Flynn JL, Goldstein MM, Chan J et al. Tumor necrosis factor-alpha is required in the protective immune response against *Mycobacterium tuberculosis* in mice. *Immunity* 1995;2:561–72.
122. Jacobs M, Samarina A, Grivennikov S et al. Reactivation of tuberculosis by tumor necrosis factor neutralization. *European Cytokine Network* 2007;18:5–13.
123. Shetty P. Twalib Ngoma: Creating cancer care in Tanzania. *Lancet* 2008;371:1657.
124. Leonardi CL, Kimball AB, Papp KA et al. Efficacy and safety of ustekinumab, a human interleukin-12/23 monoclonal antibody, in patients with psoriasis: 76-week results from a randomised, double-blind, placebo-controlled trial (PHOENIX 1). *Lancet* 2008;371:1665–74.
125. Griffiths CE, Strober BE, van de Kerkhof P et al. Comparison of ustekinumab and etanercept for moderate-to-severe psoriasis. *New England Journal of Medicine* 2010;362:118–28.
126. Paul C, Puig L, Kragballe K et al. Transition to ustekinumab in patients with moderate-to-severe psoriasis and inadequate response to methotrexate: A randomized clinical trial (TRANSIT). *British Journal of Dermatology* 2014;170:425–34.
127. Papp KA, Griffiths CE, Gordon K et al. Long-term safety of ustekinumab in patients with moderate-to-severe psoriasis: Final results from 5 years of follow-up. *British Journal of Dermatology* 2013;168:844–54.
128. Ryan C, Leonardi CL, Krueger JG et al. Association between biologic therapies for chronic plaque psoriasis and cardiovascular events: A meta-analysis of randomized controlled trials. *JAMA* 2011;306:864–71.
129. Elain G, Jeanneau K, Rutkowska A, Mir AK, Dev KK. The selective anti-IL17A monoclonal antibody secukinumab (AIN457) attenuates IL17A-induced levels of IL6 in human astrocytes. *Glia* 2014;62:725–35.
130. Maldonado-Ficco H, Perez-Alamino R, Maldonado-Cocco JA. Secukinumab: A promising therapeutic option in spondyloarthritis. *Clinical Rheumatology* 2016;35:2151–61.
131. Langley RG, Elewski BE, Lebwohl M et al. Secukinumab in plaque psoriasis—Results of two phase 3 trials. *New England Journal of Medicine* 2014;371:326–38.
132. Thaci D, Blauvelt A, Reich K et al. Secukinumab is superior to ustekinumab in clearing skin of subjects with moderate to severe plaque psoriasis: CLEAR, a randomized controlled trial. *Journal of the American Academy of Dermatology* 2015;73:400–9.
133. Griffiths CE, Reich K, Lebwohl M et al. Comparison of ixekizumab with etanercept or placebo in moderate-to-severe psoriasis (UNCOVER-2 and UNCOVER-3): Results from two phase 3 randomised trials. *Lancet* 2015;386:541–51.

134. Mease P, Genovese MC, Gladstein G et al. Abatacept in the treatment of patients with psoriatic arthritis: Results of a six-month, multicenter, randomized, double-blind, placebo-controlled, phase II trial. *Arthritis and Rheumatism* 2011;63:939–48.
135. Lebwohl M, Strober B, Menter A et al. Phase 3 studies comparing brodalumab with ustekinumab in psoriasis. *New England Journal of Medicine* 2015;373:1318–28.
136. Papp K, Thaci D, Reich K et al. Tildrakizumab (MK-3222), an anti-interleukin-23p19 monoclonal antibody, improves psoriasis in a phase IIb randomized placebo-controlled trial. *British Journal of Dermatology* 2015;173:930–9.
137. Gordon KB, Duffin KC, Bissonnette R et al. A phase 2 trial of guselkumab versus adalimumab for plaque psoriasis. *New England Journal of Medicine* 2015;373:136–44.
138. Krueger JG, Ferris LK, Menter A et al. Anti-IL-23A mAb BI 655066 for treatment of moderate-to-severe psoriasis: Safety, efficacy, pharmacokinetics, and biomarker results of a single-rising-dose, randomized, double-blind, placebo-controlled trial. *Journal of Allergy and Clinical Immunology* 2015;136:116–24 e7.

12 Management of Psoriatic Arthritis

Siba P. Raychaudhuri, Reason Wilken, Debashis Sarkar, Emanual Maverakis, and Smriti K. Raychaudhuri

CONTENTS

12.1 INTRODUCTION

Because of immunologic, genetic, and clinical phenotype overlaps, many times psoriatic arthritis (PsA) and psoriasis are grouped together as "psoriatic disease." Psoriatic disease can be a chronic, lifelong, and disabling condition [1–4]; thus, it is of utmost importance to provide patients with multispecialty care at the onset of psoriatic disease. PsA is a complex systemic inflammatory disease primarily involving the peripheral and axial joints, tendons, enthuses, skin, and nails. The involvement of different organ systems makes the clinical diagnosis and management of PsA not only difficult but also definitely very challenging. In fact, the ideal management of a patient with PsA would be to focus on its early diagnosis, correctly assess the severity of the disease, and thereafter start the right treatment of inflammatory arthritis and other PsA-related comorbidities. An appropriate screening method could help other relevant physicians for psoriatic disease, such as a general physician or a dermatologist, in making or suspecting the diagnosis of PsA, so that at a very early state of the disease, before the development of the complications of erosive arthritis, PsA patients can be referred to rheumatologists [3,4]. Once the patient is correctly screened for PsA, specific diagnostic criteria could then help one to establish the diagnosis of PsA. This process of screening methods, diagnostic aids, and disease assessment guidelines for PsA is still in its nascent stage. Right now, there are no unanimous recommended diagnostic criteria for PsA, and so PsA-specific studies are still being developed and modified [3,4]. Here, we review the currently available tools to help in the screening, diagnosis, and follow-up for PsA, and also provide a clear and vivid review of the currently available treatment or therapies, particularly the "targeted therapies," that is, anti–tumor necrosis factor (TNF) agents, biologics targeting the interleukin (IL)-23/IL-17 pathway, phosphodiesterase 4 (PDE4) inhibitors, and several other promising novel therapies for PsA. For the last several years, targeted therapies have indeed made a big breakthrough in the treatment of PsA, and in the days ahead, it tends to look even better [4–7].

12.1.1 Screening for the Early Diagnosis of Psoriatic Arthritis

Psoriasis mostly starts by the age of 25 [8]. In most of PsA patients, it is found that the earliest signs are cutaneous changes in the form of psoriasis that develop much earlier, before the development of arthritic signs and symptoms [9]. It is interesting to mention that at the moment, there are no serum biomarkers to definitely forecast which psoriasis patients will go on to develop PsA [10,11]. Rather, it usually takes a long time, sometimes several years (~10 years) for a patient with psoriasis to develop an inflammatory arthritis [12]. Thus, dermatologists and all primary care service providers should be ready to diagnose PsA in their at-risk patients with cutaneous psoriasis. In such patients, achieving a good long-term clinical outcome will depend more on the physician's ability to diagnose PsA at the earliest phase of the disease, and thus start treatment before the significant and permanent joint damage [3] has taken place. It is essential to mention that there are no well-defined diagnostic criteria for PsA. However, we do have classification criteria for PsA, the Classification Criteria for Psoriatic Arthritis (CASPAR), which are widely used for PsA (Table 12.1) [13]. Undoubtedly, early diagnosis is essential for PsA, while the disease is still in its nascent stage. The ideal diagnostic test for PsA should be highly sensitive and also highly specific. High sensitivity is, in particular, very important to ensure that patients with PsA are not missed during screening. Lately, lists of screening questionnaires for PsA have been prepared for use in primary care and dermatology offices (Table 12.2), such as the Toronto Psoriatic Arthritis Screening Questionnaire (TOPAS), the Psoriasis and

TABLE 12.1

The CASPAR consist of established inflammatory articular disease with at least 3 points from the following features:

- Current psoriasis (assigned a score of 2)
- A history of psoriasis (in the absence of current psoriasis; assigned a score of 1)
- A family history of psoriasis (in the absence of current psoriasis and a history of psoriasis; assigned a score of 1)
- Dactylitis (assigned a score of 1)
- Juxta-articular new bone formation (assigned a score of 1)
- RF negativity (assigned a score of 1)
- Nail dystrophy (assigned a score of 1)

TABLE 12.2
Psoriatic Arthritis: Early Diagnosis Screening Tools

Screening Tools	Description	Sensitivity/Specificity
PASQ	10 items + joint diagram Self-report	
PASE	Self-administered 15 items Maximum score: 75	Sensitivity 82% Specificity 73%
PEST	Self-administered 5 items + joint diagram Maximum score: NA	Sensitivity 97% Specificity 79%
TOPAS	Self-administered 11 items + pictures/diagrams Maximum score: NA	Sensitivity 86.8% Specificity 93.1%

Source: Adapted from Machado, P. M., and Raychaudhuri, S. P., *Best Pract. Res. Clin. Rheumatol.*, 28, 711–728, 2014.
Note: NA, not applicable.

Arthritis Screening Questionnaire (PASQ), the Psoriasis Epidemiology Screening Tool (PEST), and the Psoriatic Arthritis Screening and Evaluation (PASE) [14–16]. These screening questionnaires are now used internationally; the sensitivity and specificity of these questionnaires are mentioned in Table 12.2. With careful and judicious use of these tools, one can expect that PsA can be determined at the earliest stage of the onset of the disease process, and so initiating treatment in this early stage could thus minimize the joint deformities and comorbidities of PsA.

The CASPAR were determined based on the data recorded from patients with long-standing PsA and also evaluated on the basis of established diagnostic criteria for inflammatory articular disease, which were designed to include additional clinical findings specific to PsA, for example, the presence of psoriatic nail dystrophy, dactylitis, a negative rheumatoid factor (RF) test, and radiographic evidence for juxta-articular bone formation [13,17]. These were determined as PsA-specific disease manifestations by comparing 588 PsA patients with 536 controls; the data of the control group were collected mainly from patients with rheumatoid arthritis (RA) or ankylosing spondylitis. Signs specific to PsA were identified by multivariate statistical analysis of more than 50 variables. Significantly, classification criteria such as CASPAR have been designed particularly for use in the research setting to identify patients for inclusion in clinical studies. Thus, specificity is undoubtedly the most important factor. This will result in an increase in the homogeneity of the studied patient population and also ensure that individuals enrolled in a study actually have PsA. The CASPAR are believed to be highly specific (99.1%) for the diagnosis of PsA, but the sensitivity for detecting early PsA was found to be lower, at 87.4% [18,19]. Moreover, in patients with early-stage PsA, the sensitivity of the CASPAR also has some limitations. To conclude, while CASPAR have exceptional specificity for PsA, they are ideally suited to be used as a sensitive screening tool; that is, they are not so useful to determine psoriasis patients who are just developing PsA.

12.1.2 PsA Disease Severity Outcome Measures

Because patients with PsA are mostly associated with significant peripheral arthritis, we often apply the same outcome measures developed and validated for RA [20]. These include the Disease Activity Score for 28 joints (DAS28) and the American College of Rheumatology (ACR) Responder Index (ACR20) [21,22]. But, the difference in the pattern of joint involvement between PsA and RA has raised serious questions about the ability of ACR20 and DAS28 to quantify the disease activity of PsA. For example, compared with RA in PsA, there is a greater tendency for asymmetric and oligoarticular joint involvement. Moreover, the distal interphalangeal (DIP) joints are frequently involved in PsA but not in RA—a remarkable feature because the 28-joint count comprising the DAS28 *excludes* the finger (DIP) joints, as well as the ankles and feet, which are commonly affected in PsA [21]. So, in patients with oligoarthritis, use of the DAS28 can misclassify 20% of PsA patients and application of DAS28 will simply mismeasure disease activity in these patients [23]. As a result of this fallacy for PsA clinical trials, it has been recommended to do a count of 68 tender and 66 swollen joints, including the DIP joints of the hands [24].

In comparison with RA, where the major focus is peripheral arthritis, PsA disease severity also needs to be determined by measuring the severity of extra-articular manifestations, such as tendinitis, dactylitis, and severity of the psoriatic skin lesions [25]. The determination of valid, reliable, and feasible outcome measures that can be suitably employed in longitudinal cohorts and clinical trials still remains an issue of research. Several validated disease-scoring tools are listed in Table 12.3. The severity of involvement of several domains of PsA (such as joints, enthuses, skin, and nails) can vary significantly among patients with PsA and over time within the same patient, and all of the domains may have a significant effect on the patient's quality of life (QoL). So, to assess the disease activity in a condition with multiple domains for clinical active disease, such as in PsA, a composite measure may be most accurate. For PsA, this requirement has been identified in the last decade and the Group for Research and Assessment of Psoriasis and Psoriatic Arthritis (GRAPPA) has been relentlessly pursuing this task. The ultimate aim is to integrate the severity of different signs and symptoms of PsA at a specific time point [26,27]. Through the efforts by GRAPPA as a team and also by other research groups and investigators, PsA-specific composite disease measures are currently evolving. Among these, the following measures have been validated: the Disease Activity Index for Psoriatic Arthritis (DAPSA), the Composite Psoriatic Disease Activity Index (CPDAI), and the Psoriatic Arthritis Joint Activity Index (PsAJAI) [28–31]. In Table 12.4, a summary of various domains of these indices is provided.

In the CPDAI, the disease severity of PsA is categorized as mild, moderate, and severe. This outcome measure has been reported to demonstrate a remarkable correlation with patient ($r = 0.777$)

TABLE 12.3
Psoriatic Arthritis Disease Measurement Assessment Tools

Disease Phenotype/Global Disease Assessments	Disease Measurement Tools
Peripheral joint disease activity assessment	68/66 TJC/SJC, DAS, PSARC, and ACR response criteria
Axial joint disease activity assessment	BASDAI, BASFI, BASMI, ASDAS
PsA composite measures	CPDAI, PsAJAI, DAPSA
Skin assessment	BSA, PASI, target lesion, global
Enthesitis assessment	Leeds, Mander, MASES, Berlin, SPARCC
Dactylitis assessment	Leeds, present/absent, acute/chronic
Patient global	VAS (global, skin + joints)
Physician global	VAS (global, skin + joints)
Function/QoL	SF-36, HAQ, PsAQoL, DLQI

Source: Adapted from Machado, P. M., and Raychaudhuri, S. P., *Best Pract. Res. Clin. Rheumatol.*, 28, 711–728, 2014.

Note: ASDAS, Ankylosing Spondylitis Disease Activity Score; BASFI, Bath Ankylosing Spondylitis Functional Index; BASMI, Bath Ankylosing Spondylitis Metrology Index; MASES, Maastricht Ankylosing Spondylitis Enthesitis Score; SPARCC, Spondyloarthritis Research Consortium of Canada; VAS, Visual Analogue Scale; PsAQoL, Psoriatic Arthritis Quality of Life.

TABLE 12.4
Clinical Domains for Disease Activity of Psoriatic Arthritis

	Peripheral Arthritis	Pain	Patient Global Assessment	Physician Global Assessment	Skin	Enthesitis	Dactylitis	Spine Disease	HAQ	CRP
CPDAI	Yes		Yes		Yes	Yes	Yes	Yes	Yes	Yes
PsAJAI	Yes	Yes	Yes	Yes					Yes	Yes
DAPSA	Yes	Yes	Yes							Yes

Source: Adapted from Machado, P.M., and Raychaudhuri, S. P., *Best Pract. Res. Clin. Rheumatol.*, 28, 711–728, 2014.
Note: CPDAI, Composite Psoriatic Disease Activity Index; CRP, C-reactive Protein; DAPSA, Disease Activity for Psoriatic Arthritis; HAQ, Health Assessment Questionnaire; PsAJAI, Psoriatic Arthritis Joint Activity Index.

TABLE 12.5
Composite Psoriatic Disease Activity Index

Not Involved (0)	Mild (1)	Moderate (2)	Severe (3)
Peripheral arthritis	≤4 joints (swollen or tender); normal function (HAQ <0.5)[a]	≤4 joints but function impaired; or >4 joints, normal function	>4 joints and function impaired
Skin disease	PASI ≤10 and DLQI ≤10	PASI ≤10 but DLQI >10; or PASI >10 but DLQI ≤10	PASI >10 and DLQI >10
Enthesitis	≤3 sites; normal function (HAQ <0.5)[a]	≤3 sites but function impaired; or >3 sites but normal function	>3 sites and function impaired
Dactylitis	≤3 digits; normal function (HAQ <0.5)[a]	≤3 digits but function impaired; or >3 digits but normal function	>3 digits and has function impaired
Spinal disease	BASDAI <4; normal function (ASQoL <6)	BASDAI >4 but normal function; BASDAI <4 but function impaired	BASDAI >4 and function impaired

Source: Mumtaz, A. et al., *Ann. Rheum. Dis.*, 70, 272–277, 2011.
Note: CPDAI total score ranges from 0–15.
[a] HAQ only counted if clinical involvement of the domain (joint, enthesis, or dactylitis) was present.

and physician global (r = 0.809) assessments; CPDAI can differentiate between ineffectively and effectively treated patients [29]. In the CPDAI, the following five domains are evaluated: swollen joint count (SJC) of 66 joints and tender joint count (TJC) of 68 joints, skin (Psoriasis Area and Severity Index [PASI]), dactylitis, enthesitis, and spinal manifestations. Dactylitis is performed by counting the number of involved digits, enthesitis is performed by evaluating the number of tendons or fascia insertion sites, and spondylitis or spinal inflammation is measured by the Ankylosing Spondylitis Quality of Life (ASQoL) and Bath Ankylosing Spondylitis Disease Activity Index (BASDAI). All domains are scored from 0 to 3, so the total CPDAI score range is 0–15. A modified CPDAI (mCPDAI) has also been suggested [32], which includes only four domains (without the axial domain). In Table 12.5, a summary of the five domains of the CPDAI is shown.

More composite measures for the evaluation of the total disease activity in PsA are also being prepared. To assess the severity of musculoskeletal and cutaneous involvement in PsA, GRAPPA has been working on several projects, which include the minimal disease activity (MDA) criteria [33] and the GRAPPA Composite Exercise (GRACE) project [34,35]. GRAPPA has developed a composite measure for MDA, which has also been validated. MDA requires assessments of joints, entheses, skin, and physical function [33]. The GRAPPA MDA criteria can determine a low disease state of PsA, and these criteria can be used as a responder index (Table 12.6). The GRACE project has helped to develop two new composite measures for PsA disease activity evaluation: the Arithmetic Mean of Desirability Functions (AMDF) and the Psoriatic Arthritis Disease Activity Score (PASDAS) [34].

12.1.3 Treatment Recommendations for Psoriatic Arthritis

Formal treatment guidelines for PsA, meta-analysis of the drugs currently used in PsA, and treatment recommendations for PsA are now widely followed for the management of PsA [36–41]. The European League Against Rheumatism (EULAR) and GRAPPA have both made treatment recommendations for PsA [36–39]. Published in 2012, the EULAR algorithm serves as a guide for physicians in determining appropriate treatment options for psoriatic disease to optimally manage skin and joint involvement, maintain health-related QoL, and at the same time prevent or slow the progress of joint damage [36].

TABLE 12.6
Minimal Disease Activity of Psoriatic Arthritis: GRAPPA Recommendation

A patient is classified as having MDA when fulfilling 5 of the 7 following criteria:

TJC ≤1
SJC ≤1
Psoriasis Activity and Severity Index ≤1 or BSA ≤3
Patient pain visual analogue score ≤15
Patient global disease activity visual analogue score ≤20
HAQ ≤0.5
Tender entheseal points ≤1

Source: Adapted from Coates, L. C. et al. *Ann. Rheum. Dis.*, 69, 48–53, 2010.

The EULAR algorithm stresses the musculoskeletal part of the disease and recommends sequential treatment measures; the choice of medication is determined according to the disease severity (arthritis, enthesitis, and spondylitis) and response to therapy. EULAR updated its recommendations in 2015 so that currently approved therapies, such as IL-17 inhibitors, IL-12/IL-23 inhibitors, and anti-PDE4 agents can be used for PsA [38]. The EULAR algorithm is stratified into four phases, with an inadequate clinical response resulting in aggravation to the next phase (e.g., arthritis that does not respond adequately to methotrexate [Phase II] would next be treated with a TNF inhibitor [Phase III] according to the EULAR algorithm) [38]. In Figure 12.1, a schematic of the EULAR treatment algorithm for PsA is provided.

The GRAPPA treatment recommendations are based on an evidence-based literature review. In this recommendation, six key clinical domains of PsA have been considered: arthritis, enthesitis, dactylitis, spondylitis, skin, and nail disease. GRAPPA has developed a grading system to evaluate the disease severity in three groups (mild, moderate, and severe) for each clinically involved domain in PsA and the effect of these domains on physical function and QoL (Table 12.7), and disease severity was integrated into the previous GRAPPA treatment recommendations released in 2009 [39]. PsA, in addition to chronic inflammation of the cutaneous system and joints, often involves multiple extra-articular sites [40]. Thus, recommendations for treatment of PsA need to address a comprehensive management inclusive of associated conditions in PsA. In 2015, the GRAPPA treatment grid was redesigned and the distinctions between mild, moderate, and severe forms of diseases were deleted due to lack of proof to support the cutoff points between severities of grades. The revised 2015 treatment grid suggests evidence-based (GRADE) treatment guidelines (Table 12.8) for all six clinical domains, based on the strength of supporting evidence [41]. Moreover, in 2015 GRAPPA announced treatment recommendations for the major manifestations of PsA in the form of flowcharts, which include each affected clinical domain [41]. The schema provides "standard" and "expedited" treatment approaches for each clinical domain. (For example, the standard treatment for axial disease is to start with nonsteroidal anti-inflammatory drug [NSAIDs] and switch over to biologics, such as anti-TNF, IL-17, or IL 12/IL-23 antagonists, in the setting of an inadequate response, whereas the expedited option would be to initiate treatment with biologics.)

12.1.4 Comorbidities in Psoriatic Arthritis and Its Multispecialty Approach for Management

PsA is associated with an array of systemic diseases [39]; comorbidities in PsA conditions include metabolic syndrome (central obesity, insulin resistance, dyslipidemia, and hypertension), atherosclerotic cardiovascular disease (CVD), valvular heart disease, inflammatory bowel disease, fatigue,

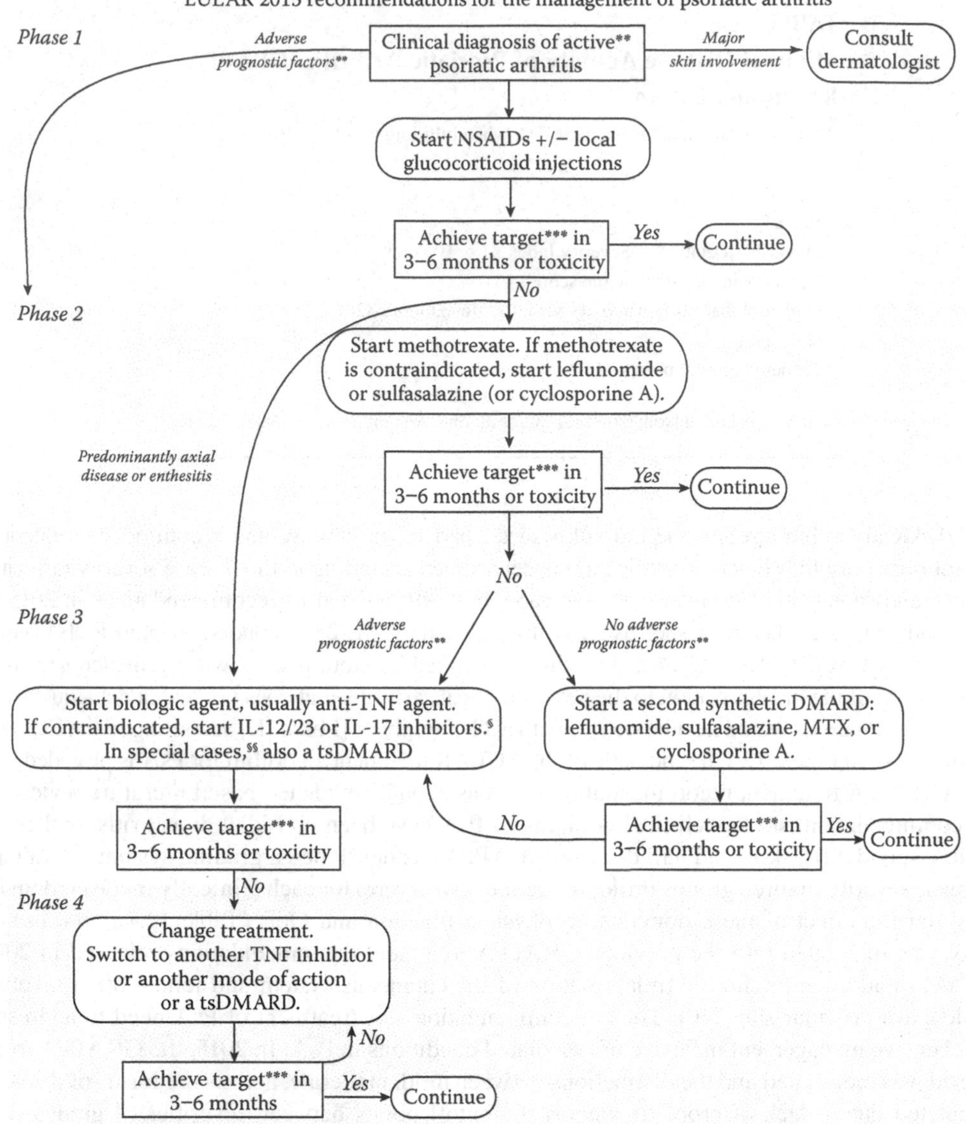

* Refer to Gossec et al. [38] for situations covered in this figure.

** Per EULAR, active disease is defined as one or more tender and inflamed joints, tender enthesis point, dactylitic digit, and/or inflammatory back pain.

** Adverse prognostic factors are defined as five or more active joints, radiographic damage, elevated acute phase reactants, extra-articular manifestations (dactylitis).

*** Treatment target is clinical remission (the absence of signs or symptoms), or low disease activity if remission is unlikely.

$ For patients with peripheral arthritis and an inadequate response to at least one csDMARD, in whom TNF inhibitors are not appropriate. With predominant spinal involvement, active enthesitis, and/or dactylitis, no csDMARD is needed—use bDMARD with preference for a TNF inhibitor.

$$ For peripheral arthritis and an inadequate response to at least one csDMARD, in whom bDMARDS are not appropriate.

FIGURE 12.1 EULAR 2015 algorithm for treatment of PsA. bDMARD, biological DMARD; csDMARD, conventional synthetic DMARD; MTX, methotrexate; tsDMARD, targeted synthetic DMARD. (Adapted from Gossec, L. et al., *Ann. Rheum. Dis.*, 75(3), 499–510, 2016.)

TABLE 12.7
GRAPPA GRID: Disease Severity of Psoriatic Arthritis

	Disease Severity		
Clinical Domains	**Mild**	**Moderate**	**Severe**
Peripheral arthritis • No. of joints • Damage on x-ray • QoL • Patient evaluation	• <5 • No damage • No • Minimal impact • Mild	• ≥5 (swollen or tender) • Moderate damage • Moderate • Moderate impact • Moderate • Inadequate response to mild Rx	• ≥5 (swollen or tender) • Severe damage • Severe • Severe impact • Severe • Inadequate response to mild–moderate Rx
Skin involvement	• BSA <5 • PASI <5 • Asymptomatic	• Nonresponse to topicals • DLQI • PASI <10	• BSA >10 • DLQI >10 • PASI >10
Spinal disease	• Mild pain • No loss of function	• Loss of function or • BASDAI >4	• Failure or response
Dactylitis	• 1–2 sites • No loss of function	• >2 sites or loss of function	• Loss of function or • >2 sites and failure of function
Enthesitis	• Pain: Absent to mild • Normal function	• Erosive disease or • Loss of function	• Failure of response

osteoporosis, uveitis, and various comorbidities secondary to chronic pain, disability, and reduced QoL [42–47]. A growing body of literature suggests that the systemic inflammatory reaction in patients with PsA imposes a higher risk for the development or rapid progression of metabolic syndrome and CVD, and thus psoriatic disease can be associated with increased morbidity and mortality [42–45]. So, PsA treatment requires a multisystem and multidisciplinary approach, and after complete physical evaluation, an individualized therapy program needs to be outlined as early as possible. The following subspecialties many times may be helpful for the proper management of PsA: dermatology, physical therapy, ophthalmology, endocrinology, cardiology, orthopedics, psychiatry, and dietary and lifestyle modification programs [41]. This will be an ideal way to treat psoriatic disease, and we have been recommending a multispecialty approach for the treatment of psoriatic disease for the last two decades [41,48].

12.2 DMARDS, NSAIDS, AND OTHER FIRST-LINE THERAPIES FOR PSORIATIC ARTHRITIS

12.2.1 Glucocorticoids

Systemic steroids, a mainstay therapy for inflammatory arthritis, are not used often to treat PsA due to the risk of aggravation of the skin manifestations of psoriasis while tapering. In addition to increasing the risk of a disease flare, glucocorticoids also have a risk for triggering pustular psoriasis, which can be seriously debilitating. There are no clinical study data to justify the use of glucocorticoids for the treatment of PsA [49].

12.2.2 Nonsteroidal Anti-Inflammatory Drugs

Patients who have minor joint involvement can be treated with NSAIDs [50–52], and simultaneously, psoriasis can be treated accordingly to its severity. However, to be very specific, NSAIDs

TABLE 12.8
GRAPPA: Treatment Recommendations for Psoriatic Arthritis

Indication	Recommended Strong	Recommended Conditionally	Not Recommended	No Recommendations due to Lack of Evidence
Peripheral arthritis, DMARD naïve	DMARDs: Methotrexate Sulfasalazine Leflunomide TNF inhibitors	NSAIDs Oral corticosteroids Intra-articular corticosteroids PDE4 inhibitors		IL-12/IL-23 inhibitors IL-17 inhibitors
Peripheral arthritis, DMARD inadequately responsive	TNF inhibitors IL-12/IL-23 inhibitors (ustekinumab) PDE4 inhibitors	NSAIDs Oral corticosteroids Intra-articular corticosteroids IL-17 inhibitors		
Peripheral arthritis, DMARD inadequately responsive	TNF inhibitors	NSAIDs Oral corticosteroids Intra-articular corticosteroids IL-12/IL-23 inhibitors IL-17 inhibitors PDE4 inhibitors		
Axial PsA, biologic naïve (based on ankylosing spondylitis literature)	NSAIDs Physiotherapy Simple analgesia TNF inhibitors	IL-17 inhibitors Sacroiliac corticosteroid injections Bisphosphonates IL-12/IL-23 inhibitors	DMARDs IL-6 inhibitors CD20 inhibitors	
Axial PsA, biologic inadequately responsive (based on ankylosing spondylitis literature)	Physiotherapy Simple analgesia	NSAIDs TNF inhibitors IL-12/IL-23 inhibitors IL-17 inhibitors		
Enthesitis	TNF inhibitors IL-12/IL-23 inhibitors	NSAIDs Physiotherapy Intra-articular corticosteroids (with caution as at risk for rupture of entheses in weight-bearing sites) PDE4 inhibitors IL-17 inhibitors		DMARDs

(*Continued*)

TABLE 12.8 (CONTINUED)
GRAPPA: Treatment Recommendations for Psoriatic Arthritis

Indication	Recommended Strong	Recommended Conditionally	Not Recommended	No Recommendations due to Lack of Evidence
Dactylitis	TNF inhibitors (infliximab, adalimumab, golimumab, certolizumab)	Intra-articular corticosteroids DMARDs (methotrexate, leflunomide, sulfsalazine) TNF inhibitors (etanercept) IL-12/IL-23 inhibitors IL-17 inhibitors (secukinumab) PDE4 inhibitors		
Psoriasis (skin)	Topical therapies Phototherapy DMARDs (methotrexate, leflunomide, cyclosporine) TNF inhibitors IL-12/IL-23 inhibitors IL-17 inhibitors PDE4 inhibitors			
Nail psoriasis	TNF inhibitors IL-12/IL-23 inhibitors	Topical therapies Procedural therapies DMARDs (methotrexate, leflunomide, cyclosporine, acitretin) IL-17 inhibitors PDE4 inhibitors		

Source: Adapted from Coates, L. C. et al., *Arthritis Rheumatol.*, 68(5), 1060–1071, 2016.

usually relieve joint pain and swelling in PsA patients, but it should be noted that they do not alter the progression of the disease process in PsA.

There are two randomized controlled trials (RCTs) that have evaluated the efficacy of NSAIDs for the treatment of PsA. A 4-week trial compared cyclooxygenase (COX) 2–selective NSAID, nimesulide, and placebo in 76 patients and demonstrated that there was significant decrease in the TJC and SJC with 200 and 400 mg daily dosing of nimesulide [51]. On the contrary, a 12-week RCT for celecoxib (a selective COX-2 inhibitor) compared the safety and efficacy of two doses of celecoxib (200 and 400 mg) daily to placebo for pain relief in PsA. At the end of the study (week 12), it was seen that there was no statistically noticeable difference in American College of Rheumatology (ACR) Responder Index (ACR20) response with celecoxib compared with the placebo groups [52].

12.2.3 Methotrexate

Methotrexate is presently U.S. Food and Drug Administration (FDA) approved for psoriasis [53]. The success of methotrexate in psoriasis is a landmark event for the treatment of many autoimmune diseases, and methotrexate has been used as a steroid-sparing agent in multiple autoimmune conditions. Methotrexate is a competitive inhibitor of the enzyme dihydrofolate reductase (DHFR), which is necessary for tetrahydrofolate synthesis. Through this pathway, methotrexate ultimately inhibits DNA, RNA, and thymidylates, and thus alters protein synthesis. Although proper clinical proof has not been found on the efficacy of methotrexate in PsA, it is usually used as a first-line treatment in PsA as a monotherapy or in combination with biologics [54]. Methotrexate in Psoriatic Arthritis (MIPA), a large RCT, compared methotrexate (target dose 15 mg weekly) with placebo and used Psoriatic Arthritis Response Criteria (PsARC) as a primary outcome measure, and secondary end points were ACR20 and DAS28. Out of 221 patients, a total of 151 patients completed the trial (74 in MTX and 77 in placebo groups). Although with MTX there was improvement in the PsARC, there was no statistically remarkable difference in the PsARC, DAS28, ACR, and erythrocyte sedimentation rate (ESR) levels, and the SJC or TJC was found between the MTX and the placebo groups [55].

The Norwegian DMARD registry study compared 430 PsA patients with 1280 RA patients and looked for the efficacy and retention rate of methotrexate in these two groups. Both the PsA and RA patients improved in most disease activity measures and patient-reported outcomes after 6 months, but this improvement was much less in PsA patients [56]. Also, two randomized placebo-controlled studies have reported marked improvement in *global* assessment in PsA patients with the use of methotrexate, but none of them showed improvement of objective measures, such as improvement in TJC and SJC [55,57]. Also, over a period of 24 months PsA patients treated with or without methotrexate did not to show any statistically noticeable difference in the radiographic progression of their joint conditions [58]. Usually, the adverse effects associated with methotrexate are hepatotoxicity, myelosuppression, and pneumonitis [59].

12.2.4 Leflunomide

Leflunomide is a pyrimidine synthesis inhibitor that blocks T-cell activation and proliferation [60]. Although it is recommended by the European Medicines Agency (EMA) for PsA, as of now the FDA has approved it only for the treatment of RA. In a 24-week randomized placebo-controlled trial carried out in 186 patients, leflunomide not only showed significant improvement in the PsARC (59% vs. 30%, respectively) but also showed better results in tender and swollen joint scores, the Health Assessment Questionnaire (HAQ), and the Dermatology Life Quality Index (DLQI) in comparison with placebo. Recently, in a randomized, double-blind, placebo-controlled clinical trials in patients with concomitant psoriasis and PsA, leflunomide seemed to display marked clinical responses in both skin and joint symptoms when compared with placebo [39,61–63]. The most common side effects of leflunomide noticed were gastrointestinal toxicity (e.g., diarrhea and nausea), elevated liver enzymes, and leukopenia [64].

12.2.5 Sulfasalazine

Sulfasalazine has been assessed in six RCTs in PsA [65–69]. Sulfasalazine is a sulfa drug that is prepared by combining salicylate and sulfapyridine through an azo bond. Its mechanism of action is not very clear; there are suggestions that sulfasalazine may work by inhibiting the 5-lipoxygenase pathway [70]. Clegg and colleagues, in a large sulfasalazine study that included 221 patients, randomized 2 g/day of sulfasalazine against a placebo [71]. The study showed that about 55% of patients in the treatment arm compared with 45% patients in the placebo arm achieved response based on PsARC. The other RCTs with sulfasalazine had fewer patients; only pain scores were considered an outcome measure; also, these studies do not have any results on radiologic progression [68,69]. Sulfasalazine can cause gastrointestinal intolerance, arthralgia, and reversible oligospermia, as well as some severe outcomes, such as leukopenia and agranulocytosis [71,72].

12.2.6 Cyclosporine A, Azathioprine, and Antimalarials

Antimalarials, for example, hydroxychloroquine, are recommended for RA but are not usually used to treat PsA because of their tendency to aggravate psoriasis or trigger an outbreak in susceptible individuals [73]. But, a case-control series of 32 patients treated with hydroxychloroquine did not show any increased risk of a psoriasis flare in the hydroxychloroquine group when compared with placebo. Moreover, a noticeable decrease in the number of actively inflamed joints was seen in the hydroxychloroquine group [74].

Three RCTs have been carried out on the safety of cyclosporine A in PsA; however, its results are only average, and the risk for serious adverse effects rightly restrains its use [75–77]. Cyclosporine A has been recommended by the FDA for the treatment of severe refractory psoriasis [72]. Cyclosporine-associated nephrotoxicity and hypertension not only deter its use for long-term therapy but also limit its feasibility for use in PsA [72].

A purine antimetabolite, azathioprine is an immunosuppressant. It is presently approved for posttransplant immunosuppression and RA. One randomized trial evaluating azathioprine for PsA has been seen in the literature, a double-blind crossover study conducted over 12 months that randomized patients to azathioprine or placebo for every 6-month period [78]. The trial showed a significant improvement in both skin and joint manifestations with azathioprine treatment. Very recently, a case series in 28 patients showed that azathioprine was well-tolerated over a period of 12 months with similar results to DMARDs, proving that it may be beneficial in methotrexate-refractory PsA and in patients where methotrexate is contraindicated [79]. The major side effects of azathioprine include myelosuppression, gastrointestinal upset, and hepatic toxicity [72].

12.3 BEYOND TRADITIONAL DMARDS: BIOLOGICS IN THE TREATMENT OF PSORIATIC ARTHRITIS

12.3.1 Anti-TNF Agents

The primary resource of TNF (cachexin or cachectin) is monocytes and macrophages and cells derived from their lineage. However, various other cells, such as the activated T cells, can secrete a large amount of TNF. TNF is involved in systemic inflammation. It is synthesized first as a transmembrane precursor protein. Then the cytoplasmic tail of this protein is cleaved to release soluble TNF. TNF's primary role is regulation of an inflammatory response. TNF requires aggregation of its three TNF monomers to form trimeric TNF for its biological activity. The trimeric TNF acts by binding on its receptors TNFR1 or TNFR2. TNFR1 and TNFR2 are known as p55 and p75, respectively. TNFR1 is expressed in most tissues and can be fully activated by both the membrane-bound and soluble trimeric forms of TNF, whereas TNFR2 is only found in cells of the immune system and responds to the membrane-bound form of the TNF homotrimer. Most information about TNF signaling is derived from TNFR1; the role of TNFR2 remains largely unknown.

TNF is seen to have a significant effect in chronic inflammatory diseases, such as psoriasis and PsA. At the moment, a number of TNF inhibitors are available, and thus it is good to have several options for their clinical use. Many of the oral inhibitors have the ability to inhibit TNF, and biologics have evolved as excellent tools to *exclusively* target TNF. Among the most commonly used biologic anti-TNF agents for psoriasis are etanercept, infliximab, and adalimumab, and relatively newer anti-TNF agents are golimumab and certolizumab [80]. Etanercept binds with only a single trimer of TNF, which is an engineered protein comprising a dimer of the human TNFR2, fused to the Fc portion of human IgG1. Etanercept also binds and inhibits other TNF receptor ligands, such as the lymphotoxin (LT) family members, which also play an important role in various types of autoimmune arthritis [81].

Infliximab is a chimeric anti-TNF monoclonal antibody (mAb) (mouse–human IgG1), whereas adalimumab and golimumab are fully humanized IgG1 anti-TNF monoclonal antibodies [80]. Unlike etancercept, the anti-TNF monoclonal antibodies have the ability to bind to both the monomer and trimer forms of TNF. Along with its soluble form, TNF is also found as a transmembrane protein (tmTNF). Adalimumab and infliximab can become directly cytotoxic to tmTNF-bearing cells by inducing complement-dependent cytotoxicity (CDC) and antibody-dependent cellular cytotoxicity (ADCC). Moreover, studies have demonstrated that once bound to TNF, both infliximab and adalimumab, but not etanercept, can bind strongly to FcγRII and FcγRIII receptors [80]. Also, etanercept cannot bind to the complement protein C1q. As a result, adalimumab and infliximab induce ADCC much more potently than etanercept. Also, differences in Fc receptor and complement C1q binding may be the reason behind the differences in efficacy among the TNF antagonists.

It is clear that TNF antagonists have made a breakthrough in the management of PsA, and their excellent clinic response in PsA has been further justified by their ability to inhibit radiographic progression of arthritis [82–92]. Among all the TNF antagonists tried, the effects in treating joint disease activity, inhibiting structural damage, and improving function and QoL appeared to be similar depending on the doses given. As far as safety issues are concerned, there is risk for infection; no additional concerns were noted in the PsA population compared with the most widely studied RA patient population. So far, the FDA has approved five specific anti-TNF agents, which are described in Table 12.9.

TABLE 12.9
Currently Available TNF-α Inhibitors for Psoriatic Arthritis

Name	Description	Half-Life	Route of Administration	Frequency of Dosing
Infliximab (Remicade®)	Mouse/human chimeric anti-TNF-α antibody	8–10 days	Intravenous infusion	• Induction with 3 doses within first 10 weeks • Every 8 weeks thereafter
Etanercept (Enbrel®)	Soluble p75 TNF-α receptor fusion protein	4–6 days	Subcutaneous injection (SQ)	Once a week
Adalimumab (Humira®)	Human monoclonal anti-TNF-α antibody	2 weeks	SQ	Once every 2 weeks
Golimumab (Simponi®)	Human monoclonal anti-TNF-α antibody	2 weeks	SQ	Once a month
Certolizumab pegol (Cimzia®)	Pegylated Fab fragment of humanized monoclonal TNF-α antibody	2 weeks	SQ	Once a month or every 2 weeks

12.3.1.1 Etanercept

In 2002, etanercept obtained approval from the FDA for the treatment of PsA. An RCT of etanercept 25 mg twice weekly (BIW) in 205 patients with PsA, in comparison with placebo, revealed significant improvement in the ACR20 response (59% vs. 15%) [87]. The etanercept group also showed remarkable regression of radiographic changes (mean adjusted change in total Sharp score of –0.38 from baseline to 2 years) when compared with the placebo group [93].

A multicenter Psoriasis Randomized Etanercept Study in Subjects with Psoriatic Arthritis (PRESTA) compared the results of two different etanercept regimens, 50 mg once weekly (QW) and 50 mg BIW, in 752 patients suffering from moderate to severe psoriasis with PsA. Over a period of 12 weeks, this trial observed that the effect of 50 mg BIW was far better than that of the doses of 50 mg QW for psoriasis. As far as joint manifestations of PSA are concerned, no remarkable differences were found in between the QW and BIW dosing schedules as assessed by the PsARC at the end of 12 weeks. Another PRESTA trial carried out on patients for a period of 12 weeks, an open-label extension of etanercept 50 mg QW versus 60 mg BIW, showed significant results in cutaneous psoriasis, as well as joint changes in both dosage groups [94].

12.3.1.2 Infliximab

Since 2005, infliximab has been used for treating PsA. Two big RCTs were carried out on patients before it was approved [83,95]: the Infliximab Multinational Psoriatic Arthritis Controlled Trial (IMPACT) and IMPACT 2 studies. The IMPACT trial, carried out over a period of 16 weeks, assessed infliximab 5 mg/kg at weeks 0, 2, 6, and 14 against placebo in 104 patients. The primary end point for this study was to identify the ACR20 response at the end of 16 weeks. ACR20 responses in the infliximab group was 65% compared with 10% in the placebo group [83].

In the IMPACT 2 study, carried out over a period of 24 weeks (randomized, $n = 200$), infliximab 5 mg/kg was compared with the placebo at weeks 0, 2, 6, 14, and 22; the primary end point was ACR20 achievement, and the secondary end points were PASI, PsARC, and dactylitis and entheseopathy assessments [95]. A total of 58% of the infliximab group, at the end of 14 weeks, obtained ACR20 and 77% obtained PsARC against 27% of patients in the placebo group [95]. Moreover, at the end of 14 and 24 weeks, active enthesopathy was significantly less in the infliximab group (18% and 20%, respectively) against the placebo cohort (30% and 37%) [95]. Radiological changes in the hands and feet of patients who completed 12-month IMPACT and IMPACT 2 trials were recorded and assigned a PsA modified van der Heijde–Sharp (vdH-S) score to determine the effect of infliximab on x-ray changes. Both the IMPACT and IMPACT 2 trials exhibited a marked effect of infliximab in retarding the progression of joint damage [84,96]. In the case of the IMPACT trial, for infliximab and placebo cohorts, average changes in the modified vdH-S scores from the beginning to week 50 were –1.95 and –1.52, respectively ($p < 0.001$) [84]. Further evaluation of the IMPACT 2 trial also revealed noticeable results ($p < 0.001$): vdH-S scores of –0.70 and 0.82 at week 24 and –0.94 and 0.53 at week 54 for infliximab and placebo groups, respectively [96].

Of late, in another trial, Remicade in Psoriatic Arthritis Patients of Methotrexate-Naïve Disease (RESPOND), the efficacy and safety of infliximab + methotrexate against methotrexate alone in 115 methotrexate-naïve patients with PsA was studied. Patients were asked to have an infliximab (5 mg/kg) infusion at 0, 2, 6, and 14 weeks, along with methotrexate (15 mg weekly), and the control group was assigned for methotrexate (15 mg/week). The primary outcome measure was an ACR20 response at the end of 16 weeks, and the secondary end points were DAS28, PASI, and actylitis and enthesitis assessments [97]. It was found that a majority of the patients (86.3%) in the infliximab–methotrexate group had an ACR20 response at week 16, against the patients who took only methotrexate (66.7%, $p < 0.0001$). The PASI-75 at week 16 was 97.1% in the combination therapy group against 54.3% patients who took only methotrexate ($p < 0.0001$). Altogether, about 46% of patients in the combination infliximab–methotrexate group had treatment-related adverse effects in the trial period against 24% in the methotrexate monotherapy cohort [97].

12.3.1.3 Adalimumab

The Adalimumab in Psoriatic Arthritis (ADEPT) trial, over a period of 24 weeks in 313 patients, compared the efficacy of adalimumab 40 mg versus placebo every alternate week in the treatment of NSAID-refractory PsA [85]. The primary end points of the ADEPT trial were ACR20 response at week 12, along with a change in the modified Sharp score for assessing structural joint changes at the end of 24 weeks. The ACR20 response at the end of 12 weeks was seen in 58% of the adalimumab-treated patients against 14% of the placebo group ($p < 0.001$). ACR20 response rates were maintained at week 24, and the average change in the modified Sharp score was –0.2 in patients taking adalimumab and 1.0 in the placebo group ($p < 0.001$) [85]. In between, evaluation of an open-label extension of the ADEPT study comprising adalimumab 40 mg every alternate week up to 120 weeks showed the presence of identical ACR20 results and improvements in joint disease after 2 years of treatment [98].

In another RCT study, the efficacy of adalimumab was also observed in a group of 100 PsA patients with a record of poor response to DMARDs for a period of 24 weeks [99]. Patients were selected to take adalimumab 40 mg or placebo on alternate weeks for 12 weeks, followed by an open-label period where all the patients received adalimumab 40 mg on the alternate week up to week 24. Altogether, 39% of adalimumab-treated patients obtained the primary end point of ACR20 at week 12, against 16% of patients in the placebo group ($p < 0.012$). In the open-label phase, all throughout improvement was found in the adalimumab group: 65% obtained ACR20 at week 24, and early signs of improvement were found in the group earlier randomized to placebo, with 57% achieving ACR20 at week 24 ($p < 0.007$) [99].

The results of adalimumab in relation to those of cyclosporine in a prospective 12-month nonrandomized open-label clinical trial were also studied wherein patients were asked to take cyclosporine (2.5–3.75 mg/kg/day), adalimumab (40 mg every other week), or both regimens [100]. Within a year, ACR20 was obtained by 65% of patients in the cyclosporine group ($p = 0.0003$ vs. combination), 85% in the adalimumab group ($p = 0.15$ vs. combination), and 95% who were given both therapies. The ACR50 rates were found to be 36% for cyclosporine, 69% for adalimumab, and 87% for combination therapy ($p < 0.0001$ and $p = 0.03$ vs. combination) [100]. Remarkably, this trial did not reveal any noticeable rise in the incidence of treatment-related side effects in the group who was on combination therapy.

12.3.1.4 Golimumab

Golimumab is a monthly anti-TNF agent. It was recommended by the FDA for PsA in 2009 after the positive results of the large Golimumab-A Randomized Evaluation of Safety and Efficacy in Subjects with Psoriatic Arthritis Using a Human Anti-TNF Monoclonal Antibody (GO-REVEAL) study [101]. The trial was carried out over a period of 24 weeks, wherein patients were randomized to get subcutaneous golimumab (50 or 100 mg) or placebo every 4 weeks for 20 weeks. On the 14th week, ACR20 were obtained by 51% of the patients in the 50 mg golimumab group, 45% in the 100 mg golimumab group, and 9% in the placebo group ($p < 0.001$). Improvement in PASI (for patients with at least a 3% body surface area [BSA] affected by psoriasis) was an additional end point of the study, and PASI-75 was seen in 40% of patients in the 50 mg golimumab arm, 58% in the 100 mg golimumab arm, and 3% in the placebo cohort ($p < 0.001$) [101]. Beneficial effects of both of these clinical end points were achieved by the 24th week. Placebo patients were given golimumab 50 mg monthly in the blinded extension of this study, and patients who were on 50 or 100 mg golimumab monthly were kept on the same regimen; clinical improvement in the ACR20 and PASI score, as observed at week 24 in the GO-REVEAL study, could be maintained in this blinded extension trial [102]. At the end of 1 year, the GO-REVEAL trial showed marked radiological changes in both golimumab groups (50 and 100 mg) compared with the placebo group [102].

An open-label extension of the GO-REVEAL trial ($n = 279$) was continued for 5 years [103]. An elaborate study of the 5-year efficacy records proved that golimumab was successful in maintaining clinical benefits in the ACR20 (62.8%–69.9% for randomized patients) and PASI-75 (60.8%–72.2% for randomized patients with >3% BSA affected by psoriasis). Also, golimumab demonstrated good results in inhibiting radiological changes. The intake of methotrexate did not significantly change the ACR20 and PASI-75 results, but did reduce the radiographic progression [103].

12.3.1.5 Certolizumab

Certolizumab received approval for treating PsA in the year 2013 [104]. In contrast to other TNF antagonists, certolizumab is a pegylated, humanized Fab′ fragment of the anti-TNF mAb. In the RAPID-PsA multicenter RCT trial ($n = 409$), certolizumab pegol (CZP) 200 mg was given to patients every 2 weeks and CZP 400 mg was given every 4 weeks, or a placebo was used [105]. The primary end points of this study were ACR20 at week 12 and modified total Sharp score (mTSS) at week 24. The ACR20 response at week 12 was remarkably greater in patients taking CZP 400 mg every 4 weeks (51.9%) or CZP 200 mg every 2 weeks (58%) in contrast to 24.3% in the placebo arm ($p < 0.001$). While evaluating mTSSs to look for radiographic progression, it appeared that most of the patients (both CZP and placebo) did not show mTSS changes over a period of 24 weeks in this study [106].

12.3.2 IL-12/IL-23 Inhibition: Ustekinumab

Psoriasis plaques overexpress IL-12, IL-17, and IL-23 [107,108]. IL-23 is necessary for regulating IL-17-secreting Th17 cells. Th17 T cells play a critical role in a number of inflammatory diseases: ankylosing spondylitis, psoriasis, and PsA [108]. In support of data in favor of IL-23's significance in psoriasis, it has been observed that long-term subcutaneous injections of IL-23 can initiate the psoriasis phenotype in mice [109].

Ustekinumab, an anti-IL-12/IL-23 mAb, is beneficial in the treatment of psoriasis. Ustekinumab has been found to be more effective than etanercept [110,111]. In PsA, a randomized, double-blind, placebo-controlled crossover study of ustekinumab has demonstrated significant positive changes in ACR response rates and marked effects on enthesitis, dactylitis, skin disease, and physical functioning [112]. The same outcome was found in a randomized placebo-controlled Phase III clinical trial with ustekinumab in PsA patients who also had anti-TNF and DMARD therapy [113]. PSUMMIT 1 is a randomized control study ($n = 615$) in which PsA patients were given ustekinumab 45 mg, ustekinumab 90 mg, or placebo at weeks 0 and 4 and then every 12 weeks. After 24 weeks, ACR20 responses were 42.4%, 49.5%, and 22.8%, respectively [113]. Improvements were also noticed in dactylitis, enthesitis, and HAQ [114]. In PsA, the same ACR20 response for ustekinumab was found in the PSUMMIT 2 trial carried out in 312 patients [115].

12.3.3 Anti-IL-17 Antagonists

IL-17 is a pro-inflammatory cytokine that plays an important part in the pathogenesis of psoriatic disease [116]. Using an IL-17A gene transfer model, investigators have reportedly proved that IL-17 singly could initiate expansion of IL-17RA + CD11b + Gr1 low osteoclast precursors and, at the same time, increase the levels of biomarkers specific to bone resorption [117]. Additionally, in the same study, IL-17 gene transfer was found to trigger cutaneous changes specific for psoriasis, such as epidermal hyperplasia, parakeratosis, and formation of Munro's microabscesses.

In recent years, the IL-17 pathway has been the primary focus for drug development of psoriatic disease. The following FDA-approved anti-IL-17 preparations are currently available:

1. Secukinumab: A fully human anti-IL-17A mAb, which has been recommended by the FDA for treating PsA, psoriasis, and ankylosing spondylitis
2. Brodalumab: A fully human IL-17 receptor (IL-17RA) mAb, approved for psoriasis
3. Ixekizumab: A humanized anti-IL-17A mAb, approved for psoriasis

Secukinumab, ixekizumab, and broadalumab are found to be useful in the treatment of psoriasis and PsA [118–126].

12.3.3.1 Secukinumab

Of late, FDA recommendations of secukinumab for treating PsA were the result of several Phase II and Phase III trials. A Phase II proof-of-concept trial was carried out over 24 weeks for secukimumab (two doses of 10 mg, spaced 3 weeks apart) against placebo in 42 patients with PsA. The primary end point in this study was an ACR20 response at week 6 [121]. In spite of nonachievement of the primary end point, 39% of secukinumab patients had an ACR20 response compared with 23% in the placebo group ($p = 0.27$). A marked decrease in the ESR ($p = 0.038$), C-reactive protein (CRP) ($p = 0.039$), Short Form Health Survey (SF-36) ($p = 0.030$), and Health Assessment Questionnaire Disability Index (HAQDI) ($p = 0.002$) were also noticed. A 48-week Phase III RCT ($n = 798$) assessed the following doses of secukinumab: 150 mg and 300 mg at weeks 1, 2, and 3 and then every 4 weeks subsequently. In this Phase III RCT, significant improvement was noticed in PASI-75 and HAQDI in the secukinumab cohort in contrast to the placebo group [127]. In the FUTURE 2 trial, a multicenter RCT compared three different dosing regimens of secukimumab in PsA ($n = 397$). The patients received 300, 150, or 75 mg QW for 4 weeks, and then every 4 weeks from week 4; in this placebo-controlled study, the primary end point was ACR20 at week 24 [128]. The number of patients achieving this end point was remarkably higher in the secukinumab cohort than in the placebo group (15%); the ACR20 responses for 300, 150, and 75 mg of secukinumab were 54% ($p < 0.0001$), 51% ($p < 0.0001$), and 29% ($p < 0.001$), respectively [128].

12.3.3.2 Brodalumab and Ixekizumab

Both broadalumab and ixekizumab have been approved by the FDA for treatment of psoriasis. Ixekizumab has been used in psoriasis (UNCOVER-2 and UNCOVER-3 Phase III trials), and trials are being conducted for use in PsA (SPIRIT-P1, Phase III) [123,129]. In the UNCOVER trials, ixekizumab (160 mg loading followed by 80 mg every 2 or 4 weeks), in contrast to etanercept (50 mg BIW) and placebo, has demonstrated excellent outcomes in psoriasis [129].

For PsA, the ongoing Phase III SPIRIT-P1 trial has been comparing ixekizumab with adalimumab; there is also a placebo arm in this study [123]. The trial period was 24 weeks, wherein patients were randomized to ixekizumab (160 mg loading dose and thereafter given 80 mg every 2 or 4 weeks), adalimumab (40 mg every other week), and the placebo group. After the RCT was over, patients were assessed for 3 years to look for the long-term efficacy and safety of brodalumab. In April 2015, the corporate sponsor (Eli Lilly) declared that the ixekizumab-treated PsA patients demonstrated a significantly better ACR20 response than those with the placebo.

The recommended doses for the above anti-IL-17 agents are given below. These preparations are given as subcutaneous injections.

- Secukinumab
  - Plaque psoriasis: 300 mg/week at weeks 0, 1, 2, 3, and 4, then 300 mg every 4 weeks
  - PsA: 150 mg/week at weeks 0, 1, 2, 3, and 4, then 150 mg every 4 weeks
- Ixekizumab
  - Plaque psoriasis: 160 mg first dose, then 80 mg at weeks 2, 4, 6, 8, 10, 12, and then 80 mg/week
  - Brodalumab: 210 mg at weeks 0, 1, and 2, then 210 mg every 2 weeks

12.3.4 Phosphodiesterase 4 Inhibition

PDE4 is a PDE isoform and is widely found in immune cells, such as neutrophils, monocytes, and T cells [130]. Apremilast is an inhibitor of PDE4 and can be given orally for the treatment of PsA. In 2014, the FDA gave its recommendation for apremilast. The PDE family of enzymes is responsible for the enzymatic degradation of cyclic AMP (cAMP). cAMP, an important second messenger of cellular signaling, regulates a number of cellular functions in almost every cell [130]. Apremilast blocks the PDE4-mediated breakdown of cAMP [131,132].

The Psoriatic Arthritis Long-Term Assessment of Clinical Efficacy (PALACE) program has assessed the efficacy of apremilast in active PsA patients. The PALACE study comprised four randomized placebo-controlled trials and open-label extensions [133–139]. The PALACE 1, PALACE 2, and PALACE 3 trials provide evidence for clinical efficacy of apremilast.

The PALACE 1 trial was carried over a period of 24 weeks where 504 patients were randomized to apremilast 30 mg twice daily (APR30), apremilast 20 mg twice daily (APR20), and placebo. The primary end point was ACR20 at week 16 [139]. It was noted that more patients in the APR30 (40%) and APR20 (31%) achieved the ACR20 response than in the placebo group (19%, $p < 0.001$) [139]. In the PALACE 2 study, 484 patients were randomized to APR30, APR20, and placebo for 52 weeks [138]. At the end of 16 weeks, the number of patients who recorded an ACR20 response was 34.4% in the APR30 group, 38.4% in the APR20 group, and 19.5% in the placebo group. Remarkable achievements of the ACR20 response were found with apremilast with longer durations: at 52 weeks, 52.9% in the APR20 group and 52.6% in the APR30 group [138]. The PALACE 4 trial compared DMARD-naïve patients with PsA, and at the 16th week, the ACR20 response figure was found to be 29% in the APR20 group ($p < 0.0235$), 32% in the APR30 group ($p < 0.0001$), and 17% in the placebo cohort [136].

12.4 EMERGING TREATMENT OPTIONS

12.4.1 Janus Kinase Inhibitors

The Janus kinase (JAK)–STAT kinase cascade plays a critical role in cell signaling induced by multiple cytokines [140]. A number of pro-inflammatory cytokine receptors utilize the JAK-STAT signal transduction pathways, which are important for the pathogenesis of psoriatic disease, such as IL-2, IL-6, IL-9, and IL-23. Tofacitinib, a small-molecule inhibitor for JAK1/JAK3, and now also established as a JAK2 inhibitor, is approved by the FDA for RA in patients who have failed DMARDs [141]. For RA, it is given orally at a 5 mg dose twice daily. Several randomized double-blind, placebo-controlled trials with tofacitinib, both Phase I and Phase II, have demonstrated a significant PASI-75 response for psoriasis [142,143]. Currently, multiple trials are going on for PsA and ankylosing spondylitis.

12.4.2 Costimulatory Blockade

Antigen-presenting cells (APCs) process and present the antigen to T cells [144]. Acting as a costimulatory molecule, CD28 induces T-cell activation by interacting with CD80/86 on the surface of APCs. CTLA4, the physiological T-cell costimulator inhibitor, controls this process by blocking the CD28-CD80/86 interaction. Abatacept (CTLA4-Ig) is synthesized to block the T-cell costimulatory signals; here CTLA4, the T-cell costimulator inhibitory molecule, is fused to the IgFc region. Thus, abatacept is a recombinant human fusion protein. When administered, abatacept is accepted to bind on CD80/86 molecules and prevents the binding of CD28 with CD80/86, and thus there is inhibited functional interaction between T cells and APCs [145]. Abatacept is given as a monthly intravenous injection. Abatacept has proven its efficacy in psoriasis and PsA [146,147]. In a Phase II trial (abatacept, 10 mg/kg IV monthly), 48% ($n = 40$) of patients with PsA achieved an ACR20 response compared with 19% in the placebo group ($p = 0.006$) [147]. But, the PASI-75 response for psoriasis was not satisfactory. Abatacept is also available as a subcutaneous preparation, and the recommended dose for RA is 125 mg subcutaneously QW.

12.5 DRUGS IN PRECLINICAL DEVELOPMENT FOR PSORIATIC ARTHRITIS

The main pathologic effects in psoriasis and PsA are also the "uncontrolled proliferation" of keratinocytes, synovial fibroblasts, endothelial cells, and T cells [1]. The mTOR signaling pathway is constitutively activated in various malignant disorders, and the efficacy of phosphatidylinositol 3-kinase (PI3K), Akt, and mTOR inhibitors in preclinical models of malignant diseases proves its role in uncontrolled cell proliferation [148]. These observations encouraged us to investigate the regulatory role of the mTOR kinase cascades in psoriasis and PsA. We have reported that mTOR signaling proteins are significantly upregulated in psoriatic disease, and further, we have demonstrated that a kinase PI3K/mTORC1 inhibitor, NVP-BEZ235, has potent antiproliferative effects on keratinocyte and synovial cells [149]. These results have been substantiated by other investigators, and currently mTOR-targeted therapies are being investigated for psoriatic disease. Numerous mTOR kinase inhibitors are nowadays in clinical development as anticancer agents, and we believe that very soon they will be evaluated in psoriatic disease. Kv1.3 is one of the two major K+ channels that are expressed in lymphocytes. These channels play a regulatory role during signal transduction in immunocytes, and they also induce proliferation and activation of immunocytes [150]. Our preclinical study recorded an increased number of Kv1.3-positive cells in psoriatic skin, as well as in the synovium of PsA [150]. In recent times, a number of Kv1.3 inhibitors are in preclinical development for psoriatic disease. And out of these small-molecule inhibitors, PAP-1 has depicted promising effects in our preclinical studies of psoriasis [150].

Nerve growth factor (NGF), a neurotrophic factor, was first identified in the nervous system, and with time, it has been identified in most of the organs. NGF acts on its two well-recognized receptors (NGF-R): tyrosine receptor kinase A (TrkA), its high-affinity receptor, and p75, the low-affinity receptor. Preclinical studies have revealed that levels of NGF are greater in synovial fluid samples from PsA and RA patients in comparison with samples from osteoarthritis patients [151]. NGF is also a pro-growth and pro-survival factor for activated T cells, fibroblast-like synovium (FLS), keratinocytes, and endothelial cells [151]. Thus, targeting NGF or its receptor may have benefits in treating psoriasis and PsA. In an in vivo study using the severe combined immunodeficient mouse–human skin model of psoriasis, we observed that treatment with K252a, a high-affinity NGF-R blocker, resulted in improvement of psoriasis [152]. NGF and TrkA targeted therapies are likely to help both the inflammatory cascades, and NGF-induced joint pain in the psoriatic arthritis [153–155].

Angiogenesis is believed to be a key pathogenic feature of psoriatic disease [156,157]. Following administration of vascular endothelial growth factor (VEGF) inhibitors (sorafenib, sunitinib, and bevacizumab) for the treatment of various malignant conditions, several case reports have demonstrated improvement of psoriasis and PsA [158,159]. Recently, we have found that bevacizumab may be very effective in PsA [159]. These results suggest VEGF as a possible target for novel therapies in psoriasis and PsA [160].

12.6 CONCLUSION

Dermatologists treating psoriasis patients have the scope for routine screening of early PsA by inquiring for evidence for joint pain, stiffness, or tenderness. PsA can also be identified at a very early stage by rapid screening questionnaires. PsA is a chronic and progressive inflammatory arthritis that is very closely associated with psoriasis, and together psoriatic disease can produce significant morbidity. Ideal interventions for active PsA should look for skin and joint involvement simultaneously. Even if conventional DMARDs may possibly work for some patients, they have not yet demonstrated the stoppage of the PsA disease process. It is extremely important to diagnose PsA at a very early stage. All efforts should be made to control the inflammatory process and prevent joint destruction and disability. Treatment should be started as discussed earlier, and depending on the severity of the disease, PsA may require aggressive treatment at the initial stage of the disease.

REFERENCES

1. Raychaudhuri SP. A cutting edge overview: Psoriatic disease. *Clin Rev Allergy Immunol* 2013;44(2):109–13.
2. Chandran V, Raychaudhuri SP. Geoepidemiology and environmental factors of psoriasis and psoriatic arthritis. *J Autoimmun* 2010;34(3):J314–21.
3. Raychaudhuri SP, Wilken R, Sukhov AC, Raychaudhuri SK, Maverakis E. Management of psoriatic arthritis: Early diagnosis, monitoring of disease severity and cutting edge therapies. *J Autoimmun* 2017;76:21–37.
4. Machado PM, Raychaudhuri SP. Disease activity measurements and monitoring in psoriatic arthritis and axial spondyloarthritis. *Best Pract Res Clin Rheumatol* 2014;28:711–28.
5. Kauffman CL, Aria N, Toichi E, McCormick TS, Cooper KD, Gottlieb AB et al. A phase I study evaluating the safety, pharmacokinetics, and clinical response of a human IL-12 p40 antibody in subjects with plaque psoriasis. *J Invest Dermatol* 2004;123:1037–44.
6. Litinsky I, Balbir-Gurman A, Wollman J, Arad U, Paran D, Caspi D et al. Ultrasound assessment of enthesis thickening in psoriatic arthritis patients treated with adalimumab compared to methotrexate. *Clin Rheumatol* 2016;35(2):363–70.
7. Atteno M, Peluso R, Costa L, Padula S, Iervolino S, Caso F et al. Comparison of effectiveness and safety of infliximab, etanercept, and adalimumab in psoriatic arthritis patients who experienced an inadequate response to previous disease-modifying antirheumatic drugs. *Clin Rheumatol* 2010;29:399–403.
8. Raychaudhuri SP, Gross J. A comparative study of pediatric onset psoriasis with adult onset psoriasis. *Pediatr Dermatol* 2000;17(3):174–8.
9. Duarte GV, Faillace C, Freire de Carvalho J. Psoriatic arthritis. *Best Pract Res Clin Rheumatol* 2012;26:147–56.
10. Hong Q, Ruhaak LR, Stroble C, Parker E, Huang J, Maverakis E et al. A method for comprehensive glycosite—Mapping and direct quantitation of serum glycoproteins. *J Proteome Res* 2015;14:5179–92.
11. Generali E, Scire CA, Favalli EG, Selmi C. Biomarkers in psoriatic arthritis: A systematic literature review. *Expert Rev Clin Immunol* 2016;12(6):651–60.
12. Girolomoni G, Gisondi P. Psoriasis and systemic inflammation: Underdiagnosed enthesopathy. *J Eur Acad Dermatol Venereol* 2009;23(Suppl. 1):3–8.
13. Taylor W, Gladman D, Helliwell P, Marchesoni A, Mease P, Mielants H et al. Classification criteria for psoriatic arthritis: Development of new criteria from a large international study. *Arthritis Rheum* 2006;54:2665–73.
14. Husni ME, Meyer KH, Cohen DS, Mody E, Qureshi AA. The PASE questionnaire: Pilot-testing a psoriatic arthritis screening and evaluation tool. *J Am Acad Dermatol* 2007;57:581–7.
15. Ibrahim GH, Buch MH, Lawson C, Waxman R, Helliwell PS. Evaluation of an existing screening tool for psoriatic arthritis in people with psoriasis and the development of a new instrument: The Psoriasis Epidemiology Screening Tool (PEST) questionnaire. *Clin Exp Rheumatol* 2009;27:469–74.
16. Chandran V, Gladman DD. Toronto Psoriatic Arthritis Screening (ToPAS) questionnaire: A report from the GRAPPA 2009 annual meeting. *J Rheumatol* 2011;38:546–7.
17. Congi L, Roussou E. Clinical application of the CASPAR criteria for psoriatic arthritis compared to other existing criteria. *Clin Exp Rheumatol* 2010;28(3):304–10.
18. Zlatkovic-Svenda M, Kerimovic-Morina D, Stojanovic RM. Psoratic arthritis classification criteria: Moll and Wright, ESSG and CASPAR—A comparative study. *Acta Reumatol Port* 2013;38:172–8.
19. Coates LC, Conaghan PG, Emery P, Green MJ, Ibrahim G, MacIver H et al. Sensitivity and specificity of the classification of psoriatic arthritis criteria in early psoriatic arthritis. *Arthritis Rheum* 2012;64:3150–5.
20. Fransen J, Antoni C, Mease PJ, Uter W, Kavanaugh A, Kalden JR et al. Performance of response criteria for assessing peripheral arthritis in patients with psoriatic arthritis: Analysis of data from randomised controlled trials of two tumour necrosis factor inhibitors. *Ann Rheum Dis* 2006;65:1373–8.
21. Felson DT, Anderson JJ, Boers M, Bombardier C, Furst D, Goldsmith C et al. American College of Rheumatology. Preliminary definition of improvement in rheumatoid arthritis. *Arthritis Rheum* 1995;38:727–35.
22. van Gestel AM, Prevoo ML, van't Hof MA, van Rijswijk MH, van de Putte LB, van Riel PL. Development and validation of the European League Against Rheumatism response criteria for rheumatoid arthritis. Comparison with the preliminary American College of Rheumatology and the World Health Organization/International League Against Rheumatism Criteria. *Arthritis Rheum* 1996;39:34–40.

23. Coates LC, FitzGerald O, Gladman DD, McHugh N, Mease P, Strand V et al. Reduced joint counts misclassify patients with oligoarticular psoriatic arthritis and miss significant numbers of patients with active disease. *Arthritis Rheum* 2013;65:1504–9.
24. Gladman DD, Mease PJ, Strand V, Healy P, Helliwell PS, Fitzgerald O et al. Consensus on a core set of domains for psoriatic arthritis. *J Rheumatol* 2007;34:1167–70.
25. Kilic G, Kilic E, Nas K, Karkucak M, Capkin E, Dagli AZ et al. Comparison of ASDAS and BASDAI as a measure of disease activity in axial psoriatic arthritis. *Clin Rheumatol* 2015;34(3):515–21.
26. Helliwell PS, Fitzgerald O, Mease PJ, Gladman DD. GRAPPA Responder Index Project (GRACE): A report from the GRAPPA 2011 annual meeting. *J Rheumatol* 2012;39:2196–7.
27. Mease PJ. Psoriatic arthritis: Update on pathophysiology, assessment and management. *Ann Rheum Dis* 2011;70(Suppl. 1):i77–84.
28. Schoels M, Aletaha D, Funovits J, Kavanaugh A, Baker D, Smolen JS. Application of the DAREA/DAPSA score for assessment of disease activity in psoriatic arthritis. *Ann Rheum Dis* 2010;69:1441–7.
29. Mumtaz A, Gallagher P, Kirby B, Waxman R, Coates LC, Veale JD et al. Development of a preliminary composite disease activity index in psoriatic arthritis. *Ann Rheum Dis* 2011;70:272–7.
30. Gladman DD, Tom BD, Mease PJ, Farewell VT. Informing response criteria for psoriatic arthritis (PsA). II. Further considerations and a proposal—The PsA joint activity index. *J Rheumatol* 2010;37:2559–65.
31. Gladman DD, Tom BD, Mease PJ, Farewell VT. Informing response criteria for psoriatic arthritis. I. Discrimination models based on data from 3 anti-tumor necrosis factor randomized studies. *J Rheumatol* 2010;37:1892–7.
32. FitzGerald O, Helliwell P, Mease P, Mumtaz A, Coates L, Pedersen R et al. Application of composite disease activity scores in psoriatic arthritis to the PRESTA data set. *Ann Rheum Dis* 2012;71:358–62.
33. Coates LC, Fransen J, Helliwell PS. Defining minimal disease activity in psoriatic arthritis: A proposed objective target for treatment. *Ann Rheum Dis* 2010;69:48–53.
34. Helliwell PS, Fitzgerald O, Strand CV, Mease PJ. Composite measures in psoriatic arthritis: A report from the GRAPPA 2009 annual meeting. *J Rheumatol* 2011;38:540–5.
35. Helliwell PS, FitzGerald O, Fransen J, Gladman DD, Kreuger GG, Callis-Duffin K et al. The development of candidate composite disease activity and responder indices for psoriatic arthritis (GRACE project). *Ann Rheum Dis* 2013;72:986–91.
36. Gossec L, Smolen JS, Gaujoux-Viala C, Ash Z, Marzo-Ortega H, van der Heijde D et al. European League Against Rheumatism recommendations for the management of psoriatic arthritis with pharmacological therapies. *Ann Rheum Dis* 2012;71:4–12.
37. Ash Z, Gaujoux-Viala C, Gossec L, Hensor EM, FitzGerald O, Winthrop K et al. A systematic literature review of drug therapies for the treatment of psoriatic arthritis: Current evidence and meta-analysis informing the EULAR recommendations for the management of psoriatic arthritis. *Ann Rheum Dis* 2012;71:319–26.
38. Gossec L, Smolen JS, Ramiro S, de Wit M, Cutolo M, Dougados M et al. European League Against Rheumatism (EULAR) recommendations for the management of psoriatic arthritis with pharmacological therapies: 2015 update. *Ann Rheum Dis* 2016;75(3):499–510.
39. Ritchlin CT, Kavanaugh A, Gladman DD, Mease PJ, Helliwell P, Boehncke WH et al. Treatment recommendations for psoriatic arthritis. *Ann Rheum Dis* 2009;68:1387–94.
40. Raychaudhuri SP. Comorbidities of psoriatic arthritis—Metabolic syndrome and prevention: A report from the GRAPPA 2010 annual meeting. *J Rheumatol* 2012;39:437–40.
41. Coates LC, Kavanaugh A, Mease PJ, Soriano ER, Laura Acosta-Felquer M, Armstrong AW et al. Group for Research and Assessment of Psoriasis and Psoriatic Arthritis 2015 treatment recommendations for psoriatic arthritis. *Arthritis Rheumatol* 2016;68(5):1060–71.
42. Gelfand JM, Neimann AL, Shin DB, Wang X, Margolis DJ, Troxel AB. Risk of myocardial infarction in patients with psoriasis. *JAMA* 2006;296:1735–41.
43. Raychaudhuri SK, Chatterjee S, Nguyen C, Kaur M, Jialal I, Raychaudhuri SP. Increased prevalence of the metabolic syndrome in patients with psoriatic arthritis. *Metab Syndr Relat Disord* 2010;8:331–4.
44. Kimhi O, Caspi D, Bornstein NM, Maharshak N, Gur A, Arbel Y et al. Prevalence and risk factors of atherosclerosis in patients with psoriatic arthritis. *Semin Arthritis Rheum* 2007;36:203–9.
45. Gladman DD, Ang M, Su L, Tom BD, Schentag CT, Farewell VT. Cardiovascular morbidity in psoriatic arthritis. *Ann Rheum Dis* 2009;68:1131–5.
46. Muna WF, Roller DH, Craft J, Shaw RK, Ross AM. Psoriatic arthritis and aortic regurgitation. *JAMA* 1980;244:363–5.
47. Khan MA. Update on spondyloarthropathies. *Ann Intern Med* 2002;136:896–907.

48. Farber EM, Raychaudhuri SP. Concept of total care: A third dimension in the treatment of psoriasis. *Cutis* 1997;59:35–9.
49. Joshi P, Dhaneshwar SS. An update on disease modifying antirheumatic drugs. *Inflamm Allergy Drug Targets* 2014;13:249–61.
50. Meyerhoff JO. Exacerbation of psoriasis with meclofenamate. *N Engl J Med* 1983;309:496.
51. Sarzi-Puttini P, Santandrea S, Boccassini L, Panni B, Caruso I. The role of NSAIDs in psoriatic arthritis: Evidence from a controlled study with nimesulide. *Clin Exp Rheumatol* 2001;19:S17–20.
52. Kivitz AJ, Espinoza LR, Sherrer YR, Liu-Dumaw M, West CR. A comparison of the efficacy and safety of celecoxib 200 mg and celecoxib 400 mg once daily in treating the signs and symptoms of psoriatic arthritis. *Semin Arthritis Rheum* 2007;37:164–73.
53. Cipriani P, Ruscitti P, Carubbi F, Liakouli V, Giacomelli R. Methotrexate: An old new drug in autoimmune disease. *Expert Rev Clin Immunol* 2014:1–12.
54. Huynh D, Kavanaugh A. Psoriatic arthritis: Current therapy and future approaches. *Rheumatology* 2015;54(1):20–28.
55. Kingsley GH, Kowalczyk A, Taylor H, Ibrahim F, Packham JC, McHugh NJ et al. A randomized placebo-controlled trial of methotrexate in psoriatic arthritis. *Rheumatology* 2012;51:1368–77.
56. Lie E, van der Heijde D, Uhlig T, Heiberg MS, Koldingsnes W, Rodevand E et al. Effectiveness and retention rates of methotrexate in psoriatic arthritis in comparison with methotrexate-treated patients with rheumatoid arthritis. *Ann Rheum Dis* 2010;69:671–6.
57. Willkens RF, Williams HJ, Ward JR, Egger MJ, Reading JC, Clements PJ et al. Randomized, double-blind, placebo controlled trial of low-dose pulse methotrexate in psoriatic arthritis. *Arthritis Rheum* 1984;27:376–81.
58. Abu-Shakra M, Gladman DD, Thorne JC, Long J, Gough J, Farewell VT. Longterm methotrexate therapy in psoriatic arthritis: Clinical and radiological outcome. *J Rheumatol* 1995;22:241–5.
59. Guidelines for monitoring drug therapy in rheumatoid arthritis. American College of Rheumatology Ad Hoc Committee on Clinical Guidelines. *Arthritis Rheum* 1996;39:723–31.
60. Breedveld FC, Dayer JM. Leflunomide: Mode of action in the treatment of rheumatoid arthritis. *Ann Rheum Dis* 2000;59:841–9.
61. Kaltwasser JP, Nash P, Gladman D, Rosen CF, Behrens F, Jones P et al. Efficacy and safety of leflunomide in the treatment of psoriatic arthritis and psoriasis: A multinational, double-blind, randomized, placebo-controlled clinical trial. *Arthritis Rheum* 2004;50:1939–50.
62. Nash P, Thaci D, Behrens F, Falk F, Kaltwasser JP. Leflunomide improves psoriasis in patients with psoriatic arthritis: An in-depth analysis of data from the TOPAS study. *Dermatology* 2006;212: 238–49.
63. Kaltwasser JP, Nash P, Gladman D, Rosen CF, Behrens F, Jones P et al. Efficacy and safety of leflunomide in the treatment of psoriatic arthritis and psoriasis: A multinational, double-blind, randomized, placebo-controlled clinical trial. *Arthritis Rheum* 2004;50:1939–50.
64. Ramiro S, Gaujoux-Viala C, Nam JL, Smolen JS, Buch M, Gossec L et al. Safety of synthetic and biological DMARDs: A systematic literature review informing the 2013 update of the EULAR recommendations for management of rheumatoid arthritis. *Ann Rheum Dis* 2014;73:529–35.
65. Combe B, Goupille P, Kuntz JL, Tebib J, Liote F, Bregeon C. Sulphasalazine in psoriatic arthritis: A randomized, multicentre, placebo-controlled study. *Br J Rheumatol* 1996;35:664–8.
66. Farr M, Kitas GD, Waterhouse L, Jubb R, Felix-Davies D, Bacon PA. Sulphasalazine in psoriatic arthritis: A double-blind placebo-controlled study. *Br J Rheumatol* 1990;29:46–9.
67. Fraser SM, Hopkins R, Hunter JA, Neumann V, Capell HA, Bird HA. Sulphasalazine in the management of psoriatic arthritis. *Br J Rheumatol* 1993;32:923–5.
68. Gupta AK, Grober JS, Hamilton TA, Ellis CN, Siegel MT, Voorhees JJ et al. Sulfasalazine therapy for psoriatic arthritis: A double blind, placebo controlled trial. *J Rheumatol* 1995;22:894–8.
69. Dougados M, vam der Linden S, Leirisalo-Repo M, Huitfeldt B, Juhlin R, Veys E et al. Sulfasalazine in the treatment of spondylarthropathy. A randomized, multicenter, double-blind, placebo-controlled study. *Arthritis Rheum* 1995;38:618–27.
70. Nielsen OH, Bukhave K, Elmgreen J, Ahnfelt-Ronne I. Inhibition of 5-lipoxygenase pathway of arachidonic acid metabolism in human neutrophils by sulfasalazine and 5-aminosalicylic acid. *Dig Dis Sci* 1987;32:577–82.
71. Clegg DO, Reda DJ, Weisman MH, Blackburn WD, Cush JJ, Cannon GW et al. Comparison of sulfasalazine and placebo in the treatment of ankylosing spondylitis. A Department of Veterans Affairs Cooperative Study. *Arthritis Rheum* 1996;39:2004–12.

72. Menter A, Korman NJ, Elmets CA, Feldman SR, Gelfand JM, Gordon KB et al. Guidelines of care for the management of psoriasis and psoriatic arthritis: Section 4. Guidelines of care for the management and treatment of psoriasis with traditional systemic agents. *J Am Acad Dermatol* 2009;61:451–85.
73. Gravani A, Gaitanis G, Zioga A, Bassukas ID. Synthetic antimalarial drugs and the triggering of psoriasis—Do we need disease-specific guidelines for the management of patients with psoriasis at risk of malaria? *Int J Dermatol* 2014;53:327–30.
74. Gladman DD, Blake R, Brubacher B, Farewell VT. Chloroquine therapy in psoriatic arthritis. *J Rheumatol* 1992;19:1724–6.
75. Fraser AD, van Kuijk AW, Westhovens R, Karim Z, Wakefield R, Gerards AH et al. A randomised, double blind, placebo controlled, multicentre trial of combination therapy with methotrexate plus ciclosporin in patients with active psoriatic arthritis. *Ann Rheum Dis* 2005;64:859–64.
76. Salvarani C, Macchioni P, Olivieri I, Marchesoni A, Cutolo M, Ferraccioli G et al. A comparison of cyclosporine, sulfasalazine, and symptomatic therapy in the treatment of psoriatic arthritis. *J Rheumatol* 2001;28:2274–82.
77. Mahrle G, Schulze HJ, Brautigam M, Mischer P, Schopf R, Jung EG et al. Anti-inflammatory efficacy of low-dose cyclosporin A in psoriatic arthritis. A prospective multicentre study. *Br J Dermatol* 1996;135:752–7.
78. Levy J, Paulus HE, Barnett EV. A double-blind controlled evaluation of azathioprine treatment in the rheumatoid arthritis and psoriatic arthritis. *Arthritis Rheum* 1972;15.
79. Lee JC, Gladman DD, Schentag CT, Cook RJ. The long-term use of azathioprine in patients with psoriatic arthritis. *J Clin Rheumatol* 2001;7:160–5.
80. Sivamani RK, Goodarzi H, Garcia MS, Raychaudhuri SP, Wehrli LN, Ono Y et al. Biologic therapies in the treatment of psoriasis: A comprehensive evidence-based basic science and clinical review and a practical guide to tuberculosis monitoring. *Clin Rev Allergy Immunol* 2013;44:121–40.
81. Neregard P, Krishnamurthy A, Revu S, Engstrom M, af Klint E, Catrina AI. Etanercept decreases synovial expression of tumour necrosis factor-alpha and lymphotoxin-alpha in rheumatoid arthritis. *Scand J Rheumatol* 2014;43:85–90.
82. Menter A, Gottlieb A, Feldman SR, Van Voorhees AS, Leonardi CL, Gordon KB et al. Guidelines of care for the management of psoriasis and psoriatic arthritis: Section 1. Overview of psoriasis and guidelines of care for the treatment of psoriasis with biologics. *J Am Acad Dermatol* 2008;58:826–50.
83. Antoni CE, Kavanaugh A, Kirkham B, Tutuncu Z, Burmester GR, Schneider U et al. Sustained benefits of infliximab therapy for dermatologic and articular manifestations of psoriatic arthritis: Results from the infliximab multinational psoriatic arthritis controlled trial (IMPACT). *Arthritis Rheum* 2005;52:1227–36.
84. Kavanaugh A, Antoni CE, Gladman D, Wassenberg S, Zhou B, Beutler A et al. The Infliximab Multinational Psoriatic Arthritis Controlled Trial (IMPACT): Results of radiographic analyses after 1 year. *Ann Rheum Dis* 2006;65:1038–43.
85. Mease PJ, Gladman DD, Ritchlin CT, Ruderman EM, Steinfeld SD, Choy EH et al. Adalimumab for the treatment of patients with moderately to severely active psoriatic arthritis: Results of a double-blind, randomized, placebo-controlled trial. *Arthritis Rheum* 2005;52:3279–89.
86. Gladman DD, Mease PJ, Ritchlin CT, Choy EH, Sharp JT, Ory PA et al. Adalimumab for long-term treatment of psoriatic arthritis: Forty-eight week data from the adalimumab effectiveness in psoriatic arthritis trial. *Arthritis Rheum* 2007;56:476–88.
87. Mease PJ, Kivitz AJ, Burch FX, Siegel EL, Cohen SB, Ory P et al. Etanercept treatment of psoriatic arthritis: Safety, efficacy, and effect on disease progression. *Arthritis Rheum* 2004;50:2264–72.
88. Saurat JH, Stingl G, Dubertret L, Papp K, Langley RG, Ortonne JP et al. Efficacy and safety results from the randomized controlled comparative study of adalimumab vs. methotrexate vs. placebo in patients with psoriasis (CHAMPION). *Br J Dermatol* 2008;158:558–66.
89. Shupack J, Abel E, Bauer E, Brown M, Drake L, Freinkel R et al. Cyclosporine as maintenance therapy in patients with severe psoriasis. *J Am Acad Dermatol* 1997;36:423–32.
90. Leonardi CL, Powers JL, Matheson RT, Goffe BS, Zitnik R, Wang A et al. Etanercept as monotherapy in patients with psoriasis. *N Engl J Med* 2003;349:2014–22.
91. Tyring S, Gottlieb A, Papp K, Gordon K, Leonardi C, Wang A et al. Etanercept and clinical outcomes, fatigue, and depression in psoriasis: Double-blind placebo-controlled randomised phase III trial. *Lancet* 2006;367:29–35.
92. Reich K, Nestle FO, Papp K, Ortonne JP, Evans R, Guzzo C et al. Infliximab induction and maintenance therapy for moderate-to-severe psoriasis: A phase III, multicentre, double-blind trial. *Lancet* 2005;366:1367–74.

93. Mease PJ, Kivitz AJ, Burch FX, Siegel EL, Cohen SB, Ory P et al. Continued inhibition of radiographic progression in patients with psoriatic arthritis following 2 years of treatment with etanercept. *J Rheumatol* 2006;33:712–21.
94. Sterry W, Ortonne JP, Kirkham B, Brocq O, Robertson D, Pedersen RD et al. Comparison of two etanercept regimens for treatment of psoriasis and psoriatic arthritis: PRESTA randomised double blind multicentre trial. *BMJ* 2010;340:c147.
95. Antoni C, Krueger GG, de Vlam K, Birbara C, Beutler A, Guzzo C et al. Infliximab improves signs and symptoms of psoriatic arthritis: Results of the IMPACT 2 trial. *Ann Rheum Dis* 2005;64:1150–7.
96. van der Heijde D, Kavanaugh A, Gladman DD, Antoni C, Krueger GG, Guzzo C et al. Infliximab inhibits progression of radiographic damage in patients with active psoriatic arthritis through one year of treatment: Results from the Induction and Maintenance Psoriatic Arthritis Clinical Trial 2. *Arthritis Rheum* 2007;56:2698–707.
97. Baranauskaite A, Raffayova H, Kungurov NV, Kubanova A, Venalis A, Helmle L et al. Infliximab plus methotrexate is superior to methotrexate alone in the treatment of psoriatic arthritis in methotrexate-naive patients: The RESPOND study. *Ann Rheum Dis* 2012;71:541–8.
98. Mease PJ, Ory P, Sharp JT, Ritchlin CT, Van den Bosch F, Wellborne F et al. Adalimumab for long-term treatment of psoriatic arthritis: 2-year data from the Adalimumab Effectiveness in Psoriatic Arthritis Trial (ADEPT). *Ann Rheum Dis* 2009;68:702–9.
99. Genovese MC, Mease PJ, Thomson GT, Kivitz AJ, Perdok RJ, Weinberg MA et al. Safety and efficacy of adalimumab in treatment of patients with psoriatic arthritis who had failed disease modifying anti-rheumatic drug therapy. *J Rheumatol* 2007;34:1040–50.
100. Karanikolas GN, Koukli EM, Katsalira A, Arida A, Petrou D, Komninou E et al. Adalimumab or cyclosporine as monotherapy and in combination in severe psoriatic arthritis: Results from a prospective 12-month nonrandomized unblinded clinical trial. *J Rheumatol* 2011;38:2466–74.
101. Kavanaugh A, McInnes I, Mease P, Krueger GG, Gladman D, Gomez-Reino J et al. Golimumab, a new human tumor necrosis factor alpha antibody, administered every four weeks as a subcutaneous injection in psoriatic arthritis: Twenty-four-week efficacy and safety results of a randomized, placebo-controlled study. *Arthritis Rheum* 2009;60:976–86.
102. Kavanaugh A, van der Heijde D, McInnes IB, Mease P, Krueger GG, Gladman DD et al. Golimumab in psoriatic arthritis: One-year clinical efficacy, radiographic, and safety results from a phase III, randomized, placebo-controlled trial. *Arthritis Rheum* 2012;64:2504–17.
103. Kavanaugh A, McInnes IB, Mease P, Krueger GG, Gladman D, van der Heijde D et al. Clinical efficacy, radiographic and safety findings through 5 years of subcutaneous golimumab treatment in patients with active psoriatic arthritis: Results from a long-term extension of a randomised, placebo-controlled trial (the GO-REVEAL study). *Ann Rheum Dis* 2014;73:1689–94.
104. Olivieri I, D'Angelo S, Palazzi C, Padula A. Advances in the management of psoriatic arthritis. *Nat Rev Rheumatol* 2014;10:531–42.
105. Mease PJ, Fleischmann R, Deodhar AA, Wollenhaupt J, Khraishi M, Kielar D et al. Effect of certolizumab pegol on signs and symptoms in patients with psoriatic arthritis: 24-week results of a phase 3 double-blind randomised placebo-controlled study (RAPID-PsA). *Ann Rheum Dis* 2014;73:48–55.
106. van der Heijde D, Fleischmann R, Wollenhaupt J, Deodhar A, Kielar D, Woltering F et al. Effect of different imputation approaches on the evaluation of radiographic progression in patients with psoriatic arthritis: Results of the RAPID-PsA 24-week phase III double-blind randomised placebo-controlled study of certolizumab pegol. *Ann Rheum Dis* 2014;73:233–7.
107. Tausend W, Downing C, Tyring S. Systematic review of interleukin-12, interleukin-17, and interleukin-23 pathway inhibitors for the treatment of moderate-to-severe chronic plaque psoriasis: Ustekinumab, briakinumab, tildrakizumab, guselkumab, secukinumab, ixekizumab, and brodalumab. *J Cutan Med Surg* 2014;18:156–69.
108. Leipe J, Grunke M, Dechant C, Reindl C, Kerzendorf U, Schulze-Koops H et al. Role of Th17 cells in human autoimmune arthritis. *Arthritis Rheum* 2010;62:2876–85.
109. Chan JR, Blumenschein W, Murphy E, Diveu C, Wiekowski M, Abbondanzo S et al. IL-23 stimulates epidermal hyperplasia via TNF and IL-20R2-dependent mechanisms with implications for psoriasis pathogenesis. *J Exp Med* 2006;203:2577–87.
110. Leonardi CL, Kimball AB, Papp KA, Yeilding N, Guzzo C, Wang Y et al. Efficacy and safety of ustekinumab, a human interleukin-12/23 monoclonal antibody, in patients with psoriasis: 76-week results from a randomised, double-blind, placebo-controlled trial (PHOENIX 1). *Lancet* 2008;371:1665–74.

111. Griffiths CE, Strober BE, van de Kerkhof P, Ho V, Fidelus-Gort R, Yeilding N et al. Comparison of ustekinumab and etanercept for moderate-to-severe psoriasis. *N Engl J Med* 2010;362:118–28.
112. Gottlieb A, Menter A, Mendelsohn A, Shen YK, Li S, Guzzo C et al. Ustekinumab, a human interleukin 12/23 monoclonal antibody, for psoriatic arthritis: Randomised, double-blind, placebo-controlled, crossover trial. *Lancet* 2009;373:633–40.
113. McInnes IB, Kavanaugh A, Gottlieb AB, Puig L, Rahman P, Ritchlin C et al. Efficacy and safety of ustekinumab in patients with active psoriatic arthritis: 1 year results of the phase 3, multicentre, double-blind, placebo-controlled PSUMMIT 1 trial. *Lancet* 2013;382:780–9.
114. Kavanaugh A, Puig L, Gottlieb A. Efficacy and safety of ustekinumab in patients with active psoriatic arthritis: 2 year results from a phase 3, multicenter, double-blind, placebo-controlled study [abstract]. *Arthritis Rheum* 2013;65(Suppl.):L10.
115. Ritchlin C, Rahman P, Kavanaugh A, McInnes IB, Puig L, Li S et al. Efficacy and safety of the anti-IL-12/23 p40 monoclonal antibody, ustekinumab, in patients with active psoriatic arthritis despite conventional non-biological and biological anti-tumour necrosis factor therapy: 6-month and 1-year results of the phase 3, multicentre, double-blind, placebo-controlled, randomised PSUMMIT 2 trial. *Ann Rheum Dis* 2014;73:990–9.
116. Raychaudhuri SP, Raychaudhuri SK, Genovese MC. IL-17 receptor and its functional significance in psoriatic arthritis. *Mol Cell Biochem* 2012;359 (1–2):419–29.
117. Adamopoulos IE, Suzuki E, Chao CC, Gorman D, Adda S, Maverakis E et al. IL-17A gene transfer induces bone loss and epidermal hyperplasia associated with psoriatic arthritis. *Ann Rheum Dis* 2015;74(6):1284–92.
118. Papp KA, Leonardi C, Menter A, Ortonne JP, Krueger JG, Kricorian G et al. Brodalumab, an anti-interleukin-17-receptor antibody for psoriasis. *N Engl J Med* 2012;366:1181–9.
119. Langley RG, Elewski BE, Lebwohl M, Reich K, Griffiths CE, Papp K et al. Secukinumab in plaque psoriasis—Results of two phase 3 trials. *N Engl J Med* 2014;371:326–38.
120. Gordon KB, Leonardi CL, Lebwohl M, Blauvelt A, Cameron GS, Braun D et al. A 52-week, open-label study of the efficacy and safety of ixekizumab, an anti-interleukin-17A monoclonal antibody, in patients with chronic plaque psoriasis. *J Am Acad Dermatol* 2014;71:1176–82.
121. McInnes IB, Sieper J, Braun J, Emery P, van der Heijde D, Isaacs JD et al. Efficacy and safety of secukinumab, a fully human anti-interleukin-17A monoclonal antibody, in patients with moderate-to-severe psoriatic arthritis: A 24-week, randomised, double-blind, placebo-controlled, phase II proof-of-concept trial. *Ann Rheum Dis* 2014;73:349–56.
122. Mease PJ, Genovese MC, Greenwald MW, Ritchlin CT, Beaulieu AD, Deodhar A et al. Brodalumab, an anti-IL17RA monoclonal antibody, in psoriatic arthritis. *N Engl J Med* 2014;370:2295–306.
123. ClinicalTrials.gov. A study of ixekizumab in participants with active psoriatic arthritis (SPIRIT-P1). Identifier: NCT01695239.
124. ClinicalTrials.gov. Study of efficacy and safety of brodalumab compared with placebo in subjects with axial spondyloarthritis. Identifier: NCT02429882.
125. ClinicalTrials.gov. Study of efficacy and safety of brodalumab compared with placebo and ustekinumab in moderate to severe plaque psoriasis subjects (AMAGINE-2). Identifier: NCT01708603.
126. ClinicalTrials.gov. Study of efficacy and safety of brodalumab in subjects with psoriatic arthritis (AMVISION-2). Identifier: NCT02024646.
127. Gottleib AB, Sigurgeirsson B, Bluvelt A, Mpfofu S, Martin R, Papavassilis C. Secukinumab shows substantial improvement in both psoriasis symptoms and physical functioning in moderate-to-severe plaque psoriasis patients with psoriatic arthritis: A subanalysis of phase 3 multicentre, double-blind, placebo-controlled study [abstract]. *Arthritis Rheum* 2013;65.
128. McInnes IB, Mease PJ, Kirkham B, Kavanaugh A, Ritchlin CT, Rahman P et al. Secukinumab, a human anti-interleukin-17A monoclonal antibody, in patients with psoriatic arthritis (FUTURE 2): A randomised, double-blind, placebo-controlled, phase 3 trial. *Lancet* 2015;386(9999):1137–46.
129. Griffiths CE, Reich K, Lebwohl M, van de Kerkhof P, Paul C, Menter A et al. Comparison of ixekizumab with etanercept or placebo in moderate-to-severe psoriasis (UNCOVER-2 and UNCOVER-3): Results from two phase 3 randomised trials. *Lancet* 2015;386(9993):541–51.
130. Houslay MD, Schafer P, Zhang KY. Keynote review: Phosphodiesterase-4 as a therapeutic target. *Drug Discov Today* 2005;10:1503–19.
131. Schafer PH, Parton A, Capone L, Cedzik D, Brady H, Evans JF et al. Apremilast is a selective PDE4 inhibitor with regulatory effects on innate immunity. *Cell Signal* 2014;26(9):2016–29.

132. Schafer PH, Parton A, Gandhi AK, Capone L, Adams M, Wu L et al. Apremilast, a cAMP phosphodiesterase-4 inhibitor, demonstrates anti-inflammatory activity in vitro and in a model of psoriasis. *Br J Pharmacol* 2010;159:842–55.
133. Mease P, Kavanaugh A, Gladman D. Long-term safety and tolerability of apremilast, an oral phosphodiesterase 4 inhibitor, in patients with psoriatic arthritis: Pooled safety analysis of three phase 3, randomized, controlled trials [abstract]. *Arthritis Rheum* 2013;65(Suppl.):131–2.
134. Cutolo M, Myerson G, Fleischmann R. Long-term (52-week) results of a phase 3, randomized, controlled trial of apremilast, an oral phosphodiesterase 4 inhibitor, in patients with psoriatic arthritis (PALACE 2) [abstract]. *Arthritis Rheum* 2013;65(Suppl.):346–7.
135. Edwards C, Blanco F. Long-term (52-week) results of a phase 3, controlled trial of apremilast, an oral phosphodiesterase 4 inhibitor, in patients with psoriatic arthritis and current skin involvement (PALACE 3) [abstract]. *Arthritis Rheum* 2013;65(Suppl.):132.
136. Wells A, Edwards C, Adebajao A. Apremilast in the treatment of DMARD naïve psoriatic arthritis patients: Results of a phase 3 randomized controlled trial (PALACE 4) [abstract]. *Arthritis Rheum* 2013;65(Suppl.):L4.
137. Schett G, Mease P, Gladman D. Apremilast, an oral phosphodiesterase 4 inhibitor, is associated with long-term (52-week) improvement in physical function in patients with psoriatic arthritis: Results from three phase 3, randomized, controlled trials [abstract]. *Arthritis Rheum* 2013;65(Suppl.):143.
138. Cutolo M, Mease P, Gladman D. Apremilast, an oral phosphodiesterase 4 inhibitor, is associated with long-term (52-week) improvement in tender and swollen joint counts in patients with psoriatic arthritis: Results from three phase 3, randomized, controlled trials [abstract]. *Arthritis Rheum* 2013;65(Suppl.):135–6.
139. Kavanaugh A, Mease PJ, Gomez-Reino JJ, Adebajo AO, Wollenhaupt J, Gladman DD et al. Treatment of psoriatic arthritis in a phase 3 randomised, placebo-controlled trial with apremilast, an oral phosphodiesterase 4 inhibitor. *Ann Rheum Dis* 2014;73:1020–6.
140. Lee EB, Fleischmann R, Hall S, Wilkinson B, Bradley JD, Gruben D et al. Tofacitinib versus methotrexate in rheumatoid arthritis. *N Engl J Med* 2014;370:2377–86.
141. van Vollenhoven RF, Fleischmann R, Cohen S, Lee EB, Garcia Meijide JA, Wagner S et al. Tofacitinib or adalimumab versus placebo in rheumatoid arthritis. *N Engl J Med* 2012;367:508–19.
142. Boy MG, Wang C, Wilkinson BE, Chow VF, Clucas AT, Krueger JG et al. Double-blind, placebo-controlled, dose-escalation study to evaluate the pharmacologic effect of CP-690,550 in patients with psoriasis. *J Invest Dermatol* 2009;129:2299–302.
143. Papp KA, Menter A, Strober B, Langley RG, Buonanno M, Wolk R et al. Efficacy and safety of tofacitinib, an oral Janus kinase inhibitor, in the treatment of psoriasis: A phase 2b randomized placebo-controlled dose-ranging study. *Br J Dermatol* 2012;167:668–77.
144. Sercarz EE, Maverakis E. MHC-guided processing: Binding of large antigen fragments. *Nat Rev Immunol* 2003;3:621–9.
145. Iannone F, Lapadula G. The inhibitor of costimulation of T cells: Abatacept. *J Rheumatol Suppl* 2012;89:100–2.
146. Abrams JR, Lebwohl MG, Guzzo CA, Jegasothy BV, Goldfarb MT, Goffe BS et al. CTLA4Ig-mediated blockade of T-cell costimulation in patients with psoriasis vulgaris. *J Clin Invest* 1999;103:1243–52.
147. Mease P, Genovese MC, Gladstein G, Kivitz AJ, Ritchlin C, Tak PP et al. Abatacept in the treatment of patients with psoriatic arthritis: Results of a six-month, multicenter, randomized, double-blind, placebo-controlled, phase II trial. *Arthritis Rheum* 2011;63:939–48.
148. Bauer TM, Patel MR, Infante JR. Targeting PI3 kinase in cancer. *Pharmacol Ther* 2015;146:53–60.
149. Kundu-Raychaudhuri S, Chen YJ, Wulff H, Raychaudhuri SP. Kv1.3 in psoriatic disease: PAP-1, a small molecule inhibitor of Kv1.3 is effective in the SCID mouse psoriasis–xenograft model. *J Autoimmun* 2014;55:63–72.
150. Raychaudhuri SK, Raychaudhuri SP. mTOR signaling cascade in psoriatic disease: Double kinase mTOR inhibitor a novel therapeutic target. *Indian J Dermatol* 2014;59:67–70.
151. Raychaudhuri SP, Raychaudhuri SK. Role of NGF and neurogenic inflammation in the pathogenesis of psoriasis. *Prog Brain Res* 2004;146:433–7.
152. Raychaudhuri SP, Sanyal M, Weltman H, Kundu-Raychaudhuri S. K252a, a high-affinity nerve growth factor receptor blocker, improves psoriasis: An in vivo study using the severe combined immunodeficient mouse-human skin model. *J Invest Dermatol* 2004;122:812–9.
153. Raychaudhuri SK, Raychaudhuri SP. NGF and its receptor system: A new dimension in the pathogenesis of psoriasis and psoriatic arthritis. *Ann N Y Acad Sci* 2009;1173:470–7.

154. Raychaudhuri SP, Raychaudhuri SK, Atkuri KR, Herzenberg LA, Herzenberg LA. Nerve growth factor: A key local regulator in the pathogenesis of inflammatory arthritis. *Arthritis Rheum* 2011;63:3243–52.
155. Raychaudhuri SP, Jiang WY, Raychaudhuri SK. Revisiting the Koebner phenomenon: Role of NGF and its receptor system in the pathogenesis of psoriasis. *Am J Pathol* 2008;172(4):961–71.
156. Leong TT, Fearon U, Veale DJ. Angiogenesis in psoriasis and psoriatic arthritis: Clues to disease pathogenesis. *Curr Rheumatol Rep* 2005;7(4):325–9.
157. Detmar M, Brown LF, Claffey KP, Yeo KT, Kocher O, Jackman RW et al. Overexpression of vascular permeability factor/vascular endothelial growth factor and its receptors in psoriasis. *J Exp Med* 1994;180:1141–6.
158. Datta-Mitra A, Riar NK, Raychaudhuri SP. Remission of psoriasis and psoriatic arthritis during bevacizumab therapy for renal cell cancer. *Indian J Dermatol* 2014;59(6):632.
159. Narayanan S, Callis-Duffin K, Batten J, Agarwal N. Improvement of psoriasis during sunitinib therapy for renal cell carcinoma. *Am J Med Sci* 2010;339:580–1.
160. Canavese M, Altruda F, Ruzicka T, Schauber J. Vascular endothelial growth factor (VEGF) in the pathogenesis of psoriasis—A possible target for novel therapies? *J Dermatol Sci* 2010;58(3):171–6.

13 Targeting IL-23/IL-17 Axis for Treatment of Psoriasis and Psoriatic Arthritis

Subhashis Banerjee and Philip Mease

CONTENTS

13.1 INTRODUCTION

Interleukin (IL) 17A was first described in 1993 as CTLA-8 isolated from activated T cells. Its function was unknown. Subsequently, other family members, IL-17B–F, were characterized that were secreted by a unique type of T cells, called TH17 cells, first described in 2005 [1,2]. These cells were distinct from hitherto defined TH1 and TH2 cells, known to be involved in adaptive immune responses leading to chronic inflammation. In contrast to TH1 or TH2 cells that were characterized by secretion of interferon γ or IL-4, respectively, TH17 cells produced a unique pattern of cytokines that included IL-17 (hence the term TH17), IL-21, IL-22, and chemokines such as CCL20. A lineage of CD8+ T cells have also been shown to secrete IL-17A (TC17) [3–5]. IL-17A has pleiotropic effects that include induction of IL-8, tumor necrosis factor (TNF), IL-6, chemokines, RANKL, and matrix metalloproteinases, from multiple target cell types, including epithelial cells, fibroblasts, macrophages, dendritic cells, endothelial cells, osteoblasts, and chondrocytes [2,6]. The discovery of IL-23, followed by elucidation in 2005 of its critical role in the terminal differentiation, proliferation, and pathogenicity of TH17 cells, advanced our understanding of the role of the IL-23/IL-17 axis in immunity and inflammation [1,2]. IL-23 is produced by keratinocytes and activated antigen-presenting cells (APCs), specifically Langerhans cells in the skin, macrophages, and dendritic cells [7].

Differentiation of TH17 cells in humans has been shown to be induced by IL-1β, as well as IL-23, and possibly transforming growth factor (TGF) (β) in the presence of inflammatory cytokines, such as IL-6, IL-21, and IL-23. IL-17A and F are involved in host defense to specific microbes, for example, *Candida*, and in inflammation, with IL-17A being more potent than IL-17F. These cytokines also play a role in neutrophil production, trafficking, and chemotaxis. IL-I7E (also known as IL-25) is involved in TH2 responses, and IL-17B–D are less well characterized in terms of their biological significance. Production of IL-17 is driven by a unique transcription factor, RORγT, in TH17 cells following signaling of the IL-23 receptor by IL-23 via JAK1/TYK2 in these cells [1,7].

There is now evidence that IL-17 may also be made by innate immune cells, including certain natural killer (NK) cells, γδ T cells, invariant natural killer T (NKT) cells, intestinal Paneth cells, neutrophils, and mast cells. Many of these cell types line body surfaces exposed to external microbes, including the gut mucosa, lung epithelia, and skin. Almost all these cell types are known to be activated by IL-23 released from macrophages and dendritic cells in response to microbial agents, such as fungi and extracellular bacteria. By production of IL-17, these cells play a role in preserving barrier function and the integrity of epithelial surfaces [1,8].

13.2 IL-23/IL-17 IN PSORIASIS AND PSORIATIC ARTHRITIS

IL-23 and IL-17 expression was found to be upregulated in skin lesions of psoriasis [1,9]. There is evidence of increased expression of IL-23 and IL-17 in spondyloarthritides, including psoriatic arthritis (PsA) and ankylosing spondylitis (AS) [8]. In PsA, increased serum levels of IL-17A and elevated expression of TH17 and TC17 cells have been shown in synovial fluid, with association of the presence of these cells with bone erosions [10]. As per the model of Lories and McInnes [11], multiple factors, such as microbial antigens, biomechanical stress, alterations in the gut microbiome, and the presence of the human leukocyte antigen (HLA)–B27, may induce local expression of IL-23 and induction of TH17 cells. IL-17 can drive inflammatory response and bone and cartilage damage in the joints, whereas IL-22 from TH17 cells can lead to osteoproliferation secondary to inflammation in periarticular tissues. This may explain the combination of articular bone destruction and periarticular new bone formation in spondyloarthritis, including PsA. Genome-wide association studies have shown that genes encoding for genetic variants of IL-23R are important risk factors for psoriasis, PsA, and AS [2,7].

13.3 AGENTS TARGETING THE IL-23/IL-17 AXIS IN PSORIASIS AND PSA

Based on the expression of IL-23, IL-17, and/or TH17 cells in serum and involved tissues, genetic evidence, and animal studies, there was rationale for testing agents that could inhibit this pathway in psoriasis and PsA [7,12,13]. Figure 13.1 illustrates the mechanism of action of various agents targeting this axis in inflammation. The efficacy of some of these agents, either recently approved or in clinical development, that target this pathway in psoriasis and PsA is described below.

13.3.1 Inhibitors of IL-23

13.3.1.1 Anti-IL-12/IL-23 p40 Antibody (Ustekinumab)

IL-12 and IL-23 share a common subunit, p40. Ustekinumab (Stelara®) is the single antagonist to IL-12/IL-23 p40 approved for psoriasis and PsA, with no other agents directed against this target in clinical development. Ustekinumab is a fully human monoclonal immunoglobulin (Ig) G1 antibody that binds to the common p40 subunit, thereby neutralizing these two cytokines, and hence TH1 and TH17 pathways, respectively [14]. Ustekinumab is now approved for the treatment of psoriasis and PsA in the United States and various parts of the world.

13.3.1.1.1 Psoriasis

Ustekinumab is approved for treatment of psoriasis in a weight-based regimen: 45 mg for patients weighing 100 kg or less and 90 mg for those who weigh more than 100 kg. It is administered subcutaneously (SC) at weeks 0 and 4 and then Q12W thereafter.

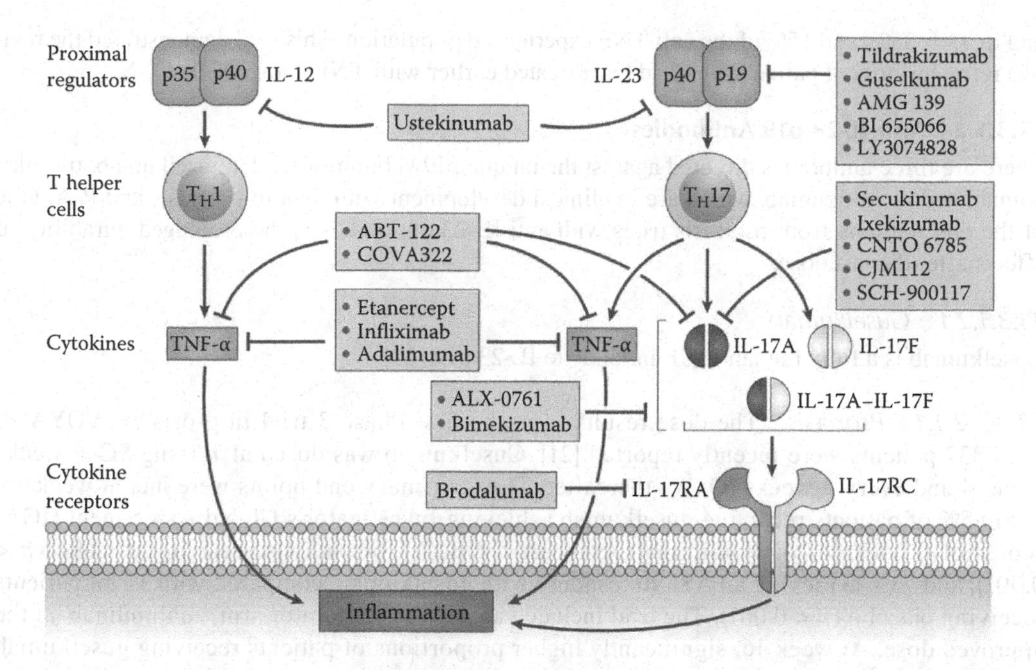

FIGURE 13.1 Targeting the IL-17/TH17 pathway. IL-17RA, interleukin 17 receptor A; IL-17RC, interleukin 17 receptor C; p19, p19 subunit of IL-23; p35, p35 subunit of IL-12; p40, p40 subunit of IL-12 or IL-23; TH1, T helper cell 1; TH17, T helper cell 17. (From Bartlett, H.S., and Million, R.P., *Nat. Rev. Drug Discov.*, 14, 11–12, 2015. Reprinted with permission from Macmillan Publishers Ltd.)

Its efficacy in psoriasis was assessed in two Phase 3 trials in psoriasis with the standard measure of Psoriasis Area and Severity Index 75% improvement (PASI 75). In the first study (PHOENIX 1), 766 patients treated with 45 mg, 90 mg, or placebo achieved PASI 75 responses at the week 12 primary end point of 67%, 66%, and 3%, respectively [15]. In the second study (PHOENIX 2), PASI 75 responses at week 12 in 1230 treated patients were 67%, 76%, and 4% in the 45 mg, 90 mg, and placebo arms, respectively [16]. Significant improvement was also seen in other measures, such as nail disease and quality of life. No major serious side effect issues emerged in these trials, and long-term data of more than 5 years failed to reveal significant safety issues [17].

13.3.1.1.2 PsA

The recommended dose for treatment of PsA in the United States is 45 mg SC initially and 4 weeks later, followed by 45 mg Q12W. For those patients with coexistent moderate to severe plaque psoriasis weighing >100 kg, the recommended dose is 90 mg initially and 4 weeks later, followed by 90 mg Q12W.

Ustekinumab was assessed in two Phase 3 trials in patients with PsA who had elevated C-reactive protein at baseline. In the first study (PSUMMIT 1), 615 patients who had an inadequate response to methotrexate inadequate responder (MTX-IR) were randomized to receive 45 or 90 mg of ustekinumab or placebo [18]. Ustekinumab was dosed SC at baseline, week 4, and Q12W thereafter. At the week 24 primary end point, the American College of Rheumatology 20% improvement (ACR20) responses in the 45 and 90 mg treated patients were 42% and 50%, respectively, which were significantly higher than the placebo response of 23%. Improvement was also noted in other clinical measures of the disease, including enthesitis, dactylitis, and skin and nail disease, as well as quality of life. The second study in PsA (PSUMMIT 2) included approximately 60% who had previously received anti-TNF agents [19]. The primary response, ACR20 at week 24, was observed in 44%, 44%, and 20% of the 45 mg, 90 mg, and placebo-treated patients in the overall population, and in 37%, 35%, and 15% of the anti-TNF experienced population. This trial demonstrated the relative refractoriness of patients who had been treated earlier with TNF antagonists.

13.3.1.2 Anti-IL-23 p19 Antibodies

There are three antibodies directed against the unique p19 subunit of IL-23, guselkumab, tildrakizumab, and risankizumab, which are in clinical development with data in psoriasis and PsA. One of the observations from psoriasis trials with anti-IL-23 antibodies is the prolonged durability of effects after the last dose.

13.3.1.2.1 Guselkumab

Guselkumab is a fully human IgG1 antibody to IL-23 p19 [20].

13.3.1.2.1.1 Psoriasis The dose results from the first Phase 3 trial in psoriasis (VOYAGE 1) in 837 patients were recently reported [21]. Guselkumab was dosed at 100 mg SC at weeks 0 and 4 and every 8 weeks (Q8W) thereafter. The coprimary end points were met at week 16, with 85% of patients receiving guselkumab achieving Investigator's Global Assessment (IGA) scores of 0 (cleared) or 1 (minimal), compared with 7% of patients receiving placebo ($p < 0.001$), and 73% achieving a PASI 90 response with guselkumab, compared with 3% of patients receiving placebo ($p < 0.001$). The trial included an active comparator arm, adalimumab, at the approved dose. At week 16, significantly higher proportions of patients receiving guselkumab achieved IGA 0/1 and PASI 90 (85% and 73%, respectively) compared with patients receiving adalimumab (66% and 50%, respectively). Higher levels of skin clearance among the guselkumab group continued through weeks 24 and 48. Similar frequencies of adverse events (AEs) were seen across the arms through week 16 (placebo [49%], guselkumab [52%], and adalimumab [51%]). Serious AEs were also comparable across arms (placebo [2%], guselkumab [2%], and adalimumab [2%]). Through week 48 of the study, AE frequencies were comparable between guselkumab (74%) and adalimumab (75%); serious AE frequencies were also similar for guselkumab (5%) and adalimumab (5%). Similar results were observed in the second Phase 3 study in psoriasis (VOYAGE 2) at week 16 [22]. Of the PASI 90 nonresponders to adalimumab who switched to guselkumab at week 28, 66% achieved a PASI 90 response at week 48 in the latter study.

13.3.1.2.1.2 PsA Guselkumab was evaluated at the above dosing in a 149-patient placebo-controlled Phase 2 trial in patients with PsA (guselkumab:placebo 2:1), >90% of whom were biologic naive [23]. At the primary end point at week 24, there was improvement in both joint and skin outcomes, with significantly higher ACR20 rates (58% vs. 18%) and PASI 90 rates (66% vs. 6%) in guselkumab versus placebo arms, respectively. Significant improvements were also noted in dactylitis and enthesitis in those patients with baseline dactylitis or enthesitis. In addition, significant improvements were observed in Health Assessment Questionnaire Disability Index (HAQ-DI) and 36-Item Short Form Health Survey (SF-36) scores. The incidence of AEs was comparable between the two groups (guselkumab 36% vs. placebo 33%), with only two serious AEs reported (knee injury and myocardial infarction).

13.3.1.2.2 Tildrakizumab

This is a humanized IgG1 antibody that neutralizes IL-23 p19 [24]. Results from two Phase 3 trials (ReSURFACE 1 and 2) in psoriasis were recently disclosed [25]. The two trials included 1862 patients with moderate to severe plaque psoriasis. In the trials, the agent dosed at weeks 0 and 4, and then quarterly at 100 or 200 mg, achieved PASI 75 response rates of 63%–64% at week 12 and 77%–80% at week 28 (placebo 3%–6%). The data further showed that more patients on tildrakizumab achieved higher skin responses (PASI 90 and 100) than those on placebo and etanercept. PASI 90 responses were achieved by 36%–37% at week 12, which increased to 54%–59% at week

28, and an average of 13% achieved PASI 100 at week 12, which increased to 24%–30% at week 28 at the two doses. The overall safety profile of tildrakizumab was consistent with previously reported studies with no significant findings. There are no available data for this agent in PsA, although there were numerical improvements in some PsA measures (Psoriatic Arthritis Screening and Evaluation [PASE], HAQ, and pain) in a small sample of patients with chronic plaque psoriasis who had concomitant PsA (18%) in the Phase 2b study [26].

13.3.1.2.3 Risankizumab

Risankizumab (BI 655066) is another antibody to IL-23 p19 that has been evaluated in psoriasis. It was tested in a small Phase 1 proof-of-concept study ($n = 39$) where patients with psoriasis achieved PASI 75 and PASI 90 at rates of 87% and 58% with a single intravenous or subcutaneous dose. Further, six of eight patients enrolled in an extension period maintained PASI 100 results over 66 weeks with that single dose [27].

New results from a Phase 2 head-to-head psoriasis study ($n = 166$) showed superior efficacy of risankizumab (90 and 180 mg) over ustekinumab (45/90 mg based on body weight), with each treatment dosed SC at weeks 0, 4, and 16 [28]. Primary end-point results showed a higher percentage of patients achieving PASI 90 after 12 weeks of treatment with 180 mg risankizumab (77%) compared with ustekinumab (40%). There was also a higher percentage of patients with PASI 100 response at week 12 with risankizumab (48%) compared with ustekinumab (18%). After 9 months, a PASI 90 response was observed in 69% patients with risankizumab 180 mg compared with 30% of patients on ustekinumab. Patients treated with risankizumab also had skin responses significantly faster (57 days vs. 113 days) and for a duration of more than 2 months longer than those on ustekinumab. In addition, a PASI 100 response was maintained after 9 months in more patients on risankizumab (43%) than on ustekinumab (15%). There was no clear difference of results with the 90 and 180 mg doses of risankizumab. Safety and tolerability were similar to those for ustekinumab with no serious drug-related side effects. There are no available data for this agent in PsA.

13.3.2 Inhibitors of IL-17

13.3.2.1 Secukinumab

Secukinumab is a human monoclonal IgG1k antibody that binds to and neutralizes IL-17A. It is approved for the treatment of psoriasis, PsA, and AS in the United States and other regions.

13.3.2.1.1 Psoriasis

Two Phase 3 trials, ERASURE and FIXTURE, of secukinumab in psoriasis have been conducted. A total of 738 (ERASURE trial) and 1306 (FIXTURE trial) patients were randomized to subcutaneous secukinumab at doses of 300 or 150 mg, or placebo, administered once weekly for 5 weeks and then Q4W thereafter [29]. In the ERASURE study, PASI 75 responses at week 12 were 82%, 72%, and 5% with 300 mg, 150 mg, and placebo, respectively. PASI 90 responses were 59%, 39%, and 1%, respectively. In the FIXTURE study, PASI 75 responses were 77%, 67%, 44%, and 5% with 300 and 150 mg of secukinumab, the anti-TNF agent etanercept (50 mg twice weekly used as comparator), and placebo, respectively. PASI 90 was met by 54%, 42%, 21%, and 2%, respectively. All responses were statistically better than those for the placebo and maintained in long-term extension periods. Improvements in nail disease, itch, and quality of life were also significant. Serious AEs were infrequent and similar in frequency across all groups. Rates of infections were similar across all active treatment arms and were numerically greater than in the placebo arm. Of note, *Candida* infections, which are of specific interest because of the role of IL-17 in host defense to *Candida*, especially at epithelial surfaces, were numerically higher in the secukinumab arms (5% with 300 mg, 2% with 150 mg) than in the etanercept arm (1%). Based on the known effects of IL-17 on neutrophils, another finding of note was Grade 3 neutropenia in 9 patients (1%) treated with secukinumab groups versus none in the etanercept or placebo arms. Rates for other AEs were similar between the two studies. Of note, there were two new cases and two exacerbations of previously known ulcerative colitis and two exacerbations of previously known Crohn's disease reported with secukinumab treatment.

13.3.2.1.2 PsA

Two Phase 3 trials of secukinumab, FUTURE 1 and FUTURE 2, were conducted in PsA [30,31]. The FUTURE 1 trial enrolled 606 patients who were randomized to an intravenous (IV) loading dose of secukinumab, 10 mg/kg at baseline, weeks 2 and 4, and then either 150 or 75 mg SC Q4W from week 8 versus placebo. At baseline, around 30% of patients had received prior anti-TNF therapy and 60% were on concomitant MTX. At 24 weeks, the ACR20, ACR50, and ACR70 responses, respectively, in the 150 mg dose arm were 50%, 35%, and 19%; in the 75 mg arm 51%, 31%, and 17%; and in the placebo arm 17%, 7%, and 2%. As observed earlier with ustekinumab, higher responses were seen in subjects who were naive to anti-TNF therapy. Key secondary measures of enthesitis, dactylitis, skin disease, radiographic evidence of inhibition of x-ray progression, function, and quality of life were all significantly better with secukinumab treatment than with placebo. The FUTURE 2 trial enrolled 397 patients to receive SC 300 mg secukinumab, 150 mg secukinumab, 75 mg secukinumab, or placebo weekly at weeks 1–4 and Q4W thereafter. The proportion of patients who had received previous anti-TNF therapy was 35%, and those on concomitant MTX were 47%. At 24 weeks, the ACR20, ACR50, and ACR70 responses, respectively, in the 300 mg dose arm were 54%, 35%, and 20%; in the 150 mg dose arm 51%, 35%, and 21%; in 75 mg arm 29%, 18%, and 6%; and in the placebo arm 15%, 7%, and 1%. The ACR, enthesitis, dactylitis, skin, function, and quality of life measures with secukinumab treatment were significantly better than with placebo. As in the FUTURE 1 trial, ACR responses were lower in tumor necrosis factor inhibitor inadequate responder (TNFi-IR) patients than in TNFi-naive patients, with lower responses seen in the 75 and 150 mg groups than in the 300 mg group. Overall, serious AEs were few and similar in frequency between the treatment and placebo arms through week 16 in both studies. The overall infection rate was slightly greater in the secukinumab arm than in placebo, with a somewhat higher incidence of candidiasis with secukinumab treatment (8 in FUTURE 1, 11 in FUTURE 2) than with placebo (none). Two cases of exacerbation of previously known inflammatory bowel disease (IBD) were reported with secukinumab treatment in PsA compared with one in the placebo arm.

As stated in the prescribing information United States Packages Insert (USPI), IBD exacerbations, in some cases serious, have occurred in patients treated with secukinumab during clinical trials in psoriasis, PsA, and AS. In addition, new-onset IBD cases, for example, ulcerative colitis (see the previous section), have occurred in clinical trials with this antibody. In an exploratory study in 59 patients with active Crohn's disease, there were trends toward greater disease activity in the secukinumab group than in the placebo group.

13.3.2.2 Ixekizumab

Ixekizumab is another IL-17A inhibitor, an IgG4 humanized monoclonal antibody (mAb) to IL-17A [32], which has been approved for treatment of psoriasis in the United States and other regions in the world.

13.3.2.2.1 Psoriasis

After a successful Phase 2 study [32] where PASI 75 responses at 12 weeks after treatment with 25, 75, or 150 mg of ixekizumab SC at weeks 0, 2, 4, and 8 were 77%, 83%, and 82%, respectively, compared with 8% in the placebo arm, and PASI 100 responses in the highest two dose groups, 150 and 75 mg, were remarkably high at 39% and 37%, respectively, three Phase 3 trials in psoriasis were conducted (UNCOVER-1, UNCOVER-2, and UNCOVER-3) [33,34]. A total of 1296 patients were dosed in the UNCOVER-1 trial, 1224 patients in the UNCOVER-2 trial, and 1346 patients in the UNCOVER-3 trial with SC placebo, 80 mg of ixekizumab Q2W after a starting dose of 160 mg (2-week dosing group), or 80 mg of ixekizumab Q4W after a starting dose of 160 mg (4-week dosing group). Additional cohorts in the UNCOVER-2 and UNCOVER-3 trials were treated with 50 mg of etanercept twice weekly. The PASI 75 responses at week 12 with placebo, ixekizumab 80 mg Q4W, and ixekizumab 80 mg Q2W in UNCOVER-1 were 4%, 83%, and 89%; in UNCOVER-2 were 2%, 78%, and 90%; and in UNCOVER-3 were 7%, 84%, and 87%, respectively. The corresponding PASI 100 responses in UNCOVER-1 were 0%, 34%, and 35%; in UNCOVER-2 were 1%, 31%, and 41%; and in UNCOVER-3 were 0%, 35%, and 38%, respectively. These responses were significantly higher than those seen with the comparator anti-TNF agent etanercept, for which the PASI 75/PASI 100 responses were 42%/5% in UNCOVER-2 and 53%/7% in UNCOVER-3. In the UNCOVER-1 and UNCOVER-2 trials, among the patients who were treated with ixekixumab Q2W for first 12 weeks and randomly reassigned at week 12 to receive 80 mg of ixekizumab Q4W, 80 mg of ixekizumab Q12W, or placebo, PASI 75 responses were maintained through week 60 by 83%, 49%, and 9% of the patients, respectively.

AEs reported during ixekizumab treatment across the three trials over 60 weeks included neutropenia, candidal infections, and IBD (14 patients across all UNCOVER trials, including 7 cases of ulcerative colitis and 7 cases of Crohn's disease).

13.3.2.2.2 PsA

Ixekizumab has been evaluated in a 417-patient Phase 3 trial in PsA (SPIRIT-P1) in patients naive to biologic therapy, at SC doses of 80 mg Q2W and Q4W, with a starting dose of 160 mg [35]. The study included an active arm with the anti-TNF antibody, adalimumab, at the approved dose. At the primary end point at week 24, there were significantly more patients treated with ixekizumab achieving an ACR20 response with ixekizumab Q2W (62%) or Q4W (58%) than placebo (30%), with responses seen as early as week 1. The ACR20 response with adalimumab (57%) was comparable to that with ixekizumab. Functional disability was improved with both ixekizumab doses versus placebo, as were dactylitis and enthesitis, and there was significantly less progression of structural damage on x-rays. The safety profile was overall consistent with that seen in psoriasis, with a few cases of mild neutropenia and two cases of candidiasis, but no cases of IBD, reported with ixekizumab treatment. A Phase 3 study of ixekizumab in PsA patients with prior exposure to biologics (SPIRIT-P2) is currently underway.

13.3.2.3 Brodalumab

Brodalumab is a fully human mAb that binds to the IL-17RA receptor subunit, thereby blocking multiple IL-17 family cytokines (IL-17A–C, E, and F) that bind to heterodimers of IL-17RA with other IL-17 receptor subunits [36,37]. It has been approved for psoriasis in the United States.

13.3.2.3.1 Psoriasis

As in the trials of the direct IL-17A inhibitors, brodalumab has demonstrated significant efficacy in psoriasis. In two Phase 3 studies (AMAGINE-2 and AMAGINE-3), patients with psoriasis were randomly assigned to receive brodalumab (210 or 140 mg SC Q2W), ustekinumab SC at approved doses, or placebo [38]. At week 12, patients receiving brodalumab were reassigned to receive it at a maintenance dose of 210 mg Q2W or 140 mg Q2W, Q4W, or Q8W; patients receiving placebo were treated with 210 mg of brodalumab Q2W. PASI 75 rates at week 12 were significantly higher with brodalumab at the 210 and 140 mg doses than with placebo (86% and 67%, respectively, vs. 8% in the AMAGINE-2 trial, and 85% and 69%, respectively, vs. 6% in the AMAGINE-3 trial); PASI 75 rates with ustekinumab were 70% and 69% in the AMAGINE-2 and AMAGINE-3 trials, respectively. The PASI 100 response rates at week 12 were significantly higher with 210 mg of brodalumab than with ustekinumab (44% vs. 22% in AMAGINE-2 and 37% vs. 19% in AMAGINE-3), with the PASI 100 response rates with 140 mg of brodalumab being 26% in AMAGINE-2 and 27% in AMAGINE-3. Using another measure of skin response, the proportion of patients with a Static Physician's Global Assessment score of 0 (clear) or 1 (almost clear) at week 52 was significantly higher in patients who had received 210 or 140 mg of brodalumab Q2W than in those who had received the other brodalumab maintenance regimens, and most patients who were switched from placebo to brodalumab had high response rates at week 52. Rates of neutropenia were higher with brodalumab than with placebo, and mild or moderate *Candida* infections were more frequent with brodalumab than with ustekinumab or placebo. One case of Crohn's disease was reported with brodalumab treatment, as were two cases of suicide. The agent has been approved with a warning for suicidality and is to be administered through a risk evaluation and mitigation strategy program in the US.

13.3.2.3.2 PsA

A Phase 2 study in 168 PsA patients has been conducted with brodalumab [39]. At the 12-week primary end point, ACR20 responses were significantly higher with brodalumab treatment (37% and 39% in the 140 and 280 mg treated arms, respectively) than with placebo (18%). These patients continued into open-label use of brodalumab, and ACR20 responses were observed to improve to 51% and 64%, respectively, in the 140 and 280 mg treated patients at 24 weeks. During the open-label extension, two events of Grade 2 neutropenia occurred.

13.3.2.4 Bimekizumab (Anti-IL-17A/F)

Bimekizumab is a humanized IgG1 mAb that binds to both IL-17A and IL-17F, in contrast to the anti-IL-17A antibodies, secukinumab and ixekizumab [40]. IL-17A and IL-17F both bind to the IL-17 receptor, a dimer of IL-17RA and IL-17RC. Both cytokines are expressed during inflammation at similar sites at different levels, and share similar functions. Bimekizumab has the potential advantage of blocking both of these cytokines without the potential negative effect of IL-17RA blockade related to potential IL-25 antagonism seen with brodalumab.

13.3.2.4.1 Psoriasis

Data from a Phase 1 single ascending dose study of IV bimekizumab in patients with mild to moderate psoriasis were reported recently [40]. Efficacy was remarkable in this trial, with complete skin clearance seen within 6 weeks with a single IV dose of 160–640 mg, with efficacy extending to around 16 weeks. A differentiating feature of bimekizumab from anti-IL-17A antibodies appears to be the durability of response—relapse occurs within 4–8 weeks of IL-17 mAb treatment withdrawal in psoriasis, while bimekizumab produced responses that lasted for at least 10 weeks after a single dose in this small study. The result of this dual targeting approach appears to be similar or show even greater efficacy than that with IL-17A blockade, but with a rapid and durable response resembling that with IL-23 mAbs. It is unclear why bimekizumab efficacy appears to be so much more durable, at least from this small study. Doses up to 640 mg in this trial were tested with a largely unremarkable safety profile.

13.3.2.4.2 PsA

Results from a proof-of-concept study of bimekizumab in PsA were recently presented, with 4 IV doses (40, 80, 160, and 320 mg, with double dose at baseline) of the drug given at 0, 3, and 6 weeks versus placebo [41]. Patients were either naive to biologics or exposed to not more than one biologic with dosing on a MTX background. The ACR20 response at week 8 at the top three doses of the agent combined ($n = 30$) was 80% versus 17% with placebo ($n = 12$), with the ACR50 response being 40% versus 8%, respectively. Durable responses were seen to at least 20 weeks. Liver enzyme elevation was reported in 20% of patients and neutropenia in 13%; otherwise, there were no significant safety issues.

13.3.2.5 ABT-122, Bispecific Anti-IL-17/TNF Antibody

ABT-122 is a bispecific dual variable domain antibody that neutralizes IL-17A and TNF, with the TNF specificity coming from the adalimumab component. Results from a recent 240-patient Phase 2 trial in MTX-IR PsA [42] showed that ACR20 responses at the primary end point of week 12 were significantly higher, with ABT-122 doses at 120 mg SC weekly (65%) and 240 mg weekly (75%), than with placebo (25%), and comparable to adalimumab at its approved dose of 40 mg SC Q2W (68%). However, the ACR50 and ACR70 responses were statistically superior with the 240 mg dose (53% and 32%, respectively) versus adalimumab (38% and 15%, respectively). The PASI 75 response was achieved by 78%, 74%, 58%, and 27% of the ABT-122 240 mg, ABT-122 120 mg, adalimumab, and placebo groups, respectively, again statistically superior in the ABT-122 240 mg group compared with adalimumab. The safety profile was acceptable, with infection rates similar to those of adalimumab. Although the high dose of ABT-122 was superior to adalimumab in ACR50, ACR70, and PASI 75 responses, the dual neutralization of IL-17A and TNF was not felt to have enough differentiated efficacy over adalimumab to proceed with further development.

13.3.3 Newer Oral Agents Targeting the IL-12/IL-23 Pathway

There are oral compounds targeting this pathway in development, for example, RORγT inhibitors [43], TyK2 (JAK family) inhibitors [44], and apilimod [45], with evidence of efficacy shown with a few of these agents in small trials in psoriasis. Results from further studies are awaited.

13.4 CONCLUSIONS

Targeting the IL-23/IL-17 axis has emerged over the past few years as an exciting approach to the treatment of psoriatic disease. The durability of response on de-escalation of dosing varies between different classes. While offering a highly efficacious option, off-treatment durability is limited, with disease flare occurring within a few weeks of discontinuation of the IL-17A mAbs, ixekizumab and secukinumab, as well as the IL-17RA mAb, brodalumab. The IL-23 blockers appear to offer efficacy that is as good as, if not better than, the IL-17 class, but with the possibility of an improved dosing regimen, at least in psoriasis. Falling somewhere between the IL-17A and IL-23 classes appears to be bimekizumab, which targets IL-17A and IL-17F, which seems to resemble more the IL-23 class than the IL-17A class in terms of efficacy and durability in early small trials. The safety of IL-17 inhibitors is consistent with the biology of IL-17 in host defense against *Candida* and neutrophil trafficking, although it is not clear if there is increased risk of development of IBD that is above the elevated background risk of IBD due to the known association and genetic linkage of psoriasis with IBD. Interestingly enough, IL-23 inhibitors have been shown to be efficacious in IBD, with ustekinumab already approved for Crohn's disease in the United States and other regions of the world.

In summary, the IL-23/IL-17 axis appears to play a critical role in the pathogenesis of psoriasis and PsA. Targeting this pathway appears to have revolutionized the treatment of psoriasis, with complete resolution of disease in many patients, and has offered efficacy that appears to be comparable to that of anti-TNF agents in PsA.

REFERENCES

1. Gaffen, S.L., Jain, R., Garg, A.V. et al. 2014. The IL-23–IL-17 immune axis: From mechanisms to therapeutic testing. *Nat. Rev. Immunol.* 14: 585–600.
2. Lubberts, E. 2015. The IL-23–IL-17 axis in inflammatory arthritis. *Nat. Rev. Rheumatol.* 11: 415–429.
3. Liang, Y., Pan, H., and Ye, D. 2015. Tc17 cells in immunity and systemic autoimmunity. *Int. Rev. Immunol.* 34 (4): 318–331.
4. Huber, M., Heink, S., Grothe, H. et al. 2009. A Th17-like developmental process leads to CD8+ Tc17 cells with reduced cytotoxic activity. *Eur. J. Immunol.* 39: 1716–1725.
5. Yen, H., Harris, T.J., Wada, S. et al. 2009. Tc17 CD8 T cells: Functional plasticity and subset diversity. *J. Immunol.* 183: 7161–7168.
6. Miossec, P., and Kolls, J.K. 2012. Targeting IL-17 and TH17 cells in chronic inflammation. *Nat. Rev. Drug Discov.* 11: 763–776.

7. Teng, M.W.L., Bowman, E.P., McElwee, J.J. et al. 2015. IL-12 and IL-23 cytokines: From discovery to targeted therapies for immune-mediated inflammatory diseases. *Nat. Med.* 21 (7): 719–729.
8. Smith, J.A., and Colbert, R.A. 2014. The interleukin-23/interleukin-17 axis in spondyloarthritis pathogenesis: Th17 and beyond. *Arthritis Rheumatol.* 66 (2): 231–241.
9. Campa, M., Mansouri, B., Warren, R. et al. 2016. A review of biologic therapies targeting IL-23 and IL-17 for use in moderate-to-severe plaque psoriasis. *Dermatol. Ther. (Heidelb.)* 6: 1–12.
10. Menon, B., Gullick, N.J., Walter, G.J. et al. 2014. Interleukin-17+CD8+ T cells are enriched in the joints of patients with psoriatic arthritis and correlate with disease activity and joint damage progression. *Arthritis Rheumatol.* 66: 1272–1281.
11. Lories, R.J., and McInnes, I.B. 2012. Primed for inflammation: Enthesis-resident T cells. *Nat. Med.* 18: 1018–1019.
12. Mease, P. 2015. Inhibition of interleukin-17, interleukin-23 and the TH17 cell pathway in the treatment of psoriatic arthritis and psoriasis. *Curr. Opin. Rheumatol.* 27 (2): 127–133.
13. Bartlett, H.S., and Million, R.P. 2015. Targeting the IL-17-Th17 pathway. *Nat. Rev. Drug Discov.* 14: 11–12.
14. Luo, J., Wu, S.J., Lacy, E.R. et al. 2010. Structural basis for the dual recognition of IL-12 and IL-23 by ustekinumab. *J. Mol. Biol.* 402: 797–812.
15. Leonardi, C.L., Kimball, A.B., Papp, K.A. et al. Efficacy and safety of ustekinumab, a human interleukin-12/23 monoclonal antibody, in patients with psoriasis: 76-week results from a randomised, double-blind, placebo-controlled trial (PHOENIX 1). *Lancet* 371: 1665–1674.
16. Papp, K.A., Langley, R.G., Lebwohl, M. et al. 2008. Efficacy and safety of ustekinumab, a human interleukin-12/23 monoclonal antibody, in patients with psoriasis: 52-week results from a randomised, double-blind, placebo-controlled trial (PHOENIX 2). *Lancet* 371: 1675–1684.
17. Papp, K.A., Griffiths, C.E.M., Gordon, K. et al. 2013. Long-term safety of ustekinumab in patients with moderate-to-severe psoriasis: Final results from 5 years of follow-up. *Br. J. Dermatol.* 168: 844–854.
18. McInnes, I.B., Kavanaugh, A., Gottlieb, A.B. et al. 2013. Efficacy and safety of ustekinumab in patients with active psoriatic arthritis: 1 year results of the phase 3, multicentre, double-blind, placebo-controlled PSUMMIT 1 trial. *Lancet* 382: 780–789.
19. Ritchlin, C., Rahman, P., Kavanaugh, A. et al. 2014. Efficacy and safety of the anti-IL-12/23 p40 monoclonal antibody, ustekinumab, in patients with active psoriatic arthritis despite conventional non-biological and biological anti-tumour necrosis factor therapy: 6-month and 1-year results of the phase 3, multicentre, double-blind, placebo controlled, randomised PSUMMIT 2 trial. *Ann. Rheum. Dis.* 73: 990–999.
20. Sofen, H., Smith, S., Matheson, R.T. et al. 2014. Guselkumab (an IL-23-specific mAb) demonstrates clinical and molecular response in patients with moderate-to-severe psoriasis. *J. Allergy Clin. Immunol.* 133: 1032–1040.
21. Blauvelt, A., Papp, K.A., Griffiths, C.E.M. et al. Efficacy and safety of guselkumab, an anti-interleukin-23 monoclonal antibody, compared with adalimumab for the continuous treatment of patients with moderate to severe psoriasis: Results from the phase III, double-blinded, placebo- and active comparator controlled VOYAGE 1 trial. *J. Am. Acad. Dermatol.* 76 (3): 405–417.
22. Reich, K., Armstrong, A.W., Foley, P. et al. 2017. Efficacy and safety of guselkumab, an anti-interleukin-23 monoclonal antibody, compared with adalimumab for the treatment of patients with moderate to severe psoriasis with randomized withdrawal and retreatment: Results from the phase III, double-blind, placebo- and active comparator controlled VOYAGE 2 trial. *J. Am. Acad. Dermatol.* 76 (3): 418–431.
23. Deodhar, A.A., Gottlieb, A.B., Boehncke, W. et al. 2016. Efficacy and safety results of guselkumab, an anti-IL23 monoclonal antibody, in patients with active psoriatic arthritis over 24 weeks: A phase 2a, randomized, double-blind, placebo-controlled study. *Arthritis Rheumatol.* 68 (Suppl. 10): abstract 4L.
24. Papp, K.A., Thaci, D., Reich, K. et al. 2015. Tildrakizumab (MK-3222), an anti-interleukin-23p19 monoclonal antibody, improves psoriasis in a phase IIb randomized placebo-controlled trial. *Br. J. Dermatol.* 173: 930–939.
25. Jancin, B. 2016. Tildrakizumab for psoriasis scores high marks in phase III. *Dermatology News (Frontline Medical News)*, October 19.
26. Langley, R., Thaçi, D., Reich, K. et al. 2016. FRI0445 tildrakizumab treatment improved measures of psoriatic arthritis in adults with chronic plaque psoriasis. *Ann. Rheum Dis.* 75: 596–597.
27. Krueger, J.G., Ferris, L.K., Menter, A. et al. 2015. Anti–IL-23A mAb BI 655066 for treatment of moderate-to-severe psoriasis: Safety, efficacy, pharmacokinetics, and biomarker results of a single-rising-dose, randomized, double-blind, placebo-controlled trial. *J. Allergy Clin. Immunol.* 136: 116–124.

28. Papp, K., Menter A, Sofen H. 2015. Onset and duration of clinical response following treatment with a selective IL-23p19 inhibitor (BI 655066) compared with ustekinumab in patients with moderate-to-severe chronic plaque psoriasis. Presented at the 24th European Academy of Dermatology and Venereology (EADV) Congress, Copenhagen, October 7–11.
29. Langley, R.G., Elewski, B.E., Lebwohl, M. et al. 2014. Secukinumab in plaque psoriasis—Results of two phase 3 trials. *N. Engl. J. Med.* 371: 326–338.
30. Mease, P.J., McInnes, I.B., Kirkham, B. et al. 2015. Secukinumab inhibition of interleukin-17A in patients with psoriatic arthritis. *N. Engl. J. Med.* 373: 1329–1339.
31. McInnes, I.B., Mease, P.J., Kirkham, B. et al. 2015. Secukinumab, a human anti-interleukin-17A monoclonal antibody, in patients with psoriatic arthritis (FUTURE 2): A randomised, double-blind, placebo-controlled, phase 3 trial. *Lancet* 386: 1137–1146.
32. Leonardi, C., Matheson, R., Zachariae, C. et al. 2012. Anti-interleukin-17 monoclonal antibody ixekizumab in chronic plaque psoriasis. *N. Engl. J. Med.* 366: 1190–1199.
33. Gordon, K.B., Blauvelt, A., Papp, K.A. et al. 2016. Phase 3 trials of ixekizumab in moderate-to-severe plaque psoriasis. *N. Engl. J. Med.* 375: 345–356.
34. Griffiths, C.E.M., Reich, K., Lebwohl, M. et al. 2015. Comparison of ixekizumab with etanercept or placebo in moderate-to-severe psoriasis (UNCOVER-2 and UNCOVER-3): Results from two phase 3 randomised trials. *Lancet* 386: 541–551.
35. Mease, P.J., Heijde, D., Ritchlin, C.T. et al. 2017. Ixekizumab, an interleukin-17A specific monoclonal antibody, for the treatment of biologic-naive patients with active psoriatic arthritis: Results from the 24-week randomised, double-blind, placebo controlled and active (adalimumab)-controlled period of the phase III trial SPIRIT-P1. *Ann. Rheum. Dis.* 76: 79–87.
36. Papp, K.A., Leonardi, C., Menter, A. et al. 2012. Brodalumab, an anti-interleukin-17-receptor antibody for psoriasis. *N. Engl. J. Med.* 366 (13): 1181–1189.
37. Ramirez-Carrozzi, V., Sambandam, A., Luis, E. et al. 2011. IL-17C regulates the innate immune function of epithelial cells in an autocrine manner. *Nat. Immunol.* 12: 1159–1167.
38. Lebwohl, M., Strober, B., Menter, A. et al. 2015. Phase 3 studies comparing brodalumab with ustekinumab in psoriasis. *N. Engl. J. Med.* 373: 1318–1328.
39. Mease, P.J., Genovese, M.C., Greenwald, M.W. et al. 2014. Brodalumab, an anti-IL17RA monoclonal antibody, in psoriatic arthritis. *N. Engl. J. Med.* 370: 2295–2306.
40. Glatt, S., Helmer, E., Haier, B. et al. 2017. First-in-human randomized study of bimekizumab, a humanized monoclonal antibody and selective dual inhibitor of IL-17A and IL-17F, in mild psoriasis. *Br. J. Clin. Pharmacol.* 83 (5): 991–1001.
41. Glatt, S., Strimenopoulou, F., Vajjah, P. et al. 2016. OP0108 bimekizumab, a monoclonal antibody that inhibits both IL-17A and IL-17F, produces a profound response in both skin and joints: Results of an early-phase, proof-of-concept study in psoriatic arthritis. *Ann. Rheum. Dis.* 75: 95–96.
42. Mease, P.J., Genovese, M.C., Weinblatt, M. et al. 2016. Safety and efficacy of ABT-122, a TNF and IL-17–targeted dual variable domain (DVD)–Ig™, in psoriatic arthritis patients with inadequate response to methotrexate: Results from a phase 2 trial. *Arthritis Rheumatol.* 68 (S10): Abstract 958.
43. Xue, X., Soroosh, P., Leon-Tabaldo, A.D. et al. 2016. Pharmacologic modulation of RORγt translates to efficacy in preclinical and translational models of psoriasis and inflammatory arthritis. *Sci. Rep.* 6: 37977.
44. Ishizaki, M., Muromoto, R., Akimoto, T. et al. 2013. Tyk2 is a therapeutic target for psoriasis-like skin inflammation. *Int. Immunol.* 26 (5): 257–267.
45. Wada, Y., Cardinale, I., Khatcherian, A. et al. 2012. Apilimod inhibits the production of IL-12 and IL-23 and reduces dendritic cell infiltration in psoriasis. *PLoS One* 7 (4): e35069.

14 DMARD Treatment in Patients with Psoriatic Arthritis

Rafael Valle Oñate and Andrea Chaparro

CONTENTS

The disease-modifying antirheumatic drugs (DMARDs) are prescribed as a first line therapy in psoriatic arthritis (PsA) especially in patients with the peripheral arthritis domain [1,2]. Different reviews and meta-analysis have demonstrated little high-quality evidence in support of the efficacy of these drugs in PsA, basically due to the small number of studies, dissimilar outcomes are being evaluated and there have been high withdrawal rates [3–7].

14.1 SULFASALAZINE

In a systematic review [5], six randomized controlled trials (RCTs) reported comparisons of sulfasalazine (SSZ) monotherapy versus placebo [8–13]. They found that SSZ was effective for the treatment of peripheral arthritis, such as pain score, number of painful and swollen joints, physician assessment, patient assessment, and other manifestation, such as morning stiffness and significant improvements in cutaneous involvement.

There was another clinical trial [14] that compared SSZ (2000 mg/day) with cyclosporine A and standard therapy (NSAIDs, analgesics, and/or prednisone ≤5 mg/day) in 99 patients with PsA; no significant differences were observed between SSZ and Standard-alone groups related to pain score, swollen joint count, tender joint count, joint or pain tenderness score, and patient and physician global assessments. However, a significant decrease was observed for the spondylitis functional index and erythrocyte sedimentation rate. Despite these results, the SSZ does not appear to halt radiographic progression in PsA. In a case-control study in which 20 patients who received SSZ for more than 3 months were compared with 20 control patients, the average change in the radiographic score at 24 months between the two groups was not statistically significant [15]. Two studies [8,10] reported no significant differences in clinical signs like dactylitis between SSZ and placebo, and one of them [8] reported no differences in the enthesitis. The latter study did not show benefits of SSZ over placebo.

In 1998, Rahman et al. [15] showed that 38% of patients discontinued SSZ within 3 months. The withdrawals and adverse drug reactions were higher in the SSZ group than in the placebo group [8], mostly related to adverse events such as gastrointestinal symptoms and rashes, which were the next most common complaints. Central nervous system symptoms, including headache, light-headedness, and confusion, were also seen, although none were judged by the investigator to be severe.

14.2 GOLD SALTS

A few RCTs were conducted to evaluate gold salts in PsA [16,17]. The evidence shows that gold salts (oral gold and intramuscular [IM] gold) were not statistically superior compared with placebo. These results were included and adjusted in a systematic review [18,19]. In order to evaluate the radiographic progression in peripheral joints, Mader et al. conducted a case-control study in 1995, in which they did not observe a statistical difference in disease progression at 24 months [20].

14.3 CYCLOSPORINE

At present, there are no RCTs comparing CsA with placebo in patients with PsA. However, there are three controlled trials that compared CsA with other disease-modifying antirheumatic drugs (DMARDs) [14,21,22]. One of them compared the effectiveness and toxicity of CsA (3–5 mg/kg/day) with a low dose of methotrexate (MTX) (maximum dose of 15 mg/weekly) over a period of 1 year in the treatment of PsA with peripheral involvement, and after 6 and 12 months, the number of painful and swollen joints, the Ritchie index, the duration of morning stiffness, grip strength, C-reactive protein (CRP), the patient's and physician's assessment of PsA activity, and the Psoriasis Area and Severity Index (PASI) were significantly improved in both treatment groups.

A second study [14] compared the efficacy and tolerability of CsA with symptomatic therapy (nonsteroidal antiinflammatory drugs, analgesics, and/or prednisone < or = 5 mg/day) alone versus with SSZ in PsA. There was a significant difference in that the CsA treatment showed changes in the pain score and a decrease in the swollen joint count, tender joint count, joint and pain tenderness score, and patient and physician global assessments.

In patients with an incomplete response to MTX, Fraser et al. [22] found that its combination with CsA resulted in significant clinical improvements when comparing the baseline in the swollen joint count and CRP synovitis detected by ultrasound and the PASI score. There is some evidence from a small study [23] that CsA had 2 years of partially controlled progression of radiographic damage in peripheral joints (60%).

The combination of adalimumab and CsA has been shown to produce improvement in both clinical and serological variables in patients with severely active PsA with inadequate response to MTX.

When the Psoriatic Arthritis Response Criteria (PsARC) or American College of Rheumatology 50% (ACR 50) response was applied after 12 months of treatment, a significantly greater mean improvement in the Health Assessment Questionnaire (HAQ) Disability Index was achieved by combination treatment compared with CsA or adalimumab alone [24]: 65% of CsA-treated, 85% of adalimumab-treated, and 95% of combination-treated patients by PsARC, and for ACR 50, the response rates were 36%, 69%, and 87%, respectively [24].

Fifty-eight percent of treated patients with CsA experienced at least one side effect [14]. The most common adverse event (28%) was mild reversible kidney dysfunction. Of particular concern, renal damage did not improve following discontinuation of therapy in some cases.

An analysis of the literature on the renal toxicity of long-term CsA exposure [25] in autoimmune diseases revealed that besides functional renal toxicity, de novo morphological kidney damage can be induced after 12 months with a low dose (≤5 mg CsA/kg/day); however, after 2 years of treatment it was light to moderate.

On the basis of all existing evidence, it can be affirmed that CsA can improve peripheral synovitis, but it has no effect on the other articular manifestations of psoriatic disease. As for the other synthetic DMARDs, the level of evidence supporting these conclusions is poor [26].

14.4 LEFLUNOMIDE

In an RCT published in 2004 [27], 190 patients with active PsA and psoriasis (at least 3% skin involvement) were randomized to receive leflunomide (LEF) (100 mg/day loading dose for 3 days, followed by 20 mg/day orally) or placebo for 24 weeks. The primary efficacy end point was the ratio of patients classified as responders according to the PsARC. The results showed 58.9% improvement in the LEF group compared with 29.7% in the placebo group. Significant differences were found in favor of LEF. Improvements were also observed in the proportion of patients achieving modified ACR 20 criteria, and in the mean changes from the baseline in PASI scores and quality of life assessments.

In a multicenter observational study [28], 514 patients were enrolled to assess the primary effectiveness of the analysis; 380 of 440 individuals (86.4%) achieved a PsARC response at 24 weeks. Significant improvements were observed in tender and swollen joint scores and counts, patient and physician global assessments, fatigue, pain, skin disease, dactylitis, and nail lesions. The withdrawal rate was 12.3%. Ninety-eight adverse drug reactions occurred in 62 (12.1%) patients; three drug reactions were serious (two increased liver enzymes and one hypertensive crisis).

In 2014, Asiri et al. [29] evaluated the effectiveness and safety of LEF as a single treatment or its combination with MTX in the treatment of PsA. The patients who continued the medication at 3 (38%), 6 (48%), and 12 (56%) months achieved a 40% or greater reduction of actively inflamed joint count. Although MTX did not modify arthritis response, psoriasis did improve. Patients taking MTX in combination with LEF were more likely to achieve a better PASI 50% response than patients with a single treatment.

There are no data on the effect of LEF on enthesitis, spondylitis, or radiographic progression. Available data suggest that in PsA, LEF has a moderate symptom-modifying effect on peripheral synovitis and might improve dactylitis. Its effects on the other articular manifestations of psoriatic disease are unknown [26].

The toxicity that leads to withdrawal is almost four times more frequent with LEF than with placebo (relative risk [RR] = 3.86; 95% confidence interval [CI] 1.2, 12.39) [30]. In a European study [28], 12.6% of patients experienced adverse events; the most frequent were diarrhea (16.3% of all adverse drug reactions), alopecia (9.2%), hypertension (8.2%), and pruritus (5.1%). The addition of LEF to concomitant DMARDs did not lead to an increase in adverse events.

14.5 METHOTREXATE

Three RCTs (n = 93 patients) comparing MTX monotherapy with placebo [31–33] and seven open or retrospective studies [34–40] of MTX in PsA were analyzed in a meta-analysis by Ash et al. [5] showing the efficacy of MTX for the treatment of peripheral arthritis and psoriasis, with a reduction in the physician global assessment. Data on radiographic progression were not conclusive, as it was only analyzed in a small case-control study [34].

The first study in 1964 [31] showed that high doses of parenteral injections of MTX appeared to be effective in suppressing skin manifestations, decreasing joint tenderness and swelling, improving joint range of motion, and decreasing the erythrocyte sedimentation rate. On the other hand, the side effects included anorexia or nausea, burning sensation in the skin, depression of the white blood cell count below 4000/cu mm, oral ulcerations, and mild hair loss, and one male patient, 39 years old, died during the period of MTX administration by myelotoxicity.

The Methotrexate in Psoriatic Arthritis (MIPA) trial [41] was performed in 221 patients who were randomized to receive MTX (target dose of 15 mg/week) or placebo. The outcomes were assessed at 6 months, with PsARC being the primary criteria. There were no differences in any of the individual outcomes (PsARC; ACR 20, 50, 70; and Disease Activity Score CRP), except for patient and physician global assessments, which were higher in the MTX group than in the placebo group. The results of this trial indicate that MTX is not effective for PsA, but several flaws in this trial emerged. First, despite the study being short in duration, only 65% and 69% of patients in the active and placebo groups, respectively, completed the trial, which might have biased the results toward a null effect. Second, patient recruitment lasted 5 years, which might reflect an element of selection bias. Third, around 35% of the patients included had oligoarticular disease, and the maximum dose of MTX was 15 mg/week, a dose achieved in only 78% of patients.

Most of the evidence to support the use of MTX in PsA is based on observational study data [42]. The efficacy of MTX was reevaluated by the University of Toronto PsA registry. They reported that patients in the 1994–2004 cohort had shorter disease duration and received higher MTX doses than the 1978–1993 cohort (16.2 vs. 10.8 mg/week, respectively) [43]. In this cohort, 68% of patients had a 40% or greater decrease in swollen joint counts and less radiographic progression than the earlier cohort, which increased the radiographic damage score assessed by the modifed Steinbrocker method, suggesting that higher MTX doses could exhibit better responses with less progression of damage. Cantini and colleagues [44,45], in 121 patients with peripheral PsA treated with MTX monotherapy, reported a remission rate (using very strict remission criteria) of 19%, and ACR 20, 50, 70 responses in 34%, 23%, and 10%, respectively.

In an open-label study, 115 patients with mild PsA were randomized to receive MTX or MTX with infliximab [46]. Although patients on the combination therapy achieved a significantly better response, patients treated with the monotherapy showed an ACR 20, 50, and 70 of 67%, 40%, and 19%, respectively.

Regarding toxicity, a meta-analysis of long-term MTX treatment studies in rheumatoid arthritis (RA) and psoriatic disease showed a threefold greater risk of hepatic fibrosis in patients with psoriatic disease [47]. The reasons for such differences could be related to higher rates of obesity and fatty liver; these results might justify the use of a different toxicity-monitoring protocol for patients with psoriatic disease.

Finally, the combination of MTX with SSZ or with an anti-tumor necrosis factor (TNF) agent could be safe; nevertheless, there is not enough consensus around the combination of MTX with LEF or CsA [48].

14.6 AZATHIOPRINE, CHLOROQUINE, D-PENICILLAMINE, FUMARIC ACID, AND COLCHICINE

Limited data are available on these agents, with no conclusive evidence for efficacy [5]. Another potential role for traditional DMARDs is their use in combination with TNF inhibitors (TNFi) [49]. The TICOPA trial [50] was the first study to assess treat to target (T2T) in each subtype of spondyloarthropathies. This trial recruited 206 patients with early psoriatic disease (<2 years of symptom duration), who had not received any treatment with DMARDs. The participants were randomized to receive either standard care or tight control. The tight control group was reviewed every 4 weeks and treated using a step-up conventional and biologic DMARD algorithm using minimal disease activity (MDA) as the target for treatment (initiating with MTX up to 25 mg/week, adding SZS, and then switching to MTX + CsA, or MTX + LEF, or MTX + TNFi) according to the number of swollen joints. The standard care group was reviewed by National Health Service (NHS) rheumatologists every 12 weeks with no restrictions or guidance on their therapeutic choices for 48 weeks. The study confirmed the benefit of this treatment approach using the MDA criteria for PsA as the treatment target. The trial showed a significant benefit in articular and skin outcomes (ACR 20, 50, 70, and PASI 75) [50].

Finally, in the management of patients with PsA, it is important to identify the commitment that the domain presents (see Algorithm 14.1). The Latin American Society and Psoriatic Arthritis Society (LAPPAS) study group conducted an online survey among Latin American rheumatologists from the Pan American League of Associations for Rheumatology (PANLAR) interested in PsA and dermatologists belonging to the Latin American Society of Society (SOLAPSO). The rheumatologists accessed the online survey (from Argentina, Bolivia, Brazil, Colombia, Costa Rica, Chile, Ecuador, El Salvador, Mexico, Panama, Peru, and Uruguay) and estimated that *enthesitis* and *oligoarthritis* are the more frequent clinical presentations upon the first clinic visit. A total of 43% estimated that PsA severity at first clinic presentation was mild, and 49% reported that MTX, NSAIDs, and topical agents are the most frequently used medications [51].

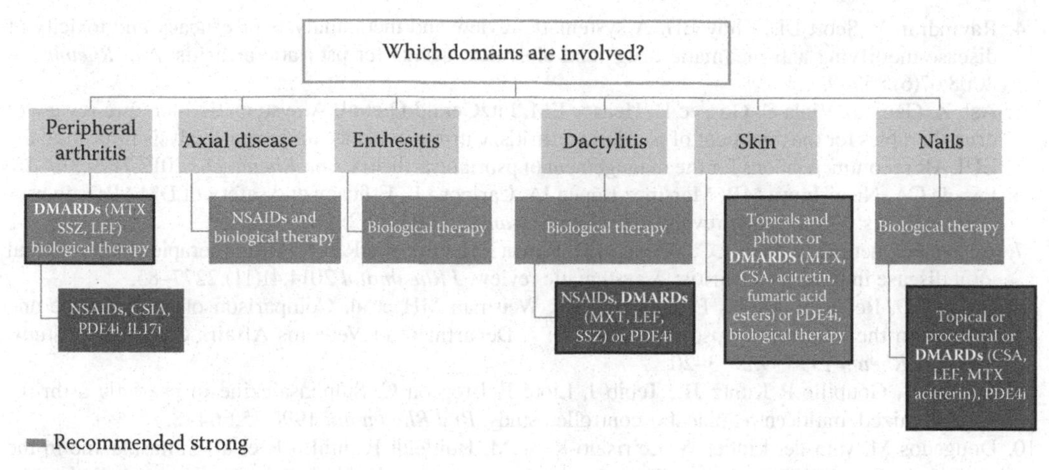

ALGORITHM 14.1 Algorithm based on treatment recommendations for PsA by GRAPPA. CS, corticosteroid; CSA, cyclosporin A; DMARDs, disease-modifying antirheumatic drugs; IA, intra-articular; LEF, leflunomide; MTX, methotrexate; NSAIDs, nonsteroidal anti-inflammatory drugs; PDE-4i, phosphodiesterase 4 inhibitor; SSZ, sulfasalazin. (From Coates, L. C. et al., *Arthritis Rheumatol.*, 68(5), 1060–1071, 2016.)

14.7 CONCLUSION

- In light of treatment strategies for PsA, the diverse nature of the clinical phenotype (peripheral arthritis, skin and nail disease, axial disease, dactylitis, and enthesitis) could complicate the therapeutic decisions considering that not all treatments are effective for all features, and patients often display a mixture of all of the features simultaneously. In both sets of recommentations (European League Against Rheumatism [EULAR] and Group for Research and Assessment of Psoriasis and Psoriatic Arthritis [GRAPPA]), the hetrogeneity of PsA is recognized and the place of various drugs in the therapeutic armamentarium is discussed [1,2].
- Traditional DMARDs remain first-line agents for PsA despite a paucity of RCT evidence. The EULAR and GRAPPA, in their recommendations, propose the use of DMARDs in patients with PsA and peripheral joint involvement (EULAR), and peripheral arthritis, skin disease, and dactylitis (GRAPPA). However, the latter is based on limited studies.
- In axial manfestations or enthesitis associated with PsA, DMARDs are not effective.
- It is very important to remember that GRAPPA recommendations include dermatological aspects in treatment, and EULAR recommendations are focused on musculoskeletal manifestations.
- The evidence observed with the treatment of DMARDs in PsA is not strong enough [52].

REFERENCES

1. Gossec L, Smolen JS, Ramiro S, de Wit M, Cutolo M et al. European League Against Rheumatism (EULAR) recommendations for the management of psoriatic arthritis with pharmacological therapies: 2015 update. *Ann Rheum Dis* 2015;75(3):499–510.
2. Coates LC, Kavanaugh A, Mease PJ, Soriano ER, Laura Acosta-Felquer M et al. Group for Research and Assessment of Psoriasis and Psoriatic Arthritis 2015 Treatment Recommendations for Psoriatic Arthritis. *Arthritis Rheumatol* 2016;68(5):1060–71.
3. Soriano ER, McHugh NJ. Therapies for peripheral joint disease in psoriatic arthritis: A systematic review. *J Rheumatol* 2006;33(7):1422–30.

4. Ravindran V, Scott DL, Choy EH. A systematic review and meta-analysis of efficacy and toxicity of disease modifying anti-rheumatic drugs and biological agents for psoriatic arthritis. *Ann Rheum Dis* 2008;67(6):855–9.
5. Ash Z, Gaujoux-Viala C, Gossec L, Hensor EM, FitzGerald O et al. A systematic literature review of drug therapies for the treatment of psoriatic arthritis: Current evidence and meta-analysis informing the EULAR recommendations for the management of psoriatic arthritis. *Ann Rheum Dis* 2012;71(3):319–26.
6. Pereda CA, Nishishinya MB, Martínez López JA, Carmona L. Efficacy and safety of DMARDs in psoriatic arthritis: A systematic review. *Clin Exp Rheumatol* 2012;30(2):282–9.
7. Acosta Felquer ML, Coates LC, Soriano ER, Ranza R, Espinoza LR et al. Drug therapies for peripheral joint disease in psoriatic arthritis: A systematic review. *J Rheumatol* 2014;41(11):2277–85.
8. Clegg DO, Reda DJ, Mejias E, Cannon GW, Weisman MH et al. Comparison of sulfasalazine and placebo in the treatment of psoriatic arthritis: A Department of Veterans Affairs Cooperative Study. *Arthritis Rheum* 1996;39:2013–20.
9. Combe B, Goupille P, Kuntz JL, Tebib J, Lioté F, Bregeon C. Sulphasalazine in psoriatic arthritis: A randomized, multicentre, placebo-controlled study. *Br J Rheumatol* 1996;35:664–8.
10. Dougados M, vam der Linden S, Leirisalo-Repo M, Huitfeldt B, Juhlin R et al. Sulfasalazine in the treatment of spondylarthropathy: A randomized, multicenter, double-blind, placebo-controlled study. *Arthritis Rheum* 1995;38:618–27.
11. Farr M, Kitas GD, Waterhouse L, Jubb R, Felix-Davies D et al. Sulphasalazine in psoriatic arthritis: A double-blind placebo-controlled study. *Br J Rheumatol* 1990;29:46–9.
12. Fraser SM, Hopkins R, Hunter JA, Neumann V, Capell HA et al. Sulphasalazine in the management of psoriatic arthritis. *Br J Rheumatol* 1993;32:923–5.
13. Gupta AK, Grober JS, Hamilton TA, Ellis CN, Siegel MT et al. Sulfasalazine therapy for psoriatic arthritis: A double blind, placebo controlled trial. *J Rheumatol* 1995;22:894–8.
14. Salvarani C, Macchioni P, Olivieri I, Marchesoni A, Cutolo M et al. A comparison of cyclosporine, sulfasalazine, and symptomatic therapy in the treatment of psoriatic arthritis. *J Rheumatol* 2001;28:2274–82.
15. Rahman P, Gladman DD, Cook RJ, Zhou Y, Young G et al. The use of sulfasalazine in psoriatic arthritis: A clinic experience. *J Rheumatol* 1998;25:1957–61.
16. Carette S, Calin A, McCafferty JP, Wallin BA. A double-blind placebo-controlled study of auranofin in patients with psoriatic arthritis. *Arthritis Rheum* 1989;32:158–65.
17. Palit J, Hill J, Capell HA, Carey J, Daunt SO et al. A multicentre double-blind comparison of auranofin, intramuscular gold thiomalate and placebo in patients with psoriatic arthritis. *Br J Rheumatol* 1990;29(4):280–3.
18. Jones G, Crotty M, Brooks P. Interventions for treating psoriatic arthritis. *Cochrane Database System Rev* 2000;(2):CD000212.
19. Jones G, Crotty M, Brooks P. Psoriatic Arthritis Meta-Analysis Study Group. Psoriatic arthritis: A quantitative overview of therapeutic options. *Br J Rheumatol* 1997;36(1):95–9.
20. Mader R, Gladman DD, Long J, Gough J, Farewell VT. Does injectable gold retard radiologic evidence of joint damage in psoriatic arthritis? *Clin Invest Med* 1995;18(2):139–43.
21. Spadaro A, Riccieri V, Sili-Scavalli A, Sensi F, Taccari E et al. Comparison of cyclosporin A and methotrexate in the treatment of psoriatic arthritis: A one-year prospective study. *Clin Exp Rheumatol* 1995;13(5):589–93.
22. Fraser AD, van Kuijk AWR, Westhovens R, Karim Z, Wakefield R et al. A randomised, double blind, placebo controlled, multicentre trial of combination therapy with methotrexate plus cyclosporin in patients with active psoriatic arthritis. *Ann Rheum Dis* 2005;64(6):859–64.
23. Macchioni P, Boiardi L, Cremonesi T, Battistel B, Casadei-Maldini M et al. The relationship between serum-soluble interleukin-2 receptor and radiological evolution in psoriatic arthritis patients treated with cyclosporin-A. *Rheumatol Int* 1998;18(1):27–33.
24. Karanikolas GN, Koukli EM, Katsalira A, Arida A, Petrou D et al. Adalimumab or cyclosporine as monotherapy and in combination in severe psoriatic arthritis: Results from a prospective 12-month nonrandomized unblinded clinical trial. *J Rheumatol* 2011;38(11):2466–74.
25. Zachariae H. Renal toxicity of long-term cyclosporin. *Scand J Rheumatol* 1999;28(2):65–8.
26. Marchesoni A, Lubrano E, Cauli A, Ricci M, Manara M. Psoriatic disease: Update on traditional disease-modifying antirheumatic drugs. *J Rheumatol Suppl* 2015;93(0):61–4.
27. Kaltwasser JP, Nash P, Gladman D, Rosen CF, Behrens F et al. Efficacy and safety of leflunomide in the treatment of psoriatic arthritis and psoriasis: A multinational, double-blind, randomized, placebo-controlled clinical trial. *Arthritis Rheum* 2004;50(6):1939–50.

28. Behrens F, Finkenwirth C, Pavelka K, Štolfa J, Šipek-Dolnicar A et al. Leflunomide in psoriatic arthritis: Results from a large European prospective observational study. *Arthritis Care Res* 2013;65(3):464–70.
29. Asiri A, Thavaneswaran A, Kalman-Lamb G, Chandran V, Gladman DD et al. The effectiveness of leflunomide in psoriatic arthritis. *Clin Exp Rheumatol* 2014;32(5):728–31.
30. Ravindran V, Scott DL, Choy EH. A systematic review and meta-analysis of efficacy and toxicity of disease modifying anti-rheumatic drugs and biological agents for psoriatic arthritis. *Ann Rheum Dis* 2008;67(6):855–9.
31. Black RL, O'Brien WM, Vanscott EJ, Auerbach R, Eisen AZ et al. Methotrexate therapy in psoriatic arthritis; double-blind study on 21 patients. *JAMA* 1964;189:743–7.
32. Scarpa R, Peluso R, Atteno M, Manguso F, Spano A et al. The effectiveness of a traditional therapeutical approach in early psoriatic arthritis: Results of a pilot randomised 6-month trial with methotrexate. *Clin Rheumatol* 2008;27(7):823–6.
33. Willkens RF, Williams HJ, Ward JR, Egger MJ, Reading JC et al. Randomized, double-blind, placebo controlled trial of low-dose pulse methotrexate in psoriatic arthritis. *Arthritis Rheum* 1984;27(4):376–81.
34. Abu-Shakra M, Gladman DD, Thorne JC, Long J, Gough J et al. Longterm methotrexate therapy in psoriatic arthritis: Clinical and radiological outcome. *J Rheumatol* 1995;22(2):241–5.
35. Espinoza LR, Zakraoui L, Espinoza CG, Gutierrez F, Jara LJ et al. Psoriatic arthritis: Clinical response and side effects to methotrexate therapy. *J Rheumatol* 1992;19(6):872–7.
36. Kane D, Gogarty M, O'Leary J, Silva I, Berminghan N et al. Reduction of synovial sublining layer inflammation and proinflammatory cytokine expression in psoriatic arthritis treated with methotrexate. *Arthritis Rheum* 2004;50(10):3286–95.
37. Kragballe K, Zachariae E, Zachariae H. Methotrexate in psoriatic arthritis: A retrospective study. *Acta Derm Venereol* 1983;63(2):165–7.
38. Ranza R, Marchesoni A, Rossetti A, Tosi S, Gibelli E. Methotrexate in psoriatic polyarthritis. *J Rheumatol* 1993;20:1804–5.
39. Ricci M, De Marco G, Desiati F, Mazzocchi D, Rotunno L et al. Long-term survival of methotrexate in psoriatic arthritis. *Reumatismo* 2009;61(2):125–31.
40. Zachariae H, Zachariae E. Methotrexate treatment of psoriatic arthritis. *Acta Derm Venereol* 1987;67:270–3.
41. Kingsley GH, Kowalczyk A, Taylor H et al. A randomized placebo-controlled trial of methotrexate in psoriatic arthritis. *Rheumatology* 2012;51(8):1368–77.
42. Ceponis A, Kavanaugh A. Use of methotrexate in patients with psoriatic arthritis. *Clin Exp Rheumatol* 2010;28(5 Suppl 61):S132–7.
43. Chandran V, Schentag CT, Gladman DD. Reappraisal of the effectiveness of methotrexate in psoriatic arthritis: Results from a longitudinal observational cohort. *J Rheumatol* 2008;35(3):469–71.
44. Cantini F, Niccoli L, Nannini C, Cassara E, Pasquetti P et al. Frequency and duration of clinical remission in patients with peripheral psoriatic arthritis requiring second-line drugs. *Rheumatology* 2008;47(6):872–6.
45. Cantini F, Niccoli L, Nannini C, Cassara E, Pasquetti P et al. Criteria, frequency, and duration of clinical remission in psoriatic arthritis patients with peripheral involvement requiring second-line drugs. *J Rheumatol Suppl* 2009;83:78–80.
46. Baranauskaite A, Raffayova H, Kungurov NV, Kubanova A, Venalis A et al. Infliximab plus methotrexate is superior to methotrexate alone in the treatment of psoriatic arthritis in methotrexate-naive patients: The RESPOND study. *Ann Rheum Dis* 2012;71(4):541–8.
47. Whiting-O'Keefe QE, Fye KH, Sack KD. Methotrexate and histologic hepatic abnormalities: A meta-analysis. *Am J Med* 1991;90(6):711–6.
48. Taylor WJ, Korendowych E, Nash P, Helliwell PS, Choy E et al. Drug use and toxicity in psoriatic disease: Focus on methotrexate. *J Rheumatol* 2008;35(7):1454–7.
49. Soriano ER. Management of psoriatic arthritis: Traditional disease-modifying rheumatic agents and targeted small molecules. *Rheum Dis Clin North Am* 2015;41(4):711–22.
50. Coates L, Moverley A, McParland L, Brown S, Navarro-Coy N et al. Effect of tight control of inflammation in early psoriatic arthritis (TICOPA): A UK multicentre, open-label, randomised controlled trial. *Lancet* 2015;386(10012):2489–98.
51. Toloza S, Valle-Oñate R, Espinoza L. Psoriatic arthritis in South and Central America. *Curr Rheumatol Rep* 2011;13(4):360–8.
52. Maese J, Díaz del Campo P, Seoane-Mato D, Guerra M, Cañete J. Eficacia de los fármacos antirreumáticos modificadores de la enfermedad sintéticos en artritis psoriásica: Una revisión sistemática. *Reumatol Clin* 2017. http://dx.doi.org/10.1016/j.reuma.2016.10.005.

15 Topical Therapies for Psoriasis

Michael Sticherling

CONTENTS

15.1 INTRODUCTION

Psoriasis is one of the most common chronic inflammatory skin diseases of man, covering a broad spectrum of clinical manifestations and affecting patients of almost any age, from early life to old age [1–3]. With partly complex health issues like comorbidities and comedication, the individually perceived impact on life quality issues varies. Whereas one-third of patients have moderate to severe disease, which should be treated systemically, two-thirds of patients have mild disease and may respond sufficiently to topical therapy. Psoriasis is not only a treatable disease, but also a disease that has to be treated. Current controlled clinical studies reflect these issues only to a limited extent, whereas disease and therapy registries give a much better and realistic impression of the disease and its impact. The common attitude of both patients and physicians that psoriasis can still not be sufficiently treated is not justified: there was an exponential growth of the scope of treatment modalities over the last decades (Figure 15.1), and in fact, more drugs are officially licensed for psoriasis than for any other dermatological disease [4–11]. It is the expertise and duty of dermatologists to choose from this broad armamentarium of topical, ultraviolet (UV), and systemic treatment modalities an individually tailored therapy [12–15] (Table 15.1). This may not be amply covered by other medical specialties that are more familiar with systemic treatment and may therefore be prone to overtreating skin diseases. On the other side, dermatologists have to be aware of systemic treatment options and use them when indicated.

1915	UV-therapy (Finsen)
1916	Cignolin
1955	Corticosteroids
1988	Ciclosporin
1992	Vitamin-D analogues
1994	Fumaderm®
2004	Biologics
2007	German S3-guide line (first edition)

FIGURE 15.1 Chronology of psoriatic treatment modalities in the twentieth century.

TABLE 15.1
Therapeutic Apremilast for Psoriasis

Topical	Systemic	Phototherapy
Corticosteroids	Fumarates	Narrowband UVB (311 nm)
Vitamin D3 analogues	Methotrexate	Photochemotherapy (PUVA)
Cignolin	Cyclosporin	Broad-spectrum UV-B
Salicylic acid	Retinoids	Balneo-phototherapy
Tazaroten	Biologics	

Clinical experience in psoriatic treatment resides on (1) solely casuistic responses at the lowest end of the evidence level, and (2) empirical and (3) evidence-based knowledge. Recent therapeutics have been developed based [1–3] on our current and advanced pathogenic ideas of psoriasis.

15.2 GENERAL ASPECTS OF TOPICAL THERAPY

These aspects set the stage for topical treatment, which is also referred to as local or external treatment [4–11]. Until today, and even more in times of very effective and well-tolerated systemic treatments, topical therapy still plays an important role either (1) as monotherapy in limited disease, (2) as combination therapy with systemic or UV treatment, or (3) when these modalities are contraindicated [12–15]. Following current treatment algorithms, mild psoriasis may be treated locally only. Mild disease is defined by a limited area of affected skin and limited disease activity, as well as the absence of relevant comorbid diseases like metabolic disorders and psoriasis arthritis. Established instruments to define severity are, for example, body surface area (BSA), the Psoriasis Area and Severity Index (PASI) (ranging from 0 to 72) [16–18], and the Dermatology Life Quality Index (DLQI) (ranging from 0, no impairment, to 30, strongest impairment) [17]. Mild psoriasis disease is defined as any of the three below 10, and moderate to severe disease as above 10–12 [19]. Some authors further divide into moderate (PASI between 10 and 20) and severe (PASI above 20) disease. However, limited disease at critical areas like the scalp, face, intertriginous areas, and nails, as well as accompanying itch [20], may become severe disease when life quality, as well as social and work issues, is affected. In these cases, systemic treatment may be advisable; however, local or national health reimbursement regulations have to be taken into account.

Although most of the currently available topical agents are effective and their clinical use is well known, their evidence levels with regard to efficacy and tolerability are partly limited (Figure 15.2).

Keratoplastic/keratinolytic

Oil baths

Salicylic acid

Urea

Anti-inflammatory

Corticosteroids

Calcineurin inhibitors

Balancing keratinization

Vitamin D analogues

Vitamin A analogues

Inhibiting keratinocyte proliferation

Cignolin

Tar

FIGURE 15.2 Therapeutic targets of topical agents.

Long-standing topical treatment on larger areas of the integument will challenge the compliance of patients, as application, up to twice daily, will consume a considerable amount of everyday life. Similarly, aspects of greasiness and stickiness, skin irritation, local adverse events, and odor and contact sensitization may deter patients from regular and continuous use [21–23] (Figure 15.3). Proper application of external therapy on 10% or more of the body surface takes 20–30 minutes daily and 100 g of ointment per week; neither is realistic in the long run. Therefore, even limited but chronic disease on around 10% of the body surface that is resistant to topical therapy may demand systemic treatment in individual cases. In addition, continuous treatment of widespread surface areas well above 20%–30% for a prolonged period of several weeks may result in relevant systemic resorption, as seen in topical corticosteroids and vitamin D analogues. Therefore, de-escalation and proactive treatment, as outlined below, should be preferred [24], or a combination of topical agents [24,25], with UV [26,27] and systemic treatment to decrease both dosage and time period of application.

Similarly, the appropriate galenic base has to be selected and adapted to the activity of skin inflammation (oil-in-water base with acute disease, water-in-oil base for subacute and chronic disease), body site (face vs. extremities, skinfolds vs. free integument), patient age (no salicylic acid in early childhood, reduce the use of urea in children), season of the year (oil-in-water base in summer,

Pros

- Mild to moderate disease
- Outpatient treatment
- Rarely systemic side efects
- Less expensive than many systemic treatments

Cons

- Local side effects (burning, contact sensitization, cosmetic restrictions)
- Time consuming
- Sometimes ineffective

FIGURE 15.3 Pros and cons of topical therapy.

water-in-oil base in winter), and skin type. The broad range of currently available topical agents will allow an individualized and tailored topical treatment of psoriasis. Various vehicles are available, from ointments and creams to lotions, gels, foams, sprays, and shampoos. Patients should be educated in the correct application of topical agents with respect to the frequency of daily application, the length of application, and the maximal BSA to be treated. The optimal amount of ointment is defined as a "fingertip unit," which is about 500 mg of cream and will cover the end of the finger to the first interphalangeal joint. This should be applied to the equivalent of one hand-sized area of skin, which is about 1% of the BSA.

The importance of the vehicle cannot be underestimated and has been examined in detail for topical corticosteroids. As a consequence, the same steroid compound may clinically be differently resorbed and differently potent depending on the formulation. This is especially important for generic and brand name products, where the potencies are not always equivalent to each other and are hardly examined in comparative studies. Variability may even exist between different generic preparations.

Even more important than with systemic treatment, aspects of patient cooperation and education have to be taken into account to guarantee correct, continuous, and motivated application of topical treatment. In this context, the term *persistence* describes the continuous and regular use of a prescribed treatment that may be influenced by various parameters. This is intimately related to *compliance*, which is the commitment of a patient's behavior to his or her physician's recommendations [28]. As *adherence* defines more precisely that the patient's behavior is based on the accepted recommendations of the physician, it is now widely used in the English literature as a substitute for *compliance* [29]. *Concordance* describes the optimal cooperation of the patient and the physician in that therapeutic recommendations are drawn in a partnership relation. Because of these important and now widely accepted aspects of therapeutic cooperation and success, patient-related outcomes (PROs), in addition to quantifiable somatic parameters, are now increasingly included in randomized clinical studies, as well as in treatment decisions in clinical practice [30].

15.3 EMOLLIENTS

As in other skin diseases, like atopic eczema and ichthyosis, skin barrier function is impaired in psoriasis, which results in increased transepidermal water loss and epidermal hyperproliferation, as well as disruption of regular keratinization. Hyperkeratosis and itch are evident clinical consequences. Therefore, skin moisturization apart from anti-inflammatory strategies is a major therapeutic approach in psoriasis. Urea is a low-molecular-weight organic compound relevant to skin hydration through its hygroscopic characteristics, and it has been used in topical formulations for decades [31,32]. Concentrations from 2% to 10% will result in rehydration of skin, as well as increase the penetration of active agents like corticosteroids. Concentrations above 10% show keratinolytic activity and may be used to remove skin hyperkeratosis and onycholytic nail plate material. Mild skin irritation, especially at sensitive sites, is the major unwanted effect. Therefore, urea at concentrations above 2% should be used cautiously, especially in young children.

Salicylic acid is mainly used as a keratinolytic agent at concentrations above 5%, and it shows antiseptic activity at lower concentrations. In modern topical combinations with corticosteroids, it is used to increase their penetration into the skin. Salicylic acid should not be used in children younger than 12 years because of possible relevant resorption and intoxication. Alternatively, keratolytic or penetration-increasing agents, like propyleglycol, dimethicon, or ethanol, may be added to topical formulations [33].

15.4 TAR

Various tar preparations are well established in medicine: wood tars have been used since ancient times and coal tar for about a hundred years [34,35]. Based on their anti-inflammatory, antipruritic, and antiproliferative activity, as well as antibacterial and antifungal activity, the major indications are chronic inflammatory skin diseases. Apart from psoriasis, these mainly are seborrheic dermatitis and atopic eczema [36]. Coal tar may be used as crude tar or more commonly as liquor carbonis detergens (LCD) [37]. This is a dark black, sticky liquid that is used in shampoos and ointments in concentrations up to 20%. It contains around 10,000 chemical compounds, only half of which have been identified so far and comprise polycyclic aromatic hydrocarbons (PAHs), phenols, and heterocyclic compounds [38]. It can be prepared from brown coal (lignite tar), bitumen (bituminous tar), and anthracite as the most metamorphosed type of coal (anthracite tar). Coal tar is mentioned among the most effective and safe medicines in the World Health Organization's List of Essential Medicines. Coal tar products are mainly sold over the counter [39,40], but they may also be used as compounded preparations (0.5%–20%) in ointment bases like petrolatum and other formulations [41]. Wood, mainly pine tars, has historically also been used for the above-mentioned purposes; nowadays, however, it is mainly sold over the counter in various formulations.

The mode of action of tar is not yet known in detail, and with regard to the numerous compounds contained, it is hard to pinpoint anyway. A reduction of DNA synthesis, as well as mitotic activity, may normalize epidermal keratinization with positive clinical results on psoriasis. For atopic eczema, skin barrier repair through an induction of the aryl hydrocarbon receptor (AHR) has been demonstrated to interfere with TH2 signaling through dephosphorylation of STAT 6 [42]. How these results compare with the clinical effects seen in psoriasis remains to be elucidated.

Crude coal tar (2%–4% in petrolatum), in combination with artificial UV radiation (either broad- or narrowband UVB), is still widely used in the United States [43–46]. It was first described by the American dermatologist William H. Goeckerman (1884–1954) and is still regarded safe and efficacious. A modified protocol, called the Ingram method, was established in 1953 by the English dermatologist John Ingram, who added topical anthralin to the Goeckerman regimen. The main side effects of tars are contact sensitization and (mild) irritation at the sites of application, folliculitis, and photosensitivity apart from odor and discoloration of the skin, as well as clothing. Possible carcinogenesis is still a matter of debate, although available data are conflicting [47–49]. Short-term use of tar preparations may still be advisable in individual cases when modern topical alternatives are either not available or applicable [50].

15.5 ANTHRALIN

Anthralin (cignolin, dithranol) is a synthetically produced derivative of a natural mixture of plant ingredients, which has been used in medicine as early as the eighteenth century [51]. The natural substance chrysarobin is derived from the araroba tree in South America. Anthralin may be used as so-called minutes or *short-contact therapy* at concentrations of 0.1%–3%, which are applied over weeks for an increasing length of time, starting with a few minutes, to be subsequently rinsed off [52]. Alternatively, anthralin may be applied as *long-contact therapy*, starting at lower concentrations of 0.01% and left on for 8–12 hours. Mild skin irritation is intended, but may limit its use at delicate locations or with children. However, contact sensitization has not been reported. As it is neither resorbed nor mutagenic or cancerogenic, it may be used in pregnancy and with ample care in children, especially in guttate psoriasis and more superficial psoriasis manifestations. Apart from possible skin irritation, other disadvantages represent dark discoloration of skin, hair, nails, and clothing, as well as sanitary fittings. Skin discoloration may be cosmetically disturbing, but will vanish within 1–2 weeks after stopping the therapy. In addition, *Woronoff's ring* or leukoderma psoriaticum may appear as white halos surrounding initial psoriatic lesions. For conservation reasons, 1% salicylic acid is regularly added to the ointment. This should be taken into account when combining with vitamin D analogues, which are sensitive to salicylic acid.

Clinical improvement up to clearing can be found in 30%–70% of patients after a 12-week treatment [52–54]. It is used mainly in a hospital setting for induction therapy of mild to moderate psoriasis [52]. Its mode of action is unknown in detail, but the generation of reactive oxygen species or intercalation in the DNA with subsequent inhibition of cell proliferation is suggested [55]. Compared with any other psoriasis treatment, anthralin appears to have the longest disease-free interval.

15.6 CORTICOSTEROIDS

Corticosteroids are steroid hormones that are produced in the adrenal cortex and play an important role in physiological and pathophysiological regulatory processes. Therapeutically, they are used as synthetic analogues of these hormones, exploiting their broad and effective anti-inflammatory capacity. The compounds bind to the intracellular glucocorticoid receptor, which after translocation to the nucleus regulates genes directly involved in inflammation. As a consequence, interleukins (IL) 1 and 8, tumor necrosis factor alpha, and interferon gamma, as well as nitric oxide, prostaglandins, and levels of leukotrienes, are reduced. The clinical availability of synthetic corticosteroid analogues by the 1950s resulted in the successful treatment of until then ill-treatable and sometimes even fatal inflammatory diseases. Both topical and systemic agents have become available; however, their initially uncritical and broad use with significant side effects, especially on prolonged and repetitive use, resulted in a negative and reluctant attitude of both patients and physicians that still persists today [56–58]. Whereas this is indeed comprehensible in the context of a chronic disease like psoriasis, topical corticosteroids are still a mainstay of treatment with regard to their immediate and reliable effects and their universal combination ability in acute and subacute disease states [12–15,59]. Topical corticosteroids have been pharmacologically improved over the years by increasing their lipophilicity through esterification, as in fluticasone proprionate, or limiting their activity to the skin organ by their inactivation within the epidermis. This holds true especially for mometasone and methylprednisolone aceponate as steroid agents or the development of novel formulations like foams and sprays. Corticosteroids are available in diverse vehicles. This allows their appropriate use at any body site, including sensitive areas like the face and folds and hard-to-reach areas like the scalp and nails, as well as in sensitive patient groups, like children, pregnant women, and elderly patients. Lotions and foam formulations are usually better accepted by patients and were shown to be more effective, like clobetasol proprionate 0.05% spray or foam, compared with ointment formulations.

Long-term data on efficacy and safety are missing; however, depending on their potency, topical corticosteroids may be used continuously for up to 8 weeks. To reduce the incidence and impact of classical corticosteroid side effects, for example, skin atrophy, vascular fragility, and localized infections, they should be used discontinuously beyond that time and be combined with other agents, like UV light. A major drawback is tachyphylaxis [60] and relapse or even rebound after (rapidly) stopping the therapy, which may be overcome by slowly tapering the application frequency, as well as steroid potency. After complete cessation of clinical symptoms, topical corticosteroids may be used over weeks or several months twice a week at the sites that were originally involved [12–15]. The steroid-sparing effect, as well as reduction of number and intensity of flares, with this so-called proactive treatment has been documented for atopic eczema in controlled clinical studies, but may work equally well in psoriasis.

The penetration of topical corticosteroids, depending on body sites and patient ages, has to be taken into account. Penetration is fourfold higher for the scrotum and eyelids than for the forehead, and 36-fold higher than for the soles and palms. Moist skin may increase penetration similar to occluded areas like skinfolds, groins, and axillae. The face and intertriginous areas are critical with respect to side effects and systemic resorption, whereas the scalp and skin of the trunk are comparatively steroid resistant. As children are more prone to side effects than adults, they should be treated with corticosteroids of lower potency. Therefore, as a general rule, halogenated corticosteroids should not be used in skinfolds or on the face [58,61]. Penetration through the skin may therapeutically be increased by application of polyurethane foils after application of corticosteroids (occlusion therapy). Short-term use and tight control for strictures, superinfection, and accumulation of body heat are, however, mandatory.

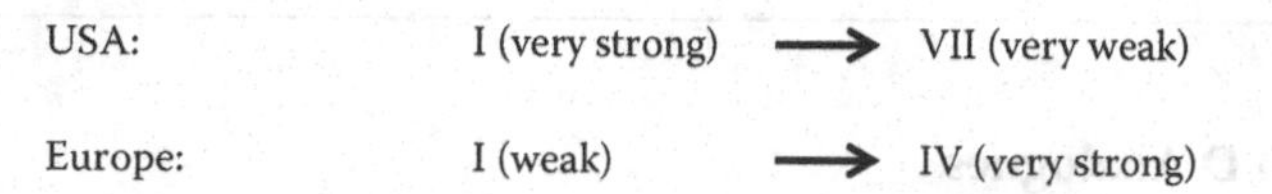

FIGURE 15.4 Potency of corticosteroids.

TABLE 15.2
Topical Corticosteroids by Their Potency

U.S. Class	European Class	Potency	Corticosteroid
I	IV	Super high	Clobetasole proprionate
II		Super potent	Halobetasol propionate
III		Very potent	Amcinonide
			Desoximetasone
			Fluocinonide
			Mometasone furoate
IV	III	Potent	Betamethasone diproprionate
V	II	Medium potent	Betamethasone valerate
			Diflucortolone valerate
			Fluocinolone acetonide
			Hydrocortisone valerate
			Triamcinolone acetonide
VI		Mild potent	Desonide
			Prednicarbate
VII	I	Mildest potent	Dexamethasone
			Flumethasone
			Hydrocortisone
			Methylprednisolone
			Prednisolone
			Fluticasone proprionate

As the potency of topical corticosteroids has been classified into three to seven classes, scientific reports and clinical recommendations have to be carefully compared. Whereas classes are numbered in Europe by increasing potency, the order is reverse in the United Stsates (Figure 15.4 and Table 15.2). As of now, clear-cut recommendations on the frequency and duration of therapy, as well as on respective body sites, are still missing.

The *German S3 guideline on plaque psoriasis* [12] includes 36 studies using topical corticosteroids, 10 of which fulfill the evidence level A2. Betamethasone dipropionate results in a complete remission in 25%–77% of cases, and mometasone in a PASI 75 between 36% and 64%, whereas the European class IV corticosteroid clobetasol 17-propionate shows a PASI 75 of 68%–89%. Topical steroids should only be used for induction therapy, be tapered quickly, and be amply combined with other topical agents. On the other side, any residual or resistant psoriasis manifestation under an otherwise effective and tolerated systemic treatment may well be tackled by additional topical steroids.

15.7 VITAMIN D ANALOGUES

Synthetic topical vitamin D analogues were introduced into clinical use for psoriasis in 1988 [62,63]. Apart from their immunomodulatory capacity, the modulation of receptor-mediated keratinocyte proliferation and differentiation is regarded as a major mode of action. The compounds

TABLE 15.3
Topical Vitamin D Analogues

Trade Name	Compound	Preparations	Application
Dovonex (United States) Daivonex (Europe)	Calcipotriol 50 µg/g	Ointment, cream, scalp solution	Initially twice daily Maintenance once daily Up to 30% of BSA Maximally 100 g/week
Dovobet (United States) Daivobet (Europe)	Calcipotriol 50 µg/g Beatamethasone dipropionate 0.5 mg/g	Ointment	Initially twice daily for 4 weeks Maximally 100 g/week
Xamiol Gel/Daivobet Gel	Calcipotriole 50 µg/g Beatamethasone dipropionate 0.5 mg/g	Scalp gel	Once daily for 4 weeks Maximally 15 g/application Up to 30% of BSA 100 g/week
Enstilar Silkis	Calcitriole 3 µg/g	Ointment	Twice daily 30 g maximal daily dose Maximally 200 g/week

bind to intracellular vitamin D receptors, which after translocation to the nucleus bind to vitamin D response elements and regulate genes directly involved in keratinocyte proliferation and keratinization, as well as epidermal inflammation. Calcipotriol (Europe and Canada; calcipotriene in the United States) is probably one of the best-studied topical agents by GCP criteria (good clinical practice) [64,65]. Monotherapy resulted in a 59% reduction of PASI 75 after 8 weeks of treatment. In head-to-head studies, calcipotriol proved superior to tar and anthralin and comparable to class II corticosteroids. In early studies, a 59% reduction of PASI 75 could be achieved after 8 weeks of treatment [12–15,66]. Vitamin D analogues are cosmetically well appreciated; however, they may cause skin irritations at locations like the face and skinfolds and result in discontinuation of treatment in 5%–10% of cases. Contact sensitization has been described in a few cases, whereas cancerogenic properties are absent. The three different agents, calcipotriol, tacalcitol [67,68], and calcitriol, are available as solution, cream, and ointment. Calcitriol at 3 µg/g ointment was shown to be equally effective as the other synthetic analogues; however, it had less irritability, especially at sensitive sites like the face and skinfolds [69,70]. Clearing or almost clearing could be seen in 34% of patients compared with the vehicle control of 12%–22%. Vitamin D analogues should only be used on less than 30% of the body surface for 8 weeks maximum because of systemic resorption with hypercalcemia and hypercalcuria (Table 15.3), and they can successfully be combined with UV light [71,72]. Long-term treatment is possible with a fixed combination of calcipotriol and betamethasone dipropionate (see the next section). As vitamin D analogues destabilize in the presence of lactic and salicylic acid, they should not be used at the same time.

15.8 VITAMIN D ANALOGUES: COMBINATION

The combination of topical corticosteroids and vitamin D analogues was shown to be superior to the monotherapy with either agent [73–75]. The fixed combination of betamethasone and calcipotriol applied once daily proved especially effective. It is currently available as a cream and a lipophilic gel (Xamiol), which was specially introduced for the scalp, but may be used on the skin as well [76–78]. In a direct comparison of Xamiol gel to Daivonex solution on the scalp, 69% of patients on the gel achieved clear or almost clear skin compared with 32% treated with the solution [12]. In the recently launched novel foam preparation (Enstilar), the agents are largely in solution, and thus clinically available, in contrast to the ointment and gel formulations, where parts of the agents are present as crystals. In a vehicle-controlled study, 53% of patients on Enstilar reached a PASI 75 after 2 weeks versus 8% on the vehicle. The application of the fixed combination of betamethasone and calcipotriol should be slowly reduced, possibly changing to calcipotriol as monotherapy. A clinical study on the proactive use of the fixed combination is ongoing.

15.9 VITAMIN A ANALOGUES

In contrast to acne, all-trans retinoic and 13-cis retinoic acid are not effective in psoriasis. However, the acetylene retinoid tazarotene is a third-generation topical retinoid that is licensed in the United States for psoriasis in adults aged above 18 years and for acne vulgaris in patients above the age of 12 [79,80]. It is no longer available in some countries. It compares well to other topical agents, like coal tar [81]. A 50% improvement was shown in 45% of patients after 6 weeks when applied in a 0.05% gel formulation twice daily [82]. Limitations are skin irritation, which is found in 23% of patients, and a maximal body surface of 10%–20% to be treated. Tazarotene was shown to bind to the retinoic acid receptors beta and gamma with a decrease of epidermal proliferation and dedifferentiation. Topical vitamin A analogues may still be used in extratemporaneous preparations on chronic and hyperproliferative (scaling) skin manifestations; however, systemic acitretin may be much more effective.

15.10 TOPICAL CALCINEURIN INHIBITORS

The topical macrolide calcineurin inhibitors pimecrolimus and tacrolimus are currently licensed for atopic eczema only [83–86]. By inhibiting the intracellular processing of calcineurin, the production of IL2, IL4, and interferon gamma by T lymphocytes is inhibited, resulting in a clinically relevant reduction of inflammatory processes. A number of case compilations and controlled studies have demonstrated good clinical effects and tolerability in plaque psoriasis [87–91], as well as in inverse locations of psoriasis, especially the face and folds [91–97]. In a double-blind, vehicle-controlled study on inverse psoriasis, twice daily application of 1% pimecrolimus resulted in a fast and significant improvement by patient and examiner evaluation [98]. At other sites, reasonable effectiveness could only be achieved under occlusion, which on the other side may increase the risk of skin irritation inherent to these compounds. However, initial burning sensations and pruritus may subside under continuous treatment. Despite a black box warning for the potential risk of lymphoma upon prolonged use of topical calcineurin inhibitors, the available long-term data do not support this possible adverse event [84,86,99]. Altogether, topical calcineurin inhibitors may represent an alternative to corticosteroids at sensitive sites and in sensitive populations like children (see below).

15.11 COMBINATIONS OF TOPICAL AGENTS

A combination of topical agents may improve their efficacy by adding or potentiating their effects seen in monotherapy while at the same time reducing side effects [12–15,25]. Apart from fixed combinations, most others lack high evidence levels, as well as licensing. In a recent systematic review, among a total of 2916 publications on topical combination therapy, 48 articles covered classical treatments [25]. The majority of combinations was at least as effective as the respective monotherapy and generally well tolerated. In this context, topical corticosteroids combined with salicylic acid, and superpotent corticosteroids with anthralin or coal tar proved most efficient. The effectiveness of topical vitamin D analogues may considerably be improved by UVB light, a combination that should be preferred in the outpatient situation [71,72]. Similarly, topical therapy may have to be followed or supported by systemic treatment when more than 10% of BSA are affected or a chronic, recalcitrant, or relapsing course is found [5,12–15].

15.12 LOCAL TREATMENT OF SPECIAL LOCATIONS

15.12.1 Scalp

Involvement of the scalp can be seen in at least two-thirds of patients and may even be the only or prominent manifestation of the disease [100,101]. A recent Cochrane systemic review included 49 randomized clinical studies with more than 11,000 participants [102]. The fixed combination of corticosteroids with vitamin D analogues and corticosteroids of high and very high potency proved better and had fewer withdrawals than vitamin D analogues as monotherapy. Although the fixed combination was better than corticosteroids alone, the difference was small. The dates only cover short-term treatment periods of less than 6 months, with insufficient reporting on quality of life issues. The effects of different vehicles have only inadequately been addressed. One recent study showed better results of corticosteroids in foam than lotion [102,103], but not in liquid. Data on other topical agents, like dithranol, tar, and tacrolimus, are limited.

15.12.2 Inverse Areas: Face and Intertriginous Areas

Inverse areas like intertriginous folds, the genital area, and the face are affected to a lesser extent than the classical predilection sites, yet may cause great distress to the afflicted patients [104–106]. At the same time, these areas show increased sensitivity to topical corticosteroids with regard to skin atrophy, increased infection rate, and in the face, steroid-induced rosacea. Furthermore, an increased irritability to topical agents like dithranol, tar, and topical calcineurin inhibitors is found. Although the face is rarely involved in adult patients, therapy is mandatory. Whereas topical corticosteroids should be used only in the short term, and at low and medium strength, calcineurin inhibitors are usually very effective and may be used over a prolonged period of time, especially as proactive therapy.

Treatment of genital and intertriginous psoriasis should first correct harmful habits like the excessive use of detergents and inappropriate cosmetic products. Fragrance-free liquid soaps should be used atraumatically, followed by careful drying. Loosely fitting underwear should be frequently changed. Whereas the vulva is relatively steroid resistant, labiocrural folds, the perineum, and perianal regions are steroid sensitive [106–108]. At these sites, care should be taken to avoid extended use of topical corticosteroids of higher strength. Whereas hydrocortisone is mostly uneffective, methylprednisolone aceponate and mometason are recommended. Clobetasol propionate will only be necessary in severe and recalcitrant cases. Similar to other sites, corticosteroids should be started at higher strength and de-escalated stepwise as quickly as possible. Proactive therapy should be continued after disappearance of skin manifestations with application 2 days weekly at originally affected sites. Alternatively, topical calcineurin inhibitors like tacrolimus and pimecrolimus can be used [92–98].

Whereas the vitamin D calcipotriol in genital folds is limited due to its irritative effect, calcitriol or tacrolimus [109] may be used alternatively. However, in severe and recalcitrant cases, mainly when accompanied by extensive skin involvement, systemic therapy may be necessary.

15.12.3 Nails

Nail involvement is seen in 30%–60% of psoriasis patients, in contrast to well above 70% of patients with psoriasis arthritis. The main manifestations are nail pitting, oil drops, and nail dystrophia with more proximal (nail fold) or distal involvement or destroying the entire nail plate. Accordingly, the clinical and patient-related effects may be minimal and more cosmetic to severely affecting the quality of life. Nail involvement may be monitored by various clinical scores. Among them, the Nail Psoriasis Severity Index (NAPSI) is well established and encompasses the number of lesions, as well as their extension. Whereas data on clinical effectiveness of novel systemic agents became available recently, similar data on topical agents are limited [12–15]. Whereas nail fold manifestations are accessible to topical and intrafocal agents, nail matrix involvement demands penetration-enhancing agents or prior onycholysis with limited efficacy. Corticosteroids and vitamin D analogues, like calcipotriol, tacrolimus, and tazarotene, are used successfully, but mainly in mild disease with less than two nails involved and with treatment periods well above 12 weeks. Procedural therapies like phototherapy, photodynamic therapy (PDT), and lasers are alternatives, yet a second choice, whereas various radiotherapeutic options should only be used with great caution. Moderate to severe nail involvement will need systemic treatment, and indeed, recent clinical studies have shown biologics to be highly effective and superior to conventional systemic agents.

15.13 LOCAL TREATMENT OF SPECIAL PATIENT GROUPS

15.13.1 Children

With a cumulative incidence of 1.4% below the age of 18 years, psoriasis is common among children and especially adolescents and has evident effects on their physical and mental development [110–112]. However, clinical studies and licensed agents are hardly available for this age group. Because psoriasis is usually milder and limited in children, topical therapy may often be sufficient. For any treatment, the clinical benefit and possible side effects have to be balanced and critically discussed with the parents and young patients, depending on their age and cooperation [112,113]. Topical corticosteroids of low and medium potency represent a mainstay of therapy, alone or in combination with vitamin D analogues, which are restricted in different age groups. As children have a higher ratio of skin surface area to body weight and are less able to metabolize corticosteroids, caution has to be taken and only lower-potency corticosteroids be used, especially in the diaper area and skinfolds. Topical calcineurin inhibitors have been studied in children and represent an alternative to corticosteroids; however, they have to be used off-label [114,115]. Vitamin D analogues were shown to be effective, safe, and well tolerated in children, but skin irritation may limit their use. Anthralin seems safe in childhood psoriasis and is especially effective in the more superficial guttate psoriasis. Short-contact therapy may often be better manageable and tolerated. Care should be taken when applying anthralin to sensitive areas like skinfolds and the anogenital area. Whereas the use of tar is generally at a very low level of evidence [12,13], the Goeckerman treatment is still an alternative, especially in the United States [116].

15.13.2 Pregnant Women

Data on the effectiveness and tolerability of topical agents in pregnancy are limited to case reports and retrospective data in women who were undeliberately treated before they realized they were pregnant. In contrast to other inflammatory skin diseases, psoriasis will improve in 50%–70% of pregnant patients, with frequent postpartum flare. Therefore, topical therapy may often suffice and even substitute systemic treatment in some cases [117,118]. Limited amounts of topical agents on limited body surfaces appear to be safe, including corticosteroids, vitamin D analogues, tar, and anthralin. The likelihood of systemic resorption is further increased by occlusion and skin barrier disruption. In the first trimester, topical corticosteroids should be restricted because of the theoretical risk of resorption and induction of cleft defects. Thereafter, mild- to moderate-potency corticosteroids may be used. Anthralin seems particularly safe, as it is not resorbed and may be used in combination with UV light.

15.13.3 Elderly Patients

As elderly patients often have thinner skin, topical corticosteroids may more easily be systemically absorbed, as well as deteriorate skin atrophy. Therefore, potent corticosteroids should be used with caution. Similarly, vitamin D analogues and anthralin may more easily induce skin irritation. In addition, adequate skin moisturization should be performed to reconstitute the disrupted skin barrier and counteract dry scaling skin [119,120].

15.14 ALTERNATIVE TOPICAL AGENTS

A huge and confusing number of alternative topical agents are available for psoriasis derived from naturopathy, anthroposophic medicine, and traditional Chinese medicine, to name a few. They are extensively referred to in the lay and alternative scientific literature and increasingly sold in Internet portals. Most of them have not been studied in controlled clinical studies for either efficacy or tolerability, nor are they standardized with regard to the integrity, purity, and amount of ingredients. Products derived from herbal medicine may in fact contain plant steroids, which explains clinical effects. However, recent clinical examinations on various compounds contained, for example, in *aloe vera* and tea tree oil show promising effectiveness on psoriasis [121,122]. Further studies, however, have to examine such effects more precisely.

Alternative agents should be applied with great caution, yet patients may use them without notice to and consent of their treating dermatologists. Physicians should, however, be open-minded and empathic toward this alternative use and discuss it both openly and critically with their patients.

15.15 NOVEL AGENTS AND SKIN DELIVERY SYSTEMS

With the advent of novel, well-tolerated, and effective systemic agents, topical therapy seemed outdated. However, as two-thirds of psoriasis patients show mild disease, for them topical therapy is still the mainstay of treatment, and systemic treatment may need supportive topical treatment to increase clinical effectiveness [5]. Over the last decade, hardly any innovations have been introduced into the market of topical agents. The new foam formulation of the fixed corticosteroid and vitamin D analogue combination (Enstilar) was the first and last to become available in recent years. However, a number of novel agents are currently in phase 2 and 3 studies, including Janus and tyrosine kinase- as well as phosphodiesterase 4 (PDE4) inhibitors [10,12]. Oral counterparts of these agents have recently been licensed for rheumatoid and psoriasis arthritis. On topical application, good therapeutic responses, together with good tolerability, have been observed. However, further and larger studies are necessary to support these limited data. Major advancements have been made to improve the penetration of antipsoriatic agents into the skin and increase their efficacy and safety, as well as increase the compliance of patients. Innovative skin drug delivery systems will be available soon [123], especially through encapsulation in nanoparticles.

REFERENCES

1. Lowes MA, Bowcock AM, Krueger JG. Pathogenesis and therapy of psoriasis. *Nature* 2007;445:866–73.
2. Griffiths CE, Barker JN. Pathogenesis and clinical features of psoriasis. *Lancet* 2007;370(9583):263–71.
3. Hebert HL, Ali FR, Bowes J, Griffiths CE, Barton A, Warren RB. Genetic susceptibility to psoriasis and psoriatic arthritis: Implications for therapy. *Br J Dermatol* 2012;166(3):474–82.
4. Mason AR, Mason J, Cork M, Dooley G, Edwards G. Topical treatments for chronic plaque psoriasis. *Cochrane Database Syst Rev* 2009;(2):CD005028. Update in *Cochrane Database Syst Rev* 2013;3:CD005028.
5. Albrecht L, Bourcier M, Ashkenas J et al. Topical psoriasis therapy in the age of biologics: Evidence-based treatment recommendations. *J Cutan Med Surg* 2011;15(6):309–21.
6. Svendsen MT, Jeyabalan J, Andersen KE, Andersen F, Johannessen H. Worldwide utilization of topical remedies in treatment of psoriasis: A systematic review. *J Dermatolog Treat* 2017;28:374–83.
7. van de Kerkhof PC. An update on topical therapies for mild-moderate psoriasis. *Dermatol Clin* 2015;33(1):73–7.

8. Samarasekera EJ, Sawyer L, Wonderling D, Tucker R, Smith CH. Topical therapies for the treatment of plaque psoriasis: Systematic review and network meta-analyses. *Br J Dermatol* 2013;168(5):954–67.
9. Kurian A, Barankin B. Current effective topical therapies in the management of psoriasis. *Skin Therapy Lett* 2011;16(1):4–7.
10. de Prost Y. New topical immunological treatments for psoriasis. *J Eur Acad Dermatol Venereol* 2006;20:80–2.
11. Laws PM, Young HS. Topical treatment of psoriasis. *Expert Opin Pharmacother* 2010;11(12):1999–2009.
12. Nast A, Boehncke WH, Mrowietz U et al. German S3-guidelines on the treatment of psoriasis vulgaris (short version). *Arch Dermatol Res* 2012;304(2):87–113.
13. Nast A, Gisondi P, Ormerod AD et al. European S3-guidelines on the systemic treatment of psoriasis vulgaris—Update 2015—Short version—EDF in cooperation with EADV and IPC. *J Eur Acad Dermatol Venereol* 2015;29(12):2277–94.
14. Menter A, Korman NJ, Elmets CA et al. Guidelines of care for the management of psoriasis and psoriatic arthritis. Section 3. Guidelines of care for the management and treatment of psoriasis with topical therapies. *J Am Acad Dermatol* 2009;60(4):643–59.
15. Zeichner JA, Lebwohl MG, Menter A et al. Optimizing topical therapies for treating psoriasis: A consensus conference. *Cutis* 2010;86(3 Suppl):5–31; quiz 32.
16. Fredrickson T, Pettersson U. Severe psoriasis: Oral therapy with a new retinoid. *Dermatologica* 1978;157:238–44.
17. Langley RG, Ellis CN. Evaluating psoriasis with Psoriasis Area and Severity Index, Psoriasis Global Assessment, and Lattice System Physician's Global Assessment. *J Am Acad Dermatol* 2004;51:563–9.
18. Finlay AY, Khan GK. Dermatology Life Quality Index (DLQI)—A simple practical measure for routine clinical use. *Clin Exp Dermatol* 1994;19:210–6.
19. Finlay AY. Current severe psoriasis and the rule of tens. *Br J Dermatol* 2005;152:861–7.
20. Dawn A, Yosipovitch G. Treating itch in psoriasis. *Dermatol Nurs* 2006;18(3):227–33.
21. Bruner CR, Feldman SR, Ventrapragada M, Fleischer AB Jr. A systematic review of adverse effects associated with topical treatments for psoriasis. *Dermatol Online J* 2003;9(1):2.
22. Prieto-Pérez R, Cabaleiro T, Daudén E, Ochoa D, Román M, Abad-Santos F. Pharmacogenetics of topical and systemic treatment of psoriasis. *Pharmacogenomics* 2013;14(13):1623–34.
23. Endzweig-Gribetz CH, Brady C, Lynde C, Sibbald D, Lebwohl M. Drug interactions in psoriasis: The pros and cons of combining topical psoriasis therapies. *J Cutan Med Surg* 2002;6(3 Suppl):12–6.
24. van de Kerkhof PC. Therapeutic strategies: Rotational therapy and combinations. *Clin Exp Dermatol* 2001;26(4):356–61.
25. Hendriks AG, Keijsers RR, de Jong EM, Seyger MM, van de Kerkhof PC. Combinations of classical time-honoured topicals in plaque psoriasis: A systematic review. *J Eur Acad Dermatol Venereol* 2013;27(4):399–410.
26. Lebwohl M, Ali S. Treatment of psoriasis. Part 1. Topical therapy and phototherapy. *J Am Acad Dermatol* 2001;45(4):487–98; quiz 499–502.
27. Nguyen T, Gattu S, Pugashetti R, Koo J. Practice of phototherapy in the treatment of moderate-to-severe psoriasis. *Curr Probl Dermatol* 2009;38:59–78.
28. Zaghloul SS, Goodfield MJ. Objective assessment of compliance with psoriasis treatment. *Arch Dermatol* 2004;140:408–14.
29. Feldman SR, Camacho FT, Krejci-Manwaring J, Carroll CL, Balkrishnan R. Adherence to topical therapy increases around the time of office visits. *J Am Acad Dermatol* 2007;57:81–3.
30. Stein Gold LF. Topical therapies for psoriasis: Improving management strategies and patient adherence. *Semin Cutan Med Surg* 2016;35(2 Suppl 2):S36–44; quiz S45.
31. Pan M, Heinecke G, Bernardo S, Tsui C, Levitt J. Urea: A comprehensive review of the clinical literature. *Dermatol Online J* 2013;19(11):20392.
32. Friedman AJ, von Grote EC, Meckfessel MH. Urea: A clinically oriented overview from bench to bedside. *J Drugs Dermatol* 2016;15(5):633–9.
33. Gelmetti C. Therapeutic moisturizers as adjuvant therapy for psoriasis patients. *Am J Clin Dermatol* 2009;10(Suppl 1):7–12.
34. Paghdal KV, Schwartz RA. Topical tar: Back to the future. *J Am Acad Dermatol* 2009;61(2):294–302.
35. Thami G, Sarkar R. Coal tar: Past, present and future. *Clin Exp Dermatol* 2002;27(2):99–103.
36. Roelofzen JH, Aben KK, van der Valk PG, van Houtum JL, van de Kerkhof PC, Kiemeney LA. Coal tar in dermatology. *J Dermatolog Treat* 2007;18(6):329–34.

37. Alora-Palli MB, Brouda I, Green B, Kimball AB. A cost-effectiveness comparison of liquor carbonis distillate solution and calcipotriol cream in the treatment of moderate chronic plaque psoriasis. *Arch Dermatol* 2010;146(8):919–22.
38. Wright CW, Later DW, Pelroy RA, Mahlum DD, Wilson BW. Comparative chemical and biological analysis of coal tar-based therapeutic agents to other coal derived materials. *J Appl Toxicol* 1985;5(2):80–8.
39. Singh P, Gupta S, Abidi A, Krishna A. Comparative evaluation of topical calcipotriol versus coal tar and salicylic acid ointment in chronic plaque psoriasis. *J Drugs Dermatol* 2013;12(8):868–73.
40. Food and Drug Administration, HHS. Dandruff, seborrheic dermatitis, and psoriasis drug products containing coal tar and menthol for over-the-counter human use; amendment to the monograph. Final rule. *Fed Regist* 2007;72(43):9849–52.
41. Cosmetic Ingredient Review Expert Panel. Final safety assessment of coal tar as used in cosmetics. *Int J Toxicol* 2008;27(Suppl 2):1–24.
42. van den Bogaard EH, Bergboer JG, Vonk-Bergers M, van Vlijmen-Willems IM, Hato SV, van der Valk PG, Schröder JM, Joosten I, Zeeuwen PL, Schalkwijk J. Coal tar induces AHR-dependent skin barrier repair in atopic dermatitis. *J Clin Invest* 2013;123(2):917–27.
43. Orseth ML, Cropley TG. What's in a name? Goeckerman therapy. *JAMA Dermatol* 2013;149(12):1409.
44. Zhu TH, Nakamura M, Farahnik B, Abrouk M, Singh RK, Lee KM, Hulse S, Koo J, Bhutani T, Liao W. The patient's guide to psoriasis treatment. Part 4: Goeckerman therapy. *Dermatol Ther (Heidelb)* 2016;6(3):333–9.
45. Davis MD, McEvoy MT, Camilleri M, Bridges AG, Gibson LE, El-Azhary RA. Goeckerman treatment: Neglected in the consensus approach for critically challenging case scenarios in moderate to severe psoriasis. *J Am Acad Dermatol* 2010;62(3):508.
46. Chern E, Yau D, Ho JC, Wu WM, Wang CY, Chang HW, Cheng YW. Positive effect of modified Goeckerman regimen on quality of life and psychosocial distress in moderate and severe psoriasis. *Acta Derm Venereol* 2011;91(4):447–51.
47. Pittelkow MR, Perry HO, Muller SA, Maughan WZ, O'Brien PC. Skin cancer in patients with psoriasis treated with coal tar. *Arch Dermatol* 1981;117:465–8.
48. Stern RS, Zierler S, Parrish JA. Skin carcinoma in patients with psoriasis treated with topical tar and artificial ultraviolet radiation. *Lancet* 1980;i:732–5.
49. Roelofzen JH, Aben KK, Oldenhof UT, Coenraads PJ, Alkemade HA, van de Kerkhof PC, van der Valk PG, Kiemeney LA. No increased risk of cancer after coal tar treatment in patients with psoriasis or eczema. *J Invest Dermatol* 2010;130(4):953–61.
50. Petrozzi JW. Goeckerman regimen for psoriatic patients refractory to biologic therapy. *J Am Acad Dermatol* 2014;71(1):195.
51. van de Kerkhof PCM. Dithranol treatment for psoriasis: After 75 years still going strong. *Eur J Dermatol* 1992;1:79–88.
52. McBride SR, Walker P, Reynolds NJ. Optimizing the frequency of outpatient short-contact dithranol treatment used in combination with broadband ultraviolet B for psoriasis: A randomized, within-patients controlled trial. *Br J Dermatol* 2003;149:1259–64.
53. Grattan CE, Christophers AP, Robinson M, Cowan MA. Double-blind comparison of a dithranol and steroid mixture with a conventional dithranol regimen for chronic plaque psoriasis. *Br J Dermatol* 1988;119:623–6.
54. Saraswat A, Agarwal R, Katare OP, Kaur I, Kumar B. A randomized, double-blind, vehicle-controlled study of a novel liposomal dithranol formulation in psoriasis. *J Dermatolog Treat* 2007;18(1):40–5.
55. Fuchs J, Nitschmann WN, Pacher L. The antipsoriatic compound anthralin influences bioenergetic parameters and redox properties of energy transducing membranes. *J Invest Dermatol* 1990;94:71–6.
56. Ruiz-Maldonado R, Zapata G, Lourdes R, Robles C. Cushing's syndrome after topical application of corticosteroids. *Am J Dis Child* 1982;136:274–5.
57. Feiwel M, Kelly WF. Adrenal unresponsiveness associated with clobetasol propionate. *Lancet* 1974;2:112–3.
58. Fisher DA. Adverse effects of topical corticosteroid use. *West J Med* 1995;162:123–6.
59. Drake L, Dinehart SM, Farmer ER et al. Guidelines of care for the use of topical glucocorticosteroids. *J Am Acad Dermatol* 1996;35:615–9.
60. Feldman SR. Tachyphylaxis to topical corticosteroids: The more you use them, the less they work. *Clin Dermatol* 2006;24:229–30.
61. Lebwohl MG, Tan MH, Meador SL, Singer G. Limited application of fluticasone propionate ointment, 0.005% in patients with psoriasis of the face and intertriginous areas. *J Am Acad Dermatol* 2001;44:77–82.

62. Kragballe K. Treatment of psoriasis by the topical application of the novel cholecalciferol analogue calcipotriol (MC903). *Arch Dermatol* 1989;125:1647–52.
63. Dubertret L, Wallach D, Souteyrand P et al. Efficacy and safety of calcipotriol (MC903) ointment in psoriasis vulgaris. *J Am Acad Dermatol* 1992;27:983–8.
64. Segaert S, Duvold LB. Calcipotriol cream: A review of its use in the management of psoriasis. *J Dermatolog Treat* 2006;17(6):327–37.
65. Ashcroft DM, Po AL, Williams HC, Griffiths CE. Systematic review of comparative efficacy and tolerability of calcipotriol in treating chronic plaque psoriasis. *BMJ* 2000;320(7240):963–7.
66. Sharma V, Kaur I, Kumar B. Calcipotriol vs coal tar: A prospective randomized study in stable psoriasis. *Int J Dermatol* 2003;42:834–8.
67. van de Kerkhof PC, Werfel T, Haustein UF et al. Tacalcitol ointment in the treatment of psoriasis vulgaris: A multicentre, placebo-controlled, double-blind study on efficacy and safety. *Br J Dermatol* 2002;135:758–65.
68. van de Kerkhof PCM, Berth Jones J, Griffiths CE et al. Long-term efficacy and safety of tacalcitol ointment in patients with chronic plaque psoriasis. *Br J Dermatol* 2002;146:414–22.
69. Barker JN, Berth Jones J, Groes R et al. Calcium homeostasis remains unaffected after 12 weeks' therapy with calcitriol 3 µg/g ointment. *J Dermatolog Treat* 2003;14:14–21.
70. Camarasa JM, Ortonne JP, Dubertret L. Calcitriol shows greater persistence of treatment effect than betamethasone diproprionate in topical psoriasis therapy. *J Dermatolog Treat* 2003;14:8–13.
71. Frappaz A, Thivolet J. Calcipotriol in combination with PUVA: A randomized double-blind placebo study in severe psoriasis. *Eur J Dermatol* 1993;3:351–354.
72. Ramsay CA, Schwartz BE, Lowson DM et al. Calcipotriol cream combined with twice weekly broad band UVB phototherapy: A safe, effective and UVB-sparing anti-psoriatic combination treatment. *Dermatology* 2000;200:17–24.
73. Kragballe J, Gjertsen BT, De Hoop DM et al. Double blind, right-left comparison of calcipotriol and betamethasone valerate in treatment of psoriasis vulgaris. *Lancet* 1991;337:193–6.
74. Cunliffe WJ, Claudy A, Fairiss GM et al. A multicenter comparative study of calcipotriol and betamethasone 17-valerate in patients with psoriasis vulgaris. *J Am Acad Dermatol* 1992;26:736–43.
75. van de Kerkhof PCM. The impact of a two compound product containing calcipotriol and betamethasone dipropionate (Daivobet/Dovobet) on the quality of life in patients with psoriasis vulgaris: A randomized controlled trial. *Br J Dermatol* 2004;151:663–8.
76. Guenther L, van de Kerkhof PC, Snellmann E et al. Efficacy and safety of a new combination of calcipotriol and betamethasone dipropionate (once or twice daily) compared to calcipotriol (twice daily) in the treatment of psoriasis vulgaris: A randomized double-blind, vehicle-controlled clinical trial. *Br J Dermatol* 2002;147:316–23.
77. Ortonne J, Kaufmann R, Lecha M, Seafield M. Efficacy of the treatment with calcipotriol/betamethasone dipropionate is followed by calcipotriol alone compared with tacalcitol for the treatment of psoriasis vulgaris: A randomized double blind trial. *Dermatology* 2004;209:308–13.
78. Kragballe K, Austad J, Barnes L et al. A 52-week randomized safety study of calcipotriol/betamethasone dipropionate two-compound product in the treatment of psoriasis. *Br J Dermatol* 2006;154:1150–60.
79. Weinstein GD. The management of psoriasis-tazarotene: The bottom line. *Cutis* 1998:61(2 Suppl):38–9.
80. Lebwohl M, Lombardi K, Tan MH. Duration of improvement in psoriasis after treatment with tazarotene 0.1% gel plus clobetasol propionate 0.05% ointment: Comparison of maintenance treatments. *Int J Dermatol* 2001;40:64–6.
81. Kumar U, Kaur I, Dogra S, De D, Kumar B. Topical tazarotene vs. coal tar in stable plaque psoriasis. *Clin Exp Dermatol* 2010;35(5):482–6.
82. Weinstein GD, Koo JY, Krueger GG et al. Tazarotene cream in the treatment of psoriasis: Two multicenter, double-blind, randomized, vehicle-controlled studies of the safety and efficacy of tazarotene creams 0.05% and 0.1% applied once daily for 12 weeks. *J Am Acad Dermatol* 2003;48:760–7.
83. Eichenfield LF, Lucky AW, Boguniewicz M, Langley RG, Cherill R, Marshall K, Bush C, Graeber M. Safety and efficacy of pimecrolimus (ASM 981) cream 1% in the treatment of mild and moderate atopic dermatitis in children and adolescents. *J Am Acad Dermatol* 2002;46:495–504.
84. Gupta AK, Chow M. Pimecrolimus: A review. *J Eur Acad Dermatol Venereol* 2003;17:493–503.
85. Azzi JR, Sayegh MH, Mallat SG. Calcineurin inhibitors: 40 years later, can't live without. *J Immunol* 2013;191(12):5785–91.
86. Malecic C, Young H. Tacrolimus for the management of psoriasis: Clinical utility and place in therapy. *Psoriasis (Auckl)* 2016;6:153–63.

87. Remitz A, Reitamo S, Erkko P, Granlund H, Lauerma AI. Tacrolimus ointment improves psoriasis in a microplaque assay. *Br J Dermatol* 1999;141:103–7.
88. Mrowietz U, Graeber M, Brautigam M et al. A novel ascomycin derivative SDZ ASM 981 is effective for psoriasis when used topically under occlusion. *Br J Dermatol* 1998;139:992–6.
89. Mrowietz U, Wustlich S, Hoexter G, Graeber M, Brautigam M, Luger T. An experimental ointment formulation of pimecrolimus is effective in psoriasis without occlusion. *Acta Derm Venereol* 2003;83:351–3.
90. Zonneveld IM, Rubins A, Jablonska S et al. Topical tacrolimus is not effective in chronic plaque psoriasis. A pilot study. *Arch Dermatol* 1998;134(9):1101–2.
91. Maloney JM, Flores J, Sheehan M, Schlessinger J. Efficacy and safety of 0.1% and 0.5% tacrolimus cream versus vehicle for treatment of mild to moderate plaque psoriasis in adults. *J Am Acad Dermatol* 2007;56(2, Suppl 2):AB10.
92. Lebwohl M, Freeman A, Chapman MS, Feldman S, Hartle J, Henning A. Proven efficacy of tacrolimus for facial and intertriginous psoriasis. *Arch Dermatol* 2005;141:1154.
93. Yamamoto T, Nishioka K. Topical tacrolimus: An effective therapy for facial psoriasis. *Eur J Dermatol* 2003;13(5):471–3.
94. Kroft EB, Erceg A, Maimets K, Vissers W, van der Valk PG, van de Kerkhof PC. Tacrolimus ointment for the treatment of severe facial plaque psoriasis. *J Eur Acad Dermatol Venereol* 2005;19(2):249–51.
95. Rallis E, Nasiopoulou A, Kouskoukis C et al. Successful treatment of genital and facial psoriasis with tacrolimus ointment 0.1%. *Drugs Exp Clin Res* 2005;31(4):141–5.
96. Martin Ezquerra G, Sanchez Regana M, Herrera Acosta E, Umbert Millet P. Topical tacrolimus for the treatment of psoriasis on the face, genitalia, intertriginous areas and corporal plaques. *J Drugs Dermatol* 2006;5(4):334–6.
97. He Y. Clinical efficacy of 0.1% tacrolimus ointment on plaque psoriasis of scalp and face. *J Clin Dermatol* 2008;37:254–5.
98. Gribetz C, Ling M, Lebwohl M et al. Pimecrolimus cream 1% in the treatment of intertriginous psoriasis: A double-blind, randomized study. *J Am Acad Dermatol* 2004;51:731–8.
99. Margolis DJ, Hoffstad O, Bilker W. Lack of association between exposure to topical calcineurin inhibitors and skin cancer in adults. *Dermatology* 2007;214:289–95.
100. Kircik LH, Kumar S. Scalp psoriasis. *J Drugs Dermatol* 2010;9(8 Suppl ODAC Conf Pt 2):s101–5.
101. van de Kerkhof PC, Franssen ME. Psoriasis of the scalp. Diagnosis and management. *Am J Clin Dermatol* 2001;2(3):159–65.
102. Schlager JG, Rosumeck S, Werner RN, Jacobs A, Schmitt J, Schlager C, Nast A. Topical treatments for scalp psoriasis. *Cochrane Database Syst Rev* 2016;2:CD009687.
103. Kircik L. The evolving role of therapeutic shampoos for targeting symptoms of inflammatory scalp disorders. *J Drugs Dermatol* 2010;9(1):41–8.
104. Omland SH, Gniadecki R. Psoriasis inversa: A separate identity or a variant of psoriasis vulgaris? *Clin Dermatol* 2015;33(4):456–61.
105. van de Kerkhof PC, Murphy GM, Austad J, Ljungberg A, Cambazard F, Duvold LB. Psoriasis of the face and flexures. *J Dermatolog Treat* 2007;18(6):351–60.
106. Meeuwis KA, de Hullu JA, Massuger LF, van de Kerkhof PC, van Rossum MM. Genital psoriasis: A systematic literature review on this hidden skin disease. *Acta Derm Venereol* 2011;91(1):5–11.
107. Kapila S, Bradford J, Fischer G. Vulvar psoriasis in adults and children: A clinical audit of 194 cases and review of the literature. *J Low Genit Tract* Dis 2012;16(4):364–71.
108. Sticherling, M. Vulvar psoriasis. In *Gynecologic Dermatology*, ed. G. Kirtschig, SM Cooper, London: JP Medical Publishers, 2016;109–114.
109. Bissonnette R, Nigen S, Bolduc C. Efficacy and tolerability of topical tacrolimus ointment for the treatment of male genital psoriasis. *J Cutan Med Surg* 2008;12(5):230–4.
110. Turnbull R. Recognising psoriasis in children. *Community Pract* 2012;85(6):39–40.
111. Leman J, Burden D. Psoriasis in children: A guide to its diagnosis and management. *Paediatr Drugs* 2001;3(9):673–80.
112. Sticherling M, Augustin M, Boehncke WH, Christophers E, Domm S, Gollnick H, Reich K, Mrowietz U. Therapy of psoriasis in childhood and adolescence—A German expert consensus. *J Dtsch Dermatol Ges* 2011;9(10):815–23.
113. Ståhle M, Atakan N, Boehncke WH et al. Juvenile psoriasis and its clinical management: A European expert group consensus. *J Dtsch Dermatol Ges* 2010;8(10):812–8.
114. Steele JA, Choi C, Kwong PC. Topical tacrolimus in the treatment of inverse psoriasis in children. *J Am Acad Dermatol* 2005;53(4):713–6.

115. Brune A, Miller DW, Lin P, Cotrim-Russi D, Paller AS. Tacrolimus ointment is effective for psoriasis on the face and intertriginous areas in pediatric patients. *Pediatric Dermatol* 2007;24(1):76–80.
116. Kortuem KR, Davis MD, Witman PM, McEvoy MT, Farmer SA. Results of Goeckerman treatment for psoriasis in children: A 21-year retrospective review. *Pediatr Dermatol* 2010;27(5):518–24.
117. Bangsgaard N, Rørbye C, Skov L. Treating psoriasis during pregnancy: Safety and efficacy of treatments. *Am J Clin Dermatol* 2015;16(5):389–98.
118. Hoffman MB, Farhangian M, Feldman SR. Psoriasis during pregnancy: Characteristics and important management recommendations. *Expert Rev Clin Immunol* 2015;11(6):709–20.
119. Wong JW, Davis SA, Feldman SR, Koo JY. Trends in older adult psoriasis outpatient health care practices in the United States. *J Drugs Dermatol* 2012;11(8):957–62.
120. Yosipovitch G, Tang MB. Practical management of psoriasis in the elderly: Epidemiology, clinical aspects, quality of life, patient education and treatment options. *Drugs Aging* 2002;19(11):847–63.
121. Feily A, Namazi MR. Aloe vera in dermatology: A brief review. *G Ital Dermatol Venereol* 2009; 144(1):85–91.
122. Pazyar N, Yaghoobi R. Tea tree oil as a novel antipsoriasis weapon. *Skin Pharmacol Physiol* 2012;25:162–3.
123. Sala M, Elaissari A, Fessi H. Advances in psoriasis physiopathology and treatments: Up to date of mechanistic insights and perspectives of novel therapies based on innovative skin drug delivery systems (ISDDS). *J Control Release* 2016;239:182–202.

16 Overview of JAK-STAT Pathways in Spondyloarthritis

Smriti K. Raychaudhuri, Sanchita Raychaudhuri, Debasis Bagchi, Anand Swaroop, and Siba P. Raychaudhuri

CONTENTS

16.1 INTRODUCTION

Spondyloarthritis (SpA) is a heterogenous group of autoimmune diseases. These inflammatory diseases exhibit overlapping genetic predisposition, clinical features, comorbidities, radiological features, and certain similar pathogenic mechanisms. Autoimmune diseases are generally characterized by persistent and chronic inflammation because of a dysregulated immune system. The pathophysiology of many inflammatory and autoimmune diseases still remains unpredictable. This may happen due to genetic, environmental, and immunologic abnormalities, along with lifestyle stresses and strains. All these underlying biologic events synergistically contribute to the pathogenesis of autoimmune diseases and disorders [1,2].

Inflammation at the tendons, or bone joints, is termed enthesitis. It is considered to be the central, characteristic feature of spondyloarthropathy. Traditionally, enthesitis has been considered an insertional disorder. Advanced imaging, along with molecular imaging, suggests that enthesitis is a diffuse process that affects the tendons, their adjacent adjacent bone, and soft tissue [3]. Continued biomechanical stress and chronic microinjury at the enthesis trigger an inflammatory response in the synovium and are also likely to be a contributing factor for synovitis. Magnetic resonance imaging (MRI) has demonstrated the ubiquitous nature of enthesitis in SpA. MRI demonstrated that enthesitis lesions may be extensive and could explain the diffuse nature of bone changes seen in some patients with spondyloarthropathies. These processes occur adjacent to synovial joints, and thus partially substantiate the mechanisms of synovitis in spondyloarthropathies [2,3]. However, the process is more complex, and how biomechanical stress interacts with the systemic immune response dysregulation in autoimmune conditions of SpA remains unclear.

Human leukocyte antigen and T-cell phenotypes, cell trafficking molecules, lesional cytokine profiles, and angiogenesis act simultaneously to develop various autoimmune pathologic events that lead to diverse clinical phenotypes for SpA [1,4,5]. Activation of T cells requires two distinct signals. In the beginning, the trimolecular complex is formed, consisting of the major histocompatibility complex (MHC) class II molecule-antigenic peptide and the T-cell receptor (TcR) [4]. Involvement of a costimulatory molecule with its respective ligand provides a "secondary signal" for the maximum activation of T cells [5]. The most important characterized T-cell costimulatory ligands are CD28 and CTLA4 (cytotoxic T-lymphocyte-associated antigen 4) (CD152), which are known to engage with CD80/CD86 receptors on antigen-presenting cells (APCs) [6].

A critical signaling process for T-cell activation is engagement of CD28 with CD80 (B7-1) and CD86 (B7-2) on APCs. The above process enhances T-cell activation by stabilizing the mRNA of the interleukin (IL) 2 cytokine and upregulation of the antiapoptotic genes [5–7], whereas CTLA4-Ig binds to CD80 (B7-1) and CD86 (B7-2) on APCs and blocks the CD28-mediated signal for T-cell activation. The activated T cells regulate the local tissue response and damage through their cytokines and an integrated interaction with multiple inflammatory cells with innate functions such as macrophages and neutrophils [1,8–10]. It is also well demonstrated that cytokines have crucial functions in the development, differentiation, and regulation of the immune cells. Therefore, by orchestrating the intercellular communication, cytokines play a crucial role in an inflammatory response and development of autoimmune disease. Cytokines propagate signals by interacting with a variety of cell surface receptors. Cytokines bind to the extracellular domain of the receptor and produce conformational changes at the intracellular domain, which leads to phosphorylation of a series of kinase proteins, and that triggers the signal transduction events.

The Janus kinases (JAKs) belong to a family of intracellular tyrosine kinases and are associated with the signaling process of several cytokines [11,12]. JAKs play a critical role in (1) hematopoiesis, (2) adaptive immunity, and (3) innate immunity [11–14]. Several JAK inhibitors have been developed; these are oral synthetic compounds. In this chapter, we describe the functional significance of the JAK-STAT (signal transducers and activators of transcription) signaling proteins in the inflammatory-proliferative cascades of SpA and potential applications of the JAK-STAT kinase inhibitors in psoriatic disease and ankylosing spondylitis (AS).

16.2 JAK-STAT KINASE PATHWAY

The JAK family consists of four members: JAK1, JAK2, JAK3, and TYK2 [11,12]. These kinase proteins are critical for cytokine signaling and are linked to inflammatory responses, and associate with the intracellular domain of receptor subunits of the class I and II receptors. The STAT family has seven members, consisting of STAT 1, 2, 3, 4, 5/5a, and 6 [13,14], that transmit signals from type I and II cytokine receptors to the nucleus. This family of STAT proteins resides in the cytosol prior to activation [11–14].

JAK-STAT activation and signal transduction have been identified in many T-cell malignancies, including SpA. Basically, JAK-STAT signaling occurs by interaction of a cytokine with its specific surface receptor on the target cells, while the cytoplasmic portion of the receptor undergoes conformational changes to phosphorylation of the JAK-associated receptor (Figure 16.1). Phosphorylation of the receptor then initiates recruitment of the STAT through their SH2 domains, and that leads to phosphorylation and dimerization of the STAT proteins. Phosphorylated STAT homodimers and heterodimers move to the cell nucleus, bind to specific sites of DNA, and thus regulate gene transcription (Figure 16.1). Cytokines that have been shown to bind to type I and II receptors are of various functional significance, such as cytokines, interferon (IFN)-like cytokines, IFNs, colony-stimulating factors, growth factors, and hormones (Figure 16.2) [15].

16.3 REGULATORY ROLE OF THE JAK-STAT SIGNALING SYSTEM IN THE PATHOGENESIS OF SPONDYLOARTHRITIS

Because of the signaling cross talks between the JAK-STAT pathway and certain cytokines associated with autoimmunity (Figure 16.2), it is expected that the JAK-STAT signaling kinase proteins are of major importance for induction of an immune-mediated inflammation.

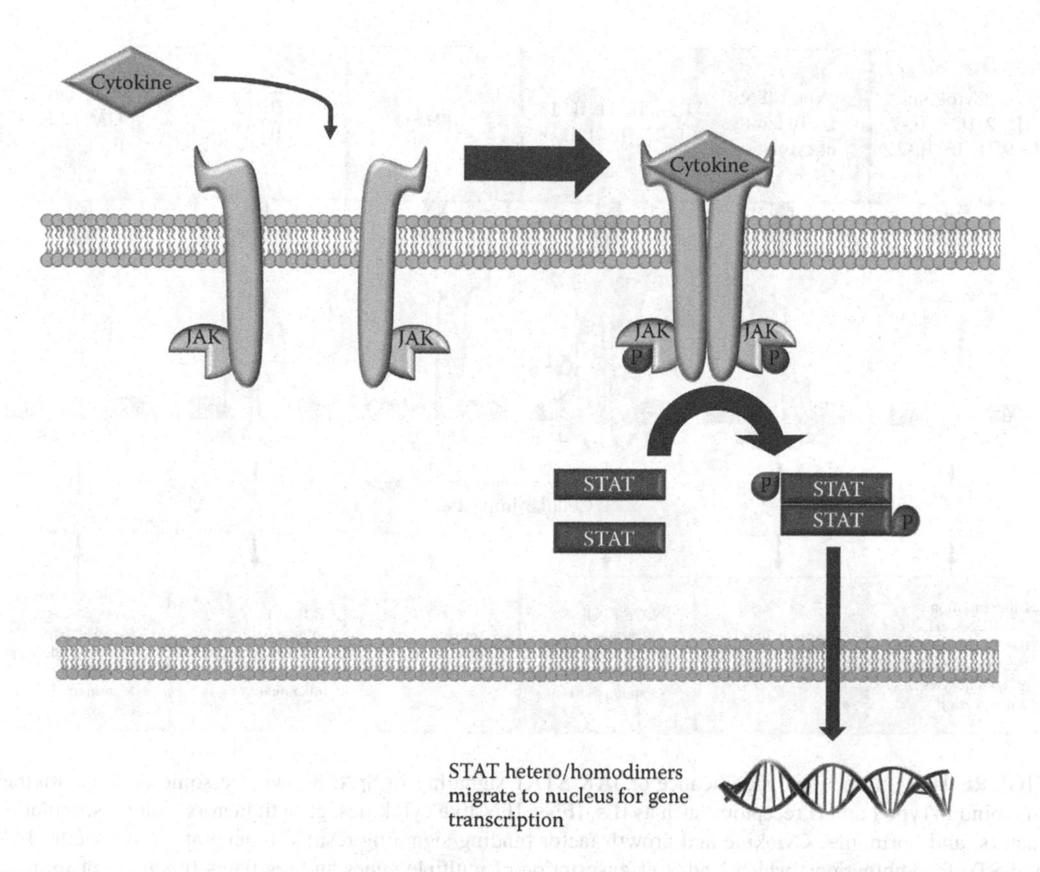

FIGURE 16.1 Cytokines and their regulation on the JAK-STAT signaling pathway. Interaction of a cytokine with its receptor on the cell surface leads to conformational changes to its intracellular domain and results in phosphorylation of the JAK proteins. Phosphorylation of the intracellular domain recruits the STATs via their SH2 domains and induces activation (phosphorylation) of the STAT proteins. The activated STAT homo- and heterodimers migrate to the nucleus and participate in gene transcriptions, which are critical for multiple biological and cellular functions for immune response, cell trafficking, and inflammation, as mentioned in Figure 16.2.

JAK1 and JAK2 have been demonstrated to play an important role in Th1 and Th17 cell differentiation, while STAT1 is critical to T-lymphocyte differentiation. STAT1 is activated by type I IFNs and IFN-γ and plays an important role in immune responses. IRF1 is the first member identified in the interferon-regulatory factor (IRF) family and is involved in innate and adaptive immune responses. Impaired or absent Th1-type immune responses favor Th2 differentiation in IRF1-deficient mice. NOS2-derived nitric oxide (NO), a key factor in immunoregulation, can inhibit Th1 as well as Th2 cytokine production and regulate the development of FoxP3+ Treg cells. JAK-STAT signaling pathway genes, including JAK1, JAK2, STAT1, IRF1, and NOS2, are strongly linked to T cells and may be involved in the pathophysiology of acute anterior uveitis (AAU), AS, psoriasis, and psoriatic arthritis (PsA).

JAK1, JAK2, and tyrosine kinase 2 are expressed ubiquitously in mammals, while JAK3 is primarily expressed by hematopoietic cells and associates with only the common γ-chain. Cytokines that signal through the common γ-chain include IL-2, IL-4, IL-7, IL-9, IL-15, and IL-21, which are integral to lymphocyte activation, proliferation, and differentiation. JAK3 is mainly expressed in the immune cells. Tofacitinib ($C_{16}H_{20}N_6O$, MW 312.370 Da), a small organic molecule, has been primarily prepared to target JAK3 with the aim to develop treatment for autoimmune arthritis and other autoimmune conditions [16].

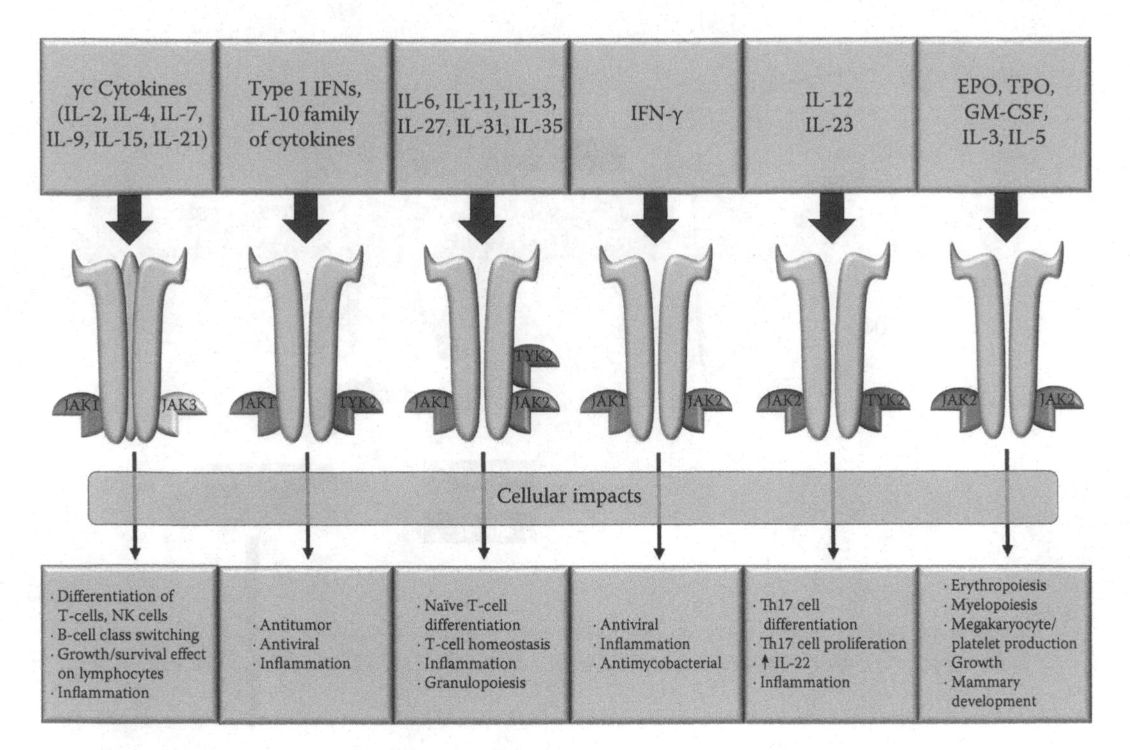

FIGURE 16.2 Functional significance of JAK-STAT signaling in SpA. Shown are some of the cytokines that bind to type I and II receptors, such as ILs, IFNs, IFN-like cytokines, growth factors, colony-stimulating factors, and hormones. Cytokine and growth factor binding signaling results in generation of specific JAK and STAT combinations, which leads to transcription of multiple genes and regulates functions of immune cells and other local lesional cells [15]. It is important to notice that in this figure, IL-2, IL-6, IL-9, IL-12, and IL-23 participate in JAK-STAT activation. Thus, all these cytokines have potential to play a critical role in an immune response, such as T-cell differentiation, proliferation, cell trafficking, and induction of an inflammation, including upregulation of IL-17/IL-22, which plays important roles in pannus formation, synovitis, bone proliferation, and bone erosion, the critical pathological events of SpA. EPO, erythropoietin; TPO, thrombopoietin; GM-CSF, granulocyte-macrophage colony-stimulating factor.

The efficacy of tofacitinib has been proposed mainly due to its regulatory role in T cells [16]. However, there are also reports suggesting that tofacitinib targets JAK1 and JAK2 with half maximal inhibitory concentration (IC50) values similar to those of JAK3 [17]. JAK1 and JAK2 are expressed in nonimmune cells, including the joint synovial cells. These findings have opened opportunities to investigate other possible cellular targets for JAK inhibitors, such as their regulating role in keratinocyte biology in psoriasis and synovial cells (fibroblast-like synoviocyte [FLS]), in PsA, and in rheumatoid arthritis (RA) [18,19].

Until now, limited studies have been conducted to understand the regulatory role of JAK-STAT kinase in FLS biology. Reports demonstrate that in PsA explants, tofacitinib can inhibit JAK1/JAK2, which in turn inhibits FLS migration and secretion of certain FLS chemokines [20].

A recent study has assessed JAK-STAT expression in psoriasis plaques and in other multiple inflammatory skin conditions [21]. JAK1 and JAK3 were overexpressed in psoriasis in the epidermal layer, and also, in an *in vitro* psoriasis model tofacitinib did inhibit phosphorylated JAK1 and JAK3 expression in keratinocytes of psoriatic lesions.

Activation of the IL-23/IL-17 cytokine axis is a pronounced abnormality in the SpA group of diseases, including in AS and PsA [8,9]. As JAK2 is recruited to the IL-23 receptor, it is expected that the JAK-STAT kinase cascade is an important signaling system in the disease process of PsA and AS. Based on these logistics, we hypothesized that (1) JAK-STAT signaling proteins regulate the Th17 cells in SpA and (2) tofacitinib, by inhibiting JAK2 signaling, will block IL-23-induced Th17 cell activation and proliferation. To substantiate these hypotheses, studies were carried out with the following aims: (1) The expression of JAK-STAT signaling proteins was evaluated in activated CD3$^+$ T cells collected from blood and the synovial fluid of PsA patients. (2) Furthermore, to elucidate the functional significance of the JAK-STAT kinase proteins, studies were conducted to determine whether the activation and proliferation of the effector memory T (TEM) cells and the Th17 cells are dependent on the signaling system of the JAK-STAT pathway [22].

It was found that in PsA, activated CD3$^+$ T cells in the presence of IL-23 had JAK2 and STAT3. Moreover, we noticed that tofacitinib significantly inhibited phosphorylation of JAK2 and STAT3. Also, tofacitinib inhibited IL-23-induced proliferation of the IL-17$^+$ TEM cells. These novel findings provide new insights for the pathogenesis of PsA and other types of SpA: (1) the generation of the pathologic IL-17$^+$ TEM cells and their proliferation are regulated by the JAK-STAT signaling proteins, and (2) a suggested mechanism of action of tofacitinib is likely to be deactivation of the IL-23/IL-17 cytokine axis through its JAK2 antagonism [22].

Polymorphisms of JAK-STAT kinases may be another plausible mode of mechanism in the etiology of spondyloarthritic diseases, and JAK2 polymorphisms have been reported to be associated with AS [23]. Nucleotide polymorphisms in the JAK-STAT signaling system have also been noticed in Crohn's disease (CD). It has been reported that the rs744166 or rs3816769 single-nucleotide polymorphisms (SNPs) in STAT3 and rs10758669 in JAK2 significantly differ in frequency in CD cases and controls [24]. The two STAT3 SNPs enhance the risk of colonic CD, while the JAK2 SNP is associated with an enhanced risk of ileocolonic disease and an increased risk for development of ileal disease complicated by stricturing.

16.4 JAK AND STAT INHIBITORS: NOVEL THERAPIES FOR PSORIATIC ARTHRITIS AND OTHER SPONDYLOARTHRITIS

The JAK-STAT pathway plays an important role in cytokine receptor-mediated signal transduction via activation of downstream signal transducers STAT, phosphoinositide 3-kinase (PI3K), and mitogen-activated protein kinase (MAPK) pathways. The novel concepts for the development of JAK inhibitors have come from several key observations. First, inhibition of JAK function leads to significant immunosuppression, as the JAK-mediated signaling mechanism involves multiple cytokines, which are relevant in immune-mediated inflammation (Figure 16.2). It is also noteworthy to mention that JAK3 is restricted to the immune cells, and it is of interest that both humans having inactive alleles and JAK3-deficient animals display a phenotype that has been observed to be restricted to the immune system [25]. These observations have encouraged scientists and pharmaceutical industries to design inhibitors for JAK3 as immunosuppressive agents, which resulted in the development of tofacitinib (CP-690,550).

It is important to mention that ruxolitinib [(R)-3-(4-(7H-pyrrolo[2,3-d]pyrimidin-4-yl)-1H-pyrazol-1-yl)-3-cyclopentylpropanenitrile phosphate], a small-molecule ATP mimetic, was the first JAK inhibitor approved by the Food and Drug Administration (FDA) in 2011. It is a potent inhibitor for both JAK1 and JAK2 and results in a dramatic decrease in levels of inflammatory cytokines, IL-6 and tumor necrosis factor (TNF) α. It has been demonstrated to be appropriate for the treatment of polycythemia vera and myelofibrosis [26].

The efficacy and safety of oral tofacitinib were first demonstrated in RA. The therapeutic use of tofacitinib 5 mg twice daily (BID) received FDA approval in 2012 for RA. Tofacitinib has also been investigated recently for the treatment of patients suffering from moderate to severe chronic plaque psoriasis. In phase 2 studies, clinical trials demonstrated safety and efficacy with BID oral dosing of tofacitinib in subjects with plaque psoriasis [27,28], and it is currently being investigated in phase 3 registration studies. A phase 2 study of tofacitinib in psoriasis patients has reported that PASI 75 response rates at week 12 were significantly higher than those for the placebo [27]. Recent data (phase 2) also suggest that baricitinib, an investigational drug, an oral JAK1/JAK2 inhibitor, is effective in psoriasis [29].

Encouraging results in RA and psoriasis have created significant enthusiasm to synthesize and investigate novel JAK-STAT inhibitors for patients with PsA and AS. Dr. Desiree van der Heijde and colleagues have conducted a very promising study. In a randomized placebo-controlled phase 2 trial (NCT01786668), these investigators demonstrated the efficacy of tofacitinib in patients suffering from active AS [30]. Subjects received BID either placebo ($n = 51$) or one of the following three dosages of tofacitinib for 12 weeks: 2 mg ($n = 52$), 5 mg ($n = 52$), or 10 mg ($n = 52$). The primary end point was an Assessment of Spondyloarthritis International Society 20% improvement (ASAS20) response rate at week 12. Secondary end points included patient-reported outcomes, disease activity, and MRI Spondyloarthritis Research Consortium of Canada (SPARCC) scores.

Patients taking tofacitinib 5 and 10 mg BID doses demonstrated better clinical efficacy than those taking the placebo. Patients with tofacitinib had a lesser degree of clinical signs and symptoms and a better end-point outcome for active AS, including improvement in MRI SPARCC scores. It was observed that patients with the 5 mg tofacitinib BID dose had an actual ASAS20 response rate of 80.8%, compared with 41.2% in the placebo arm ($p < 0.001$). The 2 mg (51.9%) and 10 mg (55.8%) BID tofacitinib groups also had a higher response, but it was not significantly significant compared with the placebo group. All tofacitinib groups exhibited ASAS40 and Bath Ankylosing Spondylitis Disease Activity Index 50% (BASDAI50) response rates and changes in the Ankylosing Spondylitis Disease Activity Score (ASDAS) of similar magnitude, and were significantly different compared with the placebo. In a recent study, Maksymowych et al. have also demonstrated that with tofacitinib, there are clinically meaningful reductions in axial MRI inflammation in subjects suffering from AS [31]. This study demonstrated that the proportion of patients achieving minimum clinically important differences (MCIDs) in sacroiliac joint (SIJ) or spine was about three times higher in the pooled tofacitinib group than in the placebo group ($p < 0.05$ for SIJ and $p < 0.01$ for spine).

Mease et al. demonstrated the efficacy and safety of tofacitinib in PsA in a randomized, multicenter, double-blind, placebo- and active-controlled against adalimumab, phase 3 study [32]. Patients with PsA were randomized 2:2:2:1:1 to tofacitinib 5 mg BID ($n = 107$), tofacitinib 10 mg BID ($n = 104$), adalimumab 40 mg subcutaneous injection every 2 weeks ($n = 106$), or placebo. At 3 months, placebo patients were rerandomized, and patients who started with placebo advanced to tofacitinib 5 mg ($n = 52$) or 10 mg ($n = 53$) BID. The study was conducted over a period of 1 year, and the primary end points were (1) the American College of Rheumatology 20% improvement (ACR20) response and (2) the Health Assessment Questionnaire Disability Index (HAQ-DI) changes at 3 months.

At baseline, demographic and disease severity were similar in the treatment and control groups. Tofacitinib exhibited significantly greater efficacy than the placebo at 3 months in both the ACR20 and HAQ-DI response rates. HAQ-DI responses were statistically significant for the tofacitinib dosing arms compared with the placebo group. ACR20 responses at 3 months for tofacitinib were 50% in the 5 mg BID group, 61% in the 10 mg BID group, and 52% in the adalimumab group, compared with only 33% in the placebo group. ACR20 responses not only could be maintained, but also, with continuation of treatment, got better in 12 months: 68%, 70%, and 60%, respectively, in the three treatment groups. Adverse event rates were similar in all treatment arms. The common adverse events were upper respiratory tract infection, nasopharyngitis, and headache.

16.5 SUMMARY

1. The JAK-STAT signaling kinase proteins play a vital role in immunity development and immune surveillance, and JAK-STAT inhibitors have demonstrated considerable therapeutic potential in autoimmune conditions, including SpA.

2. The JAK-STAT kinase cascade modulates proliferation of the effector memory T cells and is associated with a cytokine network of various T-cell subpopulations, such as Th17 cells and the IL-23/IL-17 cytokine axis.
3. As the IL-23/IL-17 cytokine axis plays a pivotal role in the pathogenesis of psoriasis, PsA, and AS, it is expected that specific JAK-STAT inhibitors will be therapeutically beneficial in diverse autoimmune diseases.
4. Encouraging findings of undergoing clinical trials with JAK inhibitors in SpA are promising and suggest that JAK inhibitors could be an effective therapeutic option.

Novel discovery of small-molecule targeted therapies represents a legendary invention in targeted therapy for autoimmune diseases owing to their ability to simultaneously block multiple signaling pathways. Tofacitinib, the first targeted JAK inhibitor approved by the FDA for use in rheumatological diseases, may be followed by a series of other JAK inhibitors. The safety profile of tofacitinib is similar to that of biologic disease-modifying antirheumatic drugs (DMARDs), and that includes risks of infections [33]. Furthermore, close monitoring is required for neutropenia, lymphopenia, liver function, renal function, and hyperlipidemia [33–38]. A higher risk of herpes zoster has been demonstrated in patients with tofacitinib compared with the placebo [36,37].

JAK inhibitors have brought another paradigm shift in the treatment for rheumatologic autoimmune diseases. In the coming years, a new chapter is going to unfold for novel applications of JAK inhibitors in diverse autoimmune and inflammatory disorders.

ACKNOWLEDGMENTS

This project was supported by the VA Sacramento Medical Center. The contents do not necessarily represent the views of the Department of Veterans Affairs or the U.S. government. The funder had no role in study design, data collection and analysis, decision to publish, or preparation of the manuscript.

REFERENCES

1. Saxena A, Raychaudhuri SK, Raychaudhuri SP. Cytokine pathways in psoriasis and psoriatic arthritis. In *Psoriatic Arthritis and Psoriasis: Pathology and Clinical Aspects* (pp. 73–82). Berlin: Springer International, 2016.
2. Chandran V, Raychaudhuri SP. Geoepidemiology and environmental factors of psoriasis and psoriatic arthritis. *J Autoimmun* 2010;34(3):J314–21.
3. Kehl AS, Corr M, Weisman MH. New Insights into pathogenesis, diagnostic modalities, and treatment. *Arthritis Rheumatol* 2016;68(2):312–22.
4. Ueda H, Morphew MK, McIntosh JR, Davis MM. CD4+ T-cell synapses involve multiple distinct stages. *Proc Natl Acad Sci U S A* 2011;108(41):17099–104.
5. Hivroz C, Chemin K, Tourret M, Bohineust A. Crosstalk between T lymphocytes and dendritic cells. *Crit Rev Immunol* 2012;32(2):139–55.
6. Raychaudhuri SP, Raychaudhuri SK, Tamura K, Masunaga T, Kubo K, Hanaoka K, Jiang WY, Herzenberg LA, Herzenberg LA. FR255734, a humanized, Fc-silent, anti-CD28 antibody improves psoriasis in the SCID mouse-psoriasis xenograft model. *J Invest Dermatol* 2008;128(8):1969–76.
7. Linsley PS, Brady W, Grosmaire L, Aruffo A, Damle NK, Ledbetter JA. Binding of the B cell activation antigen B7 to CD28 costimulates T cell proliferation and interleukin 2 mRNA accumulation. *J Exp Med* 1991;173:721–30.
8. Raychaudhuri SP, Raychaudhuri SK, Genovese MC. IL-17 receptor and its functional significance in psoriatic arthritis. *Mol Cell Biochem* 2012;359(1–2):419–29.
9. Raychaudhuri SP, Raychaudhuri SK. Mechanistic rationales for targeting interleukin-17A in spondyloarthritis. *Arthritis Res Ther* 2017 8;19(1):51. An excellent review on the role of the IL-23/IL-17 cytokine network in the pathogenesis of SpA and its therapeutic relevance.

10. Datta-Mitra A, Kundu-Raychaudhuri S, Mitra A, Raychaudhuri SP. Cross talk between neuro-regulatory molecule and monocyte: Nerve growth factor activates the inflammasome. *PLoS One* 2015;10(4):e0121626.
11. Villarino AV, Kanno Y, O'Shea JJ. Mechanisms and consequences of Jak-STAT signaling in the immune system. *Nat Immunol* 2017;18(4):374–84.
12. Schwartz DM, Bonelli M, Gadina M, O'Shea JJ. Type I/II cytokines, JAKs, and new strategies for treating autoimmune diseases. *Nat Rev Rheumatol* 2016;12(1):25–36. An excellent review on JAK-STAT signaling pathway, its relevance to autoimmune diseases, and principles for JAK-STAT-targeted therapy in autoimmune diseases.
13. Rawlings JS, Rosler KM, Harrison AD. The JAK/STAT signalling pathway. *J Cell Sci* 2004;117:1281–3.
14. Kisseleva T, Bhattacharya S, Braunstein J, Schindler CW. Signalling through the JAK/STAT pathway, recent advances and future challenges. *Gene* 2002;285:1–24.
15. Clark JD, Flanagan ME, Telliez JB. Discovery and development of Janus kinase (JAK) inhibitors for inflammatory diseases. *J Med Chem* 2014;57:5023–38.
16. Pesu M, Candotti F, Husa M et al. JAK3, severe combined immunodeficiency, and a new class of immunosuppressive drugs. *Immunol Rev* 2005;203:127–42.
17. Meyer DM, Jesson MI, Li X et al. Anti-inflammatory activity and neutrophil reductions mediated by the JAK1/JAK3 inhibitor, CP-690,550, in rat adjuvant-induced arthritis. *J Inflamm (Lond)* 2010;7:41.
18. Honma M, MinamiHori M, Takahashi H et al. Podoplanin expression in wound and hyperproliferative psoriatic epidermis: Regulation by TGFβ and STAT3 activating cytokines, IFNγ, IL6, and IL22. *J Dermatol Sci* 2012;65:134–40.
19. Boyle DL, Soma K, Hodge J et al. The JAK inhibitor tofacitinib suppresses synovial JAK1STAT signalling in rheumatoid arthritis. *Ann Rheum Dis* 2015;71:440–7.
20. Gao W, McGarry T, Orr C, McCormick J, Veale DJ, Fearon U. Tofacitinib regulates synovial inflammation in psoriatic arthritis, inhibiting STAT activation and induction of negative feedback inhibitors. *Ann Rheum Dis* 2016;75(1):311–5. This study explains the regulatory role of the JAK-STAT kinase system in synovial cell biology and synovial inflammation, and provides evidence for JAK-STAT signaling system inhibition as a therapeutic option for the treatment of PsA.
21. Alves de Medeiros AK, Speeckaert R, Desmet E, Van Gele M, De Schepper S, Lambert J. JAK3 as an emerging target for topical treatment of inflammatory skin diseases. *PLoS One* 2016;11(10):e0164080.
22. Raychaudhuri SK, Abria C, Raychaudhuri SP. Regulatory role of the JAK STAT kinase signaling system on the IL-23/IL-17 cytokine axis in psoriatic arthritis. *Ann Rheum Dis* 2017. http://dx.doi.org/10.1136/annrheumdis-2016-211046. A key article describing the functional significance of the JAK-STAT kinase signaling system in the pathogenesis of PsA and its relevance for developing novel therapies for SpA by targeting this kinase pathway.
23. Chen C, Zhang X, Wang Y. Analysis of JAK2 and STAT3 polymorphisms in patients with ankylosing spondylitis in Chinese Han population. *Clin Immunol* 2010;136:442–6.
24. Ferguson LR, Han DY, Fraser AG et al. Genetic factors in chronic inflammation: Single nucleotide polymorphisms in the STAT-JAK pathway, susceptibility to DNA damage and Crohn's disease in a New Zealand population. *Mutat Res* 2010;690:108–15.
25. O'Shea JJ, Pesu M, Borie DC, Changelian PS. A new modality for immunosuppression: Targeting the JAK/STAT pathway. *Nat Rev Drug Discov* 2004;3:555–64.
26. Verstovsek S, Kantarjian H, Mesa RA et al. Safety and efficacy of INCB018424, a JAK1 and JAK2 inhibitor, in myelofibrosis. *N Engl J Med* 2010;363:1117–27.
27. Papp KA, Menter A, Strober B et al. Efficacy and safety of tofacitinib, an oral Janus kinase inhibitor, in the treatment of psoriasis: A phase 2b randomized placebo-controlled dose-ranging study. *Br J Dermatol* 2012;167(3):668–77. A key article describing phase 2 data of tofacitinib in plaque psoriasis; tofacitinib inhibits JAK1, JAK2, and JAK3.
28. Menter A, Papp KA, Tan H et al. Efficacy of tofacitinib, an oral Janus kinase inhibitor, on clinical signs of moderate-to-severe plaque psoriasis in different body regions. *J Drugs Dermatol* 2014;13(3):252–6.
29. Papp KA, Menter MA, Raman M, Disch D, Schlichting DE, Gaich C, Macias W, Zhang X, Janes JM. A randomized phase 2b trial of baricitinib, an oral Janus kinase (JAK) 1/JAK2 inhibitor, in patients with moderate-to-severe psoriasis. *Br J Dermatol* 2016;174(6):1266–76. A key article describing phase 2 data of baricitinib in plaque psoriasis; baricitinib is a JAK1 and JAK2 inhibitor.
30. van der Heijde D, Deodhar A, Wei JC, Drescher E, Fleishaker D, Hendrikx T, Li D, Menon S, Kanik KS. Tofacitinib in patients with ankylosing spondylitis: A phase II, 16-week, randomised, placebo-controlled, dose-ranging study. *Ann Rheum Dis* 2017;76(8):1340–7. A key article describing phase 2 data of tofacitinib in AS.

31. Maksymowych W, van der Heijde D, Baraliakos X, Deodhar AA, Brown M, Sherlock S, Li D, Fleishaker D, Hendrikx T. Treatment with tofacitinib is associated with clinically meaningful reductions in axial MRI inflammation in patients with ankylosing spondylitis. *Arthritis Rheumatol* 2016;68(Suppl 10):abstract 1044.
32. Mease PJ, Hall S, FitzGerald O et al. Efficacy and safety of tofacitinib, an oral Janus kinase inhibitor, or adalimumab in patients with active psoriatic arthritis and an inadequate response to conventional synthetic DMARDs: A randomized, placebo-controlled, phase 3 trial. *Arthritis Rheumatol* 2016;68(Suppl 10):abstract 2983.
33. Strand V, Ahadieh S, French J et al. Systematic review and meta-analysis of serious infections with tofacitinib and biologic disease-modifying antirheumatic drug treatment in rheumatoid arthritis clinical trials. *Arthritis Res Ther* 2015;17:362.
34. Charles-Schoeman C, Burmester G, Nash P et al. Efficacy and safety of tofacitinib following inadequate response to conventional synthetic or biological disease-modifying antirheumatic drugs. *Ann Rheum Dis* 2016;75:1293.
35. Kremer J, Li ZG, Hall S et al. Tofacitinib in combination with nonbiologic disease-modifying antirheumatic drugs in patients with active rheumatoid arthritis: A randomized trial. *Ann Intern Med* 2013;159:253.
36. Winthrop KL, Yamanaka H, Valdez H et al. Herpes zoster and tofacitinib therapy in patients with rheumatoid arthritis. *Arthritis Rheumatol* 2014;66:2675.
37. Cohen S, Radominski SC, Gomez-Reino JJ et al. Analysis of infections and all-cause mortality in phase II, phase III, and long-term extension studies of tofacitinib in patients with rheumatoid arthritis. *Arthritis Rheumatol* 2014;66(11):2924–37.
38. Cohen SB, Koenig A, Wang L, Kwok K, Mebus CA, Riese R, Fleischmann R. Efficacy and safety of tofacitinib in US and non-US rheumatoid arthritis patients: Pooled analyses of phase II and III. *Clin Exp Rheumatol* 2016;34(1):32–6.

17 Concept of Total Care

Multidisciplinary Approach for the Management of Psoriatic Disease

Smriti K. Raychaudhuri, Debasis Bagchi, and Siba P. Raychaudhuri

CONTENTS

17.1 INTRODUCTION

Psoriatic arthritis (PsA) is a systemic inflammatory disease; in addition to chronic inflammation of the cutaneous system and joints, it often involves extra-articular sites. However, in day-to-day practice, management of PsA is focused on skin and joint symptoms, and many of these comorbidities of PsA are often neglected.

It is now well established that PsA is associated with an increased risk for cardiovascular complications and mortality, as well as with integral components of the metabolic syndrome [1–5]. The simplest explanation for increased cardiovascular complications in chronic inflammatory conditions has been proposed to be the increased prevalence of traditional cardiovascular risk factors: age, gender, smoking, and incidence of diabetes. However, in psoriasis and PsA, many studies have reported that up to 30%–50% of patients with atherosclerosis did not have these risk factors [6–8]. Thus, for an effective treatment of this patient population, an understanding of the metabolic abnormalities in psoriasis and PsA is critical. A treatment regimen should address the comorbidities associated with psoriatic disease; otherwise, it will be only partially effective. The aim of this chapter is to provide the spectrum of comorbid conditions associated with psoriatic disease, with an emphasis on atherosclerosis, intricate components of the metabolic syndrome, and general health care, including the usefulness of "wellness programs" to not only improve the underlying diseases but also reduce mortalities associated with PsA so that those with it can have a long-term healthy life.

17.2 SYSTEMIC INFLAMMATION, OBESITY, AND ATHEROSCLEROSIS: A TRIPLE PARALLEL MARCH

Obesity is now a global epidemic that is leading to excess morbidity and mortality. According to the World Health Organization projections, it is estimated that more than 1.5 billion adults are overweight and about 400 million are obese [9]. Activated white adipose tissue is an important source of pro-inflammatory cytokines, such as tumor necrosis factor (TNF) α, and other interleukins (ILs), including IL-17; also, synthesis of regulatory cytokines, such as IL-10, has been reported to be decreased [10–12]. IL-6 upregulates the hepatic production of C-reactive protein (CRP). A positive correlation has been found with abdominal obesity and CRP levels [13]. Thus, diverse pro-inflammatory conditions conferred by excess visceral adipose tissue combine to produce a tonic degree of systemic inflammation that worsens with increasing central obesity. Furthermore, pro-inflammatory cytokines stimulate adipocytes to secrete substance P (SP), a neuropeptide, and nerve growth factor (NGF); both NGF and SP have been shown to play a critical role in the pathogenesis of psoriatic disease [14]. Insulin resistance, obesity, and thus development of diabetes are also strongly influenced by multiple pro-inflammatory agents. Both insulin resistance and its associated pro-inflammatory signals may lead to endothelial dysfunction, which could be an early step for the atherogenesis process in patients with psoriasis [10].

Significant platelet activation and systemic inflammation were observed in patients with psoriasis, especially when associated with severe disease. Furthermore, increased platelet activation might be the missing link between the persistent inflammation and the development of atherosclerotic plaque, leading to the cardiovascular comorbidities seen associated with psoriasis [15].

17.3 ADIPOCYTOKINES IN PSORIATIC DISEASE

Leptin levels and leptin receptor expression are significantly high in severe psoriasis. Adipocytokines are an array of cytokines that are associated with adipose tissue; among these, the most widely studied are leptin, adiponectin, visfatin, and resistin. A contributing role of adipocytokines has been reported in obesity, insulin resistance, the induction of inflammation, and coronary heart disease [10–12,16,17]. Leptin has multiple functions, such as its regulatory role in controlling appetite and body weight, and it also may play a key role in the modulation of immune responses [10–12,17]. Serum leptin concentrations are reported to be high in obesity. Increased levels of leptin are associated with the induction of an inflammatory reaction, insulin resistance, and the onset of subclinical coronary atherosclerosis. Monocytes and macrophages, T cells, and natural killer cells express leptin receptors. In cultured monocytes and macrophages, leptin can induce secretion of TNF-α and IL-6. Compared with non-leptin-deficient mice, leptin-deficient mice are less prone to develop inflammatory diseases [16,17]. It has been well demonstrated that in patients with moderate to severe psoriasis, leptin correlates with metabolic syndrome features and inflammation, whereas resistin correlates with inflammation and disease severity [18].

Resistin, a putative adipocyte-derived signaling polypeptide, is characterized by its potential etiological link between obesity and diabetes, with a clear functional role as a pathogenic factor contributing to insulin resistance, while visfatin, another newly discovered adipocyte hormone, exerts a direct relationship with type 2 diabetes mellitus. Mechanistically, visfatin binds to the insulin receptor at a site distinct from that of insulin and causes hypoglycemia by reducing glucose release from hepatocytes and stimulating glucose utilization in adipocytes and myocytes. Visfatin is upregulated by hypoxia, inflammation, and hyperglycemia and downregulated by insulin, somatostatin, and statins. A recent clinical investigation has demonstrated increased visfatin, fetuin-A, and pentraxin 3 (PTX3) pro-inflammatory mediators in psoriasis. Okan et al. (2016) also demonstrated the positive correlation between these mediators, including serum vistafin, fetuin-A, and Psoriasis Area and Severity Index (PASI) score [19]. Incidentally, elevations in resistin and visfatin are associated with induction of inflammation, insulin resistance, and cardiovascular risk. In contrast, adiponectin is anti-inflammatory. Higher concentrations of adiponectin are inversely associated with obesity and its associated risks, such as insulin resistance and cardiovascular complications.

Because of these unique actions of adipocytokines, currently, extensive research work is going on to elucidate the regulatory role of adipocytokines in chronic inflammatory diseases, including its possible role in the inflammatory and proliferative cascades of psoriatic disease. There are reports suggesting that expressions of genes that regulate both skin and lipid metabolism are altered in skin in patients with psoriatic disease, and evidence has been provided for altered fatty acid metabolism [20] and higher levels of oxidized LDL in the skin of patients with psoriasis [21]. Furthermore, a significant spectrum of evidence suggests that leptin and resistin are likely to be associated with the pathogenesis of psoriasis in overweight individuals [22,23]. A contributing role of leptin in cardiovascular disease (CVD) is evolving, and there are reports suggesting that leptin is an independent risk factor for coronary artery disease (CAD) [24]. Similarly, contributing roles of other adipocytokines, such as resistin, gherelin, adiponectin, and cachectin, have also been reported in the pathogenesis of atherosclerotic CVD [24,25]. Thus, adipocytokines may play a key role in the pathogenesis of psoriatic disease and its underlying comorbidities, like diabetes, atherosclerosis, and hypertension [10,16–18].

17.4 LINK BETWEEN SYSTEMIC INFLAMMATORY RESPONSES AND ATHEROSCLEROSIS IN PSORIATIC DISEASE

Psoriasis is a common chronic cutaneous inflammatory disease involving the skin that is associated with serious comorbidities, including PsA, reduced quality of life, malignancy, and depression, but also a constellation of associated conditions that enhance the cardiovascular risk.

Under normal conditions, the endothelial cells of the arterial wall resist adhesion and aggregation of leukocytes and promote fibrinolysis. When activated by stimuli such as obesity, insulin resistance, hypertension, or inflammation, the endothelial cells express a series of adhesion molecules that selectively recruit various classes of leukocytes. Inflammatory cells such as blood monocytes now adhere to the "adherent" endothelial surface by binding to leukocyte adhesion molecules. After the adhesion of monocytes, pro-inflammatory proteins, including chemokines, are produced and provide a chemotactic stimulus that induces monocytes to enter the intima. Within the intima, the monocytes mature into macrophages, which express scavenger receptors. These receptors allow macrophages to engulf oxidized or modified lipoprotein particles. The macrophages also proliferate within the intima and, after being filled with lipid particles, get the frothy appearance of foam cells found in atherosclerotic lesions [26,27]. These cells also release several growth factors and cytokines, including enzymes such as metalloproteinases (MMPs) and the pro-coagulant tissue factor, which can destroy the vessel wall matrix and generation of additional signals, leading to vascular smooth muscle cell (VSMC) proliferation and migration [28].

Psoriatic disease (psoriasis and PsA) also involves increased generation of IL-1, IL-6, TNF-α, IL-17, IL-23, and other inflammatory cytokines produced in the skin and joints [29]. The IL-23/IL-17 axis is crucial in the pathogenesis of psoriatic disease. Human IL-23 is primarily produced by antigen-presenting cells and induces and maintains differentiation of Th17 and Th22 cells, a primary cellular source of pro-inflammatory cytokines such as IL-17 and IL-22, which mediate the epidermal hyperplasia, keratinocyte immune activation, and skin and joint inflammation inherent in the pathogenesis of psoriatic disease [30]. It is possible that these pro-inflammatory cytokines spill into the circulation, where they induce adhesion molecules and other pro-inflammatory molecules, such as chemokines. This leads to monocyte and leukocyte adhesion to the endothelial cells of the vessel wall, followed by the chemotaxis of these cells into vessel walls, which ultimately leads to atherosclerosis. In addition, CRP is also elevated in psoriatic disease. Vachatova et al. assessed the role of CRP and selected inflammatory and anti-inflammatory markers in the pathogenesis of metabolic syndrome and psoriasis in 74 psoriatic patients. The authors reported significantly higher body mass index (BMI) ($p < 0.05$) and diastolic blood pressure ($p < 0.05$) in these subjects. Furthermore, significantly higher CRP, lipoprotein-associated phospholipase A2 (Lp-PLA2), leptin, and resistin levels were observed in psoriatic patients. Vachatova et al. concluded that the level of Lp-PLA2 indicates the presence of subclinical atherosclerosis and higher cardiovascular risk in psoriatic patients [31]. Furthermore, CRP stimulates macrophages to produce tissue factor, an important procoagulant found in atherosclerotic plaques.

Psoriatic disease is uniquely associated with obesity, insulin resistance, and hypertension [6,32,33]. Through an array of molecular interactions, these conditions are capable of inducing inflammatory cascades on the endothelial lining to initiate the process of atherosclerosis. No physiopathological mechanism accounting for the association of the inflammatory cascades of psoriasis with atherogenesis has been demonstrated so far. The observation that psoriatic disease is a risk factor for CAD has provided us a unique opportunity to study the contributing role of systemic inflammation as an independent risk factor for atherosclerosis.

17.5 METABOLIC SYNDROME, ATHEROSCLEROSIS, AND CORONARY ARTERY DISEASE: MAJOR COMORBIDITIES IN PSORIATIC ARTHRITIS

PsA is a heterogeneous multifaceted inflammatory arthritis associated with myriad different clinical symptoms of psoriasis and exhibiting a wide range of pathologies. PsA is considered to be one of the spondyloarthritides, and as such, it has both spinal and peripheral joint involvement, as well as enthesitis and dactylitis. The severity of PsA is variable and can range from mild joint pain to debilitating polyarticular disease [34,35]. The progression of PsA can be fast, and within 2 years of onset, 50% of patients may develop erosive joint damage [36,37]. Joint damage in certain patients with the mutilating form of PsA leads to significant patient morbidity and disability.

Like other spondyloarthropathies, PsA is associated with inflammatory bowel disease [38,39], uveitis [40,41], and valvular heart disease [42,43]. PsA patients have been reported to have reduced quality of life, osteoporosis, and sleep apnea [44–47]. PsA has been reported to be associated with an array of systemic diseases. Patients with psoriatic disease suffer from associated comorbidities, including CVD, obesity and metabolic syndrome, diabetes, osteoporosis, malignancy, fatty liver disease, depression, and anxiety (Table 17.1).

In addition, as PsA is a lifelong disease, prolonged treatment with conventional disease-modifying antirheumatic drugs (DMARDs), such as methotrexate, leflunomide, and other immunosuppressives, has the potential for increased risks of infectious and malignant diseases. Similarly, the use of biologic DMARDs also has inherent risks for atypical bacterial infections, mycobacterial infections, systemic fungal infections, lymphoma, and other malignancies [48–50]. Among these comorbidities, metabolic syndrome is a silent process and leads to major cardiovascular health

TABLE 17.1
Comorbidities in Psoriatic Arthritis

- Uveitis
- Inflammatory bowel disease
- Metabolic syndrome
- Fatigue
- Valvular heart disease
- Pneumonitis/interstitial lung disease (very rare)
- Osteoporosis
- Comorbidities secondary to chronic use of topical and systemic medications and DMARDs (conventional/biologics)
- Comorbidities secondary to chronic pain/disability, such as depression, anxiety, and psychosexual problems

issues, and currently, guidelines for the management and prevention of metabolic syndrome in PsA are not available. In the next few sections, we provide some of the available information in this area and discuss a possible approach for the management of metabolic syndrome and its sequelae in PsA.

As indicated earlier, metabolic syndrome is characterized by insulin resistance, central obesity, dyslipidemia, and hypertension. It is reasonable to believe that insulin resistance is the core component of the metabolic syndrome, and thus metabolic syndrome plays a pivotal role in predisposing atherosclerosis and CAD. Patients with psoriatic disease have an increased risk of developing CVD and metabolic syndrome than controls without psoriasis [33,51]. Among the types of inflammatory arthritis, metabolic syndrome and higher risks of CVD are best documented in rheumatoid arthritis (RA) [52,53]. Metabolic syndrome is characterized by obesity, hypertension, insulin resistance, and dyslipidemia. These individual components have been reported in PsA by a number of studies. In a mortality study, among 428 Canadian patients with PsA, the leading cause of death was CVD (36.2%) [54]. The same group in a follow-up study observed that the PsA patients ($n = 648$) had a significantly higher prevalence of hypertension, angina, and myocardial infarction [55]. Overall, in this PsA cohort, 35% ($n = 227$) had cardiovascular morbidities: hypertension 206, myocardial infarction 50, angina 33, cerebrovascular accident 8, and congestive heart failure (CHF) 12. The standardized prevalence ratios (SPRs) for myocardial infarction (2.57; 95% CI 1.73–3.80), angina (1.97; 95% CI 1.24–3.12), and hypertension (1.90; 95% CI 1.59–2.27) were statistically significant. From a U.S. database in a cross-sectional comparative study of PsA patients ($n = 1843$), Han et al. reported that the prevalence of hypertension, ischemic heart disease, CHF, hyperlipidemia, atherosclerosis, and type 2 diabetes was significantly higher ($p < 0.05$) in PsA patients than in controls [1]. Kimhi et al., in 47 patients with PsA, compared with 100 healthy controls, observed that PsA patients had a higher incidence of hypertension and hyperlipidemia, and had higher levels of the erythrocyte sedimentation rate (ESR), CRP, and fibrinogen. In addition, the average intima-media wall thickness (IMT) of PsA patients was significantly higher than that of controls; the PsA patients' average IMT significantly correlated with age, BMI, duration of skin and joint disease, spine involvement, ESR, and fibrinogen [3]. A study using the Danish nationwide registries of hospitalization and drug dispensing from pharmacies has reported that the cardiovascular risk of patients with severe psoriasis or PsA can be of similar magnitude to that of diabetes patients [56].

Recently, we determined the prevalence of metabolic syndrome in 105 PsA patients [33]. We observed a higher prevalence of the metabolic syndrome in PsA patients (58.1%), compared with only 35.2% reported in the Third National Health and Nutrition Examination Survey (NHANES III) data. Among the patients with metabolic syndrome, we observed that 24.6% had CAD, 39.3% had type 2 diabetes mellitus, and 18.0% had chronic kidney disease.

17.6 CAN WE PREVENT METABOLIC SYNDROME AND CARDIOVASCULAR COMORBIDITIES OF PSORIATIC ARTHRITIS?

As mentioned earlier, PsA is a chronic inflammatory condition, and its pathogenesis involves an interaction between genetic, environmental, and immunological factors. The chronic inflammatory nature of psoriatic disease may predispose it to have an association with other inflammatory conditions, including CVDs and metabolic disorders. A growing body of literature suggests that the systemic inflammatory reaction in patients with PsA also imposes a considerable risk for the development or aggravation of CVD, metabolic disorders, and mortality. Thus, in addition to treating skin and joint pathologies in patients with PsA, it is critical to prevent and monitor risk factors of CAD. Standard care for the management and prevention of cardiovascular risk factors should be addressed in patients with PsA, including avoiding tobacco, maintaining normal blood pressure (below 140/90 mmHg), and keeping serum cholesterol below 200 mg/dL (5 mmol/L) and, more specifically, LDL cholesterol below 100 mg/dL (2.5 mmol/L). In addition, weight reduction, physical activity for at least 30 minutes a day, and a balanced healthy diet would be excellent lifestyle modifications to counter all components of the metabolic syndrome.

It has been well documented that severity of skin psoriasis is linked to blood vessel inflammation and cardiovascular risk. The National Psoriasis Foundation recommends implementing the American Heart Association guidelines [57], which recommend screening for cardiovascular risk factors (blood pressure, lipid profile, blood sugar, and BMI), smoking cessation by age 40 years, and alcohol reduction. More intensive intervention is warranted for people with risk factors, as outlined on the website of the American Heart Association: www.americanheart.org. In view of the increased risks of CVD in patients with PsA, it is reasonable to follow these guidelines for PsA. In addition, patients should be closely watched to prevent the cardiovascular risks contributed by nonsteroidal anti-inflammatory drugs and corticosteroids. It is expected that these guidelines will reduce adverse cardiovascular events and help initiate antihypertensives and statins at an appropriate time. The European League Against Rheumatism (EULAR) has issued guidelines based on a systematic literature search of cardiovascular risk management in patients with RA, ankylosing spondylitis (AS), or PsA [58]. It recommends annual screenings of PsA patients for cardiovascular risk, management of cardiovascular risk factors, and adequate control of disease activity of PsA.

In PsA patients, the severity of inflammation has been suggested to be an indicator of increased mortality. Patients with high ESR, high medication level, and rapidly progressive radiological changes had increased mortality [59]. These observations indicate that early diagnosis and aggressive treatment of the inflammatory arthritis is likely to halt the disease process and its progression, and thus likely to reduce the mortality and morbidity of PsA.

As systemic inflammation is now an established risk factor for atherogenesis of the coronary vessels, clinicians and researchers are hoping that a treatment regimen targeted to regulate the inflammation in autoimmune arthritis might be the key to prevent CAD. In support of this hypothesis, reports suggest that treatment with DMARDs, like methotrexate, can provide a substantial benefit such as reducing vascular diseases in patients with psoriasis and RA [60–63]. DMARDs have been shown to improve the lipid profile in patients with early active RA [61,62]. Furthermore, it has been demonstrated that methotrexate use is beneficial for thc RA-associated metabolic syndrome and also likely to reduce atherosclerosis [62,63].

TNF blockers have provided a new dimension for the treatment of RA, PsA, and AS. Because of its prominent anti-inflammatory action, currently the cardioprotective role of the anti-TNF agents is being investigated very closely. Two recent publications demonstrated an improvement of the arterial stiffness for etanercept in RA patients and for infliximab in AS patients [64,65]. Data from the British Biologics Registry suggest that RA patients who improved with anti-TNF therapy may have less risks for myocardial infarction [66]. This evidence justifies the usefulness of biologics in reducing or preventing certain cardiovascular comorbidities in other chronic inflammatory rheumatologic diseases inclusive of psoriasis and PsA. However, randomized controlled trials are needed to confirm the above-mentioned observations, especially in PsA patients where data are lacking.

17.7 CONCLUSION: CONCEPT OF TOTAL CARE

Given the increased prevalence of comorbidities in patients with psoriatic disease, it is essential to approach the disease as a potential multisystem disorder. A treatment regimen for PsA should include the management of its comorbidities (Table 17.1). It is understandable that for a rheumatologist, it is not possible to provide the full spectrum of health care, like a primary health care provider. However, the therapeutic approach for PsA needs a multidisciplinary approach and should include certain subspecialists on a case-to-case basis: physical therapy, endocrinology, ophthalmology, cardiology, psychiatry, and dietary and lifestyle modification programs. A rheumatologist needs to identify the potential comorbidities, work closely with the primary health care provider, and provide appropriate referrals. An ideal approach would be comprehensive and effective care as proposed for psoriasis as a "total care program" [67,68]. In PsA, it should be inclusive of exemplary care of the

TABLE 17.2
Concept of Total Care for Psoriatic Arthritis

- Thorough clinical evaluation: Systemic and cutaneous
- Educating parents and child in younger patients
- Exemplary skin care
- Cutting-edge treatment of PsA with conventional DMARDs and biologics
- Management of other clinical domains of PsA: Skin, nail, enthesitis, dactylitis, and spondylitis
- Identifying/preventing/treating
  - Comorbidities of PsA (Table 17.1)
  - Comorbidities from therapy (infection/malignancies)
- Wellness program: Exercise, diet, de-addiction, relaxation
- Building self-esteem: Support group, counseling

Source: Adopted from Raychaudhuri, S. P., *J. Rheumatol.*, 39, 437–440, 2012.

joint, skin, and associated comorbidities. Table 17.2 provides an outline in similar lines of "total care" for PsA. Recent treatment recommendations by the Group for Research and Assessment of Psoriasis and Psoriatic Arthritis (GRAPPA) provide evidence-based strategies for effective therapies, and how treatment may be affected by comorbidities in PsA [69].

REFERENCES

1. Han C, Robinson DW Jr, Hackett MV, Paramore LC, Fraeman KH, Bala MV. Cardiovascular disease and risk factors in patients with rheumatoid arthritis, psoriatic arthritis, and ankylosing spondylitis. *J Rheumatol* 2006;33:2167–72.
2. Tam LS, Shang Q, Li EK et al. Subclinical carotid atherosclerosis in patients with psoriatic arthritis. *Arthritis Rheum* 2008;59:1322–31.
3. Kimhi O, Caspi D, Bornstein NM, Maharshak N. Prevalence and risk factors of atherosclerosis in patients with psoriatic arthritis. *Semin Arthritis Rheum* 2007;36:203–9.
4. Di Minno MN, Ambrosino P, Lupoli R, Di Minno A, Tasso M, Peluso R, Tremoli E. Cardiovascular risk markers in patients with psoriatic arthritis: A meta-analysis of literature studies. *Ann Med* 2015;47(4):346–53.
5. Shen J, Shang Q, Li EK, Leung YY, Kun EW, Kwok LW, Li M, Li TK, Zhu TY, Yu CM, Tam LS. Cumulative inflammatory burden is independently associated with increased arterial stiffness in patients with psoriatic arthritis: A prospective study. *Arthritis Res Ther* 2015;17:75.
6. Gelfand JM, Neimann AL, Shin DB, Wang X, Margolis DJ, Troxel AB. Risk of myocardial infarction in patients with psoriasis. *JAMA* 2006;296:1735–41.
7. Gonzalez-Juanatey C, Llorca J, Amogo Diaz E. High prevalence of subclinical atherosclerosis in psoriatic arthritis patients without clinically evident cardiovascular disease or classic atherosclerosis risk factors. *Arthritis Rheum* 2007;57:1074–80.
8. Jamnitski A, Symmons D, Peters MJ, Sattar N, McInnes I, Nurmohamed MT. Cardiovascular comorbidities in patients with psoriatic arthritis: A systematic review. *Ann Rheum Dis* 2013;72(2):211–6.
9. World Health Organization. Obesity and overweight June 2016. http://www.who.int/mediacentre/factsheets/fs311/en/ (accessed Sept 13, 2017).
10. Siegel D, Devaraj S, Mitra A, Raychaudhuri SP, Raychaudhuri SK, Jialal I. Inflammation, atherosclerosis, and psoriasis. *Clin Rev Allergy Immunol* 2013;44:194–204.
11. Fuster JJ, Ouchi N, Gokce N, Walsh K. Obesity-induced changes in adipose tissue microenvironment and their impact on cardiovascular disease. *Circ Res* 2016;118(11):1786–807.
12. Rodríguez A, Ezquerro S, Méndez-Giménez L, Becerril S, Frühbeck G. Revisiting the adipocyte: A model for integration of cytokine signaling in the regulation of energy metabolism. *Am J Physiol Endocrinol Metab* 2015;309(8):E691–714.
13. Florez H, Castillo-Florez S, Mendez A et al. C-reactive protein is elevated in obese patients with the metabolic syndrome. *Diabetes Res Clin Pract* 2006;71(1):92–100.

14. Raychaudhuri SP, Jiang WY, Raychaudhuri SK. Revisiting the Koebner phenomenon: Role of NGF and its receptor system in the pathogenesis of psoriasis. *Am J Pathol* 2008;172(4):961–71.
15. Chandrashekar L, Rajappa M, Revathy G, Sundar I, Munisamy M, Ananthanarayanan PH, Thappa DM, Basu D. Is enhanced platelet activation the missing link leading to increased cardiovascular risk in psoriasis? *Clin Chim Acta* 2015;446:181–5.
16. Matarese G, Di Giacomo A, Sanna V et al. Requirement for leptin in the induction and progression of autoimmune encephalomyelitis. *J Immunol* 2001;166:5909–16.
17. Otero M, Lago R, Lago F, Casanueva FF, Dieguez C, Gómez-Reino JJ, Gualillo O. Leptin, from fat to inflammation: Old questions and new insights. *FEBS Lett* 2005;579:295–301.
18. Pina T, Genre F, Lopez-Mejias R, Armesto S, Ubilla B, Mijares V, Dierssen-Sotos T, Gonzalez-Lopez MA, Gonzalez-Vela MC, Blanco R, Hernández JL, Llorca J, Gonzalez-Gay MA. Relationship of leptin with adiposity and inflammation and resistin with disease severity in psoriatic patients undergoing anti-TNF-alpha therapy. *J Eur Acad Dermatol Venereol* 2015;29(10):1995–2001.
19. Okan G, Baki AM, Yorulmaz E, Dogru-Abbasoglu S, Vural P. Serum vistafin, fetuin-A, and pentraxin 3 levels in patients with psoriasis and their relation to disease severity. *J Clin Lab Anal* 2016; 30(4):284–9.
20. Romanowska M, al Yacoub N, Seidel H, Donandt S, Gerken H, Phillip S, Haritonova N, Artuc M, Schweiger S, Sterry W, Foerster J. PPARdelta enhances keratinocyte proliferation in psoriasis and induces heparin-binding EGF-like growth factor. *J Invest Dermatol* 2008;128(1):110–24.
21. Tekin NS, Tekin IO, Barut F, Sipahi EY. Accumulation of oxidized low-density lipoprotein in psoriatic skin and changes of plasma lipid levels in psoriatic patients. *Mediators Inflamm* 2007;2007:78454.
22. Zhu KJ, Zhang C, Li M, Zhu CY, Shi G, Fan YM. Leptin levels in patients with psoriasis: A meta-analysis. *Clin Exp Dermatol* 2013;38(5):478–83.
23. Johnston A, Arnadottir S, Gudjonsson JE et al. Obesity in psoriasis: Leptin and resistin as mediators of cutaneous inflammation. *Br J Dermatol* 2008;159(2):342–50.
24. Procaccini C, Pucino V, Mantzoros CS, Matarese G. Leptin in autoimmune diseases. *Metabolism* 2015;64(1):92–104.
25. Rizzo M, Rizvi AA, Rini GB, Berneis K. The therapeutic modulation of atherogenic dyslipidemis and inflammatory markers in the metabolic syndrome: What is the clinical relevance? *Acta Diabetol* 2009;46:1–11.
26. Libby P, Ridker PM, Hansson GK. Progress and challenges in translating the biology of atherosclerosis. *Nature* 2011;473(7347):317–25.
27. Worthley SG, Zhang ZY, Machac J et al. In vivo non-invasive serial monitoring of FDG-PET progression and regression in a rabbit model of atherosclerosis. *Int J Cardiovasc Imaging* 2009;25(3):251–7.
28. Kopp CW, Hölzenbein T, Steiner S et al. Inhibition of restenosis by tissue factor pathway inhibitor: In vivo and in vitro evidence for suppressed monocyte chemoattraction and reduced gelatinolytic activity. *Blood* 2004;103(5):1653–61.
29. Saxena A, Raychaudhuri SK, Raychaudhuri SP. Cytokine pathways in psoriasis and psoriatic arthritis. In *Psoriatic Arthritis and Psoriasis: Pathology and Clinical Aspects* (pp. 73–82). Berlin: Springer International, 2016.
30. Raychaudhuri SP, Raychaudhuri SK. Mechanistic rationales for targeting interleukin-17A in spondyloarthritis. *Arthritis Res Ther* 2017;19(1):51.
31. Vachatova S, Andrys C, Krejsek J, Salavec M, Ettler K, Rehacek V, Cermakova E, Malkova A, Fiala Z, Borska L. Metabolic syndrome and selective inflammatory markers in psoriatic patients. *J Immunol Res* 2016;2016:5380792.
32. Kaye JA, Li L, Jick SS. Incidence of risk factors for myocardial infarction and other vascular diseases in patients with psoriasis. *Br J Dermatol* 2008;159:895–902.
33. Raychaudhuri SK, Chatterjee S, Nguyen C, Kaur M, Jialal I, Raychaudhuri SP. Increased prevalence of the metabolic syndrome in patients with psoriatic arthritis. *Metab Syndr Relat Disord* 2010;8(4):331–4.
34. Gladman DD, Shuckett R, Russell ML et al. Psoriatic arthritis (PSA)—An analysis of 220 patients. *Q J Med* 1987;62:127–41.
35. Torre Alonso JC, Rodriguez Perez A, Arribas Castrillo JM et al. Psoriatic arthritis (PA): A clinical, immunological and radiological study of 180 patients. *Br J Rheumatol* 1991;30:245–50.
36. Queiro-Silva R, Torre-Alonso JC, Tinture-Eguren T et al. A polyarticular onset predicts erosive and deforming disease in psoriatic arthritis. *Ann Rheum Dis* 2003;62:68–70.
37. Kane D, Stafford L, Bresnihan B et al. A prospective, clinical and radiological study of early psoriatic arthritis: An early synovitis clinic experience. *Rheumatology (Oxford)* 2003;42:1460–8.

38. Moll JM, Haslock I, Macrae IF, Wright V. Associations between ankylosing spondylitis, psoriatic arthritis, Reiter's disease, the intestinal arthropathies, and Behcet's syndrome. *Medicine (Baltimore)* 1974;53(5):343–64.
39. Khan MA. Update on spondyloarthropathies. *Ann Intern Med* 2002;136(12):896–907.
40. Durrani K, Foster CS. Psoriatic uveitis: A distinct clinical entity? *Am J Ophthalmol* 2005;139:106–11.
41. Paiva ES, Macaluso DC, Edwards A et al. Characterisation of uveitis in patients with psoriatic arthritis. *Ann Rheum Dis* 2000;59:67–70.
42. Muna WF, Roller DH, Craft J, Shaw RK, Ross AM. Psoriatic arthritis and aortic regurgitation. *JAMA* 1980;244(4):363–5.
43. Kammer GM, Soter NA, Gibson DJ, Schur PH. Psoriatic arthritis: A clinical, immunologic and HLA study of 100 patients. *Semin Arthritis Rheum* 1979;9(2):75–97.
44. Gladman DD, Farewell VT, Wong K et al. Mortality studies in psoriatic arthritis: Results from a single outpatient center. II. Prognostic indicators for death. *Arthritis Rheum* 1998;41:1103–10.
45. Callis KD, Wong B, Krueger G. Sleep disturbance and medical co-morbidities in patients with psoriasis, psoriatic arthritis, and controls. Presented at the 67th Annual Meeting, San Francisco, March 6–10, 2009.
46. Husted JA, Gladman DD, Farewell VT et al. Validating the SF-36 health survey questionnaire in patients with psoriatic arthritis. *J Rheumatol* 1997;24:511–7.
47. Zachariae H, Zachariae R, Blomqvist K et al. Quality of life and prevalence of arthritis reported by 5,795 members of the Nordic Psoriasis Associations. Data from the Nordic Quality of Life Study. *Acta Derm Venereol* 2002;82:108–13.
48. Raychaudhuri SP, Nguyen CT, Raychaudhuri SK, Gershwin ME. Incidence and nature of infectious disease in patients treated with anti-TNF agents. *Autoimmun Rev* 2009;9(2):67–81.
49. Raychaudhuri SP, Wilken R, Sukhov AC, Raychaudhuri SK, Maverakis E. Management of psoriatic arthritis: Early diagnosis, monitoring of disease severity and cutting edge therapies. *J Autoimmun* 2017;76:21–37.
50. Langley RG, Strober BE, Gu Y, Rozzo SJ, Okun MM. Benefit-risk assessment of tumour necrosis factor antagonists in the treatment of psoriasis. *Br J Dermatol* 2010;162(6):1349–58.
51. Gisondi P, Tessari G, Conti A et al. Prevalence of metabolic syndrome in patients with psoriasis: A hospital-based case-control study. *Br J Dermatol* 2007;157:68–73.
52. del Rincon I, Williams K, Stern MP et al. High incidence of cardiovascular events in a rheumatoid arthritis cohort not explained by traditional cardiac risk factors. *Arthritis Rheum* 2001;44:2737–45.
53. Maradit-Kremers H, Crowson CS, Nicola PJ et al. Increased unrecognized coronary heart disease and sudden deaths in rheumatoid arthritis: A population based cohort study. *Arthritis Rheum* 2005; 52:402–11.
54. Wong K, Gladman DD, Husted J, Long JA, Farewell VT. Mortality studies in psoriatic arthritis: Results from a single outpatient clinic. I. Causes and risk of death. *Arthritis Rheum* 1997;40:1868–72.
55. Gladman DD, Ang M, Su L, Tom BDM, Schentag CT, Farewell VT. Cardiovascular morbidity in psoriatic arthritis. *Ann Rheum Dis* 2009;68:1131–5.
56. Ahlehoff O, Gislason GH, Charlot M, Jørgensen CH, Lindhardsen J, Olesen JB, Abildstrøm SZ, Skov L, Torp-Pedersen C, Hansen PR. Psoriasis is associated with clinically significant cardiovascular risk: A Danish nationwide cohort study. *J Intern Med* 2011;270(2):147–57.
57. Kimball AB, Gladman D, Gelfand JM et al. National Psoriasis Foundation clinical consensus on psoriasis comorbidities and recommendations for screening. *J Am Acad Dermatol* 2008;58:1031–42.
58. Peters MJ, Symmons DP, McCarey D et al. EULAR evidence-based recommendations for cardiovascular risk management in patients with rheumatoid arthritis and other forms of inflammatory arthritis. *Ann Rheum Dis* 2010;69:325–31.
59. Gladman DD, Farewell VT, Wong K, Husted J. Mortality studies in psoriatic arthritis: Results from a single outpatient center. II. Prognostic indicators for death. *Arthritis Rheum* 1998;41:1103–10.
60. Prodanovich S, Ma F, Taylor JR, Pezon C, Fasihi T, Kirsner RS. Methotrexate reduces incidence of vascular diseases in veterans with psoriasis or rheumatoid arthritis. *J Am Acad Dermatol* 2005;52:262–7.
61. Park YB, Choi HK, Kim MY, Lee WK, Song J, Kim DK, Lee SK. Effects of antirheumatic therapy on serum lipid levels in patients with rheumatoid arthritis: A prospective study. *Am J Med* 2002;113: 188–93.
62. Toms TE, Panoulas VF, John H, Douglas KM, Kitas GD. Methotrexate therapy associates with reduced prevalence of the metabolic syndrome in rheumatoid arthritis patients over the age of 60—More than just an anti-inflammatory effect? A cross sectional study. *Arthritis Res Ther* 2009;11:R110.

63. Westlake SL, Colebatch AN, Baird J, Kiely P, Quinn M, Choy E, Ostor AJ, Edwards CJ. The effect of methotrexate on cardiovascular disease in patients with rheumatoid arthritis: A systematic literature review. *Rheumatology* 2010;49:295–307.
64. Galarraga B, Khan F, Kumar P, Pullar T, Belch JJ. Etanercept improves inflammation-associated arterial stiffness in rheumatoid arthritis. *Rheumatology* 2009;48:1418–23.
65. van Eijk IC, Peters MJ, Serné EH, van der Horst-Bruinsma IE, Dijkmans BA, Smulders YM, Nurmohamed MT. Microvascular function is impaired in ankylosing spondylitis and improves after tumour necrosis factor-α blockade. *Ann Rheum Dis* 2009;68:362–6.
66. Dixon WG, Watson KD, Lunt M et al. Reduction in the incidence of myocardial infarction in patients with rheumatoid arthritis who respond to anti-tumor necrosis factor alpha therapy: Results from the British Society for Rheumatology Biologics Register. *Arthritis Rheum* 2007;56:2905–12.
67. Farber EM, Raychaudhuri SP. Concept of total care: A third dimension in the treatment of psoriasis. *Cutis* 1997;59:35–9.
68. Raychaudhuri SP. Comorbidities of psoriatic arthritis—Metabolic syndrome and prevention: A report from the GRAPPA 2010 annual meeting. *J Rheumatol* 2012;39:437–40.
69. Coates LC, Kavanaugh A, Mease P et al. Group for Research and Assessment of Psoriasis and Psoriatic Arthritis: Treatment recommendations for psoriatic arthritis 2015. *Arthritis Rheumatol* 2016;68(5):1060–71.

Section IV-B

Treatment Regimen

Nutraceuticals in Psoriasis

18 Nutraceutical Components in the Treatment of Psoriasis and Psoriatic Arthritis

Urmila Jarouliya and Raj K. Keservani

CONTENTS

18.1 INTRODUCTION

Psoriasis and psoriatic arthritis (PsA) are common chronic diseases of abnormal keratinocyte proliferation and differentiation, as well as localized and systemic inflammation, multisystem diseases that mainly affect the skin and joint symptoms. Lots of risk factors have been recognized in the etiology and pathological process of psoriasis, which includes family history and environmental risk factors, such as diet, obesity, smoking, stress, and alcohol consumption (Huerta et al., 2007). Recently, the pathogenesis of psoriasis and PsA has been understood by genetic and immunological factors. The treatment of PsA is aimed at controlling pain and inflammation, usually starting with nonsteroidal anti-inflammatory drugs (NSAIDs) and disease-modifying antirheumatic drugs (DMARDs) as treatment options, and slowing or blocking the progression of the disease. Furthermore, dietary factors can also affect drug absorption, bioavailability, distribution to tissues, and its metabolism in the body. Lots of single food components have been suggested to play a role indicated to act as a significant component in the treatment of psoriasis and PsA. Dietary antioxidants, such as omega-3 polyunsaturated fatty acids (PUFAs) from fish oil, some vitamins (A, E, C, and D), and minerals (iron, copper, manganese, zinc, and selenium), have the potential to reduce oxidative stress and the production of reactive oxygen species that are mainly specific in chronic systemic inflammatory diseases, like psoriasis and PsA (Millsop et al., 2014). A small number of research studies have explored the outcome of a healthy consumption pattern. In fact, the psoriatic patients regularly require dietary advice, as they usually associate too many of their health problems, including diseases of the skin, to their diet. More than 50% of psoriasis patients use some form of complementary and alternative medicine incorporating herbal medicine, which is used topically and orally. Due to such problems, more patients are nowadays found to resort to complementary and alternative medicines (CAMs), which include the use of nutraceutical as well as medicinal plants. Such an approach not only has been reported to be effective at relieving the pain symptoms associated with psoriasis and PsA, but also may prove to be safer and more effective than conventional treatment options. Nutraceuticals that have no side effects, cost less, and are more abundant help to prevent a number of chronic diseases and act as chronic fighters.

18.2 PSORIASIS

Psoriasis is an immune-related ailment in which a normal skin mistakes as a pathogen and sends an incorrect signal that causes overproduction of new skin cells. The skin connects the body and surrounding environment and continually exhibits both internal and external prooxidants, which leads to the formation of free radicals. Generated free radical causes oxidative stress, which has been associated with skin inflammation in psoriasis. Psoriatic patients have decreased plasma levels of β-carotene and α-tocopherol, as well as a reduced serum selenium level with high concentrations of malondialdehyde, which is a marker of lipid peroxidation (Azzini et al., 1995; Briganti and Picardo, 2003; Serwin et al., 2003).

It is also an inherent state, but its method of inheritance is still not foreseeable. It is a long-lasting sickness that does not have constant medication, but lots of therapy can be executed for regulating the severity of symptoms produced by it. It is also a common T-cell-mediated immune disorder characterized by circumscribed, red, thickened plaques with an overlying silver-white scale. Genetically and immunologically, psoriasis is a chronic, immune-mediated inflammatory disorder. While the genetic influence on psoriasis is well established, the role of environmental factors is less well defined. Overweight and obesity have also been identified as risk factors for psoriasis and/or a flare-up of the disease (Naldi et al., 2005). The primary immune defect in psoriasis appears to be an increase in cell signaling via chemokines and cytokines that act on upregulated gene expression and cause hyperproliferation of keratinocytes.

Recently, psoriasis was evaluated as a disorder of epidermal keratinocytes; however, it is now recognized primarily as an immune-mediated disorder. Debate continues regarding whether psoriasis is an autoimmune disorder or a T-helper 1 (Th1) immune dysfunction. The pathogenic factors, such as T-cell activation, tumor necrosis factor (TNF) α, and dendritic cells, are stimulated in response to a triggering factor, such as a physical injury, inflammation, or bacterial or viral infection. Initially, immature dendritic cells in the epidermis stimulate T cells from lymph nodes in response to an unidentified antigen (physical factors). Then T cells (CD4 and CD8) receive primary signal from an unknown antigen, and stimulate and activate the synthesis of mRNA for interleukin (IL) 2, resulting in a subsequent increase in IL-2 receptors. The elevated IL-2 from activated T cells and IL-12 from Langerhans cells ultimately regulate genes that code for the transcription of cytokines, such as interferon (IFN) γ, TNF-α, and IL-2, responsible for differentiation, maturation, and proliferation of T cells into memory effector cells. Ultimately, T cells migrate to the skin, where they accumulate around dermal blood vessels. These are the first in a series of immunologic changes that result in the formation of acute psoriatic lesions. Psoriasis is classified into several subtypes, with the chronic plaque (psoriasis vulgaris) form comprising approximately 90% of cases. Sharp differentiated erythematous silvery scaling plaques occur most commonly on the quad surface of the elbows, knees, scalp, sacral, and groin regions. Other involved areas include the ears, perianal region, and sites of repeated injury. Women and men are equally affected by this condition. Even though psoriasis can occur at any age, the average age of onset for continual plaque psoriasis is calculated at 33 years, with 75% of cases starting before age 46 (Nevitt and Hutchinson, 1996).

The major five types of psoriasis are plaque psoriasis, guttate psoriasis, inverse (flexural) psoriasis, pustular psoriasis, and erythrodermic psoriasis. Apart from these types of psoriasis, there are also nail psoriasis, which is restricted to the nails only, and PsA, which is restrained to joint and connective tissue swelling. The main characteristics of psoriasis are irritation and red and scaly dots of the skin. Other symptoms include genital sores, joint pain, thickening and browning of nails, and severe dandruff on the scalp. Dots are most frequently seen on the elbows, knees, and middle of the body, but can also be seen on the scalp and other body parts. This disorder is so serious that it usually needs long-term therapy (Jobling, 2007).

Sometimes psoriasis is caused by diverse drugs, which may cause some adverse effects leading to psoriasis or psoriasiform dermatitis. Psoriasiform drug eruption is a broad term referring to a heterogeneous group of disorders that clinically and histologically activate psoriasis. It is used to describe the presence of cellular infiltration, papillomatosis, and epidermal hyperplasia with lengthening of red ridges. The same kind of rashes can also be seen with seborrhesic dermatitis, pityriasis rubra pilaris, syphilis, and pityriasis rosea (Lionel and Baker, 2007; Grace et al., 2010).

Although little research has explored the effect of antioxidant supplementation on the symptoms of psoriasis (Wolters, 2005), the ingestion of fruits and vegetables rich in carotenoids, flavonoids, and vitamin C may be advantageous to such individuals due to their high antioxidant content. These antioxidants are useful to the prevention of imbalance between oxidative stress and antioxidant defense (Naldi et al., 1996; Wolters, 2005).

Contemporary therapies also fail to diminish the underlying pathophysiology. This can lead to more serious symptoms and cause other diseases, including PsA, cardiovascular disease, and inflammatory bowel disease (IBD). About 30% of patients with psoriasis will also develop PsA. The average time between the diagnosis of psoriasis and that of PsA is 4 years, during which irremediable joint damage can occur. Because of similar characteristics, it is usually tough to discriminate PsA from other inflammatory arthropathies, including rheumatoid arthritis (RA) and ankylosing spondylitis (AS). PsA and RA both have similar symptoms, like inflamed joints, which are often red or warm to the touch, and both are commonly found in the hands, feet, and axial skeleton. However, PsA is more likely to be asymmetric and to present with enthesopathy (inflammation frequently occurs at insertion sites, which can often cause confusion with fibromyalgia), dactylitis (inflammation of a digit), and iritis (inflammation in the eye). Some characteristic radiographic markers seen with PsA include "pencil-in-cup" changes of digital joints, especially the distal interphalangeal (DIP) joint; periostitis; joint ankyloses; osteolysis; and sacroiliac changes. However, these are more likely to be seen with advanced disease.

Traditional therapy for psoriasis is based on the severity of the disease. Mild and limited psoriasis treatment includes topical corticosteroids, tars, anthralin, calcipotriene (a vitamin D3 analog), tazarotene (a retinoid), and phototherapy. A topical combination of calcipotriene and betamethasone (Taclonex®) has shown greater efficacy in severe psoriasis than monotherapy with either alone (Kaufmann et al., 2002).

Methotrexate (MTX) is an effective agent in the treatment of psoriasis, including pustular psoriasis, psoriatic erythroderma, and PsA, as well as extensive chronic plaque psoriasis not controlled by conventional therapy. MTX, formerly known as aminopterin, has been widely used in the treatment of cancer and autoimmune diseases. MTX is one of the folic acid antagonists that is widely used in the therapy of various types of diseases, like psoriasis and PsA (Wollima et al., 2001; Thomas and Aithal, 2005).

18.2.1 Pathogenesis of Psoriasis

The pathogenesis of psoriasis and metabolic syndrome both involve inflammation. There is also evidence suggesting that there is a genetic link. A number of genes, such as PSORS2, PSORS3, and PSORS4, are associated with psoriasis susceptibility (Azfar and Gelfand, 2008). The class I region of the major histocompatibility complex (MHC) locus cluster has been correlated with psoriasis, although other factors are also involved in the pathogenesis of psoriasis. It was found that the main susceptibility locus PSORS1 (psoriasis susceptibility 1) is contained within MHC, on chromosome 6p21. Associations between psoriasis and human leukocyte antigen (HLA)–Cw6 have been reported in many different populations. Besides this, changes in the HLA-C activity are likely to influence psoriasis sensitivity because HLA-C is involved in the process of immune self-recognition. The actual role of PSORS1 is still to be confirmed; it is not clear whether PSORS1 is a classical MHC allele or a control variant. The immune system and keratinocyte separation may be adjusted by some predisposing polygenes. Chromosome 17q25 has also been associated with a family history of psoriasis. Patients suffering from psoriasis present with autosomal-dominant seborrhoea-like dermatitis and psoriasiform expression caused by alterations in zinc finger protein 750 (ZNF750). Because the alteration generally occurs in keratinocytes rather than in fibroblasts (it is rare in CD4 lymphocytes), keratinocytes should be the main site of the defect (Lowes et al., 2007) in psoriasis.

18.2.2 Therapy

For the treatment of psoriasis, four different types of therapies are included: external or topical treatments, phototherapy, systemic medication, and biological therapies. While determining the particular treatment and management in psoriatic patients, many physical and psychosocial factors should be kept in mind. The most important factors to be considered for patients are the number of lesions, phenotypical characteristics, and quality of life (Menter and Stoff, 2011). Therefore, psoriatic treatment should be individualized. This may be subject to the condition, location, impact, comorbidity, and risk factors of the disease, as well as patient compatibility with the treatment.

18.2.3 Nutritional Recommendations

- Drink lots of water.
- Have a variety of foods in your diet with adequate grain products, vegetables, and fruits. Include at least five portions of fresh fruit and vegetables per day, particularly those that are rich in β-carotene and vitamin C, for example, carrots, apricots, sweet potato, broccoli, orange, cabbage, potato, guava, tomatoes, and sweet peppers.
- Avoid sugar and white refined carbohydrates, as they feed bad bacteria in the gut and can increase toxins absorbed from the gut.
- Have a diet low in total and saturated fats. Also, limit consumption of animal fat and dairy products.
- Eat pumpkin seeds, linseeds, and sunflower seeds, as these contain a range of anti-inflammatory essential fatty acids (EFAs) and zinc, which support good skin health.
- If a patient has an allergy or sensitivity to gluten, he or she should maintain gluten-free diets, such as spelt, kamut, brown rice, buckwheat, millet, amaranth, tapioca, corn, and quinoa.

- Try alternatives to milk, including unsweetened soy milk, oat milk, and rice milk.
- Eat sources of oily fish, which contains the anti-inflammatory omega-3 fatty acid, three times per week. Oily fish include salmon, trout, herring, mackerel, anchovies, sardines, and tuna.
- Psoriatic patients should avoid consumption of alcohol, as it is known to cause sudden flare-up of psoriasis. It stimulates the release of histamine, which causes skin lesions.
- Sunbathing is helpful for psoriasis because it increases levels of vitamin D. However, avoid getting sunburned, as this can increase the risk of skin cancer.

Researchers have examined the use of topical fish oil at different eicosapentaenoic acid (EPA) concentrations. These studies have mentioned beneficial effects, including a decrease in plaque thickness and scaling (Richards et al., 2006; Zulfakar et al., 2007). In a study by Puglia et al. (2005), they observed that when fish oil extracts and ketoprofen were applied topically on psoriatic lesions, erythema reduced. Fish oil has also proven to be beneficial in autoimmune joint conditions such as RA (Cleland and James, 2000).

18.2.4 Nutritional Supplementation

18.2.4.1 Essential Fatty Acids

Metabolism of the EFAs leads to formation of eicosanoids that have many biological properties, such as regulating fluidity within the cell membrane, effecting cell transport, messenger binding, and cell communication. Linoleic acid has a major role in the maintenance of epidermal probity and prevention of transepidermal water loss. Metabolites of arachidonic acid are important agents in causing many inflammatory skin reactions with simultaneous evolution of skin diseases, such as psoriasis and atopic dermatitis. Suitable drug and dietetic control of the metabolism of arachidonic acid is a new and interesting therapeutic concept in the care of skin diseases. EFAs affect the physiopathology of psoriasis in three different ways: (1) influence the dynamics of cell membranes, (2) affect dermal and epidermal blood flow via enhancing endothelial activity, and (3) act as an immunomodulating agent through their role in eicosanoids.

18.2.4.2 Folate

Psoriasis is a chronic inflammatory skin condition that can also increase the risk of cardiovascular disease. Psoriasis patients also have lower levels of folate and higher levels of homocysteine, which in itself is a risk factor for cardiovascular disease. The supplementation of folic acid or its other active forms, like folinic acid or 5-methyltetrahydrofolate, appears to be a reasonable therapeutic option in patients affected by chronic inflammatory skin diseases, such as moderate to severe psoriasis, and in particular in those with concomitant hyperhomocysteinemia, low plasma folate, and additional cardiovascular risk factors.

18.2.4.3 Selenium

Selenium is an important trace element with an immune-modulating and antiproliferative activity; it can affect the immune response through a change in the expression of cytokines and their receptors or by creating immune cells more resistant to oxidative stress (Spallholtz et al., 1990; Roy et al., 1992; Celerier et al., 1995). Although data generated from research show that patients suffering with inflammatory skin diseases (psoriasis), skin cancer, malignant melanoma, and cutaneous T-cell lymphoma have low concentrations of selenium, Kharaeva et al. (2009) proved in their study that the fusion of conventional therapy and supplementation with vitamin E, co-enzyme Q10, and selenium resulted in an improvement in the clinical condition of patients with severe psoriasis, as well as a reduction in oxidative stress. It was also reported that supplementation with inorganic forms of selenium, such as sodium selenite and selenite, leads to clinical betterment in patients with psoriasis.

18.2.4.4 Bioactive Whey Protein

Protein extract, which is a novel dietary supplement made of bovine whey, has beneficial effects in psoriasis. It regulates the immune response by inhibiting the production of Th1 cytokines (IFN-γ, IL-2, Il-12, and TNF-α), which may make it functional in treating Th1-related disorders, such as psoriasis. In a study by Poulin et al. (2006), they patented a new dietary ingredient called XP-828L made of a protein extract obtained from bovine whey. The bioactive profile of XP-828L could be related to the presence of growth factors, active peptides, and immunoglobulins in the extract. In vitro experiments showed that XP-828L inhibits the production of Th1 cytokines (IFN-c and IL-2), suggesting that XP-828L could improve Th1-related disorders, such as psoriasis (Aattouri et al., 2004). Recently, an open-label clinical trial suggested some potential for XP-828L to reduce psoriasis severity (Poulin et al., 2006). Recently, protein complexes derived from whey have been shown to have clinically proven health benefits in cancer, hepatitis, human immunodeficiency virus (HIV), cardiovascular disease, and osteoporosis (Marshall, 2004).

18.2.4.5 Vitamin D

Epidemiological data have shown that vitamin D deficiency may be a risk for the development of other autoimmune diseases, including RA, multiple sclerosis (MS), systemic lupus erythematosus (SLE), and Crohn's disease (CD). In psoriasis, the prevalence of vitamin D deficiency varies with latitude. It is highest among residents near the poles and decreases in the tropical latitudes. Thus, there is some relationship between prevalence and latitude that may be related to sun exposure and vitamin D. Some patients with psoriasis respond to topical vitamin D analogs, which also suggests a role for the vitamin in managing the disease. It has been found that when patients were compared to age- and sex-matched controls, and also with common psoriasis, they had significantly reduced serum levels of the biologically active form of vitamin D, 1-α,25-dihydroxyvitamin D3 (1-α,25(OH)2D3; calcitriol). Vitamin D analogs (calcipotriol or calcitriol, maxacalcitol, and tacalcitol), sunlight, UVB phototherapy, and topical vitamin D analogs are effective therapy for psoriasis due to its antiproliferative and pro-differentiating effect on keratinocytes. Calcitriol binding to vitamin D receptor (VDR) in the skin regulates the production of a large number of genes, including cell cycle regulators, growth factors, and their receptors. Various forms of the VDR gene are related to psoriasis development and resistance to calcipotriol therapy (Okita et al., 2002). Several studies have revealed that in order to prevent a vitamin D deficiency, it can be taken orally in daily doses of up to 5,000 IU, with some experts recommending up to 10,000 IU daily (Grant and Holick, 2005; Hollis, 2005; Vieth et al., 2007). Some studies have demonstrated that oral and topical vitamin D, sunlight, and UVB phototherapy have shown significant efficacy in psoriasis treatment (Binkley et al., 2007).

Vitamin D performs different functions besides its well-known role in calcium-phosphorus metabolism, as indicated by the presence of VDRs and CYP271B (enzyme responsible for 25-hydroxyvitamin D [25-OHD] synthesis) in different tissues (Zehnder et al., 2001). An important regulatory role for vitamin D in the immune system is suggested by the presence of VDRs on activated T lymphocytes, the suppressive or inhibiting effect of 1,25-dihydroxyvitamin D in different autoimmune diseases, and in vitro and in vivo findings of vitamin D–induced changes in immune functions (Bhalla et al., 1983; Provvedini et al., 1983). Furthermore, dermatologists and other physicians have observed the effectiveness of vitamin D analogs to treat psoriasis plaques in daily clinical practice (Dubertret et al., 1992; Zold et al., 2011). Topical vitamin D derivatives have immunomodulatory effects on monocytes, macrophages, T cells, and dendritic cells, and are being extensively used as monotherapy or in combination with steroids for the topical treatment of psoriasis (Menter et al., 2009). Moreover, it has been proposed that narrowband (NB) UVB radiation may also mediate its beneficial effect on psoriasis by increasing endogenous vitamin D levels, as phototherapy has been shown to increase the levels of serum vitamin D in patients with psoriasis (Ryan et al., 2010).

18.2.4.6 Vitamin B12

Initial reports of therapeutic success after (mainly) parenteral administration of vitamin B12 in the treatment of psoriasis were made some 40 years ago (Ricketts et al., 2010). Ruedemann and Albany (1954) administered 1100 µg of vitamin B12 intramuscularly daily over a period of 10–20 days in 34 patients with psoriasis vulgaris. There was complete remission in 11 cases, near complete remission in a further 11 cases, and significant improvement in symptoms in 6 cases. Cohen (1958) reported on psoriasis patients who had received 1000 µg of vitamin B12 intramuscularly daily for 6 days per week over a 3-week period. In at least 50% of this collective, complete or near complete healing was achieved.

18.2.4.7 Alternative Herbal Treatment

When it comes to herbal treatment for psoriasis and PsA, conventional drugs have been shown to delay damage from the disease, but alternative therapies have not. There are many herbal remedies to get rid of the scaly patchy skin, such as *Aloe vera* gel, banana peel, apple cider vinegar, chamomile, cayenne pepper, cashew nut oil, castor oil, fish oil, and olive oil. A Chinese herbal formula (Herose® Psoria Capsule) has demonstrated safety and efficacy in the treatment of severe plaque psoriasis (Yuqi, 2005). Herose consists of Rhizoma Zingiberis, Radix Salviae Miltiorrhizae, Radix Astragali, Ramulus Cinnamomi, Radix Paeoniae Alba, Radix Codonopsis Pilosula, and Semen Coicis.

18.2.5 Recent Treatments of Psoriasis

Several topical treatments for psoriasis may provide benefits, including calcipotriene (Dovonex®; a synthetic vitamin D3 analog), tazarotene, MTX, cyclosporine, apremilast, biologic immune-modifying agents (adalimumab, etanercept, and infliximab), Berberis aquifolium cream (10%) (Psoriaflora®, Relieva®), curcumin gel (1%), *Aloe vera*, and a flavonoid-rich salve (Flavsalve®).

18.2.6 Lifestyle Involvement

It is known that lifestyle factors such as smoking, alcohol consumption, and obesity may affect psoriasis severity (Chodorowska and Kwiatek, 2004). Physical and outdoor activities are beneficial (Schiener et al., 2007). Hodak et al. (2003) observed that bathing and sunbathing at the Dead Sea over a period of 4 weeks resulted in reduction of keratinocyte hyperplasia, and almost total removal of T lymphocytes from the epidermis, with the lowest number remaining in the dermis. Stress management through yoga and meditation can also be beneficial for individuals affected with psoriasis. Finally, psychotherapy can be an essential adjunct for individuals with persistent unresolved psychological issues, such as anxiety, depression, and the psychosocial stress of this chronic skin disease.

18.3 PSORIATIC ARTHRITIS

PsA is a chronic disease that involves the inflammation of synovial tissue, entheses, and skin, and is usually seronegative for rheumatoid factor (Moll and Wright, 1973). PsA may appear in a clinical pattern very similar to that of RA, as a symmetrical small joint arthropathy involving the wrists, metacarpophalangeal joints, and proximal interphalangeal joints (Figure 18.1). In contrast, patients may develop asymmetric joint involvement, including a characteristic inflammatory arthritis of the DIP joints, often colocalized with trophic changes in the associated nail (Veale, 2013).

PsA is an inflammatory seronegative spondyloarthropathy related to psoriasis. If PsA is diagnosed, treatment should be begun to reduce signs and symptoms of PsA, inhibit structural damage, and maximize quality of life. PsA can occur at any stage of life, including childhood, but mostly it occurs between the ages of 30 and 50 years. It affects men and women equally. It is characterized

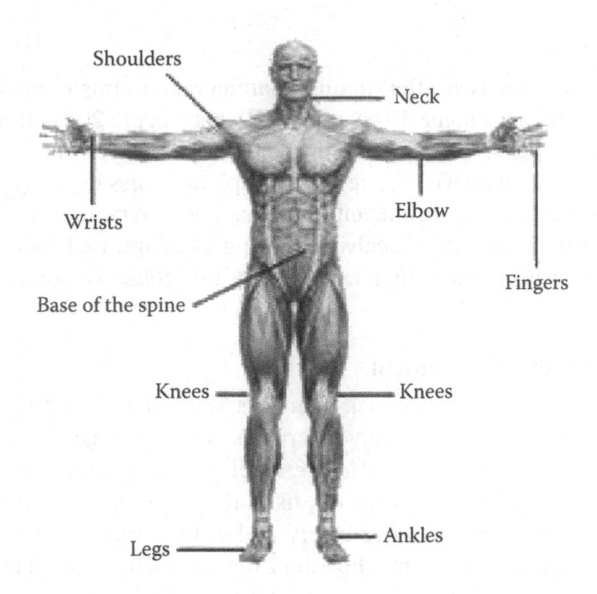

FIGURE 18.1 Joints affected in PsA.

by stiffness, pain, swelling, and tenderness of the joints and surrounding ligaments and tendons (dactylitis and enthesitis). It may start slowly with moderate signs, and in time may lead to a joint injury. Dactylitis, or "sausage digit," is a combination of enthesitis of the tendons and ligaments and synovitis involving a whole digit. Dactylitis is common among patients with PsA and most frequently influences the feet in an irregular distribution. Symptoms of PsA can range from moderate to serious. The enthesis is the anatomic location where tendon, ligament, or joint capsule fibers insert into the bone. Enthesitis may occur at any such site, although common locations include the insertion sites of the plantar fascia, the Achilles tendons, and ligamentous attachments to the ribs, spine, and pelvis. Studies from the general population indicate that PsA may have a milder course and that it is not associated with excess mortality; if it is left untreated, patients with PsA can have persistent inflammation, progressive joint damage, severe physical limitations, disability, and increased mortality.

Psoriasis and PsA are primarily mediated by T cells (rather than B cells). The histological features of psoriasis arise as a result of the interplay between T cells, dendritic cells, and keratinocytes, giving rise to an intervention loop that magnifies and sustains inflammation in lesional skin. Secretion of IL-23 and IL-12 from myeloid dendritic cell activates IL-17-producing T cells and Th22 and Th1 cells, leading to the production of inflammatory cytokines, such as IL-17, IFN-γ, TNF-α, and IL-22. These cytokines mediate effects on keratinocytes. Unlike psoriasis, the immunopathogenic features of PsA are poorly characterized, but it was mentioned that T cells work through the release of associated cytokines, TNF-α, IFN-γ, IL-12, and IL-17, and several others when compared with RA patient levels (Nakajima et al., 2011).

18.4 CONVENTIONAL DRUGS

Moderate to acute forms of the disease are initially treated with the same therapy as the mild form of the disease, but with the inclusion of some of the DMARDs (Coates et al., 2013), such as MTX and cyclosporine. The effectiveness of MTX in PsA treatment is sometimes used in combination with NSAIDs. MTX and cyclosporine treatment should be monitored carefully, as they cause hepatotoxicity (Nash and Clegg, 2005; Kivitz et al., 2007; Ash et al., 2012; Carneiro et al., 2013). Sulfasalazine can also be used in PsA treatment as a pain-relieving drug (Ash et al., 2012; Carneiro et al., 2013).

The use of biological drugs in dermatological treatment is comparatively recent and started in the early 2000s. In most countries, in order for biological treatment to be administered, specific standards should be met. The present-day treatment options for psoriasis and PsA include TNF-α blockers, IL-12 and IL-23 inhibitors, T-cell inhibitors, and B-cell inhibitors. These classes of biological drugs are characterized by their protein structure, as well as high molecular weight, and their effectiveness is evaluated based on the Psoriasis Area and Severity Index (PASI), body surface area (BSA), and Dermatology Life Quality Index (DLQI). TNF-α antagonists are one such class of biological drugs, which includes infliximab, etanercept, and adalimumab. Infliximab is a monotherapy administered in psoriasis vulgaris. Etanercept is indicated for use in both psoriasis vulgaris and PsA, and it is the only drug that can be used as a treatment for children under the age of 8 suffering with psoriasis. The drug is administered subcutaneously. Ultimately, adalimumab is a fully human monoclonal antibody that neutralizes both free and membrane-bound TNF-α and is used in the treatment of psoriasis vulgaris and PsA (Wcisło-Dziadecka et al., 2015).

Several research studies have investigated the topical application or oral administration of antioxidants and suggested them as a preventive therapy for the natural aging of skin and for cancer caused by ultraviolet rays (Briganti and Picardo, 2003).

18.5 ESSENTIAL FATTY ACIDS IN THE TREATMENT OF PSORIASIS AND PSORIATIC ARTHRITIS

18.5.1 Omega-3 Fatty Acids

Omega-3 is a group of unsaturated fatty acids, also called PUFAs, which are considered EFAs. Omega-3 fatty acids are found in fish, such as salmon, tuna, and halibut, and other seafoods, including algae and krill; nut oils; and to a lesser extent, plant leaves and some vegetable oils, such as canola. Two major omega-3 fatty acids are EPA and docosahexaenoic acid (DHA), which are plentiful in fish such as salmon, mackerel, herring, tuna, snoek, trout, sardines, and pilchards, as well as found in a few vegetarian sources, such as flaxseed oil. EPA, DHA, and α-linolenic acid have been shown to diminish inflammation by reducing the synthesis of leukotrienes that play a role in psoriasis. There are also many other therapeutic applications for omega-3 fatty acids, primarily due to their cardiovascular-enhancing and anti-inflammatory benefits. EPA and DHA have many potential health benefits, such as reducing the risk of coronary heart disease, and potential benefits in the prevention and treatment of other cardiovascular disorders, some forms of mental illness, inflammatory disorders, and insulin resistance. Supplementation of omega-3 fatty acid reduces the risk of atherosclerosis, altering cholesterol levels (elevating good HDL cholesterol and reducing bad LDL cholesterol), reducing triglyceride levels, and diminishing high blood pressure. Hence, studies have shown the potential of omega-3 fatty acid to decrease inflammation in disorders such as RA, asthma, colitis, CD, and lupus. In addition, omega-3 fatty acids have been shown to reduce the symptoms of other disorders, including angina, migraine headaches, Alzheimer's disease, dementia, and tinnitus.

Omega-3 is a precursor for several potent regulatory eicosanoids involved in bone metabolism, including prostaglandins and leukotrienes. Omega-3 fatty acid inhibits the formation of inflammatory cytokines, such as IL-1, IL-6, and TNF-α, which provide an important stimulus for osteoclastic bone resorption and prevent bone loss. It also reduces the formation of the chemoattractant protein platelet-derived growth factor (PDGF), increases the absorption of nitric oxide, and reduces the expression of adhesion molecules. The accumulative effect of these bioactive mediators is to block vascularization, or new blood vessel growth inside the psoriatic plaque, while at the same time permitting the better perfusion of dermal tissue. Supplementation with 3.6 g/day of purified omega-3 fatty acids, i.e., EPA, reduced the severity of psoriasis after 2–3 months (Kojima et al., 1989, 1991). One study showed that applying a preparation containing 10% fish oil directly to psoriatic lesions twice daily resulted in improvement after 7 weeks (Dewsbury et al., 1989). Supplementing with fish oil may also help prevent the increase in blood levels of triglycerides that occurs as a side effect of certain drugs that are used to treat psoriasis (e.g., etretinate and acitretin) (Ashley et al., 1988).

18.5.2 Vegetables and Fruits Rich in Omega-3 Fatty Acids

18.5.2.1 Flaxseed

Flaxseed (Figure 18.2a), also known as linseed, is a plant seed that is a rich source of healing compounds. It contains essential omega-3 fatty acids, dietary fibers, and various other nutrients. Omega-3 fatty acids are anti-inflammatory in nature, and they nurture the cell membranes of skin with essential fats to make the skin moist and soft and retain necessary water. These fats open blocked pores in skin cells to facilitate the detoxification of the body. In various studies, it has been found that positive changes in diet (fewer calories) and lifestyle, coupled with regular consumption of omega-3 fatty acid supplements, can heal both psoriasis and psoriasis arthritis.

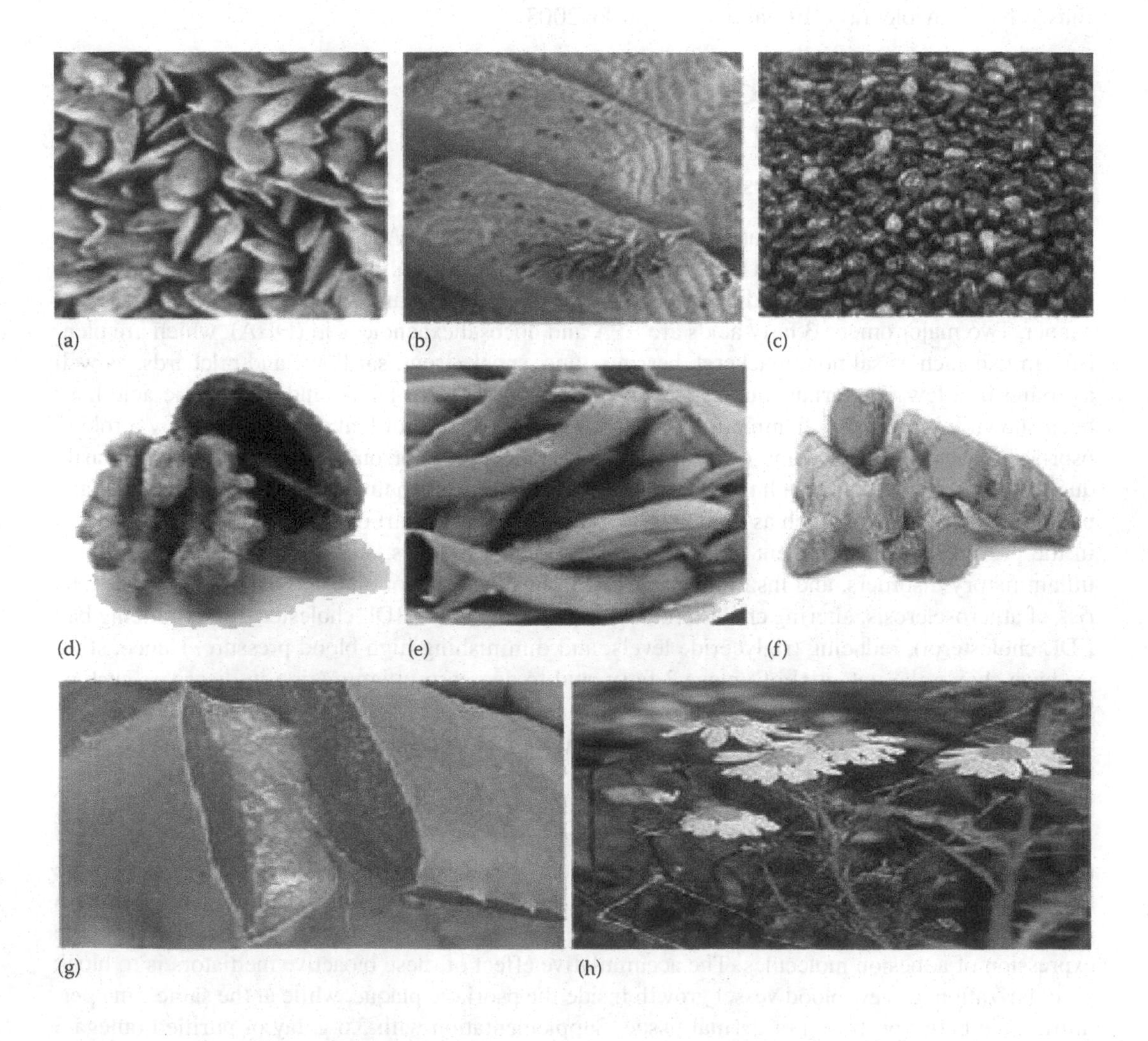

FIGURE 18.2 Vegetables and fruits used in the prevention of psoriasis and PsA: (a) flaxseed, (b) fish oil, (c) chia seed, (d) walnuts, (e) soybeans, (f) turmeric, (g) *Aloe vera*, and (h) *Matricaria recutita*.

18.5.2.2 Fish Oil

Itching, scaling, and erythema (abnormal flushing of the skin) are common features of psoriasis, a fairly common skin disorder. One of the main characteristics of psoriasis is an increased concentration of arachidonic acid and its metabolite, leukotriene B4, in and around psoriatic plaque (Escobar et al., 1992). It is well established that fish oils suppress the formation of leukotriene B4 and reduce scaling in psoriatic patients (Figure 18.2b).

18.5.2.3 Chia Seeds

Chia seeds (Figure 18.2c) are the seeds of the chia plant, *Salvia hispanica*, native to Mexico. The chia plant is in the mint family, and like other small seeds, such as flaxseed, chia seeds are nutrient rich. It is the richest plant-based source of α-linolenic acid. Chia has a soft seed coat, which makes its health-promoting fatty acids bioavailable even without grinding.

18.5.2.4 Walnuts and Walnut Oil

Walnuts (Figure 18.2d) are a rich source of omega-3 fatty acids, which is almost absent in a veggie diet. Walnuts have a high concentration of this good fat, which lowers the risks of cardiovascular diseases, promotes better cognitive function, and has anti-inflammatory properties that protect against asthma, RA, and other skin diseases related to inflammation, like psoriasis and eczema. It can lower the cholesterol level due to the nutrients it contains, like flavanoids, phenols, vitamin E, gallic acid, and ellagic acid. Research indicates that walnuts may reduce the risk of Alzheimer's disease by arresting the formation of the amyloid plaques that are found in the brains of patients who suffer from this condition.

18.5.2.5 Soybeans

Soybean (Figure 18.2e) (*Glycine max*) has been known as a golden bean (Bansal and Parle, 2010). It has been established that isoflavones are the most abundant phytoestrogens in soybean and are structurally similar to 17 β-estradiol. Genistein is considered the main isoflavone in soybean and exerts potent anti-inflammatory (Kim et al., 2011) and antioxidant properties. Because of the safety of genistein (McClain et al., 2007), its topical use might be recommended as an adjuvant, together with corticosteroids, in psoriasis management.

18.5.2.6 Turmeric

Turmeric is used as an herbal remedy for various skin infections. Its application in psoriasis is a relatively current complement. Curcumin (diferuloyl methane) is the principal curcuminoid and the most active component in turmeric. Commercial curcumin contains three major components: diferuloylmethane (82%), demethoxycurcumin (15%), and bisdemethoxycurcumin (3%), together referred to as curcuminoids. The anti-inflammatory components are thought to be contained in the curcuminoids and volatile oils that function through selective inhibition of phosphorylase kinase (PhK). PhK is an enzyme found in the epidermis. Significantly higher levels have been noted to correlate with the clinical activity of psoriasis (Figure 18.2f).

18.5.2.7 *Aloe Vera*

Aloe vera (Figure 18.2g) is one of the few herbal medicines in common usage, and it has found worldwide use in the cosmetic, pharmaceutical, and food industries. More than 75 potent active components have been recognized in *Aloe vera*, including vitamins, minerals, saccharides, amino acids, anthraquinones, enzymes, lignin, saponins, polyphenolic compounds, steroids, mucopolysaccharides, and salicylic acids. The oral application of *Aloe vera* latex is moreover used as a purgative, whereas gel and whole-leaf oral compositions have been variously suggested for use as a supplement to chemotherapy treatment and to make better various ailments, such as diabetes mellitus, infectious diseases, metastatic cancer, and ulcerative colitis. Regular ingestion of *Aloe vera* juice can be very efficient because it is a natural body cleanser, which supports its digestion activity, and is anti-inflammatory in nature. Besides this, salicylic acid, a component of *Aloe vera*, is a keratolytic, and it has been reported to contribute to the desquamation of psoriatic plaques (Choonhakarn et al., 2010; Dhanabal et al., 2012). These bioactive constituents have the ability to clear all the psoriatic plaques in almost all patients. Anthraquinone, the active compound in *Aloe vera*, acts as an analgesic, antibacterial, and antiviral, and is used for therapeutic purposes in psoriasis treatment.

18.5.2.8 *Matricaria recutita*

Matricaria recutita is commonly known as chamomile. Chamomile flowers have a long therapeutic practice in treating gastrointestinal disorders. The reason for its use in psoriasis is that chamazulene is a by-product of the nonvolatile oil extract (matricin), which is known to have an anti-inflammation function by inhibiting lipoxygenase activity and consequently leukotriene B4 production, which induces recruitment and activation of neutrophils, monocytes, and eosinophils and is able to induce the adhesion and activation of leukocytes on the endothelium, allowing them to bind to and cross into the tissue. There is proof that supports the role of elevated leukotriene B4 formation in psoriatic plaques. Chamomile oil also has antimicrobial activity against skin pathogens. The flavonoids quercetin and apigenin are also active components of the chamomile flower. Quercetin is mentioned to be a potential inhibitor of lipoxygenase and, to a lesser extent, cyclooxygenase, which shows a good skin-piercing property (Murti et al., 2012).

In a study by Eysteinsdóttir et al. (2014), they treated psoriasis with a combination of seawater baths and NB-UVB and concluded that this combination induces faster clinical and histological improvement, produces longer remission time, and permits lower NB-UVB doses than UVB therapy alone. In a study conducted by Bandara et al. (2010) on psoriasis and PsA, they used UVB irradiation to induce inflammation in mouse skin, which resulted in UVB exposure overexpressing cytokines, TNF-α, IL-6, and the adhesion molecule P-cadherin. Some research has tested the effect of two isoflavonoids, equol and a synthetic analog NV-38. Both isoflavonoids dose dependently inhibited the UVB induction of cutaneous TNF-α mRNA and protein, a cytokine critical for the initiation of psoriatic inflammation. These results suggest that isoflavonoids have potential for useful, nondangerous, and anti-inflammatory therapy in human cutaneous diseases like psoriasis (Figure 18.2h).

18.6 CONCLUSION

Psoriasis and PsA are dreadful diseases affecting the physical and mental status of the patient. A new understanding of these complex diseases has catalyzed the development of targeted biological treatments. Several dietary approaches, such as vitamins, minerals, omega-3 fatty acids, and plant products, have been proposed to play a role in the pathogenesis, management, and/or therapy of psoriasis, PsA, and some skin diseases. Phototherapy is available in a new form called NB-UVB therapy. It is more focused than other light treatments and has a lower risk of skin cancer. Another approach, called PUVA photochemotherapy, combines UVA light with a drug called psoralen, which makes skin more sensitive to light. The herbal medicines do not have more side effects than synthetic drugs. Nowadays, herbal resources play a very important role in the management of skin and inflammatory diseases. Some studies suggest that psoriasis symptoms can be relieved by a change in diet and lifestyle. Fasting from food for a period, low-energy diets, and vegetarian diets have also improved psoriasis and PsA symptoms. Thus, nutritionists should play a central role in the evaluation and management of additional studies regarding dietary manipulations, and the effect of dietary components on these skin diseases need to be studied in order to better understand and treat patients.

REFERENCES

Aattouri, N., Gauthier, S.F., Santure, M. 2004. Immunosuppressive effect of a milk-derived extract. *Clin Invest Med* 27:1–4.

Ash, Z., Gaujoux-Viala, C., Gossec, L. et al. 2012. A systematic literature review of drug therapies for the treatment of psoriatic arthritis: Current evidence and meta-analysis informing the EULAR recommendations for the management of psoriatic arthritis. *Ann Rheum Dis* 71:319–326.

Ashley, J.M., Lowe, N.J., Borok, M.E., Alfin-Slater, R.B. et al. 1988. Fish oil supplementation results in decreased hypertriglyceridemia in patients with psoriasis undergoing etretinate or acitretin therapy. *J Am Acad Dermatol* 19:76–82.

Azfar, R.S., Gelfand, J.M. 2008. Psoriasis and metabolic disease: Epidemiology and pathophysiology. *Curr Opin Rheumatol* 20(4):416–422.

Azzini, M., Girelli, D., Olivieri, O., Guarini, P., Stanzial, A.M., Frigo, A., Milanino, R., Bambara, L.M., Corrocher, R. 1995. Fatty acids and antioxidant micronutrients in psoriatic arthritis. *J Rheumatol* 22:103–108.

Bandara, M., Arun, S.J., Allanson, M., Widyarini, S., Chai, Z., Reeve, V.E. 2010. Topical isoflavonoids reduce experimental cutaneous inflammation in mice. *Immunol Cell Biol* 88:727–733.

Bansal, N., Parle, M. 2010. Effect of soybean supplementation on the memory of alprazolam-induced amnesic mice. *J Pharm Bioallied Sci* 2:144–147.

Bhalla, A.K., Amento, E.P., Clemens, T.L., Holick, M.F., Krane, S.M. 1983. Specific high-affinity receptors for 1,25-dihydroxyvitamin D3 in human peripheral blood mononuclear cells: Presence in monocytes and induction in T lymphocytes following activation. *J Clin Endocrinol Metab* 57:1308–1310.

Binkley, N., Novotny, R., Krueger, D. et al. 2007. Low vitamin D status despite abundant sun exposure. *J Clin Endocrinol Metab* 92:2130–2135.

Briganti, S., Picardo, M. 2003. Antioxidant activity, lipid peroxidation and skin disease. What's new. *J Eur Acad Dermatol Venereol* 17:663–669.

Carneiro, S., Azevedo, V.F., Bonfiglioli, R. et al. 2013. Recommendations for the management and treatment of psoriatic arthritis. *Rev Bras Reumatol* 53:227–241.

Celerier, P., Richard, A., Litoux, P., Dreno, B. 1995. Modulatory effects of selenium and atrontium salts on keratinocyte-derived inflammatory cytokines. *Arch Dermatol Res* 287(7):680–682.

Chodorowska, G., Kwiatek, J. 2004. Psoriasis and cigarette smoking. *Ann Univ Mariae Curie Sklodowska Med* 59:535–538.

Choonhakarn, C., Busaracome, P., Sripanidkulchai, B., Sarakarn, P. 2010. A prospective, randomized clinical trial comparing topical *Aloe vera* with 0.1% triamcinolone acetonide in mild to moderate plaque psoriasis. *J Eur Acad Dermatol Venereol* 24:168–172.

Cleland, L.G., James, M.J. 2000. Fish oil and rheumatoid arthritis: Antiinflammatory and collateral health benefits. *J Rheumatol* 27:2305–2307.

Coates, L.C., Tillett, W., Chandler, D. et al. 2013. The 2012 BSR and BHPR guideline for the treatment of psoriatic arthritis with biologics. *Rheumatology (Oxford)* 52:1754–1757.

Cohen, E.L. 1958. Some new treatments for psoriasis. *Practitioner* 181:618–620.

Dewsbury, C.E., Graham, P., Darley, C.R. 1989. Topical eicosapentaenoic acid (EPA) in the treatment of psoriasis. *Br J Dermatol* 120:581–584.

Dhanabal, S.P., Anand, R., Muruganantham, N. et al. 2012. Screening of *Wrightia tinctoria* leaves for anti-psoriatic activity. *Hygeia* 4:73–78.

Dubertret, L., Wallach, D., Souteyrand, P. et al. 1992. Efficacy and safety of calcipotriol (MC 903) ointment in psoriasis vulgaris: A randomized, double-blind, right/left comparative, vehicle-controlled study. *J Am Acad Dermatol* 27:983–988.

Escobar, S.O., Achenbach, R., Iannantuono, R., Torem, V. 1992. Topical fish oil in psoriasis: A controlled and blind study. *Clin Exp Dermatol* 17:159–162.

Eysteinsdóttir, J.H., Ólafsson, J.H., Agnarsson, B.A. et al. 2014. Psoriasis treatment: Faster and long-standing results after bathing in geothermal seawater. A randomized trial of three UVB phototherapy regimens. *Photodermatol Photoimmunol Photomed* 30:25–34.

Grace, K.K., James, Q., Rosso, D. 2010. Drug-provoked psoriasis: Is it drug induced or drug aggravated? Understanding pathophysiology and clinical relevance. *J Clin Aesthet Dermatol* 3:32–38.

Grant, W.B., Holick, M.F. 2005. Benefits and requirements of vitamin D for optimal health: A review. *Altern Med Rev* 10:94–111.

Hodak, E., Gottlieb, A.B., Segal, T. et al. 2003. Climatotherapy at the Dead Sea is a remittive therapy for psoriasis: Combined effects on epidermal and immunologic activation. *J Am Acad Dermatol* 49:451–457.

Hollis, B.W. 2005. Circulating 25-hydroxyvitamin D levels indicative of vitamin D sufficiency: Implications for establishing a new effective dietary intake recommendation for vitamin D. *J Nutr* 135:317–322.

Huerta, C., Rivero, E., Rodriguez, L.A. 2007. Incidence and risk factors for psoriasis in the general population. *Arch Dermatol* 143:1559–1565.

Jobling, R. 2007. A patient's journey: Psoriasis. *Br Med J* 334:953–954.

Kaufmann, R., Bibby, A.J., Bissonnette, R. et al. 2002. A new calcipotriol/betamethasone dipropionate formulation (Daivobet) is an effective once-daily treatment for psoriasis vulgaris. *Dermatology* 205:389–393.

Kharaeva, Z., Gostova, E., De Luca, C., Raskovic, D., Korkina, L. 2009. Clinical and biochemical effects of coenzyme Q10, vitamin E, and selenium supplementation to psoriasis patients. *Nutr* 25:295–302.

Kim, J.M., Uehara, Y., Choi, Y.J. et al. 2011. Mechanism of attenuation of pro-inflammatory Ang II-induced NF-kappaB activation by genistein in the kidneys of male rats during aging. *Biogerontology* 12(6): 537–550.

Kivitz, A.J., Espinoza, L.R., Sherrer, Y.R., Liu-Dumaw, M., West, C.R. 2007. A comparison of the efficacy and safety of celecoxib 200 mg and celecoxib 400 mg once daily in treating the signs and symptoms of psoriatic arthritis. *Semin Arthritis Rheum* 37:164–173.

Kojima, T., Terano, T., Tanabe, E., Okamoto, S., Tamura, Y., Yoshida, S. 1989. Effect of highly purified eicosapentaeonic acid provides improvement of psoriasis. *J Am Acad Dermatol* 21:150–151.

Kojima, T., Terano, T., Tanabe, E., Okamoto, S., Tamura, Y., Yoshida, S. 1991. Long-term administration of highly purified eicosapentaenoic acid provides improvement of psoriasis. *Dermatologica* 182:225–230.

Lionel, F., Baker, B. 2007. Triggering psoriasis: The role of infections and medications. *Clin Dermatol* 25:606–615.

Lowes, M.A., Bowcock, A.M., Krueger, J.G. 2007. Pathogenesis and therapy of psoriasis. *Nature* 445:866–873.

Marshall, K. 2004. Therapeutic applications of whey protein. *Altern Med Rev* 9:136–156.

McClain, R.M., Wolz, E., Davidovich, A., Edwards, J., Bausch, J. 2007. Reproductive safety studies with genistein in rats. *Food Chem Toxicol* 45(8):1319–1332.

Menter, A., Korman, N.J., Elmets, C.A. et al. 2009. Guidelines of care for the management of psoriasis and psoriatic arthritis. Guidelines of care for the management and treatment of psoriasis with topical therapies. *J Am Acad Dermatol* 60:643–659.

Menter, A., Stoff, B. 2011. *Psoriasis*. Boca Raton: CRC Press/Taylor & Francis Group

Millsop, J.W., Bhatia, B.K., Debbaneh, M., Koo, J., Liao, W. 2014. Diet and psoriasis, part III: Role of nutritional supplements. *J Am Acad Dermatol.* 71:561–569.

Moll, J.M., Wright, V. 1973. Psoriatic arthritis. *Semin Arthritis Rheum* 3:55–78.

Murti, K., Panchal, M.A., Gajera, V., Solanki, J. 2012. Pharmacological properties of *Matricaria recutita*: A review. *Pharmacologia* 3:348–351.

Nakajima, K., Kanda, T., Takaishi, M., Shiga, T., Miyoshi, K., Nakajima, H., Kamijima, R., Tarutani, M., Benson, J.M., Elloso, M.M., Gutshall, L.L., Naso, M.F., Iwakura, Y., DiGiovanni, J., Sano, S. 2011. Distinct roles of IL-23 and IL-17 in the development of PsO-like lesions in a mouse model. *J Immunol* 186:4481–4489.

Naldi, L., Chatenoud, L., Linder, D. et al. 2005. Cigarette smoking, body mass index, and stressful life events as risk factors for psoriasis: Results from an Italian case control study. *J Invest Dermatol* 125:61–67.

Naldi, L., Parazzini, F., Peli, L., Chatenoud, L., Cainelli, T. 1996. Dietary factors and the risk of psoriasis. Results of an Italian case-control study. *Br J Dermatol* 134:101–106.

Nash, P., Clegg, D.O. 2005. Psoriatic arthritis therapy: NSAIDs and traditional DMARDs. *Ann Rheum Dis* 64(2):ii74–ii77.

Nevitt, G.J., Hutchinson, P.E. 1996. Psoriasis in the community: Prevalence, severity and patients' beliefs and attitudes towards the disease. *Br J Dermatol* 135:533–537.

Okita, H., Ohtsuka, T., Yamakage, A., Yamazaki. S. 2002. Polymorphism of the vitamin D(3) receptor in patients with psoriasis. *Arch Dermatol Res* 294:159–162.

Poulin, Y., Pouliot, Y., Lamiot, E. et al. 2006. Safety and efficacy of a milk derived extract in the treatment of plaque psoriasis: An open-label study. *J Cutan Med Surg* 10(5):241–248.

Provvedini, D.M., Tsoukas, C.D., Deftos, L.J., Manolagas, S.C. 1983. 1,25-Dihydroxyvitamin D3 receptors in human leukocytes. *Science* 221:1181–1183.

Puglia, C., Tropea, S., Rizza, L. et al. 2005. *In vitro* percutaneous absorption studies and *in vivo* evaluation of anti-inflammatory activity of essential fatty acids (EFA) from fish oil extracts. *Int J Pharma* 299:41–48.

Richards, H., Thomas, C.P., Bowen, J.L., Heard, C.M. 2006. *In vitro* transcutaneous delivery of ketoprofen and polyunsaturated fatty acids from a pluronic lecithin organogel vehicle containing fish oil. *J Pharm Pharmacol* 58:903–908.

Ricketts, J.R., Rothe, M.J., Grant-Kels, J.M. Nutrition and psoriasis. *Clin Dermatol* 28:615–626.

Roy, M., Kiremidjan-Schumacher, L., Wishe, H.I., Cohen, M.W., Stotsky, G. 1992. Effect of selenium on the expression of high affinity interleukin 2 receptors. *Proc Soc for Exp Biol Med* 200:36–43.

Ruedemann, R., Albany, N.Y. 1954. Treatment of psoriasis with large doses of vitamin B12 1100 micrograms per cubic centimeter. *Arch Derma Syph (Chic)* 69:738.

Ryan, C., Moran, B., Mckenna, M.J. et al. 2010. The effect of narrowband UV-B treatment for psoriasis on vitamin D status during wintertime in Ireland. *Arch Dermatol* 146:836–842.

Schiener, R., Brockow, T., Franke, A. et al. 2007. Bath PUVA and saltwater baths followed by UV-B phototherapy as treatments for psoriasis: A randomized controlled trial. *Arch Dermatol* 143:586–596.

Serwin, A.B., Wasowicz, W., Gromadzinska, J., Chodynicka, B. 2003. Selenium status in psoriasis and its relation to the duration and severity of the disease. *Nutr* 19:301–304.

Spallholtz, J.E., Boylan, L.M., Larsen, H.S. 1990. Advances in understanding selenium role in the immune system. *Ann NY Acad Sci* 587:123–139.

Thomas, J.A., Aithal, G.P. 2005. Monitoring liver function during methotrexate therapy for psoriasis: Are routine biopsies necessary. *Am J Clin Dermatol* 6(6):357–363.

Veale, D.J. 2013. Psoriatic arthritis: Recent progress in pathophysiology and drug development. *Arthritis Res Ther* 15:224.

Vieth, R., Bischoff-Ferrari, H., Boucher, B.J. et al. 2007. The urgent need to recommend an intake of vitamin D that is effective. *Am J Clin Nutr* 85:649–650.

Wcisło-Dziadecka D., Zbiciak-Nylec M., Brzezińska-Wcisło L., Mazurek U. 2015. TNF-α in a molecularly targeted therapy of psoriasis and psoriatic arthritis. *Postgrad Med J* 92(1085):172–178.

Wollima, U., Stander, K., Barta, U. 2001. Toxicity of methotrexate treatment in psoriasis and psoriatic arthritis—Short- and long-term toxicity in 104 patients. *Clin Rheumatol* 20(6):406–410.

Wolters, M. 2005. Diet and psoriasis—Experimental clinical and evidence. *Br J Dermatol* 153:706–714.

Yuqi, T.T. 2005. Review of a treatment for psoriasis using Herose, a botanical formula. *J Dermatol* 32:940–945.

Zehnder, D., Bland, R., Williams, M.C. et al. 2001. Extrarenal expression of 25-hydroxyvitamin D(3)-1 alpha-hydroxylase. *J Clin Endocrinol Metab* 86:888–894.

Zold, E., Barta, Z., Bodolay, E. 2011. Vitamin D deficiency and connective tissue disease. *Vitam Horm* 86:261–286.

Zulfakar, M.H., Edwards, M., Heard, C.M. 2007. Is there a role for topically delivered eicosapentaenoic acid in the treatment of psoriasis? *Eur J Dermatol* 17:284–291.

19 Herbal Products for the Treatment of Psoriasis

Anna Herman and Andrzej P. Herman

CONTENTS

19.1 HERBAL PRODUCTS FOR THE TREATMENT OF PSORIASIS

A wide range of conventional medical therapies have been prescribed to treat psoriasis, from topical therapies to systemic medications, phototherapy, or their combinations (Rahman et al. 2012). However, most of these therapies have limited efficacy and may cause a number of side effects, including cutaneous atrophy, organ toxicity, and carcinogenic and broadband immunosuppression, limiting their long-term use (Yuqi 2005; Traub and Marshall 2007). In turn, short-term treatment of psoriasis results in remission of the disease after finishing the treatment or only relieving the patient's condition. Given the limitations of traditional pharmacological approaches in the treatment of psoriasis, patients frequently turn to complementary and alternative medicine therapies to manage their disease (Fleischer et al. 1996). Herbal products are greatly accepted by the patients because they are believed to be safer than conventional therapy. Moreover, herbal products present great structural diversity and multidirectional mechanisms of action, which is not commonly seen in the case of synthetic compounds. Therefore, herbal drugs may effectively be used in therapies for psoriasis and are characterized by low cost and a lower incidence of side or toxic effects in comparison with conventional therapies. Therefore, researchers are still looking for new herbal products and/or their active constituents, which could potentially be used in the treatment of psoriasis as alternatives for synthetic drugs.

19.1.1 Topically Used Herbal Products for the Treatment of Psoriasis

Many herbal topical formulations used for the treatment of psoriasis have been described in the scientific literature (Deng et al. 2013, 2014; Singh and Tripathy 2014; Herman and Herman 2016). The development of novel drug delivery systems for herbal products presents desirable attributes for use in extremely dehydrated and thickened psoriatic skin, which has a lipid imbalance and is sensitive to irritants (Pradhan et al. 2013; Suresh et al. 2013). For example, the use of capsaicin-containing liposomes, niosomes, emulsomes, solid lipid nanoparticles and nanostructured lipid carriers (Agrawal et al. 2013; Gupta et al. 2016), ammonium glycyrrhizinate (*Glycyrrhiza glabra*) loaded in niosomes (Marianecci et al. 2012), colchicine isolated from *Colchicum autumnale* and *Gloriosa superb* included in elastic liposomal formulations (Singh et al. 2009), a microemulsion gel-based system of babchi oil (*Psoralea corylifolia*) (Ali et al. 2008), a microemulsion system of 5% tea tree oil (Khokhra and Diwan 2011), and a nanoemulsion system loaded in 15% turmeric oil (*Curcuma longa*) (Ali et al. 2012) may be a potential approach for the topical delivery of active constituents from herbal products and at the same time bring an effective therapy for psoriasis.

19.1.1.1 Animal-Based Study

Herbal products with antipsoriasis potential tested in animal-based studies are reported in Table 19.1. Most of the studies performed in animals *in vivo* are based on the mouse tail model of psoriasis introduced by Jarrett and Spearman (1964). In this model, antipsoriatic drug activity is defined by

TABLE 19.1
Topically Used Herbal Products in the Treatment of Psoriasis: Animal Studies

Herbal Product	Animal	Model of the Study	Pharmacological Data	Effect	Reference
Cassia tora	Albino mice	UVB-induced psoriasis	• Methanolic *C. tora* extract (0.05%, 0.1%, and 0.2%) in O/W creams • Tretinoin (0.05%) in base cream • Cream base Single dose of creams with extracts/tretinoin/cream base	Reduction in epidermal thickness compared with tretinoin	Singhal and Kansara 2012
Kigelia africana	Albino mice	Mouse tail model of psoriasis	• Ointments with 200, 100, and 50 mg/mL of methanol extracts from stem, leaves, and fruit of *K. africana* • Vehicle and placebo 0.1 mL of the ointment, contact time of 2–3 h, once daily for 2 weeks	Significant orthokeratosis in parakeratotic areas of tail Significant effects on epidermal thickness	Oyedeji and Bankole-Ojo 2012
Nigella sativa	Albino mice	Mouse tail model of psoriasis	• 95% ethanolic extract of *N. sativa* dissolved in water at a 1:2 ratio • Placebo • Tazarotene gel (0.1%) Once a day for 14 days, contact time of 2 h	Epidermal differentiation in degree of orthokeratosis as tazarotene	Dwarampudi et al. 2012
Rubia cordifolia	BALB/c mice	Mouse tail model of psoriasis	• 1%, 2%, and 5% ethyl acetate fraction of ethanolic extract formulated into gel • Placebo • 1% w/w dithranol in gel Twice a day, 7 times a week for 4 consecutive weeks	Increased granular layer and epidermal thickness Keratinocyte differentiation similar to that of dithranol gel	Lin et al. 2010

(Continued)

TABLE 19.1 (CONTINUED)
Topically Used Herbal Products in the Treatment of Psoriasis: Animal Studies

Herbal Product	Animal	Model of the Study	Pharmacological Data	Effect	Reference
Scutellaria baicalensis (baicalin)	BALB/c mice	Mouse tail model of psoriasis	• Creams with 1%, 3%, and 5% baicalin • Placebo • 2,4-Dinitrofluorobenzene (induced contact hypersensitivity, CHS) • 0.1% tazarotene cream and 0.03% tacrolimus ointment Twice a day for 4 weeks	Baicalin cream inhibits CHS reaction less than tacrolimus ointment 5% baicalin cream promotes epidermal differentiation and keratinization of keratinocyte similar to that of tazarotene cream	Wu et al. 2015
Smilax china	Albino mice	Mouse tail model of psoriasis	• Methanol extract and isolated flavonoid quercetin • Retinoic acid	Significant orthokeratosis, anti-inflammatory and maximum antiproliferant activities	Vijayalakshmi et al. 2012
Thespesia populne	Wistar rats	Mouse tail model of psoriasis	• Cream with 100 mg of each extract (ethanolic, pet-ether, butanolic, and ethyl acetate) and 50 mg of each isolated compound (TpF-1 and TpF-2 as flavonoids, TpS-2 as sterole) • 0.05% tretinoin cream Once daily, 5 times in a week for 2 weeks	Pet-ether extract and TpF-2 increased orthokeratotic region	Shrivastav et al. 2009
Wrightia tinctoria	Albino mice	Mouse tail model of psoriasis	• Hydro-alcoholic extract of *W. tinctoria* leaves • Vehicle • Isoretinoic acid Once daily for 14 days	Significant degree of orthokeratosis compared with isoretinoic acid Increased the epidermal thickness compared with control	Raj et al. 2012

the increase in percentage of orthokeratotic regions after topical drug treatment of a mouse tail. Topical treatment of the mouse tail with ethanolic extract of the *Aloe vera* leaf gel (Dhanabal et al. 2012), ethanolic extract of *Nigella sativa* (Dwarampudi et al. 2012), ethanolic extract of *Rubia cordifolia* (Lin et al. 2010), methanol extract of *Smilax china* and isolated flavonoid quercetin (Vijayalakshmi et al. 2012), *Thespesia populnea* extract (Shrivastav et al. 2009), hydro-alcoholic extract of *Wrightia tinctoria* (Raj et al. 2012), and baicalin isolated from *Scutellaria baicalensis* (Wu et al. 2015) enhances orthokeratotic cell differentiation in the epidermis. Moreover, all tested herbal products exhibited the highest antipsoriatic activity compared with positive control (0.05% tretinoin, 0.1% tazarotene, 1% dithranol, 0.03% tacrolimus, and 0.05% retinoic acid). Also, topically applied methanol extract of *Kigelia africana* ointment induced a significant and dose-dependent increase in orthokeratosis in parakeratotic areas of albino mouse tail, with significant effects on epidermal thickness, compared with vehicle control (Oyedeji and Bankole-Ojo 2012).

It is worth mentioning that the experimental model of psoriasis introduced by Jarrett and Spearman is not the only *in vivo* model used for the examination of new antipsoriatic drug activity. Nagakuma et al. (1995) proposed an experimental model of psoriasis vulgaris based on the induction of dark-brown scale on the erythematous lesion after UVB irradiation on rat skin.

The antipsoriatic drug activity is defined by changes of thickness of keratinocytes at the epidermis after topical drug treatment of a rat's skin. Irradiated rat skin treated with SUEX GEL containing aqueous extract of the bark of *Pongamia pinnata* (Divakara et al. 2013), oil-in-water (O/W) creams, and crude extract containing methanolic extract of *Cassia tora* leaves (Singhal and Kansara 2012) showed a significant reduction in the total epidermal thickness and retention of the stratum granulosum compared with ointment base and 0.05% tretinoin, respectively.

19.1.1.2 Clinical Studies

The clinical trials of topically used herbal products in the treatment of psoriasis are divided into those for new herbal products (Table 19.2) and those for herbal products commercially available on the market (Table 19.3).

The clinical trials represented in Table 19.2 showed that topical application of *A. vera* extract (Choonhakarn et al. 2010) and cream with *Persea americana* oil (Stücker et al. 2001) improved

TABLE 19.2
Topically Used Herbal Products in the Treatment of Psoriasis: Clinical Studies

Herbal Product	Type of Clinical Study	Participants	Treatments	Effect	Reference
Aloe vera	Placebo-controlled, double-blind clinical trial	60 patients with slight to moderate chronic plaque psoriasis	• *A. vera* extract (0.5%) in hydrophilic cream • Base cream 3 times daily (without occlusion) for 5 consecutive days per week for 16 weeks	Significant clearing of the psoriatic plaques and decreased PASI scores	Syed et al. 1996
Aloe vera	Randomized, comparative, double-blind clinical trial	80 patients with mild to moderate plaque psoriasis	• *A. vera* cream (70% aloe mucilage) • 0.1% triamcinolone acetonide cream Twice daily for 8 weeks	More effective than triamcinolone acetonide cream	Choonhakarn et al. 2010
Baphicacanthus cusia	Vehicle-controlled clinical trial	14 patients with chronic plaque psoriasis	• Ointment with 20% *B. cusia* powder • Vehicle ointment Once daily for 8 weeks	Significant reduction of psoriasis compared with control	Lin et al. 2007
Capsicum frutescens	Comparative, vehicle-controlled, double-blind clinical trial	44 patients with moderate to severe psoriasis	• Cream with capsaicin from *C. frutescens* • Vehicle cream Once a day for 6 weeks	Significantly more effective than control	Bernstein et al. 1986

(Continued)

TABLE 19.2 (CONTINUED)
Topically Used Herbal Products in the Treatment of Psoriasis: Clinical Studies

Herbal Product	Type of Clinical Study	Participants	Treatments	Effect	Reference
Curcuma longa	Randomized, prospective intraindividual, right–left comparative, placebo-controlled, double-blind clinical trial	40 patients with mild to moderate plaque psoriasis	• Hydroalcoholic *C. longa* extract microemulgel • Vehicle ointment Twice a day for 9 weeks	Reduction of thickness In some cases significant resolution of psoriatic lesions	Sarafian et al. 2015
Hypericum perforatum	Right–left comparative, vehicle-controlled, single-blind clinical trial	10 patients with mild plaque psoriasis	• *H. perforatum* (5%) ointment • Vehicle ointment Twice daily for 4 weeks	Improvement in clinical scores compared with placebo group	Najafizadeh et al. 2012
Indigo naturalis	Randomized, vehicle-controlled, observer-blind clinical trial	42 patients with chronic plaque psoriasis	• *Indigo naturalis* (1.4%) ointment • Vehicle ointment Once a day for 12 weeks	31 of 42 patients experienced clearance of psoriasis	Lin et al. 2008
Persea americana (avocado)	Randomized, prospective, right–left comparative clinical trial	13 patients with chronic plaque psoriasis	• Cream with vitamin B12 and avocado oil • Vitamin D3 analog calcipotriol Twice daily for 12 weeks	Effective as calcipotriol cream with regard to PASI scores	Stücker et al. 2001

psoriatic treatment compared with 0.1% triamcinolone acetonide and calcipotriol analog ointment, respectively. Also, *A. vera* cream (Syed et al. 1996), *Baphicacanthus cusia* ointment (Lin et al. 2007), *C. longa* microemulgel (Sarafian et al. 2015), *Hypericum perforatum* ointment (Najafizadeh et al. 2012), *Indigo naturalis* ointment (Lin et al. 2008), and cream with capsaicin from *Capsicum frutescens* (Bernstein et al. 1986) were found to be significantly more effective than the vehicle control group. Other available literature data show that cream with 10% *Mahonia aquifolium* extract (Gulliver and Donsky 2005), 0.03% *Camptotheca acuminata* nut (Koo and Arain 1999), and oleoresin from *Copeifera langsdorffii* (5%) ointment (Gelmini et al. 2013) had significant antipsoriatic activity compared with calcipotriene, hydrocortisone, and calcipotriol ointment, respectively. In turn, *C. acuminata* nut extract in tincture, gel, and ointment (Wang et al. 1998); *I. naturalis* ointment (Lin et al. 2006); and *M. aquifolium* bark extract ointment (Wiesenauer and Lüdtke 1996) were found to be significantly more effective than the vehicle control group. There are also literature data showing no significant difference between herbal products and drug or

TABLE 19.3
Commercially Available Herbal Products Used in the Topical Treatment of Psoriasis

Herbal Product	Type of Clinical Study	Participants	Treatments	Effect	Reference
Black cumin oil, olive oil, tea tree oil, cocoa butter, vitamin A, and vitamin B12 (DurrDerma)	Case series study	12 patients with moderate to severe psoriasis	• DurrDerma preparation (>10% black cumin oil, >10% olive oil, <0.09% tea tree oil, <4% cocoa butter, <0.05% vitamin A, <0.05% vitamin B12) Twice daily for 12 weeks	PASI reduction was observed in 10 of the 12 treated patients (83%)	Michalsen et al. 2015
Indigo naturalis (Lindioil)	Randomized, vehicle-controlled, observer-blind clinical trial	31 patients with symmetrically comparable psoriatic nails	• Refined *I. naturalis* extract in oil (Lindioil) • Olive oil • Twice daily for the first 24 weeks	Reduction of NAPSI scores	Lin et al. 2014
Mahonia aquifolium (Relieva™ cream)	Placebo-controlled, double-blind clinical trial	200 patients with mild to moderate psoriasis	• Cream with 10% *M. aquifolium* extract • Placebo Twice a day for 12 weeks	Significant improvements in PASI and QLI compared with the control group	Bernstein et al. 2006
Sphaeranthus indicus (Tinefcon® cream)	Phase IIB, double-blind, randomized, placebo-controlled, multicenter clinical trial	107 patients with plaque psoriasis	• Tinefcon cream with 20% extract of *S. indicus* • Placebo group (aminoglycan cream) Twice a day for 3 months	Safe and effective in the treatment of psoriasis	Nayak et al. 2016

placebo treatment of psoriasis. The effect of *M. aquifolium* ointment appears to be less potent than that of dithranol (Augustin et al. 1999). *Aleurites moluccana* (Kukui nut oil) (Brown et al. 2005), *A. vera* gel (Paulsen et al. 2005), and as well as ointment and lotion containing 20% kunzea oil (Thomas et al. 2015) showed no significant difference between herbal product treatment and the placebo psoriasis treatment.

Table 19.3 describes herbal products commercially available on the market. DurrDerma formulation (black cumin oil, olive oil, tea tree oil, cocoa butter, vitamin A, and vitamin B12) (Michalsen et al. 2015), Lindioil (*I. naturalis* extract in oil) (Lin et al. 2014), Reliéva cream (*M. aquifolium* extract) (Bernstein et al. 2006), and Tinefcon® cream (*Strobilanthes formosanus*) (Nayak et al. 2016) showed Psoriasis Area and Severity Index (PASI), Nail Psoriasis Severity Index (NAPSI), and PASI and Quality of Life Index (QLI) reduction compared with the vehicle control group, respectively.

Some clinical studies reported significant benefits in the use of herbal medicine bath alone or in combination with phototherapy for psoriasis treatment (Yu et al. 2013). A mixture of rice starch and turmeric (*C. longa*) bath with naturopathy interventions (e.g., massage, yoga, hydrotherapy, and diet therapy) compared with naturopathy interventions alone improved PASI score reduction after 10 days of treatment and can be used as a safe and inexpensive therapy in the management of psoriasis (Shathirapathiy et al. 2015). Also, it has been reported that the combination of Chinese herbal medicine (CHM) bath with phototherapy has superior efficacy and fewer side effects because of its reduced ultraviolet (UV) dosage in comparison with phototherapy alone (Gu et al. 2009). The clinical efficacy of the combined use of narrowband ultraviolet (NB-UVB) with a Yuyin recipe bath (Cui et al. 2008) and UV irradiation with a Yinxiebing external bath formula (*Radix Cynanchi Paniculati, Fructus Cnidii, Radix Sophorae Flavescentis, Pericarpium Zanthoxyli, Herba Patriniae, Rhizoma Polygoni Cuspidati, Herba Portulacae, Radix Salviae Milti-orrhizae,* and *Rhizoma Atractylodis*) (Liu et al. 2005) possesses a good curative effect for psoriasis vulgaris with high safety and fewer side effects. The combination of a CHM bath with phototherapy appears to be safe in the short term, but there was no long-time monitoring study of the efficacy and safety of these therapies (Yu et al. 2013). Moreover, the risk of adverse events increases with topical administration and long-term use of herbal-based formulation. Only a few of the above-described clinical trials included a safety profile of herbal products. No side effects or adverse events after topical application of *C. longa* microemulgel (Sarafian et al. 2015), *H. perforatum* ointment (Najafizadeh et al. 2012), *I. naturalis* extract in oil (Lin et al. 2014), and *S. formosanus* ointment (Lin et al. 2008) were reported. Local adverse events, mainly drying up, stinging, and itching of the skin on test areas, were observed after topical application of *A. vera* gel (Paulsen et al. 2005; Choonhakarn et al. 2010). Only one clinical trial verified the possibility of acute dermal toxicity and showed that methanolic *C. tora* leaf extract incorporated into O/W creams was safe up to a dose of 2000 mg/kg (Singhal and Kansara 2012).

19.1.2 Orally Used Herbal Products for the Treatment of Psoriasis

Oral delivery is the most convenient, safe, and widely accepted route for the administration of drugs. Disadvantages include the possibility of irregular and unpredictable absorption, depending on the physiochemical properties of the drug and the anatomic and biochemical features of the gastrointestinal tract (Doshi 2007). In this route of administration, the therapeutic efficiency of herbal products depends on the liberation of active constituents, their stability, and their absorption in intestinal tract. During oral administration, the bioavailability of herbal compounds generally decreases (due to incomplete absorption and first-pass metabolism) or may vary from patient to patient. Furthermore, orally active compounds must achieve acceptable plasma levels before they can exert a clinical effect *in vivo*. Herbal product bioavailability and high exposure in plasma levels after oral administration spread to a therapeutic effect (Bhattaram et al. 2002). Curcumin from *C. longa*, often used in orally administrated product for psoriasis treatment, revealed low bioavailability due to its limited intestinal uptake and rapid metabolism (Anand et al. 2007; Yang et al. 2007). Micronized powder and liquid micellar formulation of curcumin (Schiborr et al. 2014), nanoparticle encapsulation of curcumin (Shaikh et al. 2009), curcumin-loaded solid lipid nanoparticles (Kakkar et al. 2011), and silica-coated flexible liposomes as a nanohybrid delivery system (C. Li et al. 2012) are described in literature examples for the enhancement of the oral bioavailability of curcumin. Also, glycyrrhizin (*G. glabra*) used in psoriasis treatment products has a poor oral bioavailability in both rats and humans (Isbrucker and Burdock 2006). It was found that slow conversion of glycyrrhizin into glycyrrhetic acid (major metabolite of glycyrrhizin) in the intestine, as well as poor intestinal absorption of glycyrrhetic acid, caused their low bioavailability (Takeda et al. 1996). The use of the formulation of glycyrrhizin as sodium deoxycholate–phospholipid mixed nanomicelles (Jin et al. 2012) could enhance glycyrrhizin absorption in the gastrointestinal tract and improve their bioavailability. Astilbin, flavonoid isolated from the rhizome of *Smilax glabra* (*Rhizoma Smilacis Glabrae*), is a promising immunosuppressant for immune-related diseases such as psoriasis, but is limited in clinical application due to its poor water solubility, difficult oral absorption, and low bioavailability (He et al. 2014). The self-microemulsifying drug delivery system (SMEDDS) (Mezghrani et al. 2011) and a combination of PVP K30 and Tween 80 (He et al. 2014) showed a significant enhancement of astilbin bioavailability. Unfortunately, in many cases, little is known about the bioavailability of herbal products and potentially new active compounds. A better understanding of the pharmacokinetics and bioavailability of phytopharmaceuticals becomes an important issue in linking data from pharmacological assays and clinical effects (Bhattaram et al. 2002).

19.1.2.1 Animal-Based Study

Orally used herbal products with antipsoriasis potential tested in animal-based studies are reported in Table 19.4. Di et al. (2016) investigated the effect of astilbin isolated from the rhizome of *S. glabra* on a BALB/c mice model of psoriasis. Astilbin (25–50 mg/kg) significantly reduced the thickness of the epidermis layer and imiquimod-induced proliferation of keratinocytes. Also, PSORI-CM01 tablets (*Curcuma zedoaria, Sarcandra glabra, Dark Plum Fruit, Rhizoma Smilacis Glabrae, Lithospermum erythrorhizon, Paeonia lactiflora*, and *Glycyrrhiza uralensis* at a ratio

TABLE 19.4
Orally Used Herbal Products in the Treatment of Psoriasis: Animal Studies

Herbal Product	Animal	Pharmacological Data	Effect	Reference
Astilbin (flavonoid from rhizome of *Smilax glabra*)	BALB/c mice	• Control group: Did not receive IMQ • Group I: 62.5 mg of 5% IMQ cream • Group II: 62.5 mg of 5% IMQ cream + 25 mg/kg astilbin • Group III: 62.5 mg of 5% IMQ cream +50 mg/kg astilbin • Group IV: MTX 1 mg/kg Once a day for 7 days	Reduction of inflammatory cell differentiation and cytokine secretion	Di et al. 2016
Curcuma zedoaria, Sarcandra glabra, Dark Plum Fruit, Rhizoma Smilacis Glabrae, Lithospermum erythrorhizon, Paeonia lactiflora, Glycyrrhiza uralensis (at a ratio of 3:5:5:5:2:3:2) PSORI-CM01 tablets	BALB/c mice	• Normal mice without psoriasis induced by IMQ • IMQ-induced mice with saline treatment • IMQ-induced mice receiving 6.88 mg/day glycyrrhizin • IMQ-induced mice receiving 12.5, 25.0, or 50 mg/day PSORI-CM01 tablets Oral administration of 400 μL of vehicle or drug solution daily for 20 days	Significantly inhibited epidermal hyperplasia; effect was similar to that of glycyrrhizin tablets	Wei et al. 2016
Rhinacanthus nasutus, Indigofera aspalathoides	Albino rats	• Group I: Control (5% saline) • Group II: Ethanolic extract of *R. nasutus* 1 mg/kg • Group III: Ethanolic extract of *I. aspalathoides* 1 mg/kg • Group IV: Positive control indomethacin 10 mg/kg	Significantly inhibited edema when compared with standard indomethacin	Raj et al. 2015

(Continued)

TABLE 19.4 (CONTINUED)
Orally Used Herbal Products in the Treatment of Psoriasis: Animal Studies

Herbal Product	Animal	Pharmacological Data	Effect	Reference
Tinospora cordifolia, *Curcuma longa*, *Celastrus paniculatus*, *Aloe vera*	Parkes mice strain	• Group I: Control group (vaseline cream) • Group II: Topical application of 5% IMQ cream • Group III: Oral administration of aqueous *T. cordifolia* extract • Group IV: Topical application of *C. longa* extract • Group V: Topical application of *C. paniculatus* oil • Group VI: All extracts together, *T. cordifolia* + *C. longa* + *C. paniculatus* + *A. vera*	Combination extract from all the plants was instrumental in downregulating the overexpressed cytokines	Arora et al. 2016
Wrightia tinctoria	Albino mice	• Group I: Control (water) • Group II: Positive control (isoretinoic acid 0.5 mg/kg) • Group III: Oral administration of aqueous *W. tinctoria* extract (200 mg/kg) Once daily for 14 days	Significant degree of orthokeratosis compared with control; more potent than the standard	Raj et al. 2012

Note: IMQ, imiquimod; MTX, methotrexate.

of 3:5:5:5:2:3:2, doses 12.5, 25, and 50 mg) significantly inhibited epidermal hyperplasia in the imiquimod-induced BALB/c mice model of psoriasis (Wei et al. 2016). The extracts from *Tinospora cordifolia*, *C. longa*, *Celastrus paniculatus*, and *A. vera* were instrumental in downregulating the overexpressed cytokines and can be new therapeutic strategies for psoriasis treatment (Arora et al. 2016). In particular, *C. longa* extract (150 mg/kg) caused remarkable reduction in erythema and skin thickening in psoriasis-treated mice. Also, oral administration (200 mg/kg) of the hydroalcoholic extract of *W. tinctoria* leaves was evaluated for antipsoriatic activity in the mouse tail test (Raj et al. 2012). The extract produced a significant degree of orthokeratosis compared with control and the isoretinoic acid (0.5 mg/kg) groups after 14 days of treatment. Therefore, *W. tinctoria* extract can be a useful remedy for psoriasis patients.

19.1.2.2 Clinical Studies

The clinical trials of orally used herbal products in the treatment of psoriasis are divided into those for new herbal products (Table 19.5) and those for herbal products commercially available on the market (Table 19.6).

The clinical trials represented in Table 19.5 show that oral administration of glycyrrhizin (Wang et al. 2008; Ye et al. 2009), a combination of *N. sativa* and methotrexate (Ahmed et al. 2014), and CHM with acitretin capsule (Zhang et al. 2009) had a significant improvement in the treatment of

TABLE 19.5
Orally Used Herbal Products in the Treatment of Psoriasis: Clinical Studies

Herbal Product	Type of Clinical Study	Participants	Treatments	Effect	Reference
Dandelion (10 g), *Forsythia* fruit (12 g), *Isatis* root (30 g), *Isatis* leaf (15 g), *Imperata* rhizome (30 g), honeysuckle flower (15 g), *Prunella* spike (15 g), moutan bark (15 g), red and white peony (each 15 g), *Rehmannia* root (15 g), figwort root (15 g), antelope horn powder (0.3 g)	Randomized, controlled trial	80 patients with psoriasis of blood-heat syndrome	• Oral CHM administration twice a day for 8 weeks • CHM combined with acitretin capsule (20–30 mg/day) for 8 weeks	PASI score lowered significantly after treatment in both groups	Zhang et al. 2009
Evening primrose oil	Double-blind parallel clinical trial	37 patients with chronic plaque psoriasis	• 12 capsules (430 mg evening primrose oil + 107 mg marine oil) per day + topical application (1% hydrocortisone ointment) twice daily over 24 weeks	No differences were found in clinical symptoms or plaque thickness	Oliwiecki and Burton 1994
Glycyrrhizin	Randomized, controlled trial	53 patients with psoriasis vulgaris	• Viaminate 50 mg + topical application of Elocon cream for 8 weeks • Glycyrrhizin 75 mg + the same treatment as control group for 8 weeks	Total effective rate in treatment group was significantly higher than that in control group	Ye et al. 2009
Glycyrrhizin	Comparative, controlled trial	86 patients with psoriasis vulgaris	• Conventional therapy for 3 weeks • 100 mL/day glycyrrhizin for 3 weeks	The responsive rates for treatment group and control group were 72.1% and 41.9%, respectively	Wang et al. 2008
Nigella sativa	Open-label, therapeutic, outpatient-based study	60 patients with moderate to severe plaque, palmoplantar, and guttate psoriasis	• Group 1: *N. sativa* ointment (20% w/w) 2 times daily + 500 mg *N. sativa* capsule 3 times daily • Group 2: MTX tablets 15 mg weekly • Group 3: MTX + *N. sativa* (topical + oral) Treatment: 12 weeks	*N. sativa* augments the antipsoriatic effect of MTX	Ahmed et al. 2014

Note: MTX, methotrexate.

TABLE 19.6
Commercially Available Herbal Products Used in the Oral Treatment of Psoriasis

Herbal Product	Type of Clinical Study	Participants	Treatments	Effect	Reference
Curcuminoid C3 Complex (Sabinsa Corporation, Piscataway, New Jersey)	Single-dose, noncontrolled, open-label phase II of clinical trial	18 patients with chronic plaque psoriasis; lack of placebo group	• Capsules (500 mg) of Curcuminoid C3 Complex contain 95% curcuminoids 3 times a day for 16 weeks	The response rate was low and possibly due to a placebo effect or the natural history of psoriasis	Kurd et al. 2008
Efamol Marine (Efamol Limited, Essex, United Kingdom) Evening primrose oil and fish oil	Double-blind, randomized, placebo-controlled trial	51 patients with chronic plaque psoriasis	• Control (tar and dithranol) • 12 capsules of placebo (liquid paraffin) • 12 × 500 mg capsules of Efamol Marine Once a day for 7 months	No significant difference between active and placebo groups	Strong and Hamill 1993
Efamol Marine (Efamol Limited) Evening primrose oil and fish oil	Double-blind, placebo-controlled study	38 patients with psoriatic arthritis	• 12 Efamol Marine capsules • 12 placebo (liquid paraffin) capsules Daily for 9 months	No significant change in clinical symptoms	Veale et al. 1994
Herose capsules *Miltiorrhizae* (589 mg), *Radix Astragali* (331 mg), *Ramulus Cinnamomi* (317 mg), *Radix Paeoniae Alba* (165 mg), *Radix Codonopsis Pilosula* (67 mg), *Semen Coicis* (570 mg)	Case series study	15 patients with moderate to severe chronic plaque psoriasis	• 4 Herose capsules (450 mg/capsule) 3 times a day for 10 months	Effective and safe treatment for psoriasis	Tang 2005
Meriva (Indena SpA, Milan, Italy) 20% curcuminoids in tablet	Randomized, double-blind, placebo-controlled clinical trial	63 patients with mild to moderate psoriasis vulgaris (PASI < 10)	• Topical steroids (methylprednisolone 0.1% aceponate, arm 1, once a day) + Meriva tablets (2 g/day for 12 weeks) • Topical steroids alone (arm 2, once a day) for 12 weeks	Reduction of PASI values was significantly higher than that of patients using topical steroid alone	Antiga et al. 2015
PSORI-CM01 *Radix Paeoniae Rubra*, *Rhizoma Curcumae*, *Sarcandra*, *Radix Glycytthizae*, *Fructus Mume*, *Radix Arnebiae*, *Rhizoma Smilacis Glabrae*	Double-blind, randomized, placebo-controlled trial	18 patients with moderate to severe psoriasis vulgaris	• Topical treatment: Calcipotriol 50 μg/g ointment, once daily for the first 8 weeks + betamethasone dipropionate 0.5 mg/g ointment, once daily for the remaining 4 weeks + placebo orally • Topical treatment + oral treatment PSORI-CM01 decoction (twice a day for 12 weeks)	PSORI-CM01 combined with topical treatment showed a smaller recurrence rate than placebo combined with topical therapy	Yao et al. 2016

(*Continued*)

TABLE 19.6 (CONTINUED)
Commercially Available Herbal Products Used in the Oral Treatment of Psoriasis

Herbal Product	Type of Clinical Study	Participants	Treatments	Effect	Reference
Qinzhu Liangxue decoction (30 g magnetitum, 25 g mother-of-pearl, 30 g oyster, 9 g *Scutellaria baicalensis*, 9 g *Lithospermum erythrorhizon*, 9 g *Cynanchum paniculatum*, 10 g Coix lacryma-jobi, 9 g Fang Feng, 6 g *Glycyrrhiza uralensis* Fisch)	Randomized controlled trial	72 patients with psoriasis vulgaris	• Acitretin group (30 mg daily) • Acitretin (30 mg daily) + Qinzhu Liangxue decoction group (30 mL, 2 times daily) Treatment: 8 weeks	Group treated with Qinzhu Liangxue decoction and acitretin achieved best treatment compared with the control groups	Sha et al. 2016
Tinefcon tablets Sphaeranthus indicus	Randomized, double-blind, placebo-controlled pilot study	74 patients with moderate to severe plaque psoriasis	• Placebo group • *S. indicus* extract 1.4 g/day (1 tablet of 700 mg twice daily) and 2.8 g/day (2 tablets of 700 mg twice daily) for 3 months	Tinefcon was more effective at the higher dosage of 2.8 g/day	Velaskar et al. 2016
Tinefcon tablets (methanolic extract of dried fruit and flower heads of *Sphaeranthus indicus* with no less than 28 mg of 7-hydroxy frullanolide and 9.6 mg of sphaeranthanolide)	Open-label, noncomparative, multicenter phase IV trial	401 patients with plaque psoriasis	• 700 mg Tinefcon tablets/day for 12 weeks	Reduction in severity assessed by PGA was observed in more than half of patients with moderate disease	Sharma et al. 2016
Wentong Huayu capsule *Herba ephedrae* (6 g), *Radix Aconiti Lateralis* (10 g), *Semen sinapis* (10 g), *Cortex cinnamomi* (3 g), *Rhizoma zingiberis* (3 g), *Cornu Cervi Degelatinatum* (15 g), *Radix Rehmanniae Preparata* (10 g), *Rhizoma Smilacis Glabrae* (60 g), *Cortex dictamni* (30 g), *Rhizoma imperatae* (30 g), *Radix Salviae Miltiorrhizae* (15 g), *Caulis spatholobi* (30 g), *Radix Arnebiae* (30 g), *Flos sophorae* (30 g), *Radix Glycyrrhizae* (6 g), *Indigo naturalis* (6 g)	Randomized, placebo-controlled trial	61 patients with moderate to severe plaque psoriasis	• MTX (2.5–5 mg, then increasing up to 30 mg/week) for 6 months • Wentong Huayu capsule (dose not specified) for 6 months • Treatment with placebo for 6 months	Group with MTX showed greater effectiveness than the other two groups; no significant difference was found between the TCM and placebo groups	Ho et al. 2010

(Continued)

TABLE 19.6 (CONTINUED)
Commercially Available Herbal Products Used in the Oral Treatment of Psoriasis

Herbal Product	Type of Clinical Study	Participants	Treatments	Effect	Reference
Yinxieping granule *Radix Rehmanniae*, *Radix Angelicae Formosanae*, powder of *Carapax Eretmochelydis*, *Radix Paeoniae Rubra*, *Calculus Bovis Artificial*, *Herba Schizonepetae Tenuifoliae* Xiaoyin tablet *Radix Rehmanniae*, *Paeonia suffruticosa*, *Aeonia veitchii*, *Angelica sinensis*, *Sophora flavescens*, *Lonicera japonica*, *Scrophularia ningpoensis*, *Arctium lappa*, *Cyptotympana atrata*, *Dictamnus dasycarpus*, *Saposhnikovia divaricata*	Case series study	60 patients with psoriasis vulgaris	• Yin Xie Ping granule (4.5 g), twice a day • Xiaoyin tablet, 7 tablets, 3 times a day	Statistically significant improvements for both formulations	Chang et al. 2006
YXBCM01 granule *Radix Paeoniae Rubra*, *Sarcandra Glabra*, *Rhizoma Smilacis Glabrae*, etc.	Double-blind, parallel, randomized controlled trial	600 patients with psoriasis vulgaris	• Topical treatment: Calcipotriol betamethasone for the first 4 weeks and calcipotriol ointment for the remaining 8 weeks • YXBCM01 granule (5.5 g twice daily for 12 weeks) + topical treatment • Placebo granules (5.5 g twice daily for 12 weeks) + topical treatment	High-quality evidence for the efficacy and safety of the YXBCM01 formula	Wen et al. 2014

Note: MTX, methotrexate; PGA, Physician Global Assessment; TCM, traditional Chinese medicine.

psoriasis compared with the control group. Liu and Tan (2004) described a case series of 40 patients with chronic plaque psoriasis who received an oral herbal mixture (*Radix Astragali, Radix Codonopsis, Radix Salviae Miltiorrhizae, Radix Paeoniae Rubra, Rhizoma Chuanxiong, Pheretima, Radix chyranthis Bidentatae, Radix Arnebiae seu Lithospermi,* and *Radix Glycyrrhizae*) twice a day and at the same time topically applied 10% boric acid ointment once a day for 60 days' treatment. After treatment, 60% of patients experienced almost complete clearance of lesions. In systematic review, Zhou at al. (2014) described that CHMs may have beneficial effects on the treatment of psoriasis vulgaris. For example, oral administration of Liangxue Jiedu Tang and Liangxue Huoxue Fang improved the clinical effectiveness of the treatment of psoriasis and can be strongly recommended, while Tu Ling Yin and Xiao Yin Tang received weak recommendation. The dietary supplementation of a combination of marine oil and evening primrose oil from *Oenothera biennis* in the treatment of chronic stable plaque psoriasis showed no differences in clinical symptoms or plaque thickness (Oliwiecki and Burton 1994).

Table 19.6 describes herbal products commercially available on the market, including Curcuminoid C3 Complex® (Kurd et al. 2008), Efamol Marine (Strong and Hamill 1993; Veale et al. 1994), Meriva (Antiga et al. 2015), and Tinefcon (Sharma et al. 2016; Velaskar et al. 2016), as well as Herose capsules (Tang 2005), Wentong Huayu capsules (Ho et al. 2010), PSORI-CM01 (Yao et al. 2016), Qinzhu Liangxue decoctions (Sha et al. 2016), Yinxieping granules and Xiaoyin tablets (Chang et al. 2006), and YXBCM01 granules (Wen et al. 2014). The combination of oral administration of herbal products with topical application of synthetic drugs achieved better psoriasis treatment efficacy than the use of drugs alone. This effect was observed for Meriva and 0.1% methylprednisolone aceponate (Antiga et al. 2015), PSORI-CM01 and calcipotriol 50 μg/g ointment and betamethasone dipropionate 0.5 mg/g ointment (Yao et al. 2016), Qinzhu Liangxue decoction and acitretin 30 mg (Sha et al. 2016), and YXBCM01 granule and calcipotriol betamethasone and calcipotriol ointment (Wen et al. 2014). The oral administration of Tinefcon tablets resulted in a significant improvement in the treatment of psoriasis compared with the placebo group (Velaskar et al. 2016). Also, Herose capsules (Tang 2005), Tinefcon tablets (Sharma et al. 2016), Yinxieping granules, and Xiaoyin tablets (Chang et al. 2006) support the therapeutic effect on psoriasis, but without reference to the control group. Moreover, Herose capsules (Tang 2005) and the combination of Yinxieping granules with Xiaoyin tablets (Chang et al. 2006) described in the case series study are an effective and safe treatment for psoriasis. Oral Tinefcon tablets, tested in an open-label, noncomparative, multicenter, phase IV clinical trial, showed good efficacy and had a favorable safety profile in plaque psoriasis patients (Sharma et al. 2016). In turn, Efamol Marine (Strong and Hamill 1993; Veale et al. 1994) and Wentong Huayu capsule (Ho et al. 2010) did not improve the treatment of psoriasis compared with the placebo group. Moreover, the group treated with Wentong Huayu capsules group showed less effectiveness in psoriasis treatment than the methotrexate treatment group. Curcuminoid C3 Complex, administered orally in patients with chronic plaque psoriasis, showed a low response rate, possibly due to a placebo effect or the natural history of psoriasis (Kurd et al. 2008). It is possible that oral administration of curcumin will not produce the desired clinical effect due to its low bioavailability in both animals and humans (Grant and Schneider 2000; Ireson et al. 2002). Therefore, administration of curcumin at higher doses or combining oral curcumin with agents that may enhance its absorption may result in better efficacy (Anand et al. 2007). Antiga et al. (2015) demonstrated that oral Meriva, a novel lecithin-based delivery form of curcumin, is an effective ingredient, useful for adjuvant therapy in patients with mild to moderate plaque psoriasis vulgaris treated with topical steroids (0.1% methylprednisolone aceponate).

19.2 MECHANISM OF ACTION OF HERBAL PRODUCTS USED IN THE TREATMENT OF PSORIASIS

Psoriasis is defined by a series of linked cellular changes in the skin: hyperplasia of epidermal keratinocytes, vascular hyperplasia and ectasia, and infiltration of T lymphocytes, neutrophils, and other types of leukocytes in affected skin (Krueger and Bowcock 2005). Therefore, the herbal products used in the treatment of psoriasis work directly by (1) inhibition of the keratinocyte hyperproliferation and induction of their apoptosis and (2) inhibition of immune-inflammatory reaction, as well as indirectly by (3) suppression of phosphorylase kinase (PhK) activity and (4) inhibition of the hedgehog (Hh) signaling pathway, which consequently, in both cases, affect inflammatory cells, including CD4+ and CD8+ T lymphocytes (Herman and Herman 2016).

Psoriasis is typically characterized as inflamed skin with surface scale and thickening of the epidermis (acanthosis or reduction or absence of the granular layer) caused by parakeratosis, which is a consequence of nuclei retention in stratum corneum keratinocytes caused by abnormal differentiation and hyperproliferation of epidermal keratinocytes (Johnson-Huang et al. 2012). Therefore, a number of studies have shown that inhibition of keratinocyte hyperproliferation, induction of their apoptosis, and modulation keratinocyte differentiation may be considered targets of antipsoriatic strategies. Animal-based studies support the efficacy of the herbal products for the treatment of psoriasis via inhibition of keratinocyte hyperproliferation. The ethanolic extract of *A. vera* leaf gel (Dhanabal et al. 2012) and the ethanolic extract of *N. sativa* seeds (Dwarampudi et al. 2012) produced a significant epidermal differentiation seen as orthokeratosis when compared with the control group and tazarotene (0.1%) gel, respectively. However, the most desirable herbal products for psoriasis treatment are ones that inhibit epidermal hyperplasia and inflammation simultaneously. Tuhuai extract (Man et al. 2008) and baicalin isolated from *S. baicalensis* (Wu et al. 2015) reduced epidermal hyperplasia and inflammation in mice, which makes them valuable drugs for the treatment of psoriasis. Moreover, 5% baicalin cream promotes epidermal differentiation and normal keratinization of keratinocytes in mouse skin, similar to that seen with 0.1% tazarotene cream (Wu et al. 2015). Flavonoid quercetin from the rhizome of *S. china* shows significant orthokeratosis, reduction in epidermal thickness, and anti-inflammatory and maximum antiproliferant activities compared with mice treated with retinoic acid (Vijayalakshmi et al. 2012). PSORI-CM01 (*C. zedoaria*, *S. glabra*, *Dark Plum Fruit*, *Rhizoma Smilacis Glabrae*, *L. erythrorhizon*, *P. lactiflora*, and *G. uralensis*) inhibits epidermal hyperplasia in the imiquimod-induced mouse psoriasis-form model and reduces keratinocyte proliferation *in vitro* through downregulation of cyclin B2 (Wei et al. 2016). Herbal product treatment of psoriasis through inhibition of the keratinocyte hyperproliferation was also confirmed in clinical studies. *I. naturalis* ointment modulates the proliferation (decreased proliferating marker Ki-67) and differentiation of keratinocytes in epidermis (increased levels of filaggrin), as well as inflammatory reactions by inhibiting the infiltration of T lymphocytes (decreased inflammatory marker CD3) in patients with chronic plaque psoriasis (Lin et al. 2007). Moreover, *I. naturalis*, as well as its major active constituent induribin, inhibited proliferation and abnormal differentiation of epidermal keratinocytes through decreased proliferating cell nuclear antigen (PCNA) and increased involucrin at both the mRNA and protein levels in patients with psoriatic lesions (Lin et al. 2009).

The role of the immune system and its interactive network of leukocytes and cytokines in disease pathogenesis was also described (Johnson-Huang et al. 2012). The primary immune defect in psoriasis appears to be an increase in cell signaling via chemokines and cytokines that act on upregulated gene expression and cause hyperproliferation of keratinocytes (Traub and Keri 2007). Therefore, some studies show that the inhibition of fibroblast-secreted cytokines could regulate keratinocyte proliferation and differentiation, as well as slow down the process of inflammation in psoriasis (Zhang and Gu 2007). Ethanolic extracts from *Alpinia galanga*, *C. longa*, and *Annona squamosa* (Saelee et al. 2011), as well as *C. langsdorffii* oleoresin (known as Copaiba Balsam) (Gelmini et al. 2013), exhibited anti-inflammatory activity through inhibition of NFκB signaling molecules, which may positively affect the treatment of psoriasis with inflammation and hyperproliferation. Water-soluble polysaccharide (GP-I) purified from *Gynostemma pentaphyllum* has a significant anti-proliferative effect and decreases tumor necrosis factor (TNF) α, a vital pro-inflammatory cytokine in psoriasis (X. Li et al. 2012). Methanol extracts of *Acanthus mollis*, *Achillea ligustica*, *Artemisia arborescens*, and *Inula viscosa* inhibited both 5-LOX and COX-1 activity without significant effects on the 12-LOX pathway, and NFκB activation was prevented by all extracts except *A. mollis* (Bader et al. 2015). Moreover, *A. ligustica*, *A. arborescens*, and *A. mollis* increased the biosynthesis of 15(S)-HETE, an anti-inflammatory eicosanoid. Herbal product treatment of psoriasis through inhibition of cytokines was also confirmed in animal-based studies. Topical application of an herbal extract mixture (*T. cordifolia*, *C. longa*, *C. paniculatus*, and *A. vera*) led to downregulating the overexpressed cytokines in mice initially induced with psoriasis-like dermatitis using topical application of imiquimod (Arora et al. 2015). Also, oral administration of astilbin ameliorated imiquimod-induced keratinocyte proliferation, infiltration of CD3+ cells to psoriatic lesions, and elevations in circulating CD4+ and CD8+ T cells and inflammatory cytokines (interleukin [IL] 17A, TNF-α, IL-6, interferon [IFN] γ, and IL-2) in BALB/c mice (Di et al. 2016). *In vitro*, astilbin inhibited Th17 cell differentiation and IL-17 secretion of isolated T cells, as well as inhibited Jak/Stat3 signaling in Th17 cells, while upregulating Stat3 inhibitor SCOSE3 expression in psoriatic lesions. Some animal studies have demonstrated the inhibitory effect of curcumin on NFκB (Chun et al. 2003) and downstream inflammatory cytokines, such as TNF-α and IL-6 (Gulcubuk et al. 2006; Aggarwal et al. 2013), both critical factors in the pathophysiology of psoriasis.

Some research has found that PhK enzyme is expressed at significantly higher levels in psoriatic epidermis than in normal epidermis (Heng et al. 1994). The PhK enzyme integrates multiple calcium/calmodulin-dependent signaling pathways, including those involved in cell migration and cell proliferation. Therefore, the use of a selective PhK inhibitor, such as curcumin, may be effective for the treatment of psoriasis (Heng et al. 2000). It was observed that PhK activity was highest in untreated psoriasis patients and lower in the group treated with calcipotriol and curcumin. Moreover, decreased PhK activity in psoriasis patients treated with curcumin and calcipotriol was associated with a corresponding decreased expression of keratinocyte transferrin receptor, severity of parakeratosis, and density of epidermal CD8+ T cells.

Some reports suggest that the Hh pathway is activated in lesional psoriatic skin and treatment with the Hh pathway antagonist may lead to rapid resolution of the disease (Hovhannisyan et al. 2009). Cyclopamine (Hh pathway antagonist), isolated from *Veratrum californicum*, was found to be more effective than topical clobetasol-17 propionate in the treatment of guttate and plaque-type psoriasis (Taş and Avci 2004). Besides, inflammatory cells, including CD4+ lymphocytes, were found to disappear rapidly after treatment with cyclopamine, and *hedgehog/smoothened* signaling was inhibited. On the other hand, some research found that the Hh pathway is not activated in psoriasis (Gudjonsson et al. 2009). The absence of elevated Hh target gene expression (*PTCH1* and *GLI1*) in lesional psoriatic skin indicates that the Hh pathway is not activated in this disease, which raises questions regarding the proposed use of Hh antagonists as antipsoriatic agents.

19.3 CHALLENGES AND PERSPECTIVES FOR THE TREATMENT OF PSORIASIS WITH HERBAL PRODUCTS

19.3.1 Reliable Clinical Trials

Herbal products are an important group of widely and increasingly used worldwide therapeutics. Despite the popularity of herbal products, the clinical evidence that supports the use of most herbal medicines is weak. The lack of standardization of herbal products (often unknown purity and content of active constituents) used in clinical trials, the use of different dosages of herbal medicines, and the wide variations in the duration of treatments using herbal medicines make it impossible to reconstruct the study and perform it on a larger number of volunteers. Moreover, the insufficient number of patients in most trials is inadequate for the attainment of statistical significance to support clinical evidence for herbal products. In practice, the first phase of a clinical trial usually involves 100–500 participants because only studies carried out on more than 100 patients provide opportunities for statistical analysis. Among the above-described clinical trials for topically used herbal products (Table 19.3), only two studies concerning Reliéva cream (*M. aquifolium* extract) (Bernstein et al. 2006) and Tinefcon cream (*Sphaeranthus indicus* extract) (Nayak et al. 2016), as well as clinical trials for the oral administration of herbal products (Table 19.6) such as Tinefcon tablets (*S. indicus* extract) (Sharma et al. 2016) and YXBCM01 granules (*Radix Paeoniae Rubra, S. glabra, Rhizoma Smilacis Glabrae*, etc.) (Wen et al. 2014), are representative for statistical analysis. Other clinical trials included a number of participants that were not representative, and therefore conclusions from these studies cannot be generalized to the entire population affected by psoriasis. Therefore, only well-controlled double-blind clinical trials can prove the efficacy of herbal products in psoriasis treatment.

19.3.2 Herbal Product Bioavailability

Herbal products and their active constituents may be considered effective drugs for the treatment of psoriasis if they are able to influence the biochemical mechanisms. For an herbal medicine, pharmacological activity is gained when the active agents or active metabolites reach and sustain proper levels at their sites of action, which affects their therapeutic responses. Herbal product penetration through the skin after topical application and high absorption in the intestinal tract and high exposure in plasma levels after oral administration are essential for their bioavailability. Unfortunately, for the majority of herbal medicines, data on their bioavailability and pharmacokinetic properties in human organisms are lacking or scant. There has been some research on herbal remedies, but these studies are mainly focused on a small number of herbal medicines, including St. John's wort, curcumin, ginseng, ginkgo, and ginger (He et al. 2011; Thelingwani and Masimirembwa 2014). Therefore, better understanding the pharmacokinetics and bioavailability of phytopharmaceuticals may help in designing rational dosage regimens, as well as obtaining safe herbal medicines.

19.3.3 Safety Profile of Herbal Products

The long tradition of herbal product use in the treatment of many diseases is not sufficient for considering them effective and safe drugs. It is also common knowledge that the safety of most herbal products is further compromised by the lack of suitable quality controls, inadequate labeling, and the absence of appropriate patient information (Raynor et al. 2011). The manufacturers of these products are not required to submit proof of safety and efficacy before marketing, so the adverse effects associated with remedies are largely unknown (Ekor 2014). However, various studies and researchers have highlightened their possible side effects, such as erythema, edema, allergic reactions, and photosensitization, especially if they were taken irregularly, in excessive amounts, or in combination with some medicines (Ernst 2000; De Smet 2004; Kaur et al. 2013). Moreover, tests for skin irritation performed on animals are not always predictive of what will occur in humans, but they are still the most widely used tests in toxicity research for applied topically herbal products. Furthermore, some herbal preparations can cause organ toxicity, including liver, kidneys, and heart (Stedman 2001; Dwivedi et al. 2011; Asif 2012), or possess cancerogenic properties (Bode and Dong 2015). Moreover, herbal products may contain additives or contaminants (heavy metals and pesticides) that are not listed in the formulation (Huxtable 1992; Joshi and Kaul 2001; Niggemann and Grüber 2003). Therefore, it is essential to identify the risks associated with the use of herbal medicines, and in this regard, the safety of these products has become an issue of great public health importance. With the enormous global consumption of herbal products and medicines, it is high time to include them in pharmacovigilance systems (Ekor 2014).

19.3.4 Quality Control of Herbal Products

Herbal products can make substantial contributions to drug innovation by providing novel chemical structures and/or multidirectional mechanisms of action, which are not commonly seen in synthetic compounds. Nevertheless, different parts of plants exhibit variability in composition, and different methods of preparation of herbal material may not be comparable. For this reason, maintaining quality control of raw herbs is important. The development of analytical chemistry techniques, such as high-performance liquid chromatography and gas chromatography coupled with mass spectrometry, enables progress in the assessment of the pharmacological qualities of herbal products. Moreover, the advances in analytical technology have led to the discovery of many new active constituents and an ever-increasing list of putatively active constituents.

19.3.5 Herbal Product Regulations

An increasing number of herbal products available for sale should prompt governments to introduce research regulations that should be carried out before such products are provided on the market. Unfortunately, in most countries there are no universal legal regulations that ensure the safety and activity of phytopharmaceuticals. There are no regulations governing which herbal products can be marketed for various ailments, as well as no authorities to register adverse effects (Calixto 2000). It seems that establishing a global regulatory mechanism for introducing herbal drugs to the world market is desirable and necessary. Furthermore, having scientifically proven herbal products with benefits confirmed by reliable clinical trials and standardized plant material specified by regulatory authorities will support the use of plant-based preparations in the daily clinical management of psoriasis.

REFERENCES

Aggarwal, B. B., S. C. Gupta, B. Sung. 2013. Curcumin: An orally bioavailable blocker of TNF and other pro-inflammatory biomarkers. *Br J Pharmacol* 169:1672–92.

Agrawal, U., M. Gupta, S. P. Vyas. 2013. Capsaicin delivery into the skin with lipidic nanoparticles for the treatment of psoriasis. *Artif Cells Nanomed Biotechnol* 43:33–39.

Ahmed, J. H., S. N. Kadhim, K. I. Al-Hamdi. 2014. The effectiveness of *Nigella sativa*, methotrexate and their combination in the treatment of moderate to severe psoriasis. *J Clin Exp Invest* 5:521–28.

Ali, J., N. Akhtar, Y. Sultana, S. Baboota, A. Ahuja. 2008. Antipsoriatic microemulsion gel formulations for topical drug delivery of babchi oil (*Psoralea corylifolia*). *Method Find Exp Clin* 30:277–85.

Ali, M. S., M. S. Alam, F. I. Imam, M. R. Siddiqui. 2012. Topical nanoemulsion of turmeric oil for psoriasis: Characterization, ex vivo and in vivo assessment. *Int J Drug Deliv* 4:184–97.

Anand, P., A. B. Kunnumakkara, R. A. Newman, B. B. Aggarwal. 2007. Bioavailability of curcumin: Problems and promises. *Mol Pharm* 4:807–18.

Antiga, E., V. Bonciolini, W. Volpi, E. Del Bianco, M. Caproni. 2015. Oral curcumin (Meriva) is effective as an adjuvant treatment and is able to reduce IL-22 serum levels in patients with psoriasis vulgaris. *Biomed Res Int* 2015:1–7.

Arora, N., K. Shah, S. Pandey-Rai. 2016. Inhibition of imiquimod-induced psoriasis-like dermatitis in mice by herbal extracts from some Indian medicinal plants. *Protoplasma* 253:503–15.

Asif, M. 2012. A brief study of toxic effects of some medicinal herbs on kidney. *Adv Biomed Res* 1:44.

Augustin, M., U. Andrees, H. Grimme, E. Schöpf, J. Simon. 1999. Effects of *Mahonia aquifolium* ointment on the expression of adhesion, proliferation, and activation markers in the skin of patients with psoriasis. *Forsch Komplementarmed* 6:19–21.

Bader, A., F. Martini, G. R. Schinella, J. L. Rios, J. M. Prieto. 2015. Modulation of Cox-1, 5-, 12- and 15-Lox by popular herbal remedies used in southern Italy against psoriasis and other skin diseases. *Phytother Res* 29:108–13.

Bernstein, J. E., L. C. Parish, M. Rapaport, M. M. Rosenbaum, H. H. Roenigk. 1986. Effects of topically applied capsaicin on moderate and severe psoriasis vulgaris. *J Am Acad Dermatol* 15:504–7.

Bernstein, S., H. Donsky, W. Gulliver, D. Hamilton, S. Nobel, R. Norman. 2006. Treatment of mild to moderate psoriasis with Relieva, a *Mahonia aquifolium* extract—A double-blind, placebo-controlled study. *Am J Ther* 13:121–6.

Bhattaram, V. A., U. Graefe, C. Kohlert, M. Veit, H. Derendorf. 2002. Pharmacokinetics and bioavailability of herbal medicinal products. *Phytomed* 9:1–33.

Bode, A. M., Z. Dong. 2015. Toxic phytochemicals and their potential risks for human cancer. *Cancer Prev Res* 8:1–8.

Brown, A. C., J. Koett, D. W. Johnson et al. 2005. Effectiveness of kukui nut oil as a topical treatment for psoriasis. *Int J Dermatol* 44:684–7.

Calixto, J. B. 2000. Efficacy, safety, quality control, marketing and regulatory guidelines for herbal medicines (phytotherapeutic agents). *Braz J Med Biol Res* 33:179–89.

Chang, S., Y. Liu, X. Z. Bo, A. J. Qi. 2006. Treatment of psoriasis vulgaris by oral administration of Yin Xie Ping granules—A clinical report of 60 cases. *J Trad Chin Med* 26:198–201.

Choonhakarn, C., P. Busaracome, B. Sripanidkulchai, P. A. Sarakarn. 2010. A prospective, randomized clinical trial comparing topical aloe vera with 0.1% triamcinolone acetonide in mild to moderate plaque psoriasis. *J Eur Acad Dermatol Venereol* 24:168–72.

Chun, K. S., Y. S. Keum, S. S. Han, Y. S. Song, S. H. Kim, Y. J. Surh. 2003. Curcumin inhibits phorbol ester induced expression of cyclooxygenase-2 in mouse skin through suppression of extracellular signal-regulated kinase activity and NF-kappaB activation. *Carcinogenesis* 24:1515–24.

Cui, B. N., Y. X. Sun, W. L. Liu. 2008. Clinical efficacy of narrow band ultraviolet bin combined with yuyin recipe in treating psoriasis vulgaris. *Chin J Integr Trad West Med* 28:355–7.

Deng, S., B. H. May, A. L. Zhang, C. Lu, C. C. Xue. 2013. Topical herbal medicine combined with pharmacotherapy for psoriasis: A systematic review and meta-analysis. *Arch Dermatol Res* 305:179–89.

Deng, S., B. H. May, A. L. Zhang, C. Lu, C. C. Xue. 2014. Topical herbal formulae in the management of psoriasis: Systematic review with meta-analysis of clinical studies and investigation of the pharmacological actions of the main herbs. *Phytother Res* 28:480–97.

De Smet, P. A. 2004. Health risks of herbal remedies: An update. *Clin Pharmacol Ther* 76:1–17.

Dhanabal, S. P., P. L. Dwarampudi, N. Muruganantham, R. Vadivelan. 2012. Evaluation of the antipsoriatic activity of *Aloe vera* leaf extract using a mouse tail model of psoriasis. *Phytother Res* 26:617–19.

Di, T. T., Z. T. Ruan, J. X. Zhao et al. 2016. Astilbin inhibits Th17 cell differentiation and ameliorates imiquimod-induced psoriasis-like skin lesions in BALB/c mice via Jak3/Stat3 signaling pathway. *Int Immunopharmacol* 32:32–8.

Divakara, P., B. Nagaraju, R. P. Buden, H. S. Sekhar, C. M. Ravi. 2013. Antipsoriatic activity of ayurvedic ointment containing aqueous extract of the bark of *Pongamia pinnata* using the rat ultraviolet ray photodermatitis model. *Adv Med Plant Res* 1:8–16.

Doshi, D. H. 2007. Oral drug delivery system. In *Gibaldi's Drug Delivery Systems in Pharmaceutical Care*, ed. M. Lee and A. Desai, 23–43. Bethesda, MD: ASHP.

Dwarampudi, L. P., D. Palaniswamy, M. Nithyanantham, P. S. Raghu. 2012. Antipsoriatic activity and cytotoxicity of ethanolic extract of *Nigella sativa* seeds. *Pharmacogn Mag* 8:268–72.

Dwivedi, S., A. Aggarwal, V. Sharma. 2011. Cardiotoxicity from 'safe' herbomineral formulations. *Trop Doct* 41:113–5.

Ekor, M. 2014. The growing use of herbal medicines: Issues relating to adverse reactions and challenges in monitoring safety. *Front Pharmacol* 4:177.

Ernst, E. 2000. Adverse effects of herbal drugs in dermatology. *Br J Dermatol* 143:923–9.

Fleischer, A. B., S. R. Feldman, S. R. Rapp, D. M. Reboussin, M. L. Exum, A. R. Clark. 1996. Alternative therapies commonly used within a population of patients with psoriasis. *Cutis* 58:216–20.

Gelmini, F., G. Beretta, C. Anselmi et al. 2013. GC-MS profiling of the phytochemical constituents of the oleoresin from *Copaifera langsdorffii* Desf. and a preliminary in vivo evaluation of its antipsoriatic effect. *Int J Pharm* 440:170–8.

Grant, K. L., C. D. Schneider. 2000. Turmeric. *Am J Health Syst Pharm* 57:1121–2.

Gu, Y., H. X. Liu, C. H. Zhang et al. 2009. Clinical observation of traditional Chinese medical herbs bath combined with narrowband ultraviolet B for the treatment of psoriasis vulgaris. *Chin J Dermatol Venereol* 4:243–4.

Gudjonsson, J. E., A. Aphale, M. Grachtchouk et al. 2009. Lack of evidence for activation of the hedgehog pathway in psoriasis. *J Invest Dermatol* 129:635–40.

Gulcubuk, A., K. Altunatmaz, K. Sonmez et al. 2006. Effects of curcumin on tumour necrosis factor-alpha and interleukin-6 in the late phase of experimental acute pancreatitis. *J Vet Med A Physiol Pathol Clin Med* 53:49–54.

Gulliver, W. P., H. J. Donsky. 2005. A report on three recent clinical trials using *Mahonia aquifolium* 10% topical cream and a review of the worldwide clinical experience with *Mahonia aquifolium* for the treatment of plaque psoriasis. *Am J Ther* 12:398–406.

Gupta, R., M. Gupta, S. Mangal, U. Agrawal, S. P. Vyas. 2016. Capsaicin-loaded vesicular systems designed for enhancing localized delivery for psoriasis therapy. *Artif Cells Nanomed Biotechnol* 44:825–34.

He, S. M., E. Chan, S. F. Zhou. 2011. ADME properties of herbal medicines in humans: Evidence, challenges and strategies. *Curr Pharm Design* 17:357–407.

He, Y., H. Liu, Z. Xie, Q. Liao, X. Lai, Z. Du. 2014. PVP and surfactant combined carrier as an effective absorption enhancer of poorly soluble astilbin in vitro and in vivo. *Drug Dev Ind Pharm* 40:237–43.

Heng, M. C., M. K. Song, J. Harker, M. K. Heng. 2000. Drug-induced suppression of phosphorylase kinase activity correlates with resolution of psoriasis as assessed by clinical, histological and immunohistochemical parameters. *Br J Dermatol* 143:937–49.

Heng, M. C. Y., M. K. Song, M. K. Heng. 1994. Elevated phosphorylase kinase activity in psoriatic epidermis: Correlation with increased phosphorylation and psoriatic activity. *Br J Dermatol* 130:298–306.

Herman, A., A. P. Herman. 2016. Topically used herbal products for the treatment of psoriasis—Mechanism of action, drug delivery, clinical studies. *Planta Med* 82:1447–55.

Ho, S. G. Y., C. K. Yeung, H. H. L. Chan. 2010. Methotrexate versus traditional Chinese medicine in psoriasis: A randomized, placebo-controlled trial to determine efficacy, safety and quality of life. *Clin Exp Dermatol* 35:717–22.

Hovhannisyan, A., M. Matz, R. Gebhardt. 2009. From teratogens to potential therapeutics: Natural inhibitors of the Hedgehog signaling network come of age. *Planta Med* 75:1371–80.

Huxtable, R. J. 1992. The myth of beneficent nature: The risks of herbal preparations. *Ann Intern Med* 117:165–6.

Ireson, C. R., D. J. Jones, S. Orr et al. 2002. Metabolism of the cancer chemopreventive agent curcumin in human and rat intestine. *Cancer Epidemiol Biomarkers Prev* 11:105–11.

Isbrucker, R. A., G. A. Burdock. 2006. Risk and safety assessment on the consumption of Licorice root (*Glycyrrhiza* sp.), its extract and powder as a food ingredient, with emphasis on the pharmacology and toxicology of glycyrrhizin. *Regul Toxicol Pharmacol* 46:167–92.

Jarrett, A., R. I. G. Spearman. 1964. Psoriasis. In *Histochemistry of the Skin*, ed. D. Taverner and J. Trounce, 43–53. London: University Press.

Jin, S., S. Fu, J. Han et al. 2012. Improvement of oral bioavailability of glycyrrhizin by sodium deoxycholate/phospholipid-mixed nanomicelles. *J Drug Target* 20:615–22.

Johnson-Huang, L. M., M. A. Lowes, J. G. Krueger. 2012. Putting together the psoriasis puzzle: An update on developing targeted therapies. *Dis Models Mech* 5:423–33.

Joshi, B. S., P. N. Kaul. 2001. Alternative medicine: Herbal drugs and their critical appraisal—Part I. *Prog Drug Res* 56:1–76.

Kakkar, V., S. Singh, D. Singla, I. P. Kaur. 2011. Exploring solid lipid nanoparticles to enhance the oral bioavailability of curcumin. *Mol Nutr Food Res* 55:495–503.

Kaur, J., S. Kaur, A. Mahajan. 2013. Herbal medicines: Possible risks and benefits. *Am J Phytomed Clin Ther* 1:226–39.

Khokhra, S., A. Diwan. 2011. Microemulsion based transdermal drug delivery of tea tree oil. *Int J Drug Dev Res* 3:191–8.

Koo, J., S. Arain. 1999. Traditional Chinese medicine in dermatology. *Clin Dermatol* 17:21–7.

Krueger, J. G., A. Bowcock. 2005. Psoriasis pathophysiology: Current concepts of pathogenesis. *Ann Rheumat Dis* 64:30–6.

Kurd, S. K., N. Smith, A. VanVoorhees et al. 2008. Oral curcumin in the treatment of moderate to severe psoriasis vulgaris: A prospective clinical trial. *J Am Acad Dermatol* 58:625–31.

Li, C., Y. Zhang, T. Su, L. Feng, Y. Long, Z. Chen. 2012. Silica-coated flexible liposomes as a nanohybrid delivery system for enhanced oral bioavailability of curcumin. *Int J Nanomed* 7:5995.

Li, X. L., Z. H. Wang, Y. X. Zhao et al. 2012. Purification of a polysaccharide from *Gynostemma pentaphyllum* Makino and its therapeutic advantages for psoriasis. *Carbohydrate Polymers* 89:1232–7.

Lin, Y. K., C. J. Chang, Y. C. Chang, W. R. Wong, S. C. Chang, J. H. S. Pang. 2008. Clinical assessment of patients with recalcitrant psoriasis in a randomized, observer-blind, vehicle-controlled trial using *Indigo naturalis*. *Arch Dermatol* 144:1457–64.

Lin, Y. K., Y. L. Leu, S. H. Yang, H. W. Chen, C. T. Wang, J. H. Pang. 2009. Anti-psoriatic effects of *Indigo naturalis* on the proliferation and differentiation of keratinocytes with indirubin as the active component. *J Dermatol Sci* 54:168–74.

Lin, Y. K., L. C. See, Y. H. Huang et al. 2014. Efficacy and safety of *Indigo naturalis* extract in oil (Lindioil) in treating nail psoriasis: A randomized, observer-blind, vehicle-controlled trial. *Phytomedicine* 21:1015–20.

Lin, Y. K., W. R. Wong, Y. C. Chang et al. 2007. The efficacy and safety of topically applied *Indigo naturalis* ointment in patients with plaque-type psoriasis. *Dermatology* 214:155–61.

Lin, Y. K., H. R. Yen, W. R. Wong, S. H. Yang, J. H. S. Pang. 2006. Successful treatment of pediatric psoriasis with *Indigo naturalis* composite ointment. *Pediatric Dermatol* 23:507–10.

Lin, Z. X., B. W. Jiao, C. T. Che et al. 2010. Ethyl acetate fraction of the root of *Rubia cordifolia* L. inhibits keratinocyte proliferation in vitro and promotes keratinocyte differentiation in vivo: Potential application for psoriasis treatment. *Phytother Res* 24:1056–64.

Liu, H., Q. Tan. 2004. A clinical study on treatment of senile psoriasis by replenishing qi to activate blood—A report of 40 cases. *J Trad Chin Med* 24:204–7.

Liu, H. Q., M. J. Lei, G. H. Wanc. 2005. Treatment of psoriasis vulgaris by Yinxiebing external bath formula and narrow-spectrum midwave ultraviolet irradiation: A clinical observation of 40 cases. *New J Trad Chin Med* 37:117–9.

Man, M. Q., Y. Shi, M. Man et al. 2008. Chinese herbal medicine (Tuhuai extract) exhibits topical anti-proliferative and anti-inflammatory activity in murine disease models. *Exp Dermatol* 17:681–7.

Marianecci, C., F. Rinaldi, M. Mastriota et al. 2012. Anti-inflammatory activity of novel ammonium glycyrrhizinate/niosomes delivery system: Human and murine models. *J Control Release* 164:17–25.

Mezghrani, O. K. X. B., X. Ke, N. Bourkaib, B. H. Xu. 2011. Optimized self-microemulsifying drug delivery systems (SMEDDS) for enhanced oral bioavailability of astilbin. *Die Pharmazie* 66:754–60.

Michalsen, A., O. Eddin, A. Salama. 2015. A case series of the effects of a novel composition of a traditional natural preparation for the treatment of psoriasis. *J Trad Complement Med* 6:395–8.

Nagakuma, H., T. Kambara, T. Yamamoto. 1995. Rat ultraviolet ray B photodermatitis: An experimental model of psoriasis vulgaris. *Int J Exp Pathol* 76:65–73.

Najafizadeh, P., F. Hashemian, P. Mansouri, S. Farshi, M. S. Surmaghi, R. Chalangari. 2012. The evaluation of the clinical effect of topical St Johns wort (*Hypericum perforatum* L.) in plaque type psoriasis vulgaris: A pilot study. *Aust J Dermatol* 53:131–5.

Nayak, C., V. Viswanath, R. Dhurat et al. 2016. Safety and efficacy of Tinefcon (*Sphaeranthus indicus*) cream in treatment of plaque psoriasis—A phase II B, double blind, randomized, and placebo controlled study. *Am J Dermatol Venereol* 5:25–33.

Niggemann, B., C. Grüber. 2003. Side-effects of complementary and alternative medicine. *Allergy* 58:707–16.

Oliwiecki, S., J. L. Burton. 1994. Evening primrose oil and marine oil in the treatment of psoriasis. *Clin Exp Dermatol* 19:127–9.

Oyedeji, F. O., O. S. Bankole-Ojo. 2012. Quantitative evaluation of the antipsoriatic activity of sausage tree (*Kigelia africana*). *Afr J Pure Appl Chem* 6:214–8.

Paulsen, E., L. Korsholm, F. Brandrup. 2005. A double-blind, placebo-controlled study of a commercial *Aloe vera* gel in the treatment of slight to moderate psoriasis vulgaris. *J Eur Acad Dermatol Venereol* 19:326–31.

Pradhan, M., D. Singh, M. R. Singh. 2013. Novel colloidal carriers for psoriasis: Current issues, mechanistic insight and novel delivery approaches. *J Control Release* 170:380–95.

Rahman, M., K. Alam, M. Zaki Ahmad et al. 2012. Classical to current approach for treatment of psoriasis: A review. *Endocr Metab Immune Disord Drug Targets* 12:287–302.

Raj, B. A., N. Muruganantham, T. K. Praveen, P. S. Raghu. 2012. Screening of *Wrightia tinctoria* leaves for anti psoriatic activity. *Hygeia J Drugs Med* 4:73–8.

Raj, V. B. A., K. S. Kumar, S. S. Kumar. 2015. Traditional Indian medicinal plants as a potential anti-inflammatory phytomedicine for psoriasis control. *J Pharmacog Phytochem* 4:118–122.

Raynor, D. K., R. Dickinson, P. Knapp, A. F. Long, D. J. Nicolson. 2011. Buyer beware? Does the information provided with herbal products available over the counter enable safe use? *BMC Med* 9:94.

Saelee, C., V. Thongrakard, T. Tencomnao. 2011. Effects of Thai medicinal herb extracts with anti-psoriatic activity on the expression on NF-κB signaling biomarkers in HaCaT keratinocytes. *Molecules* 16:3908–32.

Sarafian, G., M. Afshar, P. Mansouri, J. Asgarpanah, K. Raoufinejad, M. Rajabi. 2015. Topical turmeric microemulgel in the management of plaque psoriasis: A clinical evaluation. *Iran J Pharm Res* 14:865–76.

Schiborr, C., A. Kocher, D. Behnam, J. Jandasek, S. Toelstede, J. Frank. 2014. The oral bioavailability of curcumin from micronized powder and liquid micelles is significantly increased in healthy humans and differs between sexes. *Mol Nutr Food Res* 58:516–27.

Sha, H., S. Guo, Y. Liu, J. Zhao. 2016. Combination of Qinzhu Liangxue decoction and acitretin on the treatment of psoriasis vulgaris: A randomized controlled trial. *Int J Clin Exp Med* 9:7256–64.

Shaikh, J., D. D. Ankola, V. Beniwal, D. Singh, M. R. Kumar. 2009. Nanoparticle encapsulation improves oral bioavailability of curcumin by at least 9-fold when compared to curcumin administered with piperine as absorption enhancer. *Eur J Pharm Sci* 37:223–30.

Sharma, S., K. Bhatia, M. Agarwal et al. 2016. Efficacy and safety of Tinefcon® tablets in subjects with plaque psoriasis: An open label, non-comparative, multicenter, phase IV trial. *J Cosmet Dermatol Sci Appl* 6:55–66.

Shathirapathiy, G., P. M. Nair, S. Hyndavi. 2015. Effect of starch-fortified turmeric bath on psoriasis: A parallel randomised controlled trial. *Focus Altern Complement Ther* 20:125–9.

Shrivastav, S., R. Sindhu, S. Kumar, P. Kumar. 2009. Anti-psoriatic and phytochemical evaluation of *Thespesia populnea* bark extracts. *Int J Pharm Pharm Sci* 1:176–85.

Singh, H. P., P. Utreja, A. K. Tiwary, S. Jain. 2009. Elastic liposomal formulation for sustained delivery of colchicine: In vitro characterization and in vivo evaluation of anti-gout activity. *AAPS J* 11:54–64.

Singh, K. K., S. Tripathy. 2014. Natural treatment alternative for psoriasis: A review on herbal resources. *J Appl Pharm Sci* 4:114–21.

Singhal, M., N. Kansara. 2012. *Cassia tora* Linn cream inhibits ultraviolet-B-induced psoriasis in rats. *ISRN Dermatol* 2012:346510.

Stedman, C. 2001. Herbal hepatotoxicity. *Semin Liver Dis* 22:195–206.

Strong, A. M. M., E. Hamill. 1993. The effect of combined fish oil and evening primrose oil (Efamol Marine) on the remission phase of psoriasis: A 7-month double-blind randomized placebo controlled trial. *J Dermatol Treat* 4:33–6.

Stücker, M., U. Memmel, M. Hoffmann, J. Hartung, P. Altmeyer. 2001. Vitamin B(12) cream containing avocado oil in the therapy of plaque psoriasis. *Dermatology* 203:141–7.

Suresh, P. K., P. Singh, S. Saraf. 2013. Novel topical drug carriers as a tool for treatment of psoriasis: Progress and advances. *Afr J Pharm Pharmacol* 7:138–47.

Syed, T. A., S. A. Ahmad, A. H. Holt, S. A. Ahmad, S. H. Ahmad, M. Afzal. 1996. Management of psoriasis with *Aloe vera* extract in a hydrophilic cream: A placebo-controlled, double-blind study. *Trop Med Int Health* 1:505–9.

Takeda, S., K. Ishihara, Y. Wakui et al. 1996. Bioavailability study of glycyrrhetic acid after oral administration of glycyrrhizin in rats; relevance to the intestinal bacterial hydrolysis. *J Pharm Pharmacol* 48:902–5.

Tang, Y. 2005. Review of a treatment for psoriasis using herose, a botanical formula. *J Dermatol* 32:940–45.

Taş, S., O. Avci. 2004. Rapid clearance of psoriatic skin lesions induced by topical cyclopamine: A preliminary proof of concept study. *Dermatology* 209:126–31.

Thelingwani, R., C. Masimirembwa. 2014. Evaluation of herbal medicines: Value addition to traditional medicines through metabolism, pharmacokinetic and safety studies. *Curr Drug Metabol* 15:942–52.

Thomas, J., C. K. Narkowicz, G. A. Jacobson, G. M. Peterson. 2015. Safety and efficacy of kunzea oil-containing formulations for the management of psoriasis: A randomized, controlled trial. *J Clin Pharm Ther* 40:566–72.

Traub, M., K. Marshall. 2007. Psoriasis—Pathophysiology, conventional, and alternative approaches to treatment. *Altern Med Rev* 12:319–30.

Veale, D. J., H. I. Torley, I. M. Richards et al. 1994. A double-blind placebo controlled trial of Efamol Marine on skin and joint symptoms of psoriatic arthritis. *Br J Rheumatol* 33:954–8.

Velaskar, S., C. S. Nayak, R. G. Torsekar et al. 2016. Efficacy and safety of two doses of *Sphaeranthus indicus* extract in the management of plaque psoriasis: A randomized, double blind, placebo controlled phase II trial. *Am J Dermatol Venereol* 5:6–15.

Vijayalakshmi, A., V. Ravichandiran, M. Velraj, S. Nirmala, S. Jayakumari. 2012. Screening of flavonoid "quercetin" from the rhizome of *Smilax china* Linn. for anti-psoriatic activity. *Asian Pacific J Trop Biomed* 2:269–75.

Wang, A., Z. Liu, S. Liu. 1998. Treatment of psoriasis vulgaris with lacquer made of *Camptotheca acuminata* nuts. *J Clin Dermatol* 27:243–4.

Wang, M. H., J. F. Fan, F. Li, H. J. Li. 2008. Clinical observation and pharmacoeconomic evaluation on compound glycyrrhizin in the treatment of psoriasis vulgaris. *Chin J Drug Appl Monitor* 3:010.

Wei, J. A., L. Han, C. J. Lu et al. 2016. Formula PSORI-CM01 eliminates psoriasis by inhibiting the expression of keratinocyte cyclin B2. *BMC Complement Altern Med* 16:255.

Wen, Z. H., M. L. Xuan, Y. Yan et al. 2014. Chinese medicine combined with calcipotriol betamethasone and calcipotriol ointment for psoriasis vulgaris (CMCBCOP): Study protocol for a randomized controlled trial. *Trials* 15:294.

Wiesenauer, M., R. Lüdtke. 1996. *Mahonia aquifolium* in patients with psoriasis vulgaris—An intraindividual study. *Phytomedicine* 3:231–5.

Wu, J., H. Li, M. Li. 2015. Effects of baicalin cream in two mouse models: 2,4-Dinitrofluorobenzene-induced contact hypersensitivity and mouse tail test for psoriasis. *Int J Clin Exp Med* 8:2128–37.

Yang, K. Y., L. C. Lin, T. Y. Tseng, S. C. Wang, T. H. Tsai. 2007. Oral bioavailability of curcumin in rat and the herbal analysis from *Curcuma longa* by LC-MS/MS. *J Chromatogr B* 853:183–9.

Yao, D. N., C. J. Lu, Z. H. Wen et al. 2016. Oral PSORI-CM01, a Chinese herbal formula, plus topical sequential therapy for moderate-to-severe psoriasis vulgaris: Pilot study for a double-blind, randomized, placebo-controlled trial. *Trials* 17:140.

Ye, P., W. L. Huang, L. Zhen. 2009. Analysis of clinical effects of compound glycyrrhizin on treatment of 53 cases of psoriasis vulgaris. *Chongqing Med* 22:040.

Yu, J. J., C. S. Zhang, A. L. Zhang, B. May, C. C. Xue, C. Lu. 2013. Add-on effect of Chinese herbal medicine bath to phototherapy for psoriasis vulgaris: A systematic review. *J Evid Based Complementary Alt Med* 2013:2013.

Yuqi, T. T. 2005. Review of a treatment for psoriasis using herose, a botanical formula. *J Dermatol* 32:940–5.

Zhang, H., J. Gu. 2007. Progress of experimental study on treatment of psoriasis by Chinese medicinal monomer and single or compound recipe in Chinese materia medica. *Chin J Integr Med* 13:312–6.

Zhang, L. X., Y. P. Bai, P. H. Song, L. P. You, D. Q. Yang. 2009. Effect of Chinese herbal medicine combined with acitretin capsule in treating psoriasis of blood-heat syndrome type. *Chin J Integr Med* 15:141–4.

Zhou, D., W. Chen, X. Li et al. 2014. Evidence-based practice guideline of Chinese herbal medicine for psoriasis vulgaris (Bai Bi). *Eur J Integr Med* 6:135–46.

[illegible]

20 Impact of Nutrition and Dietary Supplementation on Psoriasis Pathology

Odete Mendes, Mithila Shitut, and Jayson Chen

CONTENTS

20.1 INTRODUCTION

Psoriasis is a chronic inflammatory skin disease that can have a genetic predisposition and be triggered by stress. Clinically, it is characterized by the presence of thick, tan, discolored plaques. Current oral medications can have moderate to severe side effects and usually require extensive monitoring. Published research suggests that dietary supplements, such as fish oil and vitamin D, may have a positive impact on disease progression, with the advantage of fewer negative side effects than current drug therapy (Skroza et al., 2013; Collier and Payne, 1996; Bittiner et al., 1988). Diets rich in fruits and vegetables and high in fiber, saffron tea, and slippery elm water have been reported to improve clinical psoriasis scores (Brown et al., 2004). Dietary supplementation with vitamin D, vitamin B12, selenium, and omega 3 may also have beneficial effects in psoriasis treatment.

Omega 3 fatty acids may also have a positive impact in the development of immune-mediated disease by downregulating inflammatory cytokines. Increased consumption of fish oil, rich in omega 3 fatty acids, resulted in mild to modest improvement of psoriatic symptoms. Fish oil serves as a substrate for the production of prostaglandins and leukotrienes with increased eicosapentaeonic acid (EPA) that compete with arachidonic acid and may contribute to decreased levels of cyclic GMP (cGMP) and keratinocyte proliferation. Consumption of omega 3 fatty acids, such as odd-number [OM5] prostaglandin E3 and leukotrine B5, which oppose even-numbered inflammatory mediators, decreased overall inflammation, thus having potential ameliorating effects in diseases such as psoriasis (Sicińska et al., 2015).

Topical formulations derived from vitamin D have been widely used to treat psoriasis. They have been found to have immunomodulatory properties in diseases like psoriasis via type 1 T-helper (Th) cells. The vitamin D receptor is expressed in B, T, and Langerhans cells. Vitamin D3 via the vitamin D receptor activates transcription genes that affect keratinocyte proliferation and differentiation; it can also impact dendritic cells and secretion of interferon γ (IFNγ). Vitamin D leads to *in vitro* keratinocyte proliferation at low concentrations and may inhibit that proliferation at higher concentrations. It can also act as an antioxidant when there is injury caused by ultraviolet B (UV-B) rays. In psoriasis, it decreases keratinocyte proliferation. It blocks the cathelicidin pathway and inhibits β-defensins, HDD3 and 2, and interleukin (IL)-17A, IL-1F, and IL-8 (Wadhwa et al., 2015). Other skin diseases, such as atopic dermatitis, are also associated with inflammatory phenotypes similar to psoriasis. Supplementation with vitamin D can be beneficial for patients with atopic dermatitis (Hata et al., 2014). Selenium may also have an effect in CD4+ T cells in the psoriatic plaques (Millsop et al., 2014).

Supplementation with herbal medicines and tea extracts (such as yellow saffron [*Chrhamus tinsctorus*]) may reduce inflammatory stress and, via immunomodulation, impact disease expression. For example, slippery elm (*Ulmus fulva*) may also impact mucosal inflammation and have a positive impact on disease progression (Brown et al., 2004).

Probiotic nutritional supplements may also play a potential role in disease progression by impacting immune function. *Bifidus infantis* decreases pro-inflammatory cytokines that have an impact on the development of immune-mediated diseases, such as psoriasis. It exerts immunoregulatory effects similar to commensal immune interactions, such as induction of regulatory T (Treg) cells in animal models with activity in both the gut and extraintestinal sites. It also reduced the levels of C-reactive protein (CRP) and tumor necrosis factor alpha (TNF-α) and possibly IL-6 in psoriasis patients (Groeger et al., 2013). *Lactobacillus casei* produces lactopectin that selectively degrades pro-inflammatory chemokines, reducing the immune cell infiltration and inflammation. It can also be related to impacting other microbes or modulating host functions, such as induction of IL-10-producing CD4+ T cells. Lactopectin has been shown to reduce TNF-induced secretion of IFN-γ and upregulation of IL-10 (Hörmannsperger et al., 2013).

20.2 PSORIASIS PATHOGENICITY AND PATHOLOGY

Psoriasis is an immune-mediated inflammatory skin disease. The most common form of the disease is plaque psoriasis that manifests itself as plaques of red, inflamed skin lesions (Baliwag et al., 2015). These plaques are a result of keratinocyte hyperproliferation, altered keratinocyte differentiation, and inflammation. Histologically, psoriatic plaques have three features: increased proliferation of keratinocytes, present or prominent dilated dermal blood vessels, and inflammatory infiltrates comprised of different subtypes of T cells admixed with neutrophils and macrophages (Wölfle et al., 2014). The disease is thought to be mediated by Th1-type immune cells. Changes observed in the keratinocytes are due to a perturbation of the maturation process associated with altered protein expression, loss of the mature granular cell layer, and keratinocyte nuclear retention (parakeratosis) (Baliwag et al., 2015).

Current research on psoriasis is highly dependent on the type of animal model used. There are multiple animal disease models of psoriasis, such as ones that use genetically engineered mice. Other relevant models use a UV-induced mechanism that causes histopathology lesions that mimic psoriasis and include formation of Munro's microabscesses, elongation of the rete ridges, and capillary low dilations (Singhal and Kansara, 2012). A common animal model of psoriasis consists of the application of 5% imiquimod (IMQ), which is a Toll-like receptor (TLR) 7/8 agonist and an immune cell activator (Wang et al., 2015; Klebow et al., 2016).

Initiation of the disease may involve the release of the cationic antimicrobial peptide LL37 following physical trauma (Koebner phenomenon) or infection, causing cathelicidin LL37 to bind to self-DNA or -RNA fragments, forming complexes that activate dendritic cells and releasing IFNs and inflammatory cytokines (Di Meglio et al., 2014; Mahil et al., 2016), creating an IL-23/IL-17 pro-inflammatory environment (Figure 20.1). The self-DNA/RNA–LL37 complex activates plasmocytoid dendritic cells (pDCs) that secrete type I IFN, TNF-α, IL-6, and IL-1β. In turn, these cytokines activate myeloid dendritic cells (mDCs) that secrete additional IL-23, IL-12, and IL-20 cytokines that cause, at least in part, the establishment of the Th1, Th17, and Th22 immune response. Keratinocyte injury also leads to activation of additional chemokines that, together with the cytokines mentioned above, lead to the recruitment of neutrophils and macrophages (Nedoszytko et al., 2014). In addition, a second antigen, ADAMTS–protein 5, is produced by melanocytes and also has been identified as an autoantigen involved in the inflammation mediated by CD8 T cells that release IL-17. IL-22 levels have also been correlated with disease severity by impacting keratinocyte function in multiple ways, including the production of matrix metalloproteinase (MMP) 1 and MMP3 linked to tissue degradation and further inflammatory recruitment (Diani et al., 2016).

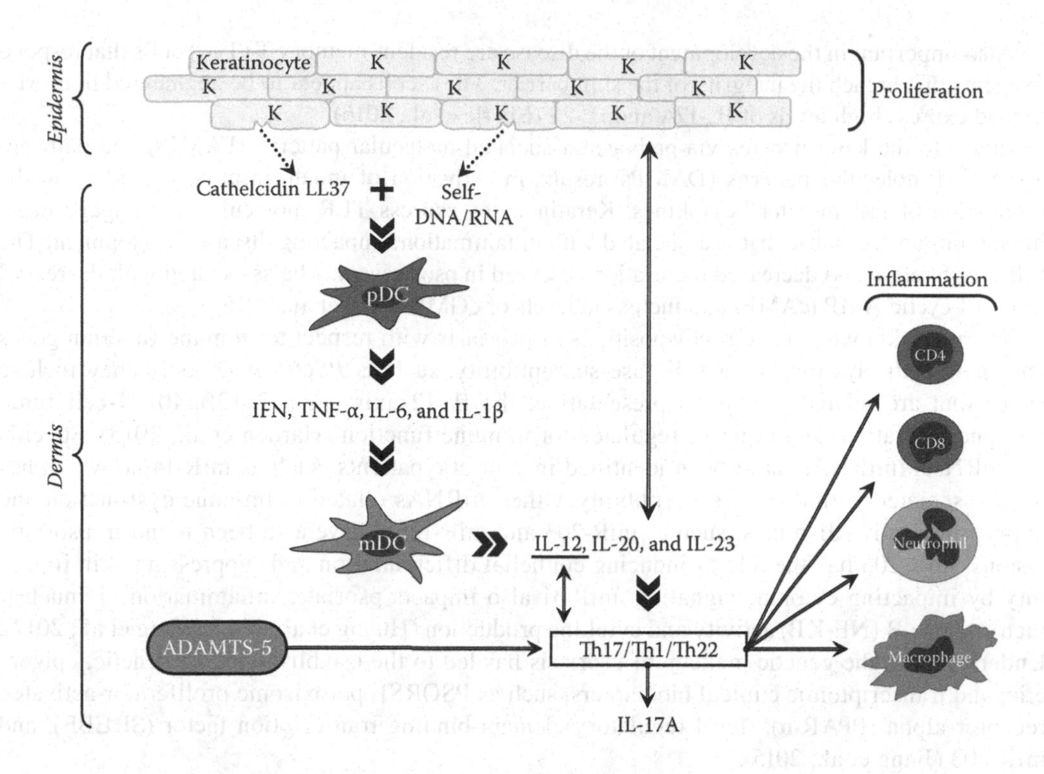

FIGURE 20.1 Brief summary of pathway components associated with psoriasis lesion development of both inflammation and keratinocyte proliferation involving pDCs and mDCs, leading to a Th17, Th1, and Th22 immune response.

The increase in Th1 pathway cytokines includes IFN-γ, IL-2, IL-6, IL-12, IL-17A and F, IL-21, IL-23, IL-12/23, granulocyte-monocyte colony-stimulating factor (GM-CSF), and inhibitors of the Janus kinase (JAK 1/2/3). Expression of IL-17A and F is regulated by signal transducer and activator of transcription 3 (STAT 3) (Eberle et al., 2016). Therefore, the disease is considered to be regarded as a T-cell-mediated immune disease with mixed Th1 and Th17 cytokine involvement. The lymphocytic infiltrate is mostly composed of a mixture of CD4 and CD8 T cells in the papillary dermis and exclusively CD8 T cells in the epidermis. There is increased expression of leukocyte adhesion molecules. T cells are activated and stimulated by an increase in IL-2, and IL-2R mRNA. Activated T cells increase secretion of IL-2 and cause increased secretion of IL-12 from Langerhans cells, which in turn regulate transcription for cytokines such as IFN-γ and TNF-α, which cause maturation and proliferation of T cells. They migrate to skin, causing acute inflammation. Inflammation causes keratinocyte stimulation, which leads to proliferation. In turn, these produce vascular endothelial growth factor (VEGF) and IL-8, which lead to an increase in vascularization. Pro-angiogenic factors, such as cytokines, MMPs, and adhesion molecules, further contribute to the development of the vascular characteristics of immune-mediated disease (Elshabrawy et al., 2015). INF-γ exerts its effects on this disease by impacting mDCs that produce CCL20 ligand for CCR6 and IL-23, which leads to the recruitment of Th17 cells. In addition to INF-γ and TNF-α, IL-1 is also overexpressed in psoriasis. It may be related to the recruitment of T cells and associated with the formation of T-cell antigen-presenting cell (APC) dermal clusters, as well as mediation of the Th17 response and the product of IL-17 (Baliwag et al., 2015). Additionally, the Th1 response can activate dendritic cells to secrete IL-12 (Feily and Namazi, 2009) and leads to IL-17-mediated increases of chemokines such as CXCL10, CCL20, CXCL1, CXCL3, and CXCL8 (Diani et al., 2016; Gladman, 2016).

Also important in the development of the disease are resident-memory T (T_{RM}) cells that respond to agents that breach the integrity of the skin barrier. These cells appear to be augmented in psoriasis and express high levels of IL-17A and IL-22 (Eberle et al., 2016).

Injury to the keratinocytes via pathogen-associated molecular patterns (PAMPs) and damage-associated molecular patterns (DAMPs) results in activation of innate immunity, leading to the production of inflammatory cytokines. Keratinocytes express TLR molecules and engage in an innate immune response that is associated with inflammation, impacting disease development. The cell proliferation and decreased maturation observed in psoriasis may be associated with decreased levels of cyclic AMP (cAMP) and increased levels of cGMP (Choi et al., 2015).

There are known genetic predispositions of psoriasis with respect to immune function genes and their pathways that impact disease susceptibility, such as *PSORS1–13* loci. They include genes that are related to antigen presentation, the IL-12 axis (e.g., IL-12Bp40), T-cell function and migration, and negative regulators of immune function (Harden et al., 2015). Specific microRNAs (miRNAs) have been identified in psoriatic patients, such as miR-146a, which has been associated with disease susceptibility. Other miRNAs related to immune dysfunction and hyperproliferative disorders, such as miR-203 and miR-125b, have also been found in psoriatic lesions. miR-203 has the role of inducing epithelial differentiation and suppressing skin immunity by impacting cytokine signaling. miR-31 also impacts psoriatic inflammation via nuclear factor-kappa B (NF-KB) activity and cytokine production (Huang et al., 2015; Wang et al., 2017). Understanding the genetic makeup of psoriasis has led to the establishment of genetic, epigenetic, and transcriptomic clinical biomarkers, such as PSORS1, peroxisome proliferator-activated receptor alpha (PPAR-α), sterol regulatory element-binding transcription factor (SREBF), and miR-203 (Jiang et al., 2015).

20.3 ANTI-INFLAMMATORY AND IMMUNOMODULATORY PROPERTIES OF HERBAL AND DIETARY SUPPLEMENTS

In the United States, herbal and dietary supplements do not require proof of efficacy and are considered safe until proven otherwise. However, a variety of psoriasis animal models have been used to investigate herbal and dietary supplements as alternatives to pharmaceutical intervention. Studies suggest that stress management, herbal medicines, omega 3, and fasting can affect psoriasis disease development (Traub and Marshall, 2007); vitamin D may help normalize the innate response and have a suppressive effect on immune-mediated skin inflammation (Hata et al., 2014).

Extensive research involving numerous plant extracts documents the potential positive impact of herbal supplements in the modulation of immunological responses in the skin, which can have ameliorating effects in the progression and outcomes of diseases such as psoriasis without some of the limiting secondary effects of current immunosuppressive and immunotoxic medicines.

One of the models for studying psoriasis consists of polyinosinic:polycytidylic (poly(I:C)) acid administration, an immunostimulant that activates TLR3 and induces an inflammatory reaction in keratinocytes. *Paeonia lactiflora* Pallas, which has long been used to treat inflammatory disorders in Eastern medicine, was demonstrated to have an inhibitory effect in poly(I:C)-induced inflammation. *P. lactiflora* Pallas extract (PE) significantly inhibited inflammasome activation, in terms of IL-1β and caspase-1 secretion, and expression of crucial psoriatic cytokines, such as IL-6, IL-8, CCL20, and TNF-α, via downregulation of the NF-KB signaling pathway (Choi et al., 2015).

A study with *Cissampelos sympodialis* leaves suggested potential effects toward decreasing the production of nitric oxide (NO) and inflammatory cytokines involved in psoriasis, while promoting the production of anti-inflammatory cytokines that ameliorate the disease. The aqueous fraction of the ethanolic extract of *C. sympodialis* leaves was shown to inhibit IL-2 and increase IL-10 production, which may contribute to cytokine downregulation and increases in cAMP levels (Feily and Namazi, 2009).

Tripterigyum wilfordii (TwHook F), an herb with the active substance triptolide (TP), can exert potent anti-inflammatory and immunosuppressive effects *in vivo* and *in vitro*, and therefore be a potential therapeutic agent for psoriasis. TP is both an anti-inflammatory and cytotoxic plant that impacts mitogen-activated protein kinase (MAPK) and NF-KB, as well as other molecules, such as IFN-γ, TNF-α, IL-1β, IL-6, and IL-8 (Han et al., 2012). TP inhibits CXCL11/I-TAC secretion induced by IFN-γ and TNF-α and decreases the infiltration of Th1 cells in the skin. It also suppresses the expression of prostaglandin E and attenuates intracellular signaling pathways, which include psoriasis-relevant TLRs (Han et al., 2012; Zhang and Ma, 2010).

Phytosphingosine is abundant in plants. It is known to prevent loss of moisture in the skin and regulate epidermal cell growth differentiation and apoptosis, in addition to having bactericidal and anti-inflammatory properties, and is associated with natural defenses of the body. Chronic intradermal injection of IL-23 into the ears of mice induces psoriaform dermatitis, which leads to increased ear thickness and edematous swelling and to decreased vascular permeability and epidermal cell proliferation. Phytosphingosine can decrease NF-KB, JAK/STAT, and ear swelling psoriasiform dermatitis in IL-23 injected mice. Phytosphingosine derivatives can suppress mRNA levels of Th17 cytokines, including CXCL1, CCL17, CCL 20, IL-17A, and IL-22, all of which are highly expressed in psoriasis. In addition, mRNA levels of pro-inflammatory mediators, such as IL-1α, IL-1β, IL-6, INF-γ, and TNF-α, can also be suppressed (Kim et al., 2014a).

Tuhuai extract (which includes *Similax glabra, Paeonia lactfolora, Radix scuttrellariae, Flos lonicerate*, and *Glyciyrrhixa uralensis*) has an antiproliferative and anti-inflammatory effect in mice models of psoriasis. Tuhai extract in 100% ethanol used in an epidermal hyperproliferative model and ear inflammation induced by application of 0.03% phorbol 12-myristate 13-acetate (TPA), caused a decrease in visible topical inflammation, epidermal hyperplasia, and keratinocyte apoptosis with an overall decrease of ear thickness. The components of the extract mixture have been reported to decrease TNF-α, lymphocyte migration, MMP2 and MMP9 activity, and levels of immunoglobulin (Ig) E and IL-4 (Man et al., 2008).

Cassia tora leaves are rich in glycosides and contain aloe emodin, which shows a protective effect in psoriasis induced by UV-B exposure. The histopathology of psoriasis lesions induced by UV-B includes the formation of Munro's microabscesses, the elongation of the rete ridges, and capillary loop dilations. These lesions decrease in severity and incidence after treatment with metholic extract of *C. tora* in a dose-dependent manner. There was also an observed decrease in epidermal thickening after treatment (Singhal and Kansara, 2012).

Givotia rottleriformis bark is a rich source of active flavonoids, rutin, quercetin, kaempferol, and lueteolin. Ethanol extracts of *G. rottleriformis* have a positive impact in UV-B-induced psoriasis in rats, reducing hyperproliferation of the keratinocytes at 200 mg/kg and achieving complete clearance at 400 mg/kg. Flavonoids are potent antioxidants and can act in multiple signaling pathways to have both antiproliferative and anti-inflammatory properties, and can also act as free radical scavengers (Vijayalakshmi and Geetha, 2014).

Hypericum perforatum (St. John's wort) components include naphtahodianthrones (hypericin) and phloroglucinos (heperforin) that have antioxidant, antiproliferative, and anti-inflammatory effects that are beneficial in skin diseases. Its effects are also attributed to inhibition of IFN-γ, strong downregulation of CXCR3, downregulation of MMP9, and a decrease in Th1-mediated inflammation. Heperforin also stimulates keratinocytes and has been associated with improved psoriasis scores (Wölfle et al., 2014).

AO is an herbal extract that contains 10 individual herbs, including Japanese creeper, Chinese honeylocust spine, woolly Dutchman's pipe, root of pubescent angelica, Cantonese buttercup, giant typhonium tuber, euphorbia, semen hyoscyami, and sesame oil. It has been shown to decrease inflammation by reducing TNF-α on macrophage cells and inhibition of oxazolone-induced inflammation in the mouse ear psoriasis model (Ye et al., 2016).

Viola tricolor has immunosuppressive and anti-inflammatory properties. It contains flavonoids, polysaccharides, phyenylcarbonic acids, salicylic acid derivatives, catechins, and cumarins, as well as macrocyclic peptides–cyclotides. Cyclotides are ribosomal synthesized plant compounds reported to have immunosuppressive properties that can impact proliferation of T lymphocytes (Grundemann et al., 2012). An aqueous extract of *V. tricolor* inhibited the secretion of IL-2 without impacting the expression of IL-R2 receptor. Additionally, it also reduced IFN-γ and TNF-α, potentially impacting disease progression (Hellinger et al., 2014).

Apigenin, a plant flavonoid, can suppress cyclooxygenase (COX) 2 and phosphatidylinositol-4,5-bisphosphate 3-kinase (PI3K). Additionally, it can sensitize T cells to apoptosis by inhibiting NF-KB-regulated B-cell lymphoma–extra large (BCL-XL), COX-2, and FLICE-like inhibitory protein expression. SNF1 mouse models of lupus treated with apigenin had suppression of Th1 and Th17 cells and B cells in lupus, demonstrating that it can have an impact on disease where both Th1 and Th17 are activated, such as psoriasis (Kang et al., 2009).

The gel of *aloe vera*, a popular plant that contains anthroquinones, steroids, saponins, mucopolysaccharides, and salicylic acid, is commonly used to treat skin diseases, including psoriasis. Recently, an ethanolic extract of the *aloe vera* gel tested in a mouse tail model of psoriasis was shown to produce a significant increase in relative epidermal thickness when compared with the control group that was treated with 0.1% tazarotene (Dhanabal et al., 2012a).

Curcumin, a polyphenolic compound isolated from the rhizome of the plant *Curcuma longa* (turmeric), has been regarded as a complementary therapy to clinical treatment of psoriasis. It has anti-inflammatory properties and the ability to decrease the expression of pro-inflammatory cytokines in keratinocytes, and it relieves IMQ-induced psoriasis, like inflammation in mice. Curcumin gel formation, when topically used in IMQ-induced epidermal hyperplasia and inflammation in the BLAB/c mouse ear skin model, produced significant inhibition of the hyperplasia and inflammation and reduction in mRNA levels of IL-17A, IL-17F, IL-22, IL-1β, IL-6, and TNF-α cytokines. Curcumin is also capable of enhancing the proliferation of epidermal γδ T cells but inhibits dermal γδ T-cell proliferation. Thus, curcumin impacts the IL-23/IL-17A axis by inhibiting IL-1β/IL-6 and then downregulates IL-17A/IL-22 production (Sun et al., 2013) (Figure 20.2).

In addition, curcumin also had anti-inflammatory effects on psoriasis developed in a keratin 14–VEGF transgenic mouse model. Oral application of curcumin significantly improved all psoriasis

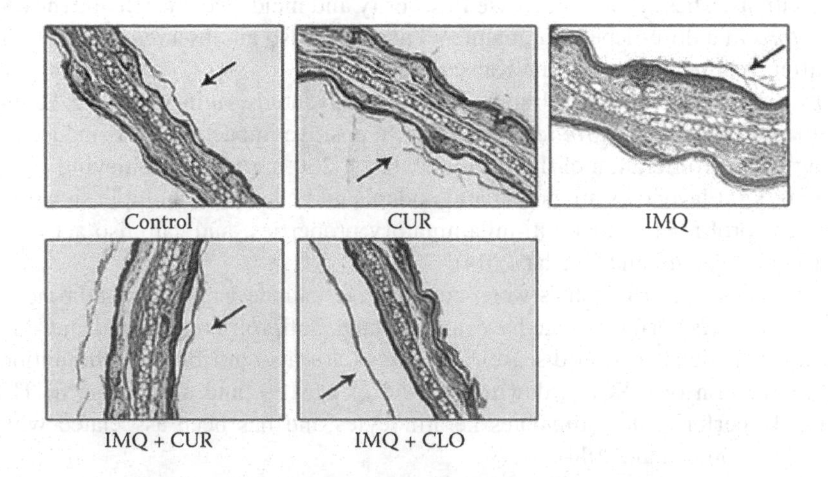

FIGURE 20.2 Curcumin inhibited IMQ-induced epidermal hyperplasia and inflammation in a BLAB/c mouse ear skin model. Hematoxylin and eosin (H&E) staining of the mouse ear skin of different treatment groups (200×). Arrowheads denote the inside of the ear skin. CUR, curcumin; CLO, clobetasol. (Copyright notice: This is an open-access article distributed under the terms of the Creative Commons Attribution License, which permits unrestricted use, distribution, and reproduction in any medium, provided the original author and source are credited: Sun, J., Zhao, Y., and Hu, J., *PLoS One*, 8(6), e67078, 2013. doi: 10.1371/journal.pone.0067078.)

indexes, including ear redness, weight, thickness, and lymph node weight, compared with severe psoriatic symptoms observed in the negative control mice. Curcumin also significantly inhibited secretion of inflammatory factors, including IL-17, IL-22, IFN-γ, IL-2, IL-8, and TNF-α in T cells *in vitro*, and decreased mouse serum levels of TNF-α, IFN-γ, IL-2, IL-12, IL-22, and IL-23 by more than 50% (Kang et al., 2016).

Andrographolide (Andro), a small-molecule compound derived from andrographis (*Andrographis paniculata*), was shown to alleviate IMQ- but not IL-23-induced psoriasis in mice with decreasing expressions of IL-23 and IL-1β in the skin. It inhibited IMQ-induced mRNA expressions of IL-23, IL-6, IL-1β, CD80, and CD86 in bone marrow–derived dendritic cells (BMDCs) from mice. In addition, Andro also controls activation of MyD88-dependent cytokines and alleviates psoriasis in mice treated with IMQ or lipopolysaccharide by inducing autophagic proteolysis of MyD88, suggesting a novel strategy to treat psoriasis (Shao et al., 2016).

The hydroalcoholic extract of *Wrightia tinctoria* leaves was evaluated for antipsoriatic activity by the mouse tail test (Dhanabal et al., 2012b). The extract produced a significant degree of orthokeratosis compared with control. The extract also showed prominent antioxidant activity and antipsoriatic activity (Antony et al., 2015).

Acanthus mollis (Acanthaceae), *Achillea ligustica*, *Artemisia arborescens*, and *Inula viscosa* (Asteraceae) are used in southern Italy for psoriasis and other skin diseases that involve imbalanced eicosanoid production. Methanol crude extracts of these herbal remedies inhibited both 5-LOX and COX-1 activities, while NF-KB activation was prevented by all extracts but *A. mollis*, *A. ligustica*, *A. arborescens*, and *A. mollis* also increased the biosynthesis of 15(S)-HETE, an anti-inflammatory eicosanoid. Their n-hexane, dichloromethane, and ethyl acetate fractions also had inhibitory effects on the leukotriene 4 (LTB4) biosynthesis (Bader et al., 2015).

The therapeutic effects of mustard seed (*Sinapis alba* Linn) were investigated for the role of NLRP3 inflammasome in IMQ-induced psoriasis-like inflammation in mice (Hu et al., 2013; Jiang et al., 2015). Mustard seed attenuated the inductions of NLRP3, ASC, caspase-1, and caspase-11 mRNA expressions; ASC and caspase-1 protein expressions; and serum levels of IL-1β and IL-18 caused by IMQ treatment. These results suggest that mustard seed can suppress inflammation induced by IL-1β and IL-18 by downregulating the expression of NLRP3 inflammasome.

Astragalus sinicus L., also known as the Chinese milkvetch, is an herbaceous and scandent perennial legume that may ameliorate chronic inflammatory skin diseases due to its antioxidant and anti-inflammatory activities (Kim et al., 2014b). Aqueous fractions isolated from *A. sinicus* L. exhibited the strong reactive oxygen species (ROS)–scavenging and anti-inflammatory activities as measured by inhibition of the intracellular ROS production, NF-KB, JAK/STAT, and PI3K/Akt signaling in cytokine-stimulated human keratinocytes. In addition, topical application of fractions suppressed the progression of psoriasis-like dermatitis and expression of pro-inflammatory mediators in IL-23-injected mouse ears.

Dillenia indica Linn. (Dilleniaceae), an evergreen tree originally from tropical Asia that is now found throughout Asia, is traditionally used to treat skin inflammation. *D. indica* fruit extracts were assessed for their healing and anti-inflammatory effects in ultraviolet radiation–induced psoriasis-like wounds in Wistar rats. The results suggested that the extracts accelerated the healing of psoriasis-like wounds and reduced inflammation, via a protective mechanism against oxidative damage to the biomolecules in the skin (Kviecinski et al., 2017).

n-3 polyunsaturated fatty acids (PUFAs) have well-recognized beneficial effects on psoriasis in both animal models and humans. A recent study provided further insight into the mechanisms involved in preventing inflammation in psoriasis-like mice by n-3 PUFAs by utilizing the fat-1 mouse, a transgenic model that can endogenously convert n-6 PUFAs into n-3 PUFAs. Fat-1 IMQ-induced mice exhibited significantly lower levels of inflammatory cell-like Th17 cells and higher levels of Treg cells in the spleen than the wild-type IMQ-induced mice. PUFAs stimulated Th17 cells to produce lower levels of inflammatory factors, including IL-17, IL-22, IL-23, and stimulated Treg cells to produce higher anti-inflammatory factors, such as Foxp3 (Qin et al., 2014).

Flowers of *Woodfordia fruticosa* (L.) Kurz, a straggling leafy shrub of family *Lythraceae*, were investigated for antipsoriatic activity of their ethanolic extract (EEWF). EEWF was observed to reduce the severity of psoriatic lesions (redness, erythema, and scales) and decrease the epidermal thickness in psoriasis models induced by complete Freund's adjuvant (CFA) and formaldehyde. The antipsoriatic activity was suggested to be the result of the rich amount of bioactive phytoconstituents (flavonoids and polyphenols) present in the EEWF (Srivastava et al., 2016).

Honokiol (HK), a biphenolic neolignan isolated from *Magnolia officinalis*, has been reported to possess anti-inflammatory and antiangiogenic activities. In a recent study, HK was found to significantly decrease the ratio of Th1/Th2 expression CD4+ T cells and inhibited TNF-α-induced activation of NF-kB. The expression of TNF-α and IFN-γ, and their corresponding mRNA levels, was downregulated; the expression of nuclear p65, VEGFR-2, and related phosphorylated proteins (p-VEGFR-2, p-ERK1/2, p-AKT, and p-p38) was also suppressed. In addition, morphology and histological features in the K14-VEGF transgenic model of psoriasis were effectively improved by HK treatment (Wen et al., 2015).

Baicalin is one of the major flavonoids and bioactive components of *Scutellaria baicalensis*, a Chinese herbal medicine that has been used for centuries to treat psoriasis. Baicalin topical cream has been formulated and evaluated *in vivo* for anti-inflammatory effects in 2,4-dinitrofluorobenzene (DNFB)-induced contact hypersensitivity (CHS) mice and keratinocyte-modulating action in the mouse tail model for psoriasis. In these models, Baicalin cream displayed a significant reduction in DNFB-induced CHS responses compared with vehicle-treated animals, and a dose-dependent increase in orthokeratosis of granular layers and a reduction of the relative epidermal thickness of mouse tail skin (Wu et al., 2015).

ABBREVIATIONS

DNFB 2,4-Dinitrofluorobenzene
Andro Andrographolide
APC Antigen-presenting cell
BCL-XL B-cell lymphoma-extra large
BMDC Bone marrow-derived dendritic cell
CRP C-reactive protein
CFA Complete Freund's adjuvant
CHS Contact hypersensitivity
cAMP Cyclic adenosine monophosphate
cGMP Cyclic guanosine monophosphate
COX Cyclooxygenase
DAMP Damage-associated molecular pattern
EEWF Ethanolic extract of *Woodfordia fruticosa*
EPA Eicosapentaeonic acid
GM-CSF Granulocyte-monocyte colony-stimulating factor
HK Honokiol
5S-HETE Hydroxyicosatetraenoic acid
IMQ Imiquimod
IFNγ Interferon gamma
IL Interleukin
JAK Janus kinase
LTB4 Leukotriene 4
MMP Matrix metalloproteinase
miR MicroRNA
MAPK Mitogen-activated protein kinase

mDC	Myeloid dendritic cell
PUFA	n-3 polyunsaturated fatty acid
NO	Nitric oxide
NF-KB	Nuclear factor-kappa B
PAMP	Pathogen-associated molecular pattern
PPAR-α	Peroxisome proliferator-activated receptor alpha
TPA	Phorbol 12-myristate 13-acetate
PI3K	Phosphatidylinositol-4,5-bisphosphate 3-kinase
pDC	Plasmocytoid dendritic cell
poly(I:C)	Polyinosinic:polycytidylic
ROS	Reactive oxygen species
Treg	Regulatory T
T_{RM}	Resident-memory T
STAT 3	Signal transducer and activator of transcription 3
SREBF	Sterol regulatory element-binding transcription factor
Th1	Type 1 T helper
TLR	Toll-like receptor
TP	Triptolide
TNF-α	Tumor necrosis factor alpha
UV-B	Ultraviolet B
VEGF	Vascular endothelial growth factor

REFERENCES

Antony J, Saikia M, Vinod V, Nath LR, Katiki MR, Murty MS, Paul A et al. DW-F5: A novel formulation against malignant melanoma from *Wrightia tinctoria*. *Sci Rep* 2015;5:11107.

Bader A, Martini F, Schinella GR, Rios JL, Prieto JM. Modulation of Cox-1, 5-, 12- and 15-Lox by popular herbal remedies used in southern Italy against psoriasis and other skin diseases. *Phytother Res* 2015;29(1):108–13.

Baliwag J, Barnes DH, Johnston A. Cytokines in psoriasis. *Cytokine* 2015;73(2):342–50.

Bittiner SB, Tucker WF, Cartwright I, Bleehen SS. A double-blind, randomised, placebo-controlled trial of fish oil in psoriasis. *Lancet* 1988;1(8582):378–80.

Brown AC, Hairfield M, Richards DG, McMillin DL, Mein EA, Nelson CD. Medical nutrition therapy as a potential complementary treatment for psoriasis–Five case reports. *Altern Med Rev* 2004;9(3): 297–307.

Choi MR, Choi DK, Sohn KC, Lim SK, Kim DI, Lee YH, Im M, Lee Y, Seo YJ, Kim CD, Lee JH. Inhibitory effect of *Paeonia lactiflora* Pallas extract (PE) on poly (I:C)-induced immune response of epidermal keratinocytes. *Int J Clin Exp Pathol* 2015;8(5):5236–41.

Collier PM, Payne CR. The dietary effect of oily fish consumption on psoriasis. *Br J Dermatol* 1996;135(5):858.

Dhanabal SP, Priyanka Dwarampudi L, Muruganantham N, Vadivelan R. Evaluation of antipsoriatic activity of *Aloe vera* leaf extract using a mouse tail model of psoriasis. *Phytother Res* 2012a;26(4):617–9.

Dhanabal SP, Raj BA, Muruganantham N, Praveen TK, Raghu PS. Screening of *Wrightia tinctoria* leaves for anti psoriatic activity. *Hygeia* 2012b;4:73–8.

Diani M, Altomare G, Reali E. T helper cell subsets in clinical manifestations of psoriasis. *J Immunol Res* 2016:7692024.

Di Meglio P, Villanova F, Nestle FO. Psoriasis. *Cold Spring Harb Perspect Med* 2014;4(8).

Eberle FC, Brück J, Holstein J, Hirahara K, Ghoreschi K. Recent advances in understanding psoriasis. *F1000Res* 2016;5. pii: F1000 Faculty Rev-770. doi: 10.12688/f1000research.7927.1.

Elshabrawy HA, Chen Z, Volin MV, Ravella S, Virupannavar S, Shahrara S. The pathogenic role of angiogenesis in rheumatoid arthritis. *Angiogenesis* 2015;18(4):433–48.

Feily A, Namazi MR. *Cissampelos sympodialis* Eichl (Menispermaceae) leaf extract as a possible novel and safe treatment for psoriasis. *Sao Paulo Med J* 2009;127(4):241–2.

Gladman DD. Recent advances in understanding and managing psoriatic arthritis [Review]. *F1000Res* 2016;5:2670.

Groeger D, O'Mahony L, Murphy EF, Bourke JF, Dinan TG, Kiely B, Shanahan F, Quigley EM. *Bifidobacterium infantis* 35624 modulates host inflammatory processes beyond the gut. *Gut Microbes* 2013;4(4):325–39.

Grundemann C, Koehbach J, Huber R, Gruber CW. Do plant cyclotides have potential as immunosuppressant peptides? *J Nat Prod* 2012;75:167–74.

Han R, Rostami-Yazdi M, Gerdes S, Mrowietz U. Triptolide in the treatment of psoriasis and other immune-mediated inflammatory diseases. *Br J Clin Pharmacol* 2012;74(3):424–36.

Harden JL, Krueger JG, Bowcock AM. The immunogenetics of psoriasis: A comprehensive review. *J Autoimmun* 2015;64:66–73.

Hata TR, Audish D, Kotol P, Coda A, Kabigting F, Miller J, Alexandrescu D et al. A randomized controlled double-blind investigation of the effects of vitamin D dietary supplementation in subjects with atopic dermatitis. *J Eur Acad Dermatol Venereol* 2014;28(6):781–9.

Hellinger R, Koehbach J, Fedchuk H, Sauer B, Huber R, Gruber CW, Gründemann C. Immunosuppressive activity of an aqueous *Viola tricolor* herbal extract. *J Ethnopharmacol* 2014;151(1):299–306.

Hörmannsperger G, von Schillde MA, Haller D. Lactocepin as a protective microbial structure in the context of IBD. *Gut Microbes* 2013;4(2):152–7.

Hu J, Yang R, Wen C, Li H, Zhao H. Expression of NLRP3 inflammasome in BALB/c mice with imiquimod-induced psoriasis-like inflammation and therapeutic effect of mustard seed (*Sinapis alba* Linn) [in Chinese]. *Nan Fang Yi Ke Da Xue Xue Bao* 2013;33(9):1394–8.

Huang RY, Li L, Wang MJ, Chen XM, Huang QC, Lu CJ. An exploration of the role of MicroRNAs in psoriasis: A systematic review of the literature. *Medicine (Baltimore)* 2015;94(45):e2030.

Jiang S, Hinchliffe TE, Wu T. Biomarkers of an autoimmune skin disease—Psoriasis. *Genomics Proteomics Bioinformatics* 2015;13(4):224–33.

Kang D, Li B, Luo L, Jiang W, Lu Q, Rong M, Lai R. Curcumin shows excellent therapeutic effect on psoriasis in mouse model. *Biochimie* 2016;123:73–80.

Kang HK, Ecklund D, Liu M, Datta SK. Apigenin, a non-mutagenic dietary flavonoid, suppresses lupus by inhibiting autoantigen presentation for expansion of autoreactive Th1 and Th17 cells. *Arthritis Res Ther* 2009;11(2):R59.

Kim BH, Lee JM, Jung YG, Kim S, Kim TY. Phytosphingosine derivatives ameliorate skin inflammation by inhibiting NF-κB and JAK/STAT signaling in keratinocytes and mice. *J Invest Dermatol* 2014a;134(4):1023–32.

Kim BH, Oh I, Kim JH, Jeon JE, Jeon B, Shin J, Kim TY. Anti-inflammatory activity of compounds isolated from *Astragalus sinicus* L. in cytokine-induced keratinocytes and skin. *Exp Mol Med* 2014b;46:e87.

Klebow S, Hahn M, Nikoalev A, Wunderlich FT, Hövelmeyer N, Karbach SH, Waisman A. IL-6 signaling in myelomonocytic cells is not crucial for the development of IMQ-induced psoriasis. *PLoS One* 2016;11(3):e0151913.

Kviecinski MR, David IM, Fernandes FS, Correa MD, Clarinda MM, Freitas AF, Silva JD et al. Healing effect of *Dillenia indica* fruit extracts standardized to betulinic acid on ultraviolet radiation-induced psoriasis-like wounds in rats. *Pharm Biol* 2017;55(1):641–648.

Mahil SK, Capon F, Barker JN. Update on psoriasis immunopathogenesis and targeted immunotherapy. *Semin Immunopathol* 2016;38(1):11–27.

Man MQ, Shi Y, Man M, Lee SH, Demerjian M, Chang S, Feingold KR, Elias PM. Chinese herbal medicine (*Tuhuai extract*) exhibits topical anti-proliferative and anti-inflammatory activity in murine disease models. *Exp Dermatol* 2008;17(8):681–7.

Millsop JW, Bhatia BK, Debbaneh M, Koo J, Liao W. Diet and psoriasis, part III: Role of nutritional supplements. *J Am Acad Dermatol* 2014;71(3):561–9.

Nedoszytko B, Sokołowska-Wojdyło M, Ruckemann-Dziurdzińska K, Roszkiewicz J, Nowicki RJ. Chemokines and cytokines network in the pathogenesis of the inflammatory skin diseases: Atopic dermatitis, psoriasis and skin mastocytosis. *Postepy Dermatol Alergol* 2014;31(2):84–91.

Qin S, Wen J, Bai XC, Chen TY, Zheng RC, Zhou GB, Ma J, Feng JY, Zhong BL, Li YM. Endogenous n-3 polyunsaturated fatty acids protect against imiquimod-induced psoriasis-like inflammation via the IL-17/IL-23 axis. *Mol Med Rep* 2014;9(6):2097–104.

Shao F, Tan T, Tan Y, Sun Y, Wu X, Xu Q. Andrographolide alleviates imiquimod-induced psoriasis in mice via inducing autophagic proteolysis of MyD88. *Biochem Pharmacol* 2016;115:94–103.

Sicińska P, Pytel E, Kurowska J, Koter-Michalak M. Supplementation with omega fatty acids in various diseases [in Polish]. *Postepy Hig Med Dosw (Online)* 2015;69:838–52.

Singhal M, Kansara N. *Cassia tora* Linn cream inhibits ultraviolet-B-induced psoriasis in rats. *ISRN Dermatol* 2012:346510.

Skroza N, Proietti I, Bernardini N, La Viola G, Nicolucci F, Pampena R, Tolino E et al. Efficacy of food supplement to improve metabolic syndrome parameters in patients affected by moderate to severe psoriasis during anti-TNFα treatment. *G Ital Dermatol Venereol* 2013;148(6):661–5.

Srivastava AK, Nagar HK, Chandel HS, Ranawat MS. Antipsoriatic activity of ethanolic extract of *Woodfordia fruticosa* (L.) Kurz flowers in a novel in vivo screening model. *Indian J Pharmacol* 2016;48(5):531–6.

Sun J, Zhao Y, Hu J. Curcumin inhibits imiquimod-induced psoriasis-like inflammation by inhibiting IL-1beta and IL-6 production in mice. *PLoS One* 2013;8(6):e67078.

Traub M, Marshall K. Psoriasis—Pathophysiology, conventional, and alternative approaches to treatment. *Altern Med Rev* 2007;12(4):319–30.

Vijayalakshmi A, Geetha M. Anti-psoriatic activity of *Givotia rottleriformis* in rats. *Indian J Pharmacol* 2014;46(4):386–90.

Wadhwa B, Relhan V, Goel K, Kochhar AM, Garg VK. Vitamin D and skin diseases: A review. *Indian J Dermatol Venereol Leprol* 2015;81(4):344–55.

Wang MJ, Xu YY, Huang RY, Chen XM, Chen HM, Han L, Yan YH, Lu CJ. Role of an imbalanced miRNAs axis in pathogenesis of psoriasis: Novel perspectives based on review of the literature. *Oncotarget* 2017;8(3):5498–507.

Wang X, Sun J, Hu J. IMQ induced K14-VEGF mouse: A stable and long-term mouse model of psoriasis-like inflammation. *PLoS One* 2015;10(12):e0145498.

Wen J, Wang X, Pei H, Xie C, Qiu N, Li S, Wang W, Cheng X, Chen L. Anti-psoriatic effects of Honokiol through the inhibition of NF-κB and VEGFR-2 in animal model of K14-VEGF transgenic mouse. *J Pharmacol Sci* 2015;128(3):116–24.

Wölfle U, Seelinger G, Schempp CM. Topical application of St. John's wort (*Hypericum perforatum*). *Planta Med* 2014;80(2–3):109–20.

Wu J, Li H, Li M. Effects of baicalin cream in two mouse models: 2,4-Dinitrofluorobenzene-induced contact hypersensitivity and mouse tail test for psoriasis. *Int J Clin Exp Med* 2015;8(2):2128–37.

Ye H, Wang Y, Jenson AB, Yan J. Identification of inflammatory factor TNFα inhibitor from medicinal herbs. *Exp Mol Pathol* 2016;100(2):307–11.

Zhang Y, Ma X. Triptolide inhibits IL-12/IL-23 expression in APCs via CCAAT/enhancer-binding protein α. *J Immunol* 2010;184(7):3866.

Commentary

Psoriasis and Psoriatic Arthritis Pathophysiology, Therapeutic Intervention, and Complementary Medicine

Smriti K. Raychaudhuri, Debasis Bagchi, and Siba P. Raychaudhuri

Immunity is the body's ability to protect against infection, disease, bacteria, or virus, and it may be inherited or acquired, while inflammation is the body's natural response to injuries or infection. In other words, infection indicates the invasion and multiplication of bacteria or pathogens within the body, while the body's protection against infection is known as inflammation, which is a complex sequelae of events involving immune cells, signaling molecules, and regulatory proteins.

Both psoriasis and psoriatic arthritis have been extensively discussed in this book. As explained, psoriasis, a chronic autoimmune disorder, begins underneath the skin and causes patches of scaly, red, or inflamed skin called plaques, while psoriatic arthritis potentiates swelling of the joints accompanied by pain, which may lead to permanent damage of the joints and their adjoining structures. The immune system is intricately associated with both psoriasis and psoriatic arthritis. However, it is important to emphasize that not everyone who suffers from psoriasis will get psoriatic arthritis, although both of these conditions have commonalities with respect to the contributing role of immunogenetics and environmental factors.

A number of susceptibility loci for both psoriasis and psoriatic arthritis have been discovered. These loci explain only a fraction of the heritability estimates. However, a model of important pathways associated with the inflammatory-proliferative cascades of psoriasis pathogenesis is emerging that explains dysfunctions in skin barrier function (LCE3B and LCE3C), innate immunity (NFκB and interferon [IFN]), the signaling pathway (TNIP1, TNFAIP3, NFKBIA, REL, IFIH1, TYK2, interleukin [IL] 23RA, and β-defensin), the TH17 pathway (IL12B, IL23R, IL23A, TRAF3IP2, and TYK2), adaptive immunity involving CD8 T cells and their signaling system (ERAP1 and ZAP70), and the TH2 pathway (IL4 and IL13). These studies illustrate the importance of keratinocytes, synovial cells (fibroblast-like synoviocytes [FLS]), and the immune system for psoriasis physiopathology. However, the association of ApoE4 gene polymorphisms points toward an important link between metabolism and psoriatic inflammation. Both psoriasis and psoriatic arthritis are uniquely associated with obesity, insulin resistance, and metabolic syndrome. There is also a possibility that the genetic factors identified will be helpful in determining disease onset, course, and severity.

Current statistics report that approximately 7.5 million Americans, 2.2% of the total population, suffer from psoriasis, while according to the World Psoriasis Day Consortium, about 125 million people worldwide, 2%–3% of the total population, suffer from psoriasis. It has been reported that about 30% of subjects with psoriasis develop psoriatic arthritis. Thus, it is very important to clearly understand the disease's epidemiology, genetics, and molecular pathophysiology; the present day's therapeutic inventions, opportunities, clinical spectrum, and manifestations; and other nutraceutical treatment options, so that a safe and efficacious treatment regimen can be identified and implemented.

The book covers the intricate aspects of psoriasis and psoriatic arthritis. Current understandings of the IL23/IL17 cytokine network, nerve growth factor (NGF) and its receptor system, JAK-STAT signaling proteins, and molecular mechanisms of angiogenesis in the pathophysiology of psoriatic disease discussed in this book should be informative and thought provoking for both the clinicians and investigators working on psoriasis and psoriatic arthritis.

In addition to conventional therapies consisting of disease-modifying antirheumatic drugs (DMARDs), topical therapies, and phototherapy, in this book we have addressed extensively cutting-edge molecular medicine approaches for the management of psoriatic disease. The IL23/IL17 cytokine axis appears to play a critical role in the pathogenesis of psoriasis and psoriatic arthritis. Targeting this pathway appears to have revolutionized the treatment of psoriasis, with complete resolution of disease in many patients, and has offered efficacy that appears to be comparable to that of anti–tumor necrosis factor (TNF) agents in psoriatic arthritis. JAK-STAT inhibitors are novel therapeutic options for autoimmune disease; here we have extensively discussed how this novel approach can be effective for psoriatic disease and spondyloarthritis.

This book also included three dedicated chapters on how novel botanicals and nutraceuticals may help in ameliorating certain symptoms of psoriasis and psoriatic arthritis.

Finally, it is very important to take comprehensive measures: a focus on lifestyle, a balanced diet and proper nutrition, exercise, stress reduction, and early cutting-edge therapeutic intervention would be an ideal approach to effectively combat psoriasis and psoriatic arthritis. The concept of total care is a novel multidisciplinary approach for the management of psoriatic disease, and it was extensively discussed in a dedicated chapter.

Index

Page numbers followed by f and t indicate figures and tables, respectively.

B

C

J

K

L

M

T

U

V

W

X

Y

Z

Printed in the United States
by Baker & Taylor Publisher Services

Printed in the United States
by Baker & Taylor Publisher Services